Workbook and Competency Evaluation Review

MOSBY'S TEXTBOOK FOR NURSING ASSISTANTS

Ninth Edition

RELDA T. KELLY, RN, MSN
Professor Emeritus, Kankakee Community College
Kankakee, Illinois;
Parish Nurse, Wesley United Methodist Church
Bradley, Illinois

Procedure Checklists by
HELEN CHIGAROS, RN, BS, MSN, CRRN, CNS
Professor Emeritus, Kankakee Community College
Director, Azzarelli Outreach Clinic, St. Teresa Roman Catholic Church
Parish Nurse, St. Teresa Roman Catholic Church
Kankakee, Illinois

ELSEVIER

ELSEVIER

3251 Riverport Lane
St. Louis, Missouri 63043

WORKBOOK AND COMPETENCY EVALUATION REVIEW   ISBN: 978-0-323-31976-8
MOSBY'S TEXTBOOK FOR NURSING ASSISTANTS, NINTH EDITION

Notices

Knowledge and best practice in this field are constantly changing. As new research and experience
broaden our understanding, changes in research methods, professional practices, or medical
treatment may become necessary.

Practitioners and researchers must always rely on their own experience and knowledge in
evaluating and using any information, methods, compounds, or experiments described herein.
In using such information or methods they should be mindful of their own safety and the safety of
others, including parties for whom they have a professional responsibility.

With respect to any drug or pharmaceutical products identified, readers are advised to check the
most current information provided (i) on procedures featured or (ii) by the manufacturer of each
product to be administered, to verify the recommended dose or formula, the method and duration
of administration, and contraindications. It is the responsibility of practitioners, relying on their
own experience and knowledge of their patients, to make diagnoses, to determine dosages and the
best treatment for each individual patient, and to take all appropriate safety precautions.

To the fullest extent of the law, neither the Publisher nor the authors, contributors, or editors,
assume any liability for any injury and/or damage to persons or property as a matter of products
liability, negligence or otherwise, or from any use or operation of any methods, products,
instructions, or ideas contained in the material herein.

International Standard Book Number: 978-0-323-31976-8

Content Strategist: Nancy O'Brien
Content Development Manager: Ellen Wurm-Cutter
Senior Content Development Specialist: Maria Broeker
Publishing Services Manager: Jeff Patterson
Senior Project Manager: Tracey Schriefer

Printed in the United States of America

Last digit is the print number: 9 8 7 6 5 4 3

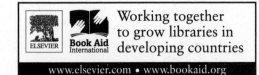

Working together
to grow libraries in
developing countries

www.elsevier.com • www.bookaid.org

PREFACE

This workbook is written to be used with Sorrentino and Remmert's *Mosby's Textbook for Nursing Assistants*, Ninth Edition. You will not need other resources to complete the exercises in this workbook.

This workbook is designed to help you apply what you have learned in each chapter of the textbook. You are encouraged to use this book as a study guide. Each chapter is thoroughly covered in the multiple-choice questions, which will help prepare you to take the NATCEP test. In addition, other exercises such as fill-in-the-blank, matching, labeling, and crossword puzzles are used in many chapters. The section titled Optional Learning Activities may be used as an alternative exercise to give you more practice in studying the materials. The Evolve Student Learning Resources also include Independent Learning Activities for each chapter that can be used to apply the information you will learn in a practical setting.

In addition, Procedure Checklists that correspond with the procedures in the textbook are provided. These checklists are designed to help you become skilled at performing procedures that affect quality of care. In addition to NATCEP skills being identified for you, icons indicate skills that are (1) in Mosby's Nursing Assistant Video Skills 4.0 and (2) on the Evolve Student Learning Resources website (video clips).

The Competency Evaluation Review includes a general review section and two practice exams with answers to help you prepare for the written certification exam. It also features a skills evaluation review to help you practice procedures required for certification.

Assistive personnel are important members of the health team. Completing the exercises in this workbook will increase your knowledge and skills. The goal is to prepare you to provide the best possible care and to encourage pride in a job well done.

Relda T. Kelly

CONTENTS

1 Introduction to Health Care Agencies

Fill in the Blank: Key Terms

Acute illness
Assisted living residence (ALR)
Case management
Chronic illness
Functional nursing
Health team
Hospice
Licensed practical nurse (LPN)
Licensed vocational nurse (LVN)
Nursing assistant
Nursing team
Patient-focused care
Primary nursing
Registered nurse (RN)
Surveyor
Team nursing
Terminal illness

1. _____ is a nursing care pattern where the RN is responsible for the person's total care.

2. A person who performs delegated nursing tasks under the supervision of an RN or LPN/LVN is a

   _____

3. An illness or injury from which the person will not likely recover is a

   _____

4. A nurse who has completed a practical nursing program and has passed a licensing test is a

   _____

5. The _____ are those who provide nursing care—RNs, LPNs/LVNs, and nursing assistants.

6. A sudden illness from which the person is expected to recover is an _____

7. When a nursing care pattern focuses on tasks and jobs, and each nursing team member has certain tasks and jobs to do, it is called _____

8. An _____ provides housing, personal care, support services, health care, and social activities in a home-like setting to persons needing help with daily activities.

9. When an illness or injury is on-going, is slow or gradual in onset, and has no known cure, it is a

   _____

10. _____ is a health care agency or program for persons who are dying.

11. LPNs are sometimes called

    _____

12. _____ is a nursing care pattern in which a case manager (an RN) coordinates a person's care from admission through discharge and into the home setting.

13. A _____ is a nurse who has completed a 2-, 3-, or 4-year nursing program and has passed a licensing test.

14. The many health care workers whose skills and knowledge focus on the person's total care are called the _____

15. _____ is a nursing care pattern in which a team of nursing staff is led by an RN who decides the amount and kind of care each person needs.

16. When services are moved from departments to the bedside, this is a nursing care pattern called

    _____

17. A person who collects information by observing and asking questions is a _____

Circle the Best Answer

18. When health care agencies offer services, the focus of care is always
    A. To cure illness
    B. To give daily personal care
    C. The person
    D. To provide care after surgery or injury

19. Health promotion includes
    A. Immunizations against infectious diseases
    B. Respiratory, physical, and occupational therapies
    C. Learning skills needed to live, work, and enjoy life
    D. Learning about healthy living

20. Diagnostic tests, physical exams, surgery, emergency care, and drugs are used in
    A. Health promotion
    B. Detection and treatment of disease
    C. Rehabilitation and restorative care
    D. Disease prevention

21. The goal of rehabilitation and restorative care is
    A. Teaching the person about healthy living
    B. Returning persons to their highest possible level of physical and psychological functioning
    C. Returning the person completely to normal functioning
    D. Treating the illness with diet, exercise, and medications

22. A person with an acute illness will probably be treated in
    A. A hospital
    B. A long-term care center
    C. An assisted living facility
    D. A rehabilitation agency

23. Sub-acute care is needed when the person needs
    A. Minor surgery
    B. Care that falls between hospital care and long-term care
    C. Help with personal care and drugs
    D. Care at the end of life when the person is dying

24. Persons in a long-term care center
    A. Need hospital care
    B. Are acutely ill
    C. May be older with chronic diseases, poor nutrition, or poor health
    D. Are never able to return home

25. Skilled nursing facilities
    A. Provide nursing care needed until death
    B. Provide more complex care than do nursing centers
    C. Provide care in the person's home
    D. Provide out-patient care

26. A person may have an apartment and receive help with personal care when living in
    A. A long-term care center
    B. An assisted living facility
    C. A rehabilitation care agency
    D. A skilled nursing facility

27. Persons who have problems dealing with life events may be treated in a
    A. Mental health center   C. Long-term care center
    B. Skilled care facility   D. Hospice

28. Home care agencies provide
    A. More complex care than nursing centers
    B. Care for persons who have problems with life events
    C. Physical therapy, rehabilitation, and food services
    D. Care that falls between hospital care and long-term care

29. Hospices
    A. Provide short-term care until the person recovers
    B. Give care only in the home
    C. Provide care to persons who no longer respond to treatments aimed at cures
    D. Provide care only to meet the person's physical needs

30. Health care systems are
    A. Agencies that join together as 1 provider of care
    B. Members of the health team that give bedside care
    C. Members of the health team that work in a hospital
    D. The hospitals in a community

31. All of these are members of the health team *except*
    A. Occupational therapist   C. Social worker
    B. Janitor   D. Cleric

32. The person responsible for nursing service is
    A. A medical doctor
    B. An RN with a bachelor's or master's degree (DON)
    C. A person with many years' experience in giving nursing care
    D. The board of trustees

33. Nursing education staff may teach all of these *except*
    A. Basic nursing skills needed to begin employment as a nurse
    B. How to use new equipment
    C. New employee orientation programs
    D. New and changing information for the nursing team

34. A registered nurse who completes a university program will be in school for
    A. 2 years   C. 3 years
    B. 1 year   D. 4 years

35. An RN
    A. Assesses, makes nursing diagnoses, plans, implements, and evaluates nursing care
    B. Is supervised by licensed doctors and licensed dentists
    C. Gives care only when the person's condition is stable and care is simple
    D. Is always able to diagnose diseases or illnesses

36. An LPN/LVN
    A. Prescribes medications
    B. Assists RNs in caring for acutely ill persons and with complex procedures
    C. Assesses, makes nursing diagnoses, plans, implements, and evaluates care
    D. Is supervised by nursing assistants

37. When a team leader delegates the care of certain persons to other nurses, the nursing care pattern is called
    A. Patient-focused care   C. Functional nursing
    B. Team nursing   D. Primary nursing

38. An example of functional nursing is
    A. An RN coordinates a person's care from admission through discharge
    B. Nursing tasks and procedures are delegated to nursing assistants
    C. One nurse gives all treatments
    D. Services are moved from departments to the bedside

39. When the number of people caring for each person is reduced, this nursing care pattern is
    A. Functional nursing   C. Patient-focused care
    B. Case management   D. Team nursing

40. Medicare
    A. Is bought by individuals and families from an insurance company
    B. Helps to pay medical costs for low-income families
    C. May be provided by an employer
    D. Is a federal health insurance program for person 65 years and older

41. The Patient Protection and Affordable Care Act
    A. Replaces Medicare and Medicaid
    B. Requires everyone to have health insurance
    C. Is only for those who can afford health insurance
    D. Will not insure those who have chronic illnesses

42. In a prospective payment system (PPS)
    A. The patient may choose any doctor
    B. The focus is on preventing disease and maintaining health
    C. The amount paid for services is determined before giving care
    D. Doctors or hospitals may charge whatever is necessary

43. When a health care agency is accredited
    A. It is voluntary and signals quality and excellence
    B. The agency is licensed by the state to operate and provide care
    C. It allows the agency to receive Medicare and Medicaid funds
    D. The agency meets standards set by the federal and state governments

44. If a deficiency is found during a survey of a health care agency, the agency
    A. Usually is given 60 days to correct it
    B. Will be closed immediately
    C. Can decide whether or not to correct the deficiency
    D. Can sue the survey team

45. When you are asked questions by a surveyor, you should
    A. Explain that you are not allowed to answer any questions
    B. Answer the questions honestly and completely
    C. Tell the surveyor you are busy and cannot talk now
    D. Tell the surveyor you do not know the answers and he or she will have to ask someone else

Matching

Match the type of health care agency with the service provided.

A. hospital
B. rehabilitation agency
C. long-term care center
D. mental health center
E. home care agency
F. hospice
G. skilled nursing facility
H. assisted living residence

46. _____ Serves people who are dying

47. _____ Provides complex care while the person recovers from illness or surgery before returning home

48. _____ Provides services to persons who do not need hospital care but cannot care for themselves at home

49. _____ Serves people of all ages for acute, chronic, or terminal illnesses

50. _____ Treats people who may have difficulty dealing with events in life

51. _____ Provides housing, personal care, and other services in a home-like setting

52. _____ Serves people who do not need hospital care but need complex equipment and care measures

53. _____ Provides care to persons at home

Fill in the Blank

54. Write out the abbreviations.
    A. DON _____
    B. LPN _____
    C. LVN _____
    D. RN _____
    E. SNF _____

Write the name of the health team member described.

55. _____ Supervises LPNs/LVNs and assistive personnel

56. _____ Diagnoses and treats diseases and injuries

57. _____ Collects samples and performs laboratory tests on blood, urine, and other body fluids and secretions

58. _____ Takes x-rays and processes film for viewing

59. _____ Gives respiratory treatments and therapies

60. _____ Assesses and plans for nutritional needs

61. _____ Assists persons with movement and pain management

62. _____ Assists persons to learn or retain skills needed to perform activities of daily living

63. _____ Treats persons with speech, voice, hearing, communication, and swallowing disorders

64. _____ Assists persons with their spiritual needs

65. _____ Helps patients and families with social, emotional, and environmental issues affecting illness and recovery

66. _____ Tests hearing and prescribes hearing aids

Use the FOCUS ON PRIDE section to complete these statements.

67. The word PRIDE used in the chapter stands for:
    P _____
    R _____
    I _____
    D _____
    E _____

68. When you work in health care, your work affects the person's _____.

69. When you carefully plan career choices, it shows respect for _____, those _____, and _____.

70. Positive interactions with others promotes _____ for you.

71. When you offer to help team members, it shows that you are _____ and value _____.

72. To protect yourself and others, you should know the limits of _____ in your state and agency.

Labeling

73. Fill in members of nursing service on the organizational chart (A–F).

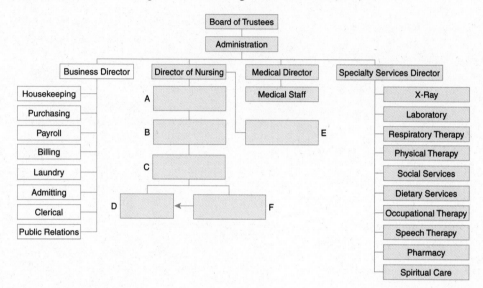

74. The nursing assistant reports to 2 groups of nursing service. They are

    A. _____

    B. _____

Optional Learning Exercises

Name the member of the health team who provides the service described.

75. Mr. Williams needs assistance to regain skills to dress, shave, and feed himself (ADL). He is assisted by the _____

76. Mrs. Young needs the corns on her feet treated. The nurse notifies the _____.

77. Ms. Stewart has the responsibility of doing physical examinations, health assessments, and health educations in the center where she works. She is a _____

78. Mr. Gomez keeps turning up the volume of his TV. His hearing is tested by the _____.

79. The _____ meets with a new resident and his family to discuss his nutritional needs.

80. Mr. Fox had a stroke and has weakness on his left side. The _____ assists him by developing a plan that focuses on restoring function and preventing disability from his illness.

81. The doctor orders x-rays after Mr. Jackson falls. The x-rays are done by the _____.

82. Mr. Ling has chronic lung disease and needs respiratory treatments. These are given by the _____

83. Ms. Walker plans the recreational needs of a nursing center. She is an _____.

84. After a stroke, Mr. Stubbs has difficulty swallowing. He is evaluated by the _____.

85. When the doctor orders blood tests, the samples are collected by the _____.

Name the nursing care pattern described in the following examples.

86. Ms. Hines works with Dr. Hogan. When his patient, Harry Forbes, is admitted to the hospital, Ms. Hines coordinates his care from admission to discharge. She also communicates with the insurance company and community agencies involved in Mr. Forbes' care. This is an example of _____.

87. When Mr. Holcomb reports for work as a nursing assistant, he is assigned to make all beds on the unit. The RN gives all drugs and the LPN gives all treatments. This nursing care pattern is _____

88. Ms. Conroy works on the same nursing unit each day. She has a group of patients and she gives total care to each of them. She teaches and counsels the person and family and plans for home care or long-term care when needed. This is an example of _____.

89. Ms. Ryan is a nursing assistant. She gives care that is delegated by an RN. The RN leads a team of nursing staff members and she decides the amount and kind of care each person needs. This is called _____.

90. Mrs. Young receives her care and physical therapy on the nursing unit. She does not have to go to different departments to receive treatments and care. This care is provided by the nursing team instead of by other health team members. This is called

_____

Fill in the Blank: Key Terms

Involuntary seclusion   Ombudsman   Representative   Treatment

1. A _____ is any person who has the legal right to act on the resident's behalf when he or she cannot do so for himself or herself.

2. Separating a person from others against his or her will, keeping the person to a certain area, or keeping the person away from his or her room without consent is _____.

3. The care provided to maintain or restore health, improve function, or relieve symptoms is _____.

4. An _____ is someone who supports or promotes the needs and interests of another person.

Circle the Best Answer

5. Which of these is a part of the Patient Care Partnership?
   A. The person must follow all recommended treatments or plans of care.
   B. The doctor does not need to share all of the information about his or her treatments.
   C. The person should know when students or other trainees are involved in his or her care.
   D. Hospital charges are not given to the person, only to the insurance companies.

6. Resident rights include all of the following rights except
   A. The right to have a private room in which to live
   B. The right to have and use personal items and clothing
   C. The right to personal privacy and confidentiality
   D. The right to refuse treatment

7. Under OBRA, if a resident is incompetent (not able) to exercise his or her rights, who can exercise these rights for the person?
   A. The doctor
   B. A representative such as a partner, adult child, or court-appointed guardian
   C. The charge nurse
   D. A neighbor

8. If a resident refuses treatment, what should you do?
   A. Avoid giving any care to the person and move on to other duties.
   B. Report the refusal to the nurse.
   C. Tell the resident the treatment must be done and continue to carry out the treatment.
   D. Tell the resident's family so they can make him accept the treatment.

9. A student wants to observe a treatment but the resident does not want her to be present. What is the correct action?
   A. The student cannot watch as this violates the resident's right to privacy.
   B. The student may observe from the doorway where the resident cannot see her.
   C. The staff nurse tells the resident he must allow the student to watch.
   D. The nurse calls the resident's wife to get her permission.

10. The resident should be given personal choice whenever it
    A. Is safely possible
    B. Does not interfere with scheduled activities
    C. Is approved by the director of nursing
    D. Is ordered by the doctor

11. If a resident voices concerns about care and the center promptly tries to correct the situation, this action meets the resident's right to
    A. Participate in a resident group
    B. Voice a dispute or grievance
    C. Personal choice
    D. Freedom from abuse, mistreatment, and neglect

12. A resident volunteers to take care of houseplants at the center. This is an acceptable part of the following except
    A. The care plan
    B. A requirement to receive care or care items
    C. The resident's regular activity
    D. Rehabilitation

13. When residents and their families plan activities together, this meets the resident's right to
    A. Privacy
    B. Freedom from restraint
    C. Freedom from mistreatment
    D. Participate in resident and family groups

14. The resident you are caring for has many old holiday decorations covering her nightstand. If you throw away these items without her permission, you are denying her right to
    A. Privacy
    B. Work
    C. Keep and use personal items
    D. Freedom from abuse

15. A staff member tells a resident he cannot leave his room because he talks too much. This action denies the resident
    A. Freedom from abuse, mistreatment, and neglect (involuntary seclusion)
    B. Freedom from restraint
    C. Care and security of personal possessions
    D. Personal choice

16. When a resident is given certain drugs that affect his mood, behavior, or mental function, it may deny his right to
    A. Freedom from abuse, mistreatment, and neglect
    B. Personal choice
    C. Privacy
    D. Freedom from restraint

17. Which of these actions will promote courteous and dignified care?
    A. Calling the resident by a nickname he does not choose
    B. Assisting with dressing the resident in clothing appropriate to the time of day
    C. Changing the resident's hairstyle without her permission
    D. Leaving the bathroom door open so you can see the resident

18. You ask a resident if you may touch him. This is an example of
    A. Courteous and dignified interaction
    B. Courteous and dignified care
    C. Providing privacy and self-determination
    D. Maintaining personal choice and independence

19. Assisting a resident to ambulate without interfering with her independence is an example of
    A. Courteous and dignified interaction
    B. Courteous and dignified care
    C. Providing privacy and self-determination
    D. Maintaining personal choice and independence

20. You provide privacy and self-determination for a resident when you
    A. Knock on the door before entering and wait to be asked in
    B. Allow her to smoke in designated areas
    C. Listen with interest to what the person is saying
    D. Groom his beard as he wishes

21. You allow the resident to maintain personal choice and independence when you
    A. Obtain her attention before interacting with her
    B. Provide extra clothing for warmth such as a sweater or lap robe
    C. Assist him to take part in activities according to his interests
    D. Use curtains or screens during personal care and procedures

22. Which of these activities would be carried out by an ombudsman?
    A. Organize activities for a group of residents
    B. Accompany residents to a religious service at a house of worship
    C. Investigate and resolve complaints made by a resident
    D. Assist the resident to choose friends

Fill in the Blank
23. CMS _____
24. OBRA _____

25. According to the Patient Care Partnership, in order for the patient to make informed decisions with his or her doctor, the person needs to understand
    A. _____
    B. _____
    C. _____
    D. _____
    E. _____
    F. _____

26. According the resident's rights, what should the nursing center do if a resident refuses treatment?
    A. _____
    B. _____
    C. _____
    D. _____

27. You are responsible for the care you give. To provide quality care
    A. _____
    B. _____
    C. _____
    D. _____
    E. _____
    F. _____

28. When a person refuses treatment, the health team offers _____.

29. You can encourage social interaction by telling about _____ and offering _____ activities.

30. You help to keep a person's personal information private when you discuss the person's treatment only with staff _____.

Optional Learning Activities
OBRA-Required Actions to Promote Dignity and Privacy (Box 2-3)

Match the action to promote dignity and privacy with the example.
A. Courteous and dignified interaction
B. Courteous and dignified care
C. Privacy and self-determination
D. Maintain personal choice and independence

31. _____ File fingernails and apply polish as the resident requests.
32. _____ Cover the resident with a blanket during a bath.
33. _____ Gain the person's attention before giving care.
34. _____ Show interest when a resident tells stories about his past.
35. _____ Open containers and arrange food at meal times to assist the resident.
36. _____ Close the door when the person asks for privacy.
37. _____ Allow a resident to smoke in a designated area.
38. _____ Make sure the resident is wearing his dentures when he goes to the dining room.
39. _____ Take the resident to her weekly card game.

3 The Nursing Assistant

Fill in the Blank: Key Terms

Certification   Endorsement   Equivalency   Job description   Nursing task   Reciprocity

1. A _____ is nursing care or a nursing procedure, activity, or work that can be delegated to nursing assistants when it does not require an RN's professional knowledge or judgment.

2. When a state recognizes the certificate, license, or registration issued by another state it is _____. This is also called reciprocity or equivalency.

3. A _____ is a document that describes what the agency expects you to do.

4. Another name for equivalency or endorsement is _____

5. Official recognition by a state that standards or requirements have been met is _____.

6. _____ is also called endorsement or reciprocity.

Circle the Best Answer

7. Until the 1980s, nursing assistants
   A. Attended nursing assistant classes approved by the state
   B. Were not used to provide basic nursing care
   C. Received on-the-job training from nurses
   D. Only worked in hospitals

8. Efforts to reduce health care costs include
   A. Nursing shortages
   B. Changes made by the Omnibus Budget Reconciliation Act of 1987 (OBRA)
   C. Hospital closings and mergers
   D. Changes in the nurse practice acts

9. When staff members are given training to perform basic skills that are provided by other health team members, it is called
   A. Staff mixing
   B. Cross-training
   C. Managed care
   D. Scope of practice

10. An example of cross-training would be
    A. A nursing assistant is delegated to give basic care to a patient
    B. Blood is drawn by a medical technician sent from the laboratory
    C. An RN gives medications to a group of patients
    D. A member of the nursing team draws blood when the order is given

11. Nurse practice acts
    A. Only affect RNs and LPNs/LVNs
    B. Teach classes for nurses and nursing assistants
    C. Define RNs and LPNs/LVNs and sometimes also regulate nursing assistants
    D. Are exactly the same in every state

12. _____ decides what nursing assistants can do.
    A. Joint Commission of Hospital Accreditation
    B. The nurse practice act
    C. The state medical society
    D. The hospital board of directors

13. If you do something beyond the legal limits of your role, you could be
    A. Protected by the nurse practice act
    B. Practicing nursing without a license
    C. Protected by the nurse who supervises your work
    D. Accused of a criminal act

14. Nursing assistants can have their certification, license, or registration denied, revoked, or suspended for
    A. Being absent from work frequently
    B. Failing to maintain the confidentiality of patient or resident information
    C. Refusing to care for a certain patient
    D. Having frequent arguments with co-workers

15. OBRA requires that the nursing assistant training and competency evaluation program have at least _____ hours of instruction.
    A. 16   C. 120
    B. 75   D. 200

16. Which of these areas of study is *not* included in a training program for nursing assistants?
    A. Communication
    B. Elimination procedures
    C. Resident rights
    D. Phlebotomy (drawing blood)

17. The competency evaluation for nursing assistants has two parts. They are
    A. Written test and skills test
    B. Multiple-choice test and true-false test
    C. Skills test and complete bed bath demonstration
    D. Written test and oral questions-and-answers test

18. If you fail the competency evaluation the first time you take it, you
    A. May retest a second time
    B. Can retest two more times for a total of three times
    C. Must repeat your training program
    D. Can retest as often as necessary, free of charge

19. All of the following information is contained in the nursing assistant registry *except*
    A. Information about findings of abuse or neglect and of dishonest use of property
    B. Date of birth
    C. Number of dependents
    D. Date the competency test was passed

20. OBRA requires that re-training and a new competency evaluation test must be taken if you have not worked as a certified nursing assistant for
    A. 24 months   C. 1 year
    B. 5 years   D. 6 months

21. If you want to work in another state, the state agency will require all of these *except*
    A. Proof of full-time employment within the last month
    B. Proof of successfully completing a NATCEP
    C. Written registry verification from the state in which you are currently certified
    D. Fingerprints
22. Your work as a nursing assistant is supervised by
    A. A licensed nurse
    B. A doctor or dentist
    C. The director of nursing
    D. A nursing assistant with more experience than you
23. As a nursing assistant, you never give medications unless
    A. The nurse is busy and asks you to give the medications
    B. The person is in the shower and the nurse leaves the medications at the bedside
    C. You have completed a state-approved medication assistant training program
    D. You are feeding the person and the nurse asks you to mix the medications with the food
24. You are alone in the nurses' station and you answer the phone. Dr. Smith begins to give you verbal orders. You should
    A. Hang up the phone
    B. Politely give her your name and title and ask her to wait while you get the nurse
    C. Quickly write down the orders and give them to the nurse
    D. Politely give her your name and title and tell her to call back later when the nurse is there
25. The nurse asks you to assist him as he changes sterile dressings. You should
    A. Assist him as needed
    B. Tell him you cannot assist in performing any sterile procedures
    C. Tell him you will change the dressings yourself, so that he can carry out duties
    D. Report his request to the director of nursing
26. Who can tell the person or family a diagnosis or prescribe treatments?
    A. Director of nursing
    B. RN
    C. Doctor
    D. Experienced nursing assistant
27. The nurse asks you carry out a task that you do not know how to do. You should
    A. Ignore the order because it would not be safe for you to carry out the task
    B. Promptly explain to the nurse why you cannot carry out the task
    C. Perform the task as well as you can
    D. Ask another nursing assistant to show you how to carry out the task
28. The nurse knows you are an EMT in addition to being a CNA. She is very busy and asks if you will start an IV on a patient. You should
    A. Politely tell her that you cannot start an IV as a CNA
    B. Start the IV since you start IVs routinely as an EMT
    C. Ask her to spend a few minutes supervising you as you start the IV
    D. Report her to the state board of nursing
29. If you are giving care in a home, you may be expected to
    A. Give medications
    B. Provide personal care and prepare meals
    C. Move heavy furniture
    D. Drive the person's car so the person can shop or run errands
30. When you read a job description, you should not take a job if it requires you to
    A. Carry out duties you do not like to do
    B. Function beyond your training limits
    C. Maintain required certification
    D. Attend in-service training

Fill in the Blank

31. Write out the abbreviations.
    A. CNA _____
    B. LNA _____
    C. LPN _____
    D. LVN _____
    E. OBRA _____
    F. NATCEP _____
    G. NCSBN _____
    H. RN _____
    I. RNA _____
    J. SRNA _____
    K. STNA _____
32. When hospitals make an effort to reduce costs with a staffing mix, nursing care is given by a mix of
    A. _____
    B. _____
    C. _____
33. A nurse practice act
    A. Defines _____ and describes their _____
    B. Describes the education and _____
    C. Protects the public from _____
34. The nursing assistant registry has this information about each nursing assistant:
    A. _____
    B. _____
    C. _____
    D. _____
    E. _____
    F. _____
    G. _____
35. Why does OBRA require 12 hours of educational programs and performance reviews each year for every nursing assistant? _____

36. A surveyor may
    A. Check to see if nursing assistants have completed
       a _____
    B. Ask nursing assistants where they received
       _____
    C. Observe if nursing assistants are able to observe,
       describe, and report _____
    D. Transfer the person from the _____

37. When a nursing assistant applies for reciprocity in
    another state, the application review results in 1 or
    more of these actions:
    A. _____
    B. _____
    C. _____

38. What are tasks you should never do as a nursing
    assistant?
    A. _____
    B. _____
    C. _____
    D. _____
    E. _____
    F. _____
    G. _____
    H. _____

39. Do not take a job that requires you to
    A. _____
    B. _____
    C. _____

**Use the FOCUS ON PRIDE section to complete these
statements.**

40. During and after your training you should make an
    effort to develop personal and _____
    _____.

41. If a patient refuses to have a student care for him, you
    should kindly _____ the person's
    rights to choose who is involved in his care.

42. Practicing skills in the classroom or laboratory will
    make you feel more _____.

Optional Learning Exercises
OBRA requirements related to the nursing assistant.

43. OBRA requires _____ hours of instruction.
    _____ hours must be supervised practical
    training. Where can the practical training take place?
    _____ or _____

44. OBRA requires 14 areas of study. Write the area of
    study where you learn the skill used in each example.
    A. _____ You make a bed.
    B. _____ You close
       Mr. Smith's door to give him privacy.
    C. _____ You tell Mrs. Forbes
       the time of day and the day of the week frequently
       because she is mildly confused.
    D. _____ You apply lotion to a resident's skin.
    E. _____ You assist
       a person to put on his shirt.
    F. _____ When assigned to a new unit,
       you check the location of the fire alarm.
    G. _____ You practice hand
       hygiene before and after giving care.
    H. _____ You get help to move
       a person from his bed to the chair.
    I. _____ When speaking to
       Mr. Jackson, you maintain good eye contact.
    J. _____ The nurse tells you to
       exercise a person's extremities (limbs).
    K. _____ You position a urinal
       for a resident in bed.
    L. _____ You assist Mrs.
       Young to walk in the hall.
    M. _____ You notice that Mrs. Peck
       has an elevated temperature and her skin is warm.
    N. _____ You cut up the meat
       on Mr. Sanyo's plate before helping him to eat.

Working in another state.

45. To work in another state, you must meet that state's
    _____.

46. To find the state agency responsible for NATCEPs and
    the nursing assistant registry, you will
    A. _____
    B. _____

47. When the state determines that you may work in that
    state as a nursing assistant, the state may use these
    terms.
    A. _____
    B. _____
    C. _____

48. When you apply to work in another state, expect to
    A. _____
    B. _____
    C. _____
    D. _____
    E. _____

Job description.
Refer to Figure 3-2 in the textbook to answer these questions.

49. The nursing assistant notifies appropriate _____ staff when a resident complains _____.

50. Takes and records _____, _____, _____, _____, _____, and _____.

51. Participates in _____ activities on the unit.

52. Must be able to follow _____, both _____ and oral, and work _____ with other staff members.

53. Maintains personal _____ to prevent _____ from work due to health problems.

54. Completes annual _____ requirements.

55. Reports to work _____ and as _____, and completes work within _____ times.

4 Delegation

Fill in the Blank: Key Terms

Accountable   Competent   Delegate   Nursing task   Responsibility

1. Being responsible for one's actions and the actions of others who perform delegated tasks is being

   _____.

2. To _____ means to authorize another person to perform a nursing task in a certain situation.

3. A _____ is nursing care or a nursing procedure, activity, or work that can be delegated to nursing assistants when it does not require an RN's professional knowledge or judgment.

4. _____ is the duty or obligation to perform some act or function.

5. _____ means having the necessary ability, knowledge, or skill to perform a task safely and successfully.

Circle the Best Answer

6. Which of the following is *not* acceptable?
   A. An RN delegates a task to an LPN/LVN.
   B. An RN delegates a task to a nursing assistant.
   C. An LPN/LVN delegates a task to a nursing assistant.
   D. A nursing assistant delegates a task to another nursing assistant.

7. When a nurse decides how to delegate tasks, the decision depends on
   A. What is best for the person at the time
   B. How well the nurse likes the nursing assistant
   C. How busy the nurse is that day
   D. Whether the nurse likes the person receiving the care

8. You have been caring for Mr. Watson for several weeks. The nurse tells you that she will give his care today. Her delegation decision is based on
   A. How well you gave his care in the past
   B. Changes in Mr. Watson's condition today
   C. How well she knows you
   D. How much supervision you need

9. At which step of the delegation process would you tell the nurse you have not performed a task before or often?
   A. Assess and plan
   B. Communication
   C. Surveillance and supervision
   D. Evaluation and feedback

10. When the nurse supervises the nursing assistant, she
   A. Tells the nursing assistant how to perform and complete the task
   B. Determines what knowledge and skills are needed to safely perform the nursing task
   C. Observes the care that the nursing assistant gives
   D. Decides whether the care plan needs to change

11. Which of the following is *not* a right of delegation?
   A. The right task
   B. The right time
   C. The right person
   D. The right supervision

12. Which of these tasks cannot be delegated to a nursing assistant?
   A. Give perineal care
   B. Supervise others
   C. Assist with coughing and deep-breathing exercises
   D. Collect specimens

13. You have the right to refuse a task if
   A. You have never cared for the person before
   B. You have too much to do and do not have time to carry out the task
   C. The task is not in your job description
   D. You do not like to do the task

Fill in the Blank

14. Write out the abbreviations.
   A. LPN _____
   B. LVN _____
   C. NCSBN _____
   D. RN _____

15. Nursing assistants cannot delegate. This means you cannot
   A. Delegate any task to other _____
      or any other _____
   B. You cannot _____ or
      _____ someone else to do your work
   C. You cannot re-delegate a task to another
      _____

16. You must refuse a delegated task that is
   A. _____
   B. _____
   C. _____

17. What directions must be given when the nurse communicates with the nursing assistant about a delegated task?
   A. _____
   B. _____
   C. _____
   D. _____
   E. _____
   F. _____

18. During Step 4 of the delegation process, the nurse will give feedback. What 2 things will occur during feedback?

    A. The nurse will tell you what you did _____ and _____.

    B. It is a way for you to _____ and _____.

19. What are the five rights of delegation?

    A. _____

    B. _____

    C. _____

    D. _____

    E. _____

Use the FOCUS ON PRIDE section to complete these statements.

20. You show responsibility when you refuse a task to protect _____.

21. With corrective feedback, you should

    A. _____

    B. _____

    C. _____

    D. _____

    E. _____

22. Delegation experiences are positive when the staff

    A. _____

    B. _____

    C. _____

    D. _____

Optional Learning Experiences

23. What are the 4 steps in the delegation process described by the National Council of State Boards of Nursing (NCSBN)?

    A. Step 1 _____

    B. Step 2 _____

    C. Step 3 _____

    D. Step 4 _____

24. Read the following statements and for each indicate which of the four steps of the delegation process it describes.

    A. The nurse makes sure that you complete the task correctly. _____

    B. Asking, how will delegating the task help the person and what are the risks to the person.

    _____

    C. The nurse tells you when to report observations.

    _____

    D. Asking, was the outcome the desired result and was the outcome good or bad. _____

25. Look at the *Five Rights of Delegation for Nursing Assistants* in Box 4-2. List the right in which each of these questions is listed.

    A. Did you review the task with the nurse?

    _____

    B. Were you trained to do the task? _____

    C. Do you have concerns about performing the task?

    _____

    D. Is the nurse available if the person's condition changes or if problems occur? _____

    E. Do you have the equipment and supplies to safely complete the task? _____

Fill in the Blank: Key Terms

Abuse
Assault
Battery
Boundary crossing
Boundary sign
Boundary violation
Child abuse and neglect
Civil law
Code of ethics

Crime
Criminal law
Defamation
Elder abuse
Ethics
False imprisonment
Fraud
Intimate partner violence
Invasion of privacy

Law
Libel
Malpractice
Neglect
Negligence
Professional boundary
Professional sexual
  misconduct

Protected health
  information
Self-neglect
Slander
Standard of care
Tort
Vulnerable adult
Will

1. Physical, sexual, or psychological abuse by a current of former partner or spouse is

   _____.

2. Any knowing, intentional, or negligent act by a caregiver or any other person to an older adult is

   _____.

3. A rule of conduct made by a government body is a

   _____.

4. _____ is injuring a person's name and reputation by making false statements to a third person.

5. An act, behavior, or comment that is sexual in nature is _____.

6. Touching a person's body without his or her consent is _____.

7. _____ are laws concerned with offenses against the public and society in general.

8. Failure to provide the person with the goods or services needed to avoid physical harm, mental anguish, or mental illness is _____.

9. _____ are rules, or standards of conduct, for group members to follow.

10. An act, behavior, or thought that warns of a boundary crossing or violation is a _____.

11. _____ is the skills, care, and judgments required by a health team member under similar conditions.

12. A _____ is a legal document of how a person wants property distributed after death.

13. _____ is saying or doing something to trick, fool, or deceive a person.

14. The intentional mistreatment or harm of another person is _____.

15. An unintentional wrong in which a person did not act in a reasonable and careful manner and causes harm to a person or to the person's property is

   _____.

16. _____ is a person's behaviors and way of living that threaten his or her health, safety, and well-being.

17. A wrong committed against a person or the person's property is a _____.

18. _____ is a brief act or behavior outside of the helpful zone.

19. Making false statements in print, writing, or through pictures or drawings is _____.

20. A _____ is an act that violates a criminal law.

21. _____ is knowledge of what is right conduct and wrong conduct.

22. Violating a person's right not to have his or her name, photo, or private affairs exposed or made public without giving consent is an _____.

23. Identifying information and information about the person's health care is _____.

24. A _____ is a person 18 years old or older who has a disability or condition that makes him or her at risk to be wounded, attacked, or damaged.

25. A _____ is an act or behavior that meets your needs, not the person's.

26. Negligence by a professional person is

   _____.

27. Making false statements orally is _____.

28. _____ are laws concerned with relationships between people.

29. _____ is that which separates helpful behaviors from behaviors that are not helpful.

30. Unlawful restraint or restriction of a person's freedom of movement is _____.

31. _____ is intentionally attempting or threatening to touch a person's body without the person's consent.

32. The intentional harm or mistreatment of a child under 18 years old is _____.

Circle the Best Answer

33. Which situation is unethical behavior for a nursing assistant?
    A. A person of another race is given personal care as delegated by the nurse.
    B. The nursing assistant avoids giving care to a person with body piercings.
    C. The nursing assistant reports that an elderly patient says her son sometimes hits her.
    D. The nursing assistant gives good care to a man who does not want life-saving measures, even though the nursing assistant disagrees with his decision.

34. What should the nursing assistant do if he finds a co-worker drinking alcohol at work?
    A. Report this behavior to the nurse
    B. Tell the co-worker that he will report this behavior unless the person pays him not to
    C. Give the co-worker information about a program for alcoholics
    D. Ignore the behavior to be loyal to his co-worker

35. Which code of conduct for nursing assistants is followed when you schedule your lunch to finish giving personal care to a person?
    A. Perform no act that will cause the person harm
    B. Know the limits of your role and knowledge
    C. Consider the person's needs to be more important than your own
    D. Protect the person's privacy

36. An example of boundary crossing would be all of these *except*
    A. Telling a person you are caring for details about your family
    B. Hugging the person each time you see him
    C. Comforting the person with a hug when you find her crying one day
    D. Accepting cash from the person

37. You may be accused of negligence when giving care if you
    A. Tell the nurse that you know the person you are assigned to care for
    B. Assist a person to the bathroom and make sure the call light is available for her to call you
    C. Give the wrong care to the wrong person because they both have the same name
    D. Report to the nurse that the person is complaining of chest pain

38. You tell another nursing assistant that you think the housekeeper is stealing money from the staff. This is an example of
    A. Defamation
    B. Boundary crossing
    C. Invasion of privacy
    D. Libel

39. In the cafeteria, you overhear two nursing assistants talking about a person they are caring for. This is an example of
    A. Defamation
    B. Libel
    C. Boundary crossing
    D. Invasion of privacy

40. If you begin to give care to a person without asking permission, you may be guilty of
    A. Battery
    B. Assault
    C. Invasion of privacy
    D. Defamation

41. A person *cannot* give informed consent for treatment or care if
    A. He or she is over legal age (usually 18 years)
    B. He or she clearly understands what will be done
    C. He or she is sedated
    D. He or she is mentally competent

42. If you are asked to witness the signing of a consent, you
    A. Must know the agency policy on whether you may do this
    B. Should always refuse as it is not legal to do this
    C. Cannot ethically or legally witness a will
    D. Cannot refuse as it is part of your responsibility

43. If you are convicted of abuse, neglect, or mistreatment, this information will be
    A. In your nursing assistant registry information
    B. In the nurse's notes
    C. In the court records only
    D. Destroyed as soon as the abused person leaves the agency

44. You notice a home care patient has no food in the house and the water has been turned off. This could be a sign of
    A. Self-neglect
    B. Physical abuse
    C. Involuntary seclusion
    D. Emotional abuse

45. If you suspect an elderly person is being abused, you should
    A. Ask the person to tell you who is abusing him or her
    B. Discuss the abuse with the caregiver
    C. Call the police
    D. Discuss the matter and your observations with the nurse

46. A child who shows great affection to others may be a victim of
    A. Physical abuse
    B. Neglect
    C. Sexual abuse
    D. Emotional abuse

47. If you suspect a child is being abused
    A. Ask the child whether he or she is being abused
    B. Share your concerns with the nurse
    C. Call the local child welfare agency
    D. Talk to the parents

Matching

Match the statements to the correct topic.
A. Rules for maintaining professional boundaries
B. Boundary signs
C. Boundary crossing
D. Boundary violation

48. _____ Keep the person's information confidential.

49. _____ You borrow money from a patient's family.

50. _____ Do not date a current patient or resident or family members of a current patient or resident.

51. _____ You believe you are the only person who understands the person and his needs.

52. _____ You hug a person because he or she is crying.

53. _____ You tell a person about your personal relationships or problems.

54. _____ You select what you report and record. You do not give complete information.

55. _____ You trade assignments with other nursing assistants so you can provide the person's care.

Fill in the Blank

56. Write out the meaning of the abbreviations.
    A. CDC _____
    B. HIPAA _____
    C. IPV _____
    D. OBRA _____

57. When you judge a person based on your values and standards, you are not using _____ behavior.

58. It violates rules for _____ if you accept a gift from a patient, resident, or his or her family.

59. If you cause harm to a person because you did not act in a reasonable and careful manner, you may be found _____.

60. When giving care, you must follow standards of care. Standards of care come from
    A. _____
    B. _____
    C. _____
    D. _____
    E. _____
    F. _____
    G. _____

61. If you injure a person's name and reputation by making false statements to a third person, you can be accused of _____. Explain the difference between two forms of this offense.
    A. Libel _____
    B. Slander _____

62. When you get a person's consent to give him or her a shower, you protect yourself from being accused of _____ and _____.

63. When using electronic communications, you should never
    A. Take _____ or _____ of the person or any part of the person's body
    B. Identify the patients or residents by _____

64. As a nursing assistant, you are never responsible for obtaining written _____.

65. What problems would cause a person to be considered a vulnerable adult?
    A. _____
    B. _____
    C. _____

66. If an elderly person is deprived of a basic need, such as food or clothing, this would be _____ abuse and _____.

67. You accept an assignment to give care to an elderly person. You do not report off to a staff member who will assume responsibility for the person. You will be accused of _____.

68. Name the type of child abuse described in these examples.
    A. The child is injured mentally.
    _____
    B. The child was left in circumstances where the child suffers serious harm. _____
    C. The child has been kicked, burned, or bitten.
    _____
    D. The child has engaged in sexual activity with a family member. _____
    E. Drug activity has taken place when the child is present. _____

69. What kinds of violence are considered intimate partner violence?
    A. _____
    B. _____
    C. _____
    D. _____

70. When a domestic partner controls friendships and other relationships of the other person, this is _____ violence.

Use the FOCUS ON PRIDE section to complete these statements.

71. Health care providers are mandatory reporters. This means they must report suspected abuse or neglect of

_____, _____,

and _____.

72. If you suspect a person is being abused, tell

_____

73. To maintain professional boundaries, you can

A. Follow the _____

B. Obey the _____

C. Monitor for _____

D. Ask the _____

74. Accepting a task beyond the legal limits of your role

can lead to _____

Optional Learning Exercises

Which rule in the Code of Conduct for Nursing Assistants applies to the situations in the next 5 questions?

75. A nursing assistant has back pain and takes her

mother's medication to treat it. _____

_____

76. A nursing assistant is caring for a person her sister knows. The sister asks for information about the

person. _____

77. A nursing assistant changes her lunch time because her assigned patient needs unexpected care.

_____

78. The nursing assistant tells the nurse that he recorded

information on the wrong patient. _____

_____

79. The nursing assistant knows that she is not allowed to

carry out sterile procedures by herself. _____

_____

80. If a nursing assistant causes unintentional harm to a

person, it is called _____. If a nurse or

other professional person causes unintentional harm,

it is called _____.

81. If you are giving care in a home and you notice the person is not taking needed drugs, you think this is

a sign of _____. What should you do

about this situation? _____

82. When you are working in a long-term care center, you notice another nursing assistant forcing food into a 90-year-old person's mouth. When you ask about her actions, she laughs and says, "That's the only way I can get done with my assignments, so I can go to

lunch." This is an example of _____.

What should you do? _____

_____

6 Student and Work Ethics

Fill in the Blank: Key Terms

Bullying
Burnout
Confidentiality

Conflict
Courtesy
Gossip

Harassment
Priority
Professionalism

Stress
Stressor

Teamwork
Work ethics

1. A clash between opposing interests or ideas is

   _____.

2. _____ is job stress resulting in being physically or mentally exhausted.

3. Following laws, being ethical, having good work ethics, and having the skills to do your work is

   _____.

4. A _____ is the event or factor that causes stress.

5. The most important thing at the time is the

   _____

6. Trusting others with personal and private information is _____.

7. _____ is behavior in the workplace.

8. _____ is to spread rumors or talk about the private matters of others.

9. The response or change in the body caused by any emotional, physical, social, or economic factor is

   _____.

10. _____ is a polite, considerate, or helpful comment or act.

11. _____ means to trouble, torment, offend, or worry a person by one's behavior or comments.

12. When staff members work together as a group it is called _____.

13. Repeated attacks or threats of fear, distress, or harm by a bully toward a victim is _____.

Circle the Best Answer

14. Work ethics involve
    A. How well you do your skills
    B. What religion you practice
    C. How you treat others and work with others
    D. Cultural beliefs and attitudes

15. Your diet will maintain your weight if
    A. You avoid salty and sweet foods
    B. You take in fewer calories than your energy needs require
    C. It includes foods with fats and oils
    D. You balance the number of calories taken in with your energy needs

16. Adults need about _____ hours of sleep daily.
    A. 7 to 8
    B. 10 to 11
    C. Less than 6
    D. 12

17. Exercise is needed
    A. For rest and sleep
    B. To help you feel better physically and mentally
    C. To have good body mechanics
    D. To improve your nutrition

18. Smoking odors
    A. Disappear quickly when the person finishes smoking
    B. Can be covered up by chewing gum
    C. Are noticed only by the smoker
    D. Stay on the person's breath, hands, clothing, and hair

19. The most important reason a person should not work under the influence of alcohol or drugs is that it
    A. Affects the person's safety and yours
    B. Causes the person to be disorganized
    C. Makes co-workers angry
    D. Is not allowed by your nursing center

20. Tattoos should be covered when working because they
    A. May offend persons you care for, their families, and co-workers
    B. Can become infected
    C. May confuse persons
    D. Increase the risk of skin injuries

21. When working, the nursing assistant may wear
    A. Jewelry in pierced eyebrow, nose, lips, or tongue
    B. Wedding and engagement rings
    C. Multiple earrings in each ear
    D. Nail polish

22. When working, the nursing assistant *should not* wear
    A. A beard or mustache that is clean and trimmed
    B. Hair that is off the collar and away from the face
    C. Perfume, cologne, or after-shave
    D. A wristwatch with a second hand

23. When in school or working, the most important reason to plan good childcare and transportation in advance is it will
    A. Make your instructor or employer like you
    B. Show you are a responsible student or employee
    C. Prevent stress
    D. Show you are a good parent

24. What is a common reason for losing a job?
    A. Not knowing how to perform a task
    B. Absences and tardiness
    C. Being disorganized
    D. Lacking self-confidence

25. When you are scheduled to begin work at 3 PM, you should
    A. Plan to arrive by 2:30 PM
    B. Arrive at exactly 3 PM
    C. Plan to arrive a few minutes early and be ready to work at 3 PM
    D. Arrive within a few minutes before or after 3 PM

26. Which of these statements would signal you have a good attitude?
    A. "I will do that right away."
    B. "It's not my turn. I did that yesterday."
    C. "That's not my patient."
    D. "It's not my fault."

27. You can avoid being part of gossip by
    A. Remaining quiet when you are in a group where gossip is occurring
    B. Talking about persons and family members only to co-workers
    C. Repeating comments only in writing
    D. Removing yourself from a group or situation where gossip is occurring

28. The person's information can be shared
    A. With the person's family
    B. Only among staff involved in his or her care
    C. With your family
    D. With friends who know the person

29. Slang or swearing should not be used at work because
    A. Words used with family and friends may offend persons and family members
    B. The person may not understand you
    C. The person may have difficulty hearing
    D. Co-workers may over-hear it

30. You should say "please" and "thank you" to others because
    A. Courtesies mean so much to people; it can brighten someone's day
    B. It shows respect to the person
    C. It is required by your job
    D. It shows you like the person

31. It is acceptable at work if you
    A. Take a pen to use at home
    B. Sell cookies for your child's school project
    C. Use a pay phone or wireless phone on your break to call your child
    D. Make a copy of a letter on the copier in the nurses' station

32. When you leave and return to the unit for breaks or lunch, you should
    A. Tell each person you see
    B. Tell any family members present
    C. Tell the nurse
    D. Tell your best friend

33. Safety practices are important to follow because
    A. They help you to be more organized
    B. Negligent behavior affects the safety of others
    C. They save the center money
    D. You will get promoted more quickly

34. Which of these would *not* be a good safety practice?
    A. Know the contents and policies in personnel and procedure manuals
    B. Question unclear instructions and things you do not understand
    C. Do not tell anyone when you make a mistake
    D. Ask for any training you might need

35. When setting priorities they are planned around
    A. Your break and lunch time
    B. The person's needs
    C. Co-workers' schedules
    D. The time scheduled by the nurse

36. Stress occurs
    A. Only when you have unpleasant situations in your life
    B. Because you do not handle your problems well
    C. Because you are in the wrong job
    D. Every minute of every day and in everything you do

37. What physical effects of stress can be life-threatening?
    A. High blood pressure, heart attack, strokes, ulcers
    B. Increased heart rate, faster and deeper breathing
    C. Anxiety, fear, anger, depression
    D. Headaches, insomnia, muscle tension

38. When you are dealing with a conflict, the first step to resolve the problem is
    A. Talk to my supervisor
    B. Quit my job
    C. Define the problem
    D. Identify possible solutions

39. Burnout
    A. Occurs in every life situation
    B. Occurs when you are happy with your job or school
    C. Can lead to physical and mental health problems
    D. Will improve if you just ignore the symptoms

40. Which of these actions is harassment?
    A. Offending others with gestures or remarks
    B. Gossiping about a patient or his family
    C. Having doubts about your abilities
    D. Ignoring a conflict among staff members

41. If you resign from a job, it is good practice to give
    A. One week's notice
    B. Two weeks' notice
    C. Four weeks' notice
    D. No notice

Matching

Match the qualities and characteristics of good work ethics with the examples.

A. Caring
B. Dependable
C. Considerate
D. Cheerful
E. Empathy
F. Trustworthy
G. Respectful
H. Courteous
I. Conscientious
J. Honest
K. Cooperative
L. Enthusiasm
M. Self-aware
N. Patience

42. _____ While working with Mr. Smith, you try to understand and feel what it must be like to be paralyzed on one side.

43. _____ You realize you are very good at giving basic care. You know you need to improve your communication skills.

44. _____ When caring for elderly residents, you try to do small things to make them happy or to find ways to ease their pain.

45. _____ You thank co-workers when they help you and remember to wish residents happy birthday as appropriate.

46. _____ When Mrs. Gibson is upset and angry, you remember to respect her feelings and to be kind.

47. _____ You report the blood pressure and temperature readings accurately to the nurse.

48. _____ You realize giving care to residents is important and you are excited about your work.

49. _____ Your supervisor tells you she knows she can count on you because you are always on time and perform delegated tasks as assigned.

50. _____ Even though Mr. Acevado has different cultural and religious views than yours, you value his feelings and beliefs.

51. _____ Before you left home today you had an argument with your child. When you get to work you make every effort to put that aside and be pleasant and happy.

52. _____ The nurse discusses a resident problem with you and states she knows you will keep the information confidential.

53. _____ When you are assigned to give care to a resident, you make sure his or her care is done thoroughly and exactly as instructed.

54. _____ Your co-worker says she needs help to turn her resident and you cheerfully offer to help.

55. _____ You adjust your schedule when your patient has a visitor and you cannot give care when you planned.

Fill in the Blank

56. NATCEP means _____.

57. Work ethics involves

   A. _____
   B. _____
   C. _____
   D. _____
   E. _____

58. Personal health is important when you are on the job and caring for other persons. For each of the following examples, name the related health, hygiene, or appearance factor.

   A. _____ Hand-washing and good personal hygiene are needed to remove odors on your breath, hands, clothing, and hair.

   B. _____ If you have fatigue, lack of energy, and irritability, it may mean you need more of this.

   C. _____ You will feel better physically and mentally if you walk, run, swim, or bike regularly.

   D. _____ Some of these affect thinking, feeling, behavior, and function. This may affect the person's safety.

   E. _____ Avoid foods from the fats, oils, and sweets group. Also avoid salty foods and crash diets.

   F. _____ You may not be able to read instructions and take measurements accurately if you do not have these checked.

   G. _____ Practice this when you bend, carry heavy objects, and lift, move, and turn persons.

   H. _____ This substance depresses the brain and affects thinking, balance, coordination, and mental alertness.

59. What should you do if you will be late or cannot work or attend school? _____ and know the _____.

60. How can you promote teamwork and manage your time when someone is late or does not show up for work?

   A. _____
   B. _____
   C. _____

61. You hear a co-worker say, "It's not my turn. I did it yesterday." This is an example of having a

   _____

62. If you make or repeat any comment that you do not know to be true, or a comment that can hurt a person or family member, you are _____

63. You are caring for a friend of your mother and your mother asks for information about her friend's illness and care. If you repeat this information to your mother, you will violate the person's

_____ and

_____.

64. If your friends or family need to visit with you when you are working, they must meet you

_____.

65. Setting priorities involves deciding
    A. _____
    B. _____
    C. _____
    D. _____
    E. _____
    F. _____
    G. _____
    H. _____

66. What physical symptoms may occur when a person has stress?
    A. _____
    B. _____
    C. _____
    D. _____
    E. _____

67. When you have a conflict with another person, what are steps to take when resolving the conflict?
    A. Step 1 _____
    B. Step 2 _____
    C. Step 3 _____
    D. Step 4 _____
    E. Step 5 _____
    F. Step 6 _____

68. What are the causes of burnout?
    A. _____
    B. _____
    C. _____
    D. _____
    E. _____
    F. _____
    G. _____
    H. _____

69. When you resign from a job, you tell the employer by doing 1 of the following:
    A. _____
    B. _____
    C. _____

Use the FOCUS ON PRIDE section to complete these statements.

70. Patients, residents, families, visitors, and co-workers depend on you to give safe and effective care. They trust that you will
    A. _____
    B. _____
    C. _____
    D. _____
    E. _____
    F. _____

71. When you greet patients and residents and politely introduce yourself, you are displaying good social

_____.

72. When you offer to help others, ask the nurse if you can help others, and return from breaks on time, you are displaying actions that help build a strong

_____.

Optional Learning Exercises

73. Use Box 6-2, Practices for a Professional Appearance, in the text to answer these questions.
    A. It is best to wear your name badge

    _____

    B. Why should undergarments be the correct color for your skin tone?

    _____

    C. You should follow the dress code for jewelry and not wear necklaces or dangling earrings because

    _____

    D. Chipped nail polish may provide a

    _____.

    E. Perfume, cologne, or after-shave lotion scents may

    _____

Fill in the Blank: Key Terms

Abbreviation	Dorsal	Medial	Recording
Anterior	Electronic health record	Medical record	Reporting
Chart	Electronic medical record	Posterior	Root
Clinical record	End-of-shift report	Prefix	Suffix
Communication	Kardex	Progress note	Ventral
Distal	Lateral	Proximal	Word element

1. An electronic version of a person's medical record is _____; also called electronic medical record.

2. Another term for medical record is _____.

3. At or toward the front of the body or body part is ventral or _____.

4. A _____ is a word element placed after a root; it changes the meaning of the word.

5. At the side of the body or body part is _____.

6. An _____ is a shortened form of a word or phrase.

7. A part of a word is a _____.

8. A _____ is a type of card file that summarizes information found in the medical record.

9. The medical record is also called the _____.

10. The part nearest to the center or the point of origin is _____.

11. _____ is the exchange of information—a message sent is received and interpreted by the intended person.

12. Another term for anterior is _____.

13. A written account of a person's condition and response to treatment and care is the chart or _____.

14. _____ is at or toward the back of the body or body part; posterior.

15. The oral account of care and observations is _____.

16. _____ is the part farthest from the center or from the point of attachment.

17. A word element placed before a root is the _____. It changes the meaning of the word.

18. A word element containing the basic meaning of the word is the _____.

19. Another word for dorsal is _____.

20. _____ is the written account of care and observations.

21. _____ is at or near the middle or mid-line of the body or body part.

22. _____ describes the care given and the person's response and progress.

23. Another name for an electronic health record is _____.

24. A report that the nurse gives at the end of the shift to the on-coming staff is _____.

Circle the Best Answer

25. When health team members communicate, they share all of this information *except*
    A. Gossip about the person and his family
    B. What was done for the person
    C. What needs to be done for the person
    D. The person's response to treatment

26. A nursing assistant tells the nurse that Mr. Jones ate a small amount of his lunch. The nurse
    A. Knows this means Mr. Jones ate one half of his meal
    B. Thinks Mr. Jones ate two or three bites of food
    C. Thinks Mr. Jones ate only 25% of his meal
    D. Asks for further information because words may have different meanings to different people

27. When giving information to another health team member
    A. Be brief and concise to reduce omitting important details
    B. Use terms that may or may not be familiar to others
    C. Give many details unrelated to the information
    D. Use general terms instead of facts

28. The medical record or chart is
    A. A temporary record of the person
    B. Discarded when the person leaves the agency
    C. A permanent legal document
    D. Given to the person when he or she is discharged

29. Which of these is not included in the person's chart?
    A. The daily menu
    B. X-ray reports
    C. Special consents
    D. Health history

30. A nursing assistant
    A. May read the charts in all health care agencies
    B. Is never allowed to read the person's chart
    C. Must know the agency policy before reading the chart
    D. Is allowed to tell the person what is recorded in the chart

31. If a person asks to see his or her record, the nursing assistant
    A. Reports the request to the nurse
    B. Checks the agency policy to see if this is allowed
    C. Gives the chart to the person's legal representative
    D. Gives the chart to the person

32. The admission record contains
    A. Doctor's orders
    B. The name, birth date, age, and gender of the person
    C. Test results
    D. Special diet information

33. The health history is completed
    A. When the person is discharged
    B. When the person is admitted
    C. By the doctor
    D. By the nursing assistant

34. The nurse records the person's reason for seeking health care in the
    A. Health history   C. Progress notes
    B. Graphic sheet   D. Kardex

35. Vital signs taken every shift are recorded in the
    A. Health history   C. Flow sheet
    B. Graphic sheet   D. Progress notes

36. In long-term care, OBRA requires a written summary of the person
    A. Each shift   C. Every month
    B. Each day   D. Every 3 months

37. A weekly care record that has boxes for each day of the week is used in
    A. Home care   C. Long-term care
    B. Hospitals   D. Special care units

38. The Kardex is
    A. Used to record visits by health team members
    B. A sheet used to record vital signs taken every 15 minutes
    C. A record of the person's family history
    D. A quick, easy source of information about the person

39. The nursing assistant reports information about the person
    A. After the end of the shift
    B. When there is a change in the person's condition
    C. Each time care is given
    D. Only in writing

40. During the end-of-shift report, call lights, care, and routine tasks are usually done
    A. After the report is finished
    B. By the staff going off duty
    C. By the staff coming on duty
    D. By the person assigned by the charge nurse to carry out the task

41. The general rules for recording include all of these *except*
    A. Include the date and time for every recording
    B. Use ditto marks if needed
    C. Sign all entries with your name and title as required by the agency
    D. Record only what you observed and did yourself

42. If you are recording using the 24-hour clock, which of these is correct?
    A. 8 AM   C. 1300
    B. 1 PM   D. 5:30 PM

In questions 43-47, choose the correct spelling of the medical term

43. Slow heart rate
    A. Bradecardia   C. Bradacordia
    B. Bradycardia   D. Bradicardia

44. Difficulty urinating
    A. Dysuria   C. Dysuira
    B. Dysurya   D. Disuria

45. Blue color or condition
    A. Cyonosis   C. Cyanosis
    B. Cyinosis   D. Cianosys

46. Rapid breathing
    A. Tachepnea   C. Tachypnea
    B. Tachypinea   D. Tachypnia

47. Opening into the trachea
    A. Tracheastomy   C. Tracheostome
    B. Trachiostomy   D. Tracheostomy

48. If a person points to the left side of his body below the umbilicus and tells you he has pain, you will tell the nurse he has pain in the
    A. Right upper quadrant
    B. Left lower quadrant
    C. Left upper quadrant
    D. Right lower quadrant

49. When describing the position of body parts, the hands and fingers are
    A. Medial   C. Proximal
    B. Distal   D. Posterior

50. When you are given a computer password, you
    A. Must never change it
    B. Can share it with a co-worker
    C. Should never tell anyone your password
    D. Can use another person's password when entering the computer

51. The agency computers should not be used to
    A. Send messages and reports to the nursing unit
    B. Store resident records and care plans
    C. Send e-mails that require immediate reporting
    D. Monitor blood pressures, temperatures, and heart rates

52. Privacy is protected when you
    A. Turn the screen toward a public area
    B. Prevent others from seeing what is on the screen
    C. Throw computer-printed worksheets in the trash
    D. Share your password with a co-worker

53. When you answer the telephone, do not put the caller on hold if
    A. The person has an emergency
    B. The caller is a doctor
    C. The call needs to be transferred to another unit
    D. You are too busy to find the nurse

54. When you answer a phone when giving home care, you should
    A. Give your name, title, and location
    B. Simply answer with "Hello"
    C. Explain that you are there to give care to the person who lives in the home
    D. Not speak to the caller and hand the receiver to the person in the home

Matching
Match the word with the correct definition.

A. arthroscope
B. bronchoscope
C. cholecystectomy
D. colostomy
E. cyanotic
F. dermatology
G. dysuria
H. enteritis
I. gastrostomy
J. gastritis
K. glossitis
L. nephritis
M. neuralgia
N. oophorectomy
O. proctoscopy

55. _____ Difficulty urinating
56. _____ Inflammation of kidneys
57. _____ Pertaining to blue coloration
58. _____ Joint examination with a scope
59. _____ Study of the skin
60. _____ Incision into large intestine
61. _____ Instrument used to examine bronchi
62. _____ Inflammation of the tongue
63. _____ Nerve pain
64. _____ Examination of rectum with instrument
65. _____ Excision of gallbladder
66. _____ Excision of ovary
67. _____ Incision into stomach
68. _____ Inflammation of stomach
69. _____ Inflammation of intestine

Fill in the Blank
70. Write out the meaning of these abbreviations. They are found on the inside of the back textbook cover.
    A. ADL _____
    B. CBC _____
    C. FBS _____
    D. LOC _____
    E. ROM _____

71. Next to each time, write the time using the 24-hour clock.
    A. _____ 11:00 AM   G. _____ 3:00 AM
    B. _____ 8:00 AM   H. _____ 4:50 AM
    C. _____ 4:00 PM   I. _____ 5:30 PM
    D. _____ 7:30 AM   J. _____ 10:45 PM
    E. _____ 6:45 PM   K. _____ 11:55 PM
    F. _____ 12 NOON   L. _____ 9:15 PM

Write the definition of each prefix.

72. auto- _____
73. brady- _____
74. dys- _____
75. ecto- _____
76. leuk- _____
77. macro- _____
78. neo- _____
79. supra- _____
80. uni- _____

Write the definition of each root word.

81. adeno _____
82. angio _____
83. broncho _____
84. cranio _____
85. duodeno _____
86. entero _____
87. gyneco _____
88. masto _____
89. pyo _____

Write the definition of each suffix.

90. -asis _____
91. -genic _____
92. -oma _____
93. -phasia _____
94. -ptosis _____
95. -plegia _____
96. -megaly _____
97. -scopy _____
98. -stasis _____

Write the correct abbreviations.

99. Before meals _____
100. After meals _____

101. With _____

102. Cancer _____

103. Intake and output _____

104. Lower left quadrant _____

105. Temperature, Pulse, Respiration

_____

106. Urinary tract infection _____

Use the FOCUS ON PRIDE section to complete these statements.

107. If your agency allows nursing assistants to chart, you have a professional responsibility to

A. _____

B. _____

C. _____

D. _____

108. When filling out a survey, you should

A. _____

B. _____

C. _____

109. When the delegating nurse asks what was done and what was not done, you can show you are accountable by

A. _____

B. _____

C. _____

D. _____

110. If charting is not truthful, _____ can be taken against the person who records false information.

Labeling

For questions 111-120, convert the times from military time to standard time and from standard time to military time. Use the figure as a guide.

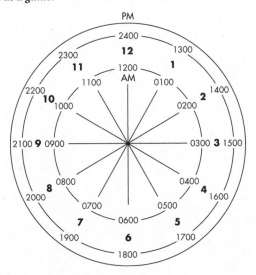

111. 2:00 AM = _____

112. 10:30 AM = _____

113. 5:00 AM = _____

114. 9:30 AM = _____

115. 5:45 PM = _____

116. 10:45 PM = _____

117. 0600 = _____ AM/PM

118. 1145 = _____ AM/PM

119. 1800 = _____ AM/PM

120. 2200 = _____ AM/PM

121. Label the 4 abdominal regions. Use RUQ, LUQ, RLQ, LLQ to label.

A. _____

B. _____

C. _____

D. _____

Optional Learning Exercises

Class Experiment

It is often difficult to describe fluids in a clear and precise manner. Set up the following examples that imitate situations where you need to describe intake, output, or drainage. Describe as accurately as possible what you see in terms of amounts, colors, and textures. Compare your notes with classmates to see if you are using words that all have the same meaning. What words were used that were clear to understand? What words were used that had more than one meaning?

1. Bloody drainage: Mix a teaspoon of ketchup and a teaspoon of water. Pour onto the center of a paper napkin.
2. Urine: Pour a tablespoon of tea into the center of a paper towel.

3. Bleeding: Smear a teaspoon of red jelly in the center of a paper towel.

4. Broth: Pour 4 ounces of tea into a bowl.

Class Experiment	
Substance	Observations
Bloody drainage	
Urine	
Bleeding	
Broth	

Case Study

Mr. Larsen was admitted to a sub-acute care center after his abdominal surgery 1 week ago. This morning the nursing assistant gave Mr. Larsen a shower and assisted him to sit in a comfortable chair. The nursing assistant noticed that he sat there very still and held his arms across his abdomen. He asked for a pillow and held it tightly against his abdomen.

Imagine you are the patient and answer these questions.
- What would you like the nursing assistant to ask you?
- How would you communicate your feelings to the nursing assistant?
- How could you let the nursing assistant know that you had pain without telling her?

Imagine you are the nursing assistant and answer these questions.
- As the nursing assistant, what observations would be important to make about Mr. Larsen?
- What questions could you ask Mr. Larsen?
- What nonverbal communication would give you information about Mr. Larsen?

Case Study

Mrs. Miller was admitted to the health care center since you last worked 3 days ago. You have just started your shift and have been assigned to Mrs. Miller.
- What information would you need to know before giving care? Why?
- What information would be important to provide to the on-coming shift?
- What methods would you use to communicate this information?

8 Assisting With the Nursing Process

Fill in the Blank: Key Terms

Assessment Implementation Nursing diagnosis Objective data Signs
Evaluation Medical diagnosis Nursing intervention Observation Subjective data
Goal Nursing care plan Nursing process Planning Symptoms

1. _____ are things a person tells you about that you cannot observe through your senses; symptoms.

2. _____ is to perform or carry out measures in the care plan; a step in the nursing process.

3. The method RNs use to plan and deliver nursing care is the _____.

4. Another name for subjective data is _____.

5. A written guide about the person's care is the _____.

6. _____ is collecting information about the person; a step in the nursing process.

7. Another name for objective data is _____.

8. The _____ describes a health problem that can be treated by nursing measures; a step in the nursing process.

9. Information that is seen, heard, felt, or smelled is _____ or signs.

10. A step in the nursing process that is used to measure if goals in the planning step were met is called _____.

11. _____ is setting priorities and goals; a step in the nursing process.

12. A _____ is an action or measure taken by the nursing team to help the person reach a goal.

13. A _____ is that which is desired in or by the person as a result of nursing care.

14. Using the senses of sight, hearing, touch, and smell to collect information is _____.

15. The identification of a disease or condition by a doctor is a _____.

Circle the Best Answer

16. Which of these *is not* a step in the nursing process?
    A. Assessment
    B. Objective data
    C. Planning
    D. Evaluation

17. The nursing process focuses on
    A. The doctor's orders
    B. The person's nursing needs
    C. Tasks and procedures that are needed
    D. Reducing the cost of health care

18. The nursing process
    A. Stays the same from admission to discharge
    B. Is used in all health care settings
    C. Cannot be used in home care
    D. Can be used only for adults

19. When you observe by using your senses, you assist the nurse to
    A. Assess the person
    B. Plan for care
    C. Implement care for the person
    D. Evaluate the person

20. Which of these is an example of objective data you can collect?
    A. Mrs. Hewitt complains of pain and nausea.
    B. Mr. Stewart tells you he has a dull ache in his stomach.
    C. You are taking Mrs. Jensen's blood pressure and you notice her skin is hot and moist.
    D. Mrs. Murano tells you she is tired because she could not sleep last night.

21. When you take Mr. Young's blood pressure, you notice it is 50 points higher than when you took it in the morning. You
    A. Chart the results on the graphic sheet
    B. Tell the nurse when you report off at the end of your shift
    C. Tell the nurse at once
    D. Call the doctor

22. A Minimum Data Set (MDS) is used
    A. For nursing center residents
    B. In all health care settings
    C. In acute care settings
    D. In home care

23. The MDS is updated
    A. Only once a year
    B. Every month
    C. Before each care conference
    D. Once every 2 months

24. A nursing diagnosis
    A. Identifies a disease or condition
    B. Helps to identify drugs or therapies used by the doctor
    C. Describes a health problem that can be treated by nursing measures
    D. Identifies only physical problems

25. When a nurse uses the nursing process, the person is given
    A. Only one nursing diagnosis
    B. No more than 5 nursing diagnoses
    C. As many nursing diagnoses as are needed
    D. Nursing diagnoses that involve only physical needs

26. Planning involves all of these *except*
    A. Setting priorities and goals
    B. Choosing nursing actions to help the person meet goals
    C. Writing the nursing care plan
    D. Measuring whether all goals are met

27. A problem-focused conference is held
    A. Once a month for each person
    B. To meet agency guidelines
    C. When one problem affects the person's care
    D. To implement the care plan

28. CMS requires a comprehensive care plan. It is a
    A. Conference held to update care plan
    B. Written guide about the person's care
    C. Conference held when one problem affects a person's care
    D. Conference held regularly to review and update care plans

29. What part of the nursing process is being carried out when you give personal care to a person?
    A. Assessing   C. Implementation
    B. Planning   D. Evaluation

30. Nurses will measure if goals in the planning steps are met during
    A. Assessing   C. Implementation
    B. Planning   D. Evaluation

Fill in the Blank

31. Write out the meaning of the abbreviations.
    A. BMs _____
    B. CAA _____
    C. CMS _____
    D. IDCP _____
    E. MDS _____
    F. OASIS _____
    G. RN _____

32. When you make observations while you give care, what senses are used?
    A. _____
    B. _____
    C. _____
    D. _____

33. Name the body system or other area you are observing in each of these examples (from Box 8-2, Basic Observations).
    A. Is the abdomen firm or soft?

    _____

    B. Is the person sensitive to bright lights?

    _____

    C. Are sores or reddened areas present?

    _____

    D. What is the frequency of the person's cough?

    _____

    E. Can the person bathe without help?

    _____

    F. Can the person swallow food and fluids?

    _____

    G. What is the position of comfort?

    _____

    H. Does the person answer questions correctly?

    _____

    I. Does the person complain of stiff or painful joints?

    _____

34. An assessment and screening tool completed when the person is admitted to a long-term care center is called

    _____.

    A. The form is updated before each

    _____.

    B. A new form is completed _____
       and whenever _____.

35. When planning care, needs that are required for life and survival must be met before _____.

36. Name the two resident care conferences used in long-term care.
    A. The _____ is held regularly to develop, review, and update care plans.
    B. _____
       are held when one problem affects a person's care.

37. The assignment sheet tells you about
    A. _____
    B. _____
    C. _____

38. You have a key role in the nursing process. How do you assist the nurse?
    A. The nurse uses your observations for

    _____ and

    _____.

    B. You may help develop the _____.

    C. In the _____ step, you perform nursing actions and measures.

    D. Your observations are used for the

    _____ step.

Use the FOCUS ON PRIDE section to complete these statements.

39. When you learn skills and practice until you are comfortable performing the skills, it shows you take _____ in learning to do your job well.

40. To encourage independence and to help the person feel involved in his or her care, you can

    A. _____
    B. _____
    C. _____

41. When you keep your assignment sheets with you at all times and place them in the wastebasket for shredding at the end of your shift, it shows that you take pride in protecting the _____ _____.

Optional Learning Exercises

List at least three Nursing Interventions for each of these Nursing Diagnoses and Goals.

42. Nursing Diagnosis: Feeding Self Care Deficit related to weakness in right arm

    Goal: Patient will eat 75% of each meal by 2/1

    Nursing Interventions:

    A. _____
    B. _____
    C. _____

43. Nursing Diagnosis: Hygiene Self Care Deficit related to forgetfulness

    Goal: Patient will be assisted to maintain good hygiene throughout hospital stay

    Nursing Interventions:

    A. _____
    B. _____
    C. _____

9 Understanding the Person

Fill in the Blank: Key Terms

Bariatrics
Body language
Comatose
Culture
Disability

Esteem
Geriatrics
Holism
Morbid
    obesity

Need
Nonverbal
    communication
Obesity
Obstetrics

Optimal level of
    functioning
Paraphrasing
Pediatrics
Psychiatry

Religion
Self-actualization
Self-esteem
Verbal
    communication

1. When a person's weight is 20% or more above what is considered normal for that person's height and age, he or she has _____.

2. _____ is the characteristics of a group of people—language, values, beliefs, habits, likes, dislikes, customs—passed from one generation to the next.

3. Communication that uses written or spoken word is _____.

4. _____ is re-stating the person's message in your own words.

5. The branch of medicine concerned with the problems and diseases of old age and older persons is _____.

6. Messages sent through facial expressions, gestures, posture, hand and body movements, gait, eye contact, and appearance is _____.

7. The field of medicine focused on the treatment and control of obesity is _____.

8. The worth, value, or opinion one has of a person is _____.

9. _____ is communication that does not use words.

10. The branch of medicine concerned with mental health disorders is _____.

11. Thinking well of oneself and seeing oneself as useful and having value is _____.

12. _____ is a concept that considers the whole person; physical, social, psychological, and spiritual parts are woven together and cannot be separated.

13. A lost, absent, or impaired physical or mental function is a _____.

14. The branch of medicine concerned with the care of women during pregnancy, labor, and childbirth and for 6 to 8 weeks after birth is _____.

15. _____ is experiencing one's potential.

16. _____ is the branch of medicine concerned with the growth, development, and care of children who range in age from newborn to teenagers.

17. A _____ is something necessary or desired for maintaining life and well-being.

18. _____ is spiritual beliefs, needs, and practices.

19. Being unable to respond to verbal stimuli is called a _____.

20. _____ is a person's highest potential for mental and physical performance.

21. The person has _____ when he or she weighs 100 pounds or more over his or her normal weight.

Circle the Best Answer

22. Who is the most important person in the health care agency?
    A. The patient or resident
    B. The doctor
    C. The director of nursing
    D. The administrator

23. When you are caring for a person, you should
    A. Consider only the physical problems the person has
    B. Treat the physical, social, psychological, and spiritual parts separately
    C. Ignore the person's experiences, life-style, culture, joys, sorrows, and needs
    D. Consider the whole person—physical, social, psychological, and spiritual parts

24. You can show you see the person as a whole person by which of these statements?
    A. "I need to give a bath to the gallbladder in 205."
    B. "The old guy in 220 needs something for pain."
    C. "Mrs. Jones is complaining of a lot of pain in her leg this morning."
    D. "Room 235 needs something for pain."

25. The lowest-level basic needs are
    A. Physical needs
    B. Safety and security needs
    C. Love and belonging needs
    D. Self-esteem needs

26. Oxygen, food, water, elimination, rest, and shelter needs
    A. Relate to feeling safe from harm, danger, and fear
    B. Are needed to survive
    C. Relate to love, closeness, and affection
    D. Relate to the worth, value, or opinion one has of a person

27. It is important to tell a person why a procedure is needed because it
    A. Helps the person feel more safe and secure
    B. Makes the person feel loved
    C. Is required by law
    D. Increases the person's self-esteem

28. You may need to repeat information many times to a person admitted to a long-term care nursing center because the person
    A. May have a hearing loss
    B. Is senile and cannot remember anything
    C. Is in a strange place with strange routines
    D. Is not able to understand what you are saying

29. Meeting love and belonging needs is important because
    A. It helps a person think well of himself or herself
    B. Some people become weaker or die from the lack of love and belonging
    C. The person will feel more safe and secure
    D. It helps the person experience his or her potential

30. A need that is rarely, if ever, totally met is
    A. Safety and security
    B. Love and belonging
    C. Self-actualization
    D. Self-esteem

31. When you are caring for a person from a different culture or religion than your own, you must
    A. Judge the person's behavior according to your own practices
    B. Assume that the person's behavior will not be influenced by culture or religion
    C. Give needed care and not worry about culture or religious beliefs
    D. Respect and accept the person's culture and religion

32. A culture that believes hot and cold imbalances cause disease is from
    A. Mexico
    B. England
    C. The United States
    D. Russia

33. When a person does not follow all beliefs and practices of his or her religion, you
    A. Assume the person is not religious
    B. Know each person is unique
    C. Can call a spiritual leader to help the person follow the beliefs
    D. Should not be concerned about the person's religion when giving care

34. When people are ill, they
    A. Will feel better if you keep talking to them all the time
    B. May fear death, disability, chronic illness, and loss of function
    C. Want to be left alone, so avoid entering their room
    D. Want someone to do everything for them

35. A person who is having the appendix removed is
    A. An adult with medical problems
    B. A person having surgery
    C. A person with mental health disorders
    D. A person needing sub-acute care or rehabilitation

36. Which of these persons would need the care of a branch of medicine called pediatrics?
    A. A woman who had a new baby today
    B. An older person with problems and diseases of old age
    C. A 7-year-old child with pneumonia
    D. A person receiving kidney dialysis

37. A person who weighs 600 pounds would need
    A. Sub-acute care
    B. Bariatric care
    C. Care in a special care unit
    D. Geriatric care

38. Which of these persons *would not* receive care in a long-term care center?
    A. A man who is recovering from minor surgery
    B. An alert person with a chronic illness who requires help with personal care
    C. A 25-year-old who is unable to care for himself due to injuries
    D. A person with a terminal illness

39. Which of these would *not* help effective communication?
    A. Use words that have the same meaning to both you and the person.
    B. Communicate in a logical and orderly manner.
    C. Give specific and factual information.
    D. Use medical terminology when talking to the person.

40. When using verbal communication, a rule to follow is
    A. Ask one question at a time, then wait for an answer
    B. Speak in a loud voice so the person can hear you
    C. Ask several questions at a time, then wait for answers
    D. Use slang words to make the person comfortable

41. Mrs. Stevens cannot speak. How does she use verbal communication?
    A. She may use touch.
    B. Her body language sends messages.
    C. She can use gestures to communicate.
    D. She may write messages on a pad of paper.

42. When you use touch to communicate, it is important to
    A. Be aware of the person's culture and practices about touch
    B. Write a note to the person to ask if touch is permitted
    C. Check the doctor's order to see if touch is ordered
    D. Touch the person before you speak

43. Which of these would be a sign that Mrs. Green is not happy or is not feeling well?
    A. Her hair is well groomed.
    B. She has a slumped posture.
    C. She smiles when you come into the room.
    D. She has applied her make-up.

44. All of these would show you listen effectively *except* when you
    A. Face the resident and have good eye contact
    B. Lean back and cross your arms
    C. Respond to the resident by asking questions
    D. Use words the person can understand

45. Which of these is paraphrasing?
    A. "You don't know how long you will be here."
    B. "Do you want to take a tub bath or a shower?"
    C. "Tell me about living on a farm."
    D. "Can you explain what you mean?"

46. When you say, "Mr. Davis, have you taken a shower this morning?" you are
    A. Paraphrasing his thoughts
    B. Asking a direct question
    C. Focusing his thoughts
    D. Asking an open-ended question

47. Responses to open-ended questions generally
    A. Invite the person to share thoughts, feelings, or ideas
    B. Are "yes" or "no" answers
    C. Are able to make sure you understand the message
    D. Focus on dealing with a certain topic

48. When you do not understand the message, you may
    A. Ask the person an open-ended question
    B. Make a statement to clarify what he is saying
    C. Use nonverbal communication
    D. Use silence to show you do not understand

49. Mr. Parker often rambles and tells long stories where his thoughts wander. You need to know if he had a bowel movement today, so you will
    A. Make a clarifying statement
    B. Ask an open-ended question
    C. Ask a focusing question
    D. Paraphrase his thoughts

50. What is best if the person takes long pauses between statements?
    A. Just being there shows you care.
    B. Try to cheer the person up by talking.
    C. Leave the room.
    D. Find another resident to talk with him.

51. A barrier to communication would be
    A. Asking a clarifying question
    B. Giving your opinion
    C. Remaining silent when the person is silent
    D. Paraphrasing the person's message

52. When you care for a person who is comatose, you
    A. Explain what you are going to do
    B. Remain silent so you do not disturb the person
    C. Enter the room quietly so you do not startle the person
    D. Speak in a loud voice to make sure the person hears you

53. Mrs. Duke has visitors and you need to give care. What would you do?
    A. Give the care while visitors are present.
    B. Politely ask the visitors to leave the room until you are finished.
    C. Ask the visitors to give the care.
    D. Tell the visitors that they must leave the nursing center.

54. When you are caring for a person who becomes angry, you should
    A. Avoid answering call lights
    B. Tell the person what you are going to do and when
    C. Explain to the person why he or she should not be angry
    D. Tell the person to stop being angry

55. If a person hits, pinches, or bites you when you are giving care, you should
    A. Protect the person, others, and yourself from harm
    B. Stop giving care to the person
    C. Firmly tell the person to stop acting like that
    D. Refuse to care for the person when he or she is assigned to you

Fill in the Blank

56. What are the parts of the person you consider when you use the concept of holism?
    A. _____
    B. _____
    C. _____
    D. _____

57. List the basic needs in order, starting with the lowest level.
    A. _____
    B. _____
    C. _____
    D. _____
    E. _____

58. Name the culture that may follow the listed belief or custom.
    A. _____ or _____ Food and medicine is given to restore the hot–cold balance
    B. _____ Folk healers called *yerbero* use herbs and spices to prevent or cure disease.
    C. In Vietnam or _____, men shake hands with other men but do not touch women they do not know.
    D. _____ Eyes are rolled upward to express disapproval.
    E. _____ Facial expressions may mean the opposite of what the person is feeling. Negative emotions may be concealed with a smile.
    F. In _____ and Asian cultures, eye contact is impolite and an invasion of privacy.

G. In some _____ cultures, silence is a sign of respect, particularly toward an older person.

H. In _____, family members are involved in the person's care.

59. When you use verbal communication, words are _____ or _____.

60. Written words are used when a person cannot _____ or _____.

61. If a person can hear but cannot speak or read, ask questions that have _____.

62. Nonverbal communication messages reflect a person's _____ more accurately than words do.

63. Body language is nonverbal communication that is shown with

A. _____

B. _____

C. _____

D. _____

E. _____

F. _____

G. _____

64. When you listen, you follow these guidelines.

A. _____

B. _____

C. _____

D. _____

E. _____

65. When you fail to listen, you can miss complaints of

_____

_____

Use the FOCUS ON PRIDE section to complete these statements.

66. To promote a sense of identity, worth, and belonging when communicating, you should

A. _____

B. _____

C. _____

D. _____

E. _____

F. _____

G. _____

67. When you care for persons with different ideas, values, and lifestyles, it is not ethical to

A. _____

B. _____

C. _____

Crossword

Fill in the crossword by answering the clues below with the words from this list:

Clarifying	Direct	Holism	Paraphrasing	Touch
Comatose	Esteem	Need	Silence	Verbal
Culture	Focusing	Nonverbal		

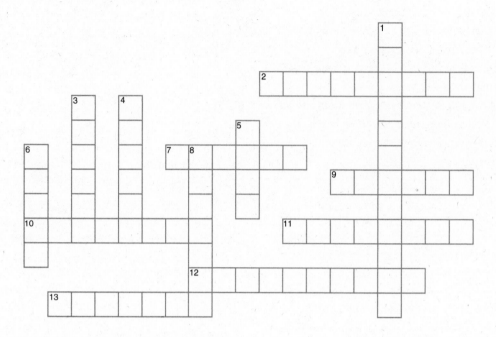

Across

2. Communication expressed with gestures, facial expressions, posture, body movements, touch, and smell

7. The worth, value, or opinion one has of a person

9. Communication in which the words are spoken or written

10. An unconscious person who cannot respond to others

11. A communication method that is useful when a person rambles or wanders in thought

12. A communication method in which you can ask the person to repeat the message, say you do not understand, or restate the message

13. The characteristics of a group of people—language, values, beliefs, habits, likes, dislikes, customs—passed from one generation to another

Down

1. Restating the person's message in your own words

3. A concept that considers the whole person—physical, social, psychological, and spiritual parts

4. A question that focuses on certain information and may require a "yes" or "no" answer or more information

5. Something necessary or desired for maintaining life and mental well-being

6. Nonverbal communication that conveys comfort, caring, loving, affection, interest, concern, and reassurance

8. Communicating by not saying anything

Optional Learning Exercises

Basic Needs

Physical Needs

68. What are the six physical needs required for survival?

    A. _____

    B. _____

    C. _____

    D. _____

    E. _____

    F. _____

69. Physical needs must be met before the _____ needs.

Safety and Security

70. Safety and security needs relate to protection from

    A. _____

    B. _____

    C. _____

71. When a person is in a health care agency, you can help meet safety and security needs when you explain the following for every task.

    A. _____

    B. _____

    C. _____

    D. _____

Love and Belonging

72. The need for love and belonging relates to

    A. _____

    B. _____

    C. _____

Self-Esteem

73. Self-esteem means to

    A. Think _____

    B. See _____

    C. See oneself as having _____

74. Why is it important to encourage residents to do as much as possible for themselves? _____

Self-Actualization

75. What does self-actualization involve?

    A. _____

    B. _____

    C. _____

76. What happens if self-actualization is postponed? _____

Culture and Religion Practices

Religion

77. How can you help a resident observe religious practices if services are held in the nursing center?

    _____

78. If the resident wants a spiritual leader or advisor to visit in the room, you should tell the nurse and

    A. _____

    B. _____

    C. _____

Cultural Health Care Beliefs

79. People from Mexico or Vietnam believe that illness occurs by _____.

Cultural Sick Practices

80. How do Vietnamese folk practices treat these illnesses?

    A. Common cold _____

    B. Headache and sore throat _____

81. What illnesses do these Russian folk practices treat?

    A. _____ An ointment placed behind the ears and temples and also on the back of the neck

    B. _____ Placing a dough made of dark rye flour and honey on the spinal column

Cultural Touch Practices

82. What is the meaning of touch to some people from Mexico? _____

83. If you are caring for a resident from India, what might you notice about his practice of shaking hands?

    _____

84. Residents from some countries may not like to be touched, especially by those they do not know. Name two examples of these countries.

    _____

Eye Contact Practices

85. Why would you avoid making direct eye contact with a resident from Mexico?

    _____

86. If a resident from Vietnam blinks when you explain a procedure, it probably means that the message

    _____

87. Eye contact in the American culture signals

    _____

Family Roles in Sick Care

88. You are caring for a resident from China. You might expect the family members to provide _____, _____, and _____ to the person.

Using Communication Methods

You have completed your duties for the morning and have some free time. Mr. Harry Donal is a resident of the nursing center. He rarely has visitors and you try to spend time with him when you can. Answer the following questions about communication techniques you use when you visit with Mr. Donal.

89. You sit in a chair next to Mr. Donal so you can see each other. This position will help you to have better

    _____

90. You should lean _____ Mr. Donal to show interest.

91. Mr. Donal says, "I know this is the best place for me but I miss my flower garden at home." You respond, "You miss your home." This is an example of

    _____

92. You ask Mr. Donal, "You told me you did not sleep well last night. Can you tell me why?" He replies, "There was a lot of noise in the hall." This is an

    example of a _____ question.

93. You say to Mr. Donal, "Tell me about your flower garden at home." This is an _____ question.

94. When you say, "Can you explain what that means?" you are asking a person to _____.

95. Mr. Donal says he "hurts all over" and then begins to talk about the weather. You say, "Tell me more about where you hurt. You said you hurt all over." This statement helps in _____ the topic.

96. Mr. Donal begins to cry when he talks about his flower garden. How can you show caring and respect for his situation and feelings? _____

    _____

97. When Mr. Donal begins to cry, you quickly begin to talk about the activities planned this morning. Changing the subject is a _____

    _____

10 Body Structure and Function

Fill in the Blank: Key Terms

Artery	Digestion	Immunity	Organ	System
Capillary	Hemoglobin	Menstruation	Peristalsis	Tissue
Cell	Hormone	Metabolism	Respiration	Vein

1. The substance in red blood cells that carries oxygen and gives blood its color is _____.

2. _____ is protection against a disease or condition.

3. The process of supplying the cells with oxygen and removing carbon dioxide from them is _____

4. The process of physically and chemically breaking down food so that it can be absorbed for use by the cells is _____

5. _____ is the burning of food for heat and energy by the cells.

6. A blood vessel that carries blood away from the heart is an _____.

7. _____ is the involuntary muscle contractions in the digestive system that move food through the alimentary canal.

8. Organs that work together to perform special functions form a _____.

9. The basic unit of body structure is a _____

10. Groups of tissues with the same function form an _____

11. A _____ is a tiny blood vessel.

12. A group of cells with similar function is _____

13. _____ is the process in which the lining of the uterus breaks up and is discharged from the body through the vagina.

14. A chemical substance secreted by the glands into the bloodstream is a _____.

15. A _____ is a blood vessel that carries blood back to the heart.

Circle the Best Answer

16. A cell
    A. Is only found in muscles
    B. Is the basic unit of body structure
    C. Can live without oxygen
    D. Is a group of tissues

17. The control center of a cell is the
    A. Membrane   C. Cytoplasm
    B. Protoplasm   D. Nucleus

18. Genes control
    A. Cell division
    B. Tissues
    C. Physical and chemical traits inherited by children
    D. Organs

19. Connective tissue
    A. Covers internal and external body surface
    B. Receives and carries impulses to the brain and back to body parts
    C. Anchors, connects, and supports other body tissues
    D. Allows the body to move by stretching and contracting

20. Living cells of the epidermis contain
    A. Blood vessels and many nerves
    B. Sweat and oil glands
    C. Pigment that gives skin color
    D. Hair roots

21. Sweat glands help
    A. The body regulate temperature
    B. Keep the hair and skin soft and shiny
    C. Protect the nose from dust, insects, and other foreign objects
    D. The skin sense pleasant and unpleasant sensations

22. Long bones
    A. Allow skill and ease in movement
    B. Bear the weight of the body
    C. Protect organs
    D. Allow various degrees of movement and flexion

23. Blood cells are manufactured in
    A. The heart   C. Blood vessels
    B. The liver   D. Bone marrow

24. Joints move smoothly because of
    A. Cartilage   C. Muscle
    B. Synovial fluid D. Ligaments

25. A joint that moves in all directions is a
    A. Ball and socket C. Pivot
    B. Hinge   D. All of the above

26. Voluntary muscles are
    A. Found in the stomach and intestines
    B. Attached to bones
    C. Cardiac muscle
    D. Tendons

27. Muscles produce heat by
    A. Contracting   C. Maintaining posture
    B. Relaxing   D. Working automatically

28. The central nervous system consists of
    A. A myelin sheath
    B. Nerves throughout the body
    C. The brain and spinal column
    D. Cranial nerves

29. The medulla controls
    A. Muscle contraction and relaxation
    B. Heart rate, breathing, blood vessel size, and swallowing
    C. Reasoning, memory, and consciousness
    D. Hearing and vision

30. Cerebrospinal fluid
    A. Cushions shocks that could injure structures of the brain and spinal cord
    B. Controls voluntary muscles
    C. Lubricates movement
    D. Controls involuntary muscles

31. Cranial nerves conduct impulses between the
    A. Brain and the head, neck, chest, and abdomen
    B. Brain and the skin and extremities
    C. Brain and internal body structures
    D. Spinal cord and lower extremities

32. When you are frightened, the _____ nervous system is stimulated.
    A. Sympathetic   C. Central
    B. Parasympathetic   D. Cranial

33. Receptors for vision and nerve fibers of the optic nerve are found in the
    A. Sclera   C. Retina
    B. Choroids   D. Cornea

34. What structure of the ear is involved in balance?
    A. Malleus   C. Tympanic membranes
    B. Auditory canal   D. Semicircular canals

35. Hemoglobin in red blood cells gives blood its red color and carries _____ to the cells.
    A. Oxygen   C. Waste products
    B. Food   D. Water

36. Red blood cells live for
    A. About 9 days   C. 4 days
    B. 3 or 4 months   D. A year

37. White blood cells or leukocytes
    A. Protect the body against infection
    B. Are necessary for blood clotting
    C. Carry food, hormones, chemicals, and waste products
    D. Pick up carbon dioxide

38. The left atrium of the heart
    A. Receives blood from the lungs
    B. Receives blood from the body tissues
    C. Pumps blood to the lungs
    D. Pumps blood to all parts of the body

39. Arteries
    A. Return blood to the heart
    B. Pass food, oxygen, and other substances into the cells
    C. Pick up waste products, including carbon dioxide, from the cells
    D. Carry blood away from the heart

40. In the lungs, oxygen and carbon dioxide are exchanged
    A. In the epiglottis
    B. Between the right bronchus and the left bronchus
    C. By the bronchioles
    D. Between the aveoli and capillaries

41. The lungs are protected by
    A. The diaphragm
    B. The pleura
    C. A bony framework of the ribs, sternum, and vertebrae
    D. The lobes

42. Food is moved through the alimentary canal (GI tract) by
    A. Chyme   C. Swallowing
    B. Peristalsis   D. Bile

43. Water is absorbed from chyme in the
    A. Small intestine   C. Esophagus
    B. Stomach   D. Large intestine

44. Digested food is absorbed through tiny projections called
    A. Jejunum   C. Villi
    B. Ileum   D. Colon

45. A function of the urinary system is to
    A. Remove waste products from the blood
    B. Rid the body of solid waste
    C. Rid the body of carbon dioxide
    D. Burn food for energy

46. A person feels the need to urinate when the bladder contains about
    A. 1000 mL of urine   C. 250 mL of urine
    B. 500 mL of urine   D. 125 mL of urine

47. Testosterone is needed for
    A. Male secondary sex characteristics
    B. Female secondary sex characteristics
    C. Sperm to be produced
    D. Ova to be produced

48. The prostate gland lies
    A. In the scrotum
    B. In the testes
    C. Just below the bladder
    D. In the penis

49. The ovaries secrete progesterone and
    A. Estrogen   C. Ova
    B. Testosterone   D. Semen

50. When an ovum is released from an ovary, it travels first through the
    A. Uterus   C. Endometrium
    B. Fallopian tubes   D. Vagina

51. Menstruation occurs when
    A. The hymen is ruptured
    B. The ovary releases an ovum
    C. The endometrium breaks up
    D. Fertilization occurs

52. A fertilized cell implants in the
    A. Ovary   C. Endometrium
    B. Fallopian tubes   D. Vagina

53. The master gland is the
   A. Thyroid gland
   B. Parathyroid gland
   C. Adrenal gland
   D. Pituitary gland
54. Thyroid hormone regulates
   A. Growth
   B. Metabolism
   C. Proper functioning of nerves and muscles
   D. Energy produced during energy
55. If too little insulin is produced by the pancreas, the person has
   A. Tetany
   B. Slow growth
   C. Diabetes mellitus
   D. Slowed metabolism
56. When antigens enter the body, they are attacked and destroyed by
   A. Antibodies
   B. Lymphocytes
   C. B cells
   D. T cells

Fill in the Blank

57. Write out these abbreviations.
   A. CNS _____
   B. GI _____
   C. mL _____
   D. RBC _____
   E. WBC _____

Use the FOCUS ON PRIDE section to complete these statements.

58. To care for others, you need a strong and healthy body. You can stay healthy by
   A. Seeing your doctor at least _____
   B. Keeping your _____ up to date
   C. Protecting your bones and muscles from injury by
   _____
   D. Practicing good hand _____
59. You can help a person maintain his or her optimal level of function when you
   A. _____
   B. _____
   C. _____
   D. _____
   E. _____

Matching

Match the terms with the descriptions.

Musculo-skeletal
A. Periosteum
B. Joint
C. Cartilage
D. Synovial fluid
E. Striated muscle
F. Smooth muscle
G. Cardiac muscle
H. Tendons

60. _____ Connective tissue at end of long bones
61. _____ Skeletal muscle
62. _____ Membrane that covers bone
63. _____ Connects muscle to bone
64. _____ Point at which two or more bones meet
65. _____ Heart muscle
66. _____ Involuntary muscle
67. _____ Acts as a lubricant so the joint can move smoothly

Nervous System
A. Sclera
B. Cornea
C. Retina
D. Cerumen
E. Middle ear
F. Inner ear
G. Brainstem
H. Cerebral cortex
I. Autonomic nervous system
J. Peripheral nervous system

68. _____ Contains eustachian tubes and ossicles
69. _____ Has 12 pairs of cranial nerves and 31 pairs of spinal nerves
70. _____ White of the eye
71. _____ Outside of cerebrum; controls highest function of brain
72. _____ Inner layer of eye; receptors for vision are contained here
73. _____ Controls involuntary muscles, heart beat, blood pressure, and other functions
74. _____ Light enters eye through this structure
75. _____ Contain midbrain, pons, and medulla
76. _____ Waxy substance secreted in auditory canal
77. _____ Contains semicircular canal and cochlea

Circulatory System
A. Plasma
B. Erythrocytes
C. Hemoglobin
D. Leukocytes
E. Thrombocytes
F. Pericardium
G. Myocardium
H. Endocardium
I. Arteries
J. Veins
K. Capillaries

78. _____ Liquid part of blood
79. _____ Thin sac covering the heart
80. _____ Very tiny blood vessels
81. _____ Substance in blood that picks up oxygen
82. _____ Carry blood away from heart
83. _____ White blood cells
84. _____ Carry blood toward heart
85. _____ Red blood cells
86. _____ Thick muscular portion of heart
87. _____ Platelets; necessary for clotting
88. _____ Membrane lining inner surface of heart

Respiratory System

A. Epiglottis   D. Trachea   F. Diaphragm
B. Larynx   E. Aveoli   G. Pleura
C. Bronchiole

89. _____ Air passes from larynx into this structure

90. _____ A two-layered sac that covers the lungs

91. _____ Piece of cartilage that acts like a lid over larynx

92. _____ Separates lungs from the abdominal cavity

93. _____ The voice box

94. _____ Several small branches that divide from the bronchus

95. _____ Tiny one-celled air sacs

Digestive System

A. Liver   D. Duodenum   G. Pancreas
B. Chyme   E. Jejunum   H. Gallbladder
C. Colon   F. Saliva

96. _____ Structure that adds more digestive juices to chyme

97. _____ Semi-liquid food mixture formed in stomach

98. _____ Portion of GI tract that absorbs food

99. _____ Stores bile

100. _____ Portion of GI tract that absorbs water

101. _____ Produces bile

102. _____ Moistens food particles in the mouth

103. _____ Produces digestive juices

Urinary System

A. Bladder   D. Meatus   G. Ureter
B. Glomerulus   E. Nephrons   H. Urethra
C. Kidney   F. Tubules

104. _____ Basic working unit of the kidney

105. _____ Bean-shaped structure that produces urine

106. _____ A cluster of capillaries in Bowman's capsule

107. _____ Structure that allows urine to pass from the bladder

108. _____ A tube attached to the renal pelvis of the kidney

109. _____ Hollow muscular sac that stores urine

110. _____ Opening at the end of the urethra

111. _____ Fluid and waste products form urine in this structure

Reproductive System

A. Scrotum   D. Gonads   G. Labia
B. Testes   E. Fallopian tubes H. Vulva
C. Seminal vesicle F. Endometrium

112. _____ Male or female sex organs

113. _____ Two folds of tissue on each side of the vagina

114. _____ Sac between thighs that contains testes

115. _____ External genitalia of female

116. _____ Testicles; sperm produced here

117. _____ Attached to uterus; ovum travel through this structure

118. _____ Stores sperm and produces semen

119. _____ Tissue lining the uterus

Endocrine System

A. Epinephrine   D. Parathormone
B. Estrogen   E. Testosterone
C. Insulin   F. Thyroxine

120. _____ Released by pancreas; regulates sugar in blood

121. _____ Sex hormone secreted by testes

122. _____ Sex hormone secreted by ovaries

123. _____ Regulates metabolism

124. _____ Regulates calcium levels in the body

125. _____ Stimulates the body to produce energy during emergencies

Immune System

A. Antibodies   D. Lymphocytes
B. Antigens   E. B cells
C. Phagocytes   F. T cells

126. _____ Normal body substances that recognize abnormal or unwanted substances

127. _____ Type of cell that destroys invading cells

128. _____ Type of white blood cell that digests and destroys microorganisms

129. _____ Type of cell that causes production of antibodies

130. _____ An abnormal or unwanted substance

131. _____ Type of white blood cell that produces antibodies

Labeling

132. Name the parts of the cell in the figure.

A. _____

B. _____

C. _____

133. Name each type of joint in the figures.

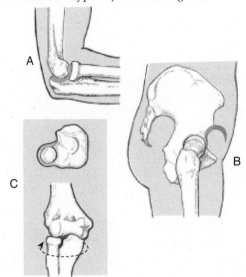

A. _____
B. _____
C. _____

134. Name the parts of the brain in the figure.

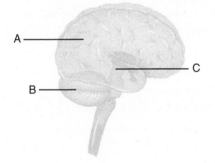

A. _____
B. _____
C. _____

135. Name the four chambers of the heart in the figure.

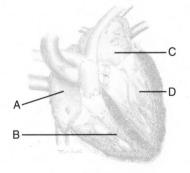

A. _____
B. _____
C. _____
D. _____

136. Name the structures of the respiratory system in the figure.

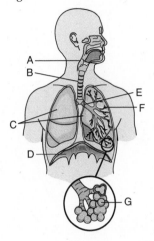

A. _____
B. _____
C. _____
D. _____
E. _____
F. _____
G. _____

137. Name the structures of the digestive system in the figure.

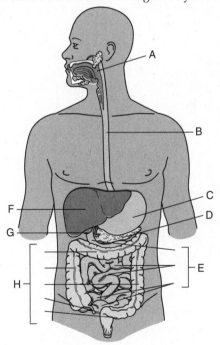

A. _____
B. _____
C. _____
D. _____
E. _____
F. _____
G. _____
H. _____

138. Name the structures of the urinary system in the figure.

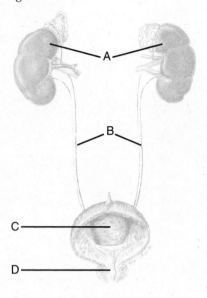

C ———
D ———

A. _____
B. _____
C. _____
D. _____

139. Name the structures of the male reproductive system in the figure.

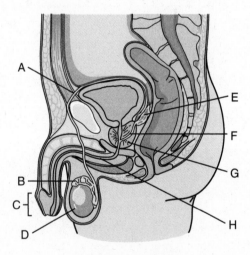

A. _____
B. _____
C. _____
D. _____
E. _____
F. _____
G. _____
H. _____

140. Name the external female genitalia in the figure.

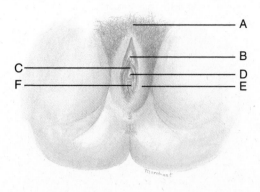

A. _____
B. _____
C. _____
D. _____
E. _____
F. _____

Optional Learning Exercises

141. Explain the function of each part of the cell.
    A. Cell membrane _____
    B. Nucleus _____
    C. Cytoplasm _____
    D. Protoplasm _____
    E. Chromosomes _____
    F. Genes _____

142. List what structures are contained in the two skin layers.
    A. Epidermis _____
    B. Dermis _____

143. Explain the function of the types of bone.
    A. Long bones _____
    B. Short bones _____
    C. Flat bones _____
    D. Irregular bones _____

144. Describe how each type of joint moves and give an example of each type.
    A. Ball and socket _____
        Ex. _____
    B. Hinge _____
        Ex. _____
    C. Pivot _____
        Ex. _____

145. Explain what happens when muscles contract.

_____

_____

_____

146. Explain the function of the three main parts of the brain. Include the function of the cerbral cortex and the midbrain, pons, and medulla.
    A. Cerebrum _____

    _____

    B. Cerebral cortex _____

    _____

    C. Cerebellum _____

    _____

    D. Brainstem _____
    E. Midbrain and pons _____

    _____

    F. Medulla _____

147. Explain how the sympathetic and parasympathetic nervous systems balance each other.

    _____

    _____

148. Explain what happens to each of these structures when light enters the eye.
    A. Choroid _____
    B. Cornea _____
    C. Lens _____
    D. Retina _____

149. Explain how each of these structures helps to carry sound in the ear.
    A. Ossicles _____
    B. Cochlea _____
    C. Acoustic nerve _____

150. Where are red blood cells destroyed as they wear out? _____

151. When an infection occurs, what do white blood cells do? _____

    _____

152. Explain the function of the four atria of the heart.
    A. Right atrium _____
    B. Left atrium _____
    C. Right ventricle _____
    D. Left ventricle _____

153. Explain where each of these veins carries blood.
    A. Inferior vena cava

    _____

    B. Superior vena cava

    _____

154. Explain what happens in the aveoli.

    _____

    _____

155. After food is swallowed, explain what happens in each of these parts of the digestive tract.
    A. Stomach _____
    B. Duodenum _____
    C. Jejunum and ileum _____
    D. Colon _____
    E. Rectum _____
    F. Anus _____

156. Explain what happens in these structures of the kidney.
    A. Glomerulus _____
    B. Collecting tubules _____
    C. Ureters _____
    D. Urethra _____
    E. Meatus _____

157. Sperm is produced in the testicles. What happens to the sperm in each of these structures?
    A. Testes _____
    B. Vas deferens _____
    C. Seminal vesicle _____
    D. Ejaculatory duct _____
    E. Prostate gland _____
    F. Urethra _____

158. What is the function of the endometrium?

    _____

    _____

159. Menstruation occurs about every _____ days.
    Ovulation usually occurs on or about day _____ of the cycle.

160. What is the function of each of these pituitary hormones?
    A. Growth hormone _____
    B. Thyroid-stimulating hormone ____
    C. Adrenocorticotropic hormone ____
    D. Antidiuretic hormone _____
    E. Oxytocin _____

161. What is the function of insulin?

    _____

    _____

162. What happens if too little insulin is produced?

    _____

    _____

163. What happens when the body senses an antigen?

    _____

    _____

11 Growth and Development

Fill in the Blank: Key Terms

Adolescence	Ejaculation	Menarche	Primary caregiver	Sexual orientation
Development	Growth	Menopause	Puberty	Teen dating violence
Developmental task	Infancy	Peer	Reflex	

1. The first menstruation and the start of menstrual cycles is _____.

2. _____ is the time between puberty and adulthood; a time of rapid growth and physical and social maturity.

3. The release of semen is _____.

4. The period when reproductive organs begin to function and secondary sex characteristics appear is _____.

5. _____ is the first year of life.

6. Changes in mental, emotional, and social function is _____.

7. An involuntary movement is a _____.

8. _____ is the physical changes that can be measured and that occur in a steady, orderly manner.

9. The person mainly responsible for providing or assisting with the child's basic needs is the _____.

10. A skill that must be completed during a stage of development is a _____.

11. _____ is the time when menstruation stops and menstrual cycles end.

12. A person of the same age-group and background is a _____.

13. _____ refers to sexual arousal or romantic attraction to persons of the other gender, the same gender, or both genders.

14. _____ is the physical, sexual, psychological, or emotional violence within a dating relationship as well as stalking.

Circle the Best Answer

15. Growth is measured all of these ways *except*
    A. The ways a person behaves and thinks
    B. Height and weight
    C. By changes in appearance
    D. By changes in body functions

16. Growth and development begin
    A. At fertilization
    B. At birth
    C. When the baby sits up
    D. When children have growth spurts

17. The process of growth and development
    A. Occurs in a random order or pattern
    B. Progresses at a steady pace in each stage
    C. Occurs from the center of the body outward
    D. From the foot to the head

18. Movements in the newborn are uncoordinated and lack purpose because
    A. The baby has not been taught to move in a pattern
    B. The central nervous system is not well developed
    C. The baby moves only with reflexes
    D. The baby has skipped a developmental task

19. The birth weight of a newborn
    A. Doubles in the first year
    B. Triples in the first year
    C. Doubles in the first 3 months
    D. Triples in the first 6 months

20. Reflexes present in newborns
    A. Are learned behaviors
    B. Remain active through the first year
    C. Are an abnormal developmental task
    D. Decline and then disappear as the central nervous system develops

21. Infants can play peek-a-boo by
    A. 2 to 3 months   C. 8 to 9 months
    B. 4 to 5 months   D. The first birthday

22. During toddlerhood, the child may have temper tantrums and say "no" to
    A. Assert independence
    B. Show more dependence on the primary caregiver
    C. Develop language skills
    D. Increase coordination

23. A major task for toddlers is
    A. Learning to walk
    B. Learning to feed themselves
    C. Learning to share toys with others
    D. Toilet training

24. Toddlers learn to feel secure when
    A. Primary caregivers are consistently present when needed
    B. Long periods of separation from primary caregivers are planned
    C. Needs are not met quickly
    D. They are allowed to be alone for long periods of time

25. Three-year-olds are able to
    A. Play simple games and learn simple rules
    B. Use a pencil well to print letters, numbers, and their first names
    C. Hop, skip, and throw and catch a ball
    D. Be more responsible and truthful

26. During the pre-school years, children grow
    A. Much more rapidly than during infancy
    B. 2 to 3 inches per year and gain about 5 pounds per year
    C. Very slowly, if at all
    D. 6 to 7 inches per year and gain about 10 pounds per year

27. Baby teeth are lost and permanent teeth erupt at about
    A. 2 years of age
    B. The end of the first year
    C. 6 years of age
    D. 9 or 10 years of age

28. Reading, writing, grammar, and math skills develop during
    A. Toddlerhood
    B. Pre-school years
    C. School-age years
    D. Late childhood

29. Girls have a growth spurt during
    A. School-age years
    B. Late childhood
    C. Adolescence
    D. Young adulthood

30. During late childhood, children
    A. Accept adult standards and rules without question
    B. Increase math and language skills
    C. Are not yet interested in sexual information
    D. Become more awkward and clumsy

31. Girls reach puberty
    A. When menarche occurs
    B. Between the ages of 12 and 16
    C. When they stop growing
    D. Later than boys

32. Coordination and graceful movements develop in adolescence as
    A. Growth spurts occur
    B. Puberty is reached
    C. All growth stops
    D. Muscle and bone growth even out

33. Adolescents need guidance and discipline because
    A. They need to remain dependent on parents
    B. Judgment and reasoning are not always sound
    C. They are just learning right from wrong
    D. They make bad decisions without strict rules

34. Teens usually do not understand why parents worry about sexual activities, pregnancy, and sexually transmitted diseases because
    A. They are emotionally unstable at this stage
    B. Independence from adults is important
    C. They may have trouble controlling sexual urges and considering the consequences of sexual activity
    D. They do not have a sense of right and wrong, or good and bad

35. Development ends
    A. When puberty occurs
    B. When all physical growth is complete
    C. At young adulthood
    D. At death

36. Young adulthood includes all of these tasks *except*
    A. Adjusting to physical changes
    B. Learning to live with a partner
    C. Developing a satisfactory sex life
    D. Choosing education and a career

37. A developmental task of middle adulthood is
    A. Developing leisure-time activities
    B. Coping with a partner's death
    C. Preparing for one's own death
    D. Learning to live with a partner

Fill in the Blank

38. Write out the meaning of the abbreviations
    A. CDC _____
    B. CNS _____
    C. IPV _____

Use the FOCUS ON PRIDE section to complete these statements.

39. When caring for a 1-year old, you can gain the child's trust while checking the pulse when you
    A. Ask _____
    B. Show _____
    C. Let _____
    D. Talk _____

40. You show respect for different family situations when you
    A. Do not _____
    B. Treat them as _____
    C. Take pride in not allowing _____

41. When children become emancipated minors, it means they are able to make their _____.

42. A child can become emanicipated by
    A. _____
    B. _____
    C. _____
    D. In some states, _____

Matching

Match the description with the correct reflex of a newborn.
A. Moro (startle) reflex   D. Grasp (palmar) reflex
B. Rooting reflex   E. Step reflex
C. Sucking reflex

43. _____ Legs extend and then flex

44. _____ Occurs when baby is held upright and the feet touch a surface

45. _____ Guides baby's mouth to the nipple

46. _____ Occurs when lips are touched

47. _____ Fingers close firmly around the object

Match the developmental task with the correct age-group.
A. Infancy (birth–1 year)
B. Toddler (1–3 years)
C. Preschooler (3–6 years)
D. School Age (6–9 or 10 years)
E. Late Childhood (9 or 10–12 years)
F. Adolescence (12–18 years)
G. Young Adulthood (18–40 years)
H. Middle Adulthood (40–65 years)
I. Late Adulthood (65 years and older)

48. _____ Accepting changes in body and appearance

49. _____ Developing leisure-time activities

50. _____ Gaining control of bowel and bladder functions

51. _____ Becoming independent from parents and adults

52. _____ Learning to eat solid foods

53. _____ Adjusting to decreased strength and loss of health

54. _____ Learning how to study

55. _____ Learning how to get along with peers

56. _____ Increasing ability to communicate and understand others

57. _____ Tolerating separation from primary caregiver

58. _____ Learning to live with a partner

59. _____ Developing moral or ethical behavior

60. _____ Learning basic reading, writing, and arithmetic skills

61. _____ Developing stable sleep and feeding patterns

62. _____ Performing self-care

63. _____ Using words to communicate with others

64. _____ Adjusting to aging parents

65. _____ Accepting male or female role appropriate for one's age

66. _____ Beginning to talk and communicate with others

67. _____ Choosing education and a career

Optional Learning Exercises

Infancy

68. You are observing a newborn. You know the neonate
    A. Sleeps _____ a day
    B. Can turn the head from _____

69. Between 1 month and 1 year
    A. The Moro, rooting, and grasp reflexes disappear by _____ months
    B. The baby can roll from front to back by _____ months
    C. The baby can learn to drink from a cup with handles by _____ months
    D. Walking skills increase by _____ months

Toddlerhood

70. During toddlerhood, the developmental tasks are
    A. _____
    B. _____
    C. _____
    D. _____

71. Toilet training starts with _____.

72. Bladder control during the _____ occurs before bladder control at _____.

Preschool

73. What personal skills can be done by 3-year-olds?
    A. Put on _____
    B. Manage _____
    C. Wash _____
    D. Brush _____

74. Four-year-olds prefer the primary caregiver of the _____ sex.

75. Communication skills increase in 5-year-olds.
    A. They can speak in _____.
    B. Questions have more _____.
    C. The child wants words _____.

School-Age

76. Play activities in school-age children have a _____.
    A. They like household tasks such as _____ _____.
    B. Rewards are important, such as _____ _____.

Late Childhood

77. The developmental tasks of late childhood are like those for _____ _____. The tasks are
    A. _____
    B. _____
    C. _____
    D. _____
    E. _____
    F. _____

Adolescence

78. The developmental tasks of adolescence are

    A. _____

    B. _____

    C. _____

    D. _____

    E. _____

    F. _____

    G. _____

79. During adolescence, girls and boys need about

    _____ hours of sleep at

    night because of _____.

80. Girls usually complete development by age

    _____. Boys usually stop

    growing between _____ years.

81. Teen dating violence often begins with

    _____

    and _____.

Young Adulthood

82. During young adulthood, little physical growth

    occurs but _____

    and _____ development

    continues.

83. Many factors affect the selection of a partner during
    young adulthood. They include

    A. _____

    B. _____

    C. _____

    D. _____

    E. _____

    F. _____

    G. _____

Middle Adulthood

84. During middle adulthood, weight control becomes a

    problem because _____.

85. People in middle adulthood may have parents who

    are _____

    and _____. Many also

    deal with the _____ of

    parents.

Late Adulthood

86. The developmental tasks of late adulthood are

    A. _____

    B. _____

    C. _____

    D. _____

    E. _____

Crossword

Fill in the crossword by answering the clues below with the words from this list:

Development	Menopause	Neonatal	Puberty	Step
Grasp	Moro	Pre-adolescence	Rooting	Sucking
Growth				

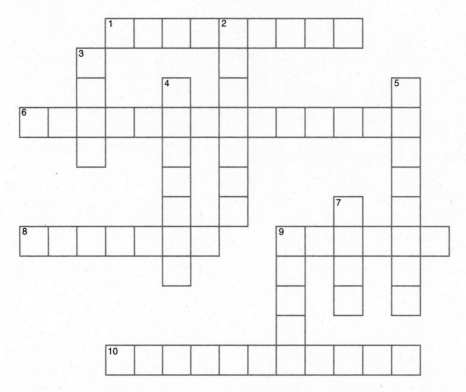

Across

1. Event that occurs to women between ages 40 and 55
6. Time between childhood and adolescence (late childhood)
8. Reflex that occurs when the lips are touched
9. Physical changes that can be measured and that occur in a steady, orderly manner
10. Changes in mental, emotional, and social function

Down

2. Period between ages 9 and 15 years that girls reach; period between ages 12 and 16 years that boys reach
3. Reflex in which the feet move up and down as in stepping motions
4. Reflex that occurs when the cheek is touched near the mouth
5. Period of infancy from birth to 1 month of age
7. Reflex that occurs when a loud noise, a sudden movement, or the head falling back startles the baby
9. Reflex that occurs when the palm is stroked

12 Care of the Older Person

Fill in the Blank: Key Terms

Atrophy   Gerontology
Geriatrics

1. _____ is the care of aging people.

2. Another word for shrink is _____.

3. The study of the aging process is _____

Circle the Best Answer

4. Most older people live
   A. In a nursing center   C. In a family setting
   B. Alone   D. With non-relatives

5. The oldest-old are
   A. 65 to 74 years   C. 60 to 65 years
   B. 75 to 84 years   D. 85 years and older

6. As aging occurs
   A. Disability always results
   B. Changes are often slow
   C. Most people adapt poorly
   D. Mental function declines

7. A myth about aging is
   A. Many older people enjoy a fulfilling sex life
   B. Mental function declines with age
   C. Many older persons have jobs
   D. Most older persons have frequent contact with their children

8. Social changes of aging include
   A. Graying hair
   B. Disabilities
   C. Retirement and deaths of loved ones
   D. Decreased physical strength

9. All of these are benefits of retiring except
   A. The person can do whatever he or she wants
   B. Travel and leisure-time activities are possible
   C. The person can relax and enjoy life
   D. The person may have reduced income, which affects life-style

10. Money problems can result with retirement because
    A. Income is reduced
    B. Expenses increase
    C. The person is unable to work
    D. The person planned for retirement

11. Loneliness may be a bigger problem for foreign-born persons because
    A. Families from other cultures do not care about older persons
    B. The person is not accepted by native-born persons
    C. They may not have anyone to talk to in their own language
    D. They have more chronic illnesses

12. An older person can adjust to social relationship changes by doing all of these except
    A. Stay at home alone to save money
    B. Find new friends
    C. Develop hobbies and church and community activities
    D. Have regular contact with family

13. A benefit when children care for older parents may be
    A. The older person may feel unwanted and useless
    B. The older person may feel more secure
    C. Tension may develop among the children and the family
    D. Parents and children change roles

14. When a partner dies, the older person
    A. Accepts this as part of life
    B. May develop serious physical and mental problems
    C. Forms new friendships easily
    D. Usually has prepared for this change

15. What causes wrinkles to appear on an older person?
    A. Decreases in oil and sweat gland secretions
    B. Fewer nerve endings
    C. Loss of elasticity, strength, and fatty tissue layer
    D. Poor circulation

16. Healing in older people is delayed because of
    A. Poor nutrition
    B. Fragile blood vessels in the skin
    C. Fewer nerve endings
    D. Loss of fatty tissue

17. Hot water bottles and heating pads are not used with older persons because
    A. They generally complain of being too warm
    B. The skin is dry
    C. Burns are a risk because of decreased sensing of heat and cold
    D. Blood vessels decrease in number

18. Older persons can prevent bone loss and loss of muscle strength by
    A. Activity, exercise, and diet
    B. Taking hormones
    C. Resting with feet elevated
    D. Taking vitamins

19. Bones may break easily because
    A. Joints become stiff and painful
    B. Joints become slightly flexed
    C. Bones lose strength and become brittle
    D. Vertebrae shorten

20. Dizziness may increase in older people because
    A. They have difficulty sleeping
    B. Blood flow to the brain is reduced
    C. Nerve cells are lost
    D. Brain cells are lost

21. Older persons
    A. Have longer memories
    B. Often remember events from long ago better than recent events
    C. May remember more recent events better than events of long ago
    D. Always become confused as aging progresses

22. Painful injuries and disease may go unnoticed because
    A. The person is confused
    B. Touch and sensitivity to pain are reduced
    C. Memory is shorter
    D. The blood flow is reduced

23. Older people often complain that food has no taste because
    A. Of memory loss
    B. The appetite decreases
    C. Taste buds decrease in number
    D. They cannot sense heat and cold

24. Eyes become irritated easily because
    A. The lens yellows
    B. The eye takes longer to adjust to changes in light
    C. Tear secretion is less
    D. The person becomes farsighted

25. An older person may have difficulty in hearing
    A. Loud music   C. High-pitched sounds
    B. Low-pitched sounds   D. All sounds

26. When severe circulatory changes occur, the person
    A. May be encouraged to walk long distances
    B. May need to rest during the day
    C. Should not do any kind of exercise
    D. Should exercise only once a week

27. When a person has difficulty breathing, it is easier to breathe when
    A. Lying flat in bed
    B. Covered with heavy bed linens
    C. Allowed to be on bedrest
    D. Resting in the semi-Fowler's position

28. Dulled taste and smell decreases
    A. Peristalsis   C. Saliva
    B. Appetite   D. Swallowing

29. Older persons need
    A. Fewer calories   C. More calories
    B. Less fluids   D. Low-protein diets

30. Many older persons have to urinate several times during the night because
    A. Bladder infections are common
    B. Urine is more concentrated
    C. The bladder stores less urine
    D. Urinary incontinence may occur

31. An older woman may find intercourse uncomfortable or painful because
    A. Her partner does not achieve an erection easily
    B. There is vaginal dryness
    C. Arousal takes longer
    D. Orgasm is less intense

32. All of these are advantages of an older person living with family *except*
    A. It provides companionship
    B. The family can provide care
    C. They can share living expenses
    D. Sleeping plans may need to change

33. Adult day-care centers
    A. Provide meals, supervision, and activities for older persons
    B. Accept only self-care persons and those who can walk without help
    C. Provide complete care
    D. Provide respite care

34. When an older person rents an apartment, it allows the person to
    A. Remain independent
    B. Share common meals with others
    C. Enjoy gardening and yard work
    D. Repair appliances and maintain the property

35. Elder Cottage Housing Opportunity or accessory dwelling units allow the person to
    A. Have meals with other people
    B. Have supervision and activities
    C. Live independently but near friends and family
    D. Receive medical care in the home

36. Senior citizen housing is available to
    A. Only those who can afford the rent
    B. Those who have no disabilities
    C. Older and disabled persons
    D. Families who live with an older person

37. Home-sharing is a way to avoid
    A. Living alone
    B. Paying rent
    C. Doing housework or yard work
    D. Disabilities

38. Assisted living facilities are for persons who
    A. Need daily nursing care
    B. Need help getting in and out of bed
    C. Need help with daily living
    D. Are dependent on others for all care

39. Continuing care retirement communities (CCRCs)
    A. Only have independent living units
    B. Only have 24-hour nursing care
    C. Add services as the person's needs change
    D. Require the person to leave when health care needs increase

40. Nursing centers are housing options for older persons who
    A. Need companionship only
    B. Cannot care for themselves
    C. Need care during the day-time while family works
    D. Are developmentally disabled

41. A quality nursing center must meet OBRA and CMS requirements to
    A. Be approved by the medical society
    B. Receive Medicare and Medicaid funds
    C. Give care
    D. Be licensed by the local health department

42. A quality nursing center would *not* be required to have
    A. An activity area for residents' use
    B. Common areas, resident rooms, and doorways that are designed for wheelchair use
    C. Toilet facilities that allow wheelchair use
    D. An area where residents may have private gardens

43. A feature of a quality nursing center is
    A. Hand rails are provided in hallways
    B. Each resident must have a private bathroom
    C. Residents are expected to provide furniture for their rooms
    D. Tablecloths and cloth napkins are used in the dining room.

Matching

Match physical changes during the aging process with the body system affected.

A. Integumentary
B. Musculo-skeletal
C. Nervous
D. Cardiovascular
E. Respiratory
F. Digestive
G. Urinary

44. _____ Reduced blood flow to kidneys

45. _____ Arteries narrow and are less elastic

46. _____ Forgetfulness

47. _____ Gradual loss of height

48. _____ Decreased strength for coughing

49. _____ Decreased secretion of oil and sweat glands

50. _____ Difficulty digesting fried and fatty foods

51. _____ Heart pumps with less force

52. _____ Bladder muscles weaken

53. _____ Difficulty seeing green and blue colors

54. _____ Difficulty swallowing

55. _____ Lung tissue less elastic

56. _____ Bone mass decreases

57. _____ Facial hair in some women

Fill in the Blank

58. Write out the meaning of the abbreviations.
    A. ADU _____
    B. CCRC _____
    C. CMS _____
    D. ECHO _____

59. What changes can be made in the bathroom to make it safer for a person with poor eyesight?
    A. _____ flooring
    B. Grab bars by _____
    C. _____
       surfaces in showers and tubs
    D. Rugs with _____
    E. _____
       devices on faucets and shower-heads
    F. Toilet with raised _____ or
       toilet _____
    G. _____ lighting

60. Name the housing options described in each of the following:
    A. A small portable home that can be placed in the yard of a single-family home _____
    B. Provides meals, supervision, activities, and sometimes rehabilitation to elderly during day-time _____
    C. The elderly person lives with older brothers, sisters, or cousins for companionship or to share living expenses _____
    D. The elderly person pays rent and utility bills but does not need to do maintenance, yard work, or snow removal _____
    E. The elderly person who needs help with activities of daily living but does not need nursing care may live in a _____.
    F. A _____ meets the changing needs of older persons. Services change as the person's needs change.

Use the FOCUS ON PRIDE section to complete these statements.

61. It is your responsibility to avoid believing myths about aging. These myths are
    A. _____
    B. _____
    C. _____
    D. _____
    E. _____
    F. _____

62. You can promote social interaction when caring for an older person when you
    A. Encourage _____
    B. Ask _____
    C. Use _____
    D. Take _____

Optional Learning Exercises

63. When bathing an older person, what kind of soap should be used? _____

    Often no soap is used on the _____.

64. What can happen if a nick or cut occurs on the feet?

    _____

    Why can this happen?

    _____

65. Because bone mass decreases, why is it important to turn an older person carefully?

    _____

66. Why does an older person often have a gradual loss of height? _____

    _____

67. What types of exercise help prevent bone loss and loss of muscle strength? _____

    _____

68. Older people have changes in the nervous system. When the changes listed occur, what can happen?
    A. Nerve conduction and reflexes are slower.

    _____

    B. Blood flow to brain is reduced.

    _____

    C. Touch and sensitivity to pain and pressure are reduced.

    _____

69. When you are eating with an older person, you notice she puts salt on vegetables that taste fine to you. What may be a reason she does this?

    _____

70. What exercises will help a person with circulation changes who must stay in bed?

    _____

71. What can the nursing assistant do to prevent respiratory complications from bedrest?

    _____

72. The stomach and colon empty slower and flatulence and constipation are common in the older person. What causes these problems?

    _____

73. How will good oral hygiene and denture care improve food intake? _____

74. How can a nursing assistant help prevent urinary tract infections in an older person?

    _____

75. Why should you plan to give most fluids to the older person before 1700 (5:00 PM)?

    _____

13 Safety

Fill in the Blank: Key Terms

Coma
Dementia
Disaster
Electrical shock

Elopement
Ground
Hazard
Hazardous chemical

Hemiplegia
Incident
Paralysis

Paraplegia
Poison
Quadraplegia

Suffocation
Tetraplegia
Workplace violence

1. When a patient or resident leaves the agency without staff knowledge it is __elopement__.

2. The loss of cognitive and social function caused by changes in the brain is __dementia__.

3. __Workplace violence__ are violent acts (including assault or threat of assault) directed toward persons at work or while on duty.

4. Paralysis from the neck down is __quadriplegia__

5. __Hazardous chemical__ is any chemical that is a physical hazard or a health hazard.

6. A __disaster__ is a sudden catastrophic event in which many people are injured and killed and property is destroyed.

7. __Suffocation__ occurs when breathing stops from the lack of oxygen.

8. Paralysis on one side of the body is __Hemiplegia__

9. A __coma__ is a state of being unaware of one's surroundings and being unable to react or respond to people, places, or things.

10. That which carries leaking electricity to the earth and away from an electrical appliance is a __ground__.

11. __Paraplegia__ is paralysis from the waist down.

12. __electrical shock__ occurs when electrical current passes through the body.

13. Any event that has harmed or could harm a patient, resident, visitor, or staff member is an __incident__.

14. __Paralysis__ means loss of muscle function, loss of sensation, or loss of both muscle function and sensation.

15. __Poison__ is any substance harmful to the body when ingested, inhaled, injected, or absorbed through the skin.

16. Another term for quadraplegia is __tetraplegia__

17. A __Hazard__ is anything in the person's setting that could cause injury or illness.

Circle the Best Answer

18. Safety measures needed by a person can be found
    A. In the doctor's orders
    B. In the person's care plan
    C. By talking to the family
    D. By asking the person

19. When checking for safety issues, a survey team will observe
    A. How well you give care
    B. For actual or potential hazards
    C. How quickly you can answer a question
    D. Whether the staff is well groomed — prepare.

20. A reason drugs can be an accident risk factor is because they
    A. Affect hearing
    B. Reduce ability to sense heat and cold
    C. Can cause loss of balance or lack of coordination
    D. Can cause hemiplegia

21. Children are at risk of injury because they
    A. Have not learned the difference between safety and danger
    B. Have not learned right from wrong
    C. Have problems sensing heat and cold
    D. Have poor vision

22. When a person has dementia, he or she is at risk for injury because
    A. He or she may not detect smoke or gas odors
    B. Judgment is poor
    C. He or she cannot move out of the way to safety
    D. He or she is more sensitive to hazardous materials

23. Identifying persons is most important because
    A. Life and health are threatened if the wrong care is given
    B. Visitors may ask for your help to find someone
    C. You need to call the person by the right name
    D. You will have to give care to 2 people if you give it to the wrong person first

24. Which of these is not a reliable way to identify the person?
    A. Check the identification bracelet.
    B. Use the person's picture to compare it with the person.
    C. If the person is alert and oriented, follow center policy to identify him or her.
    D. Just call the person by name.

25. A leading cause of death, especially among children and older persons, is
    A. Falls   C. Accidental poisoning
    B. Burns   D. Suffocation

26. When children are in the kitchen
    A. Use the stove's back burners
    B. Turn pot and pan handles so they point outward
    C. Let children help you cook at the stove
    D. Leave cooking utensils in pots and pans

27. Burns can be avoided if oven mitts and pot-holders are kept dry because
    A. They conduct heat better
    B. Water conducts heat and can cause burns
    C. Moisture allows bacteria to move through the cloth
    D. The mitts fit around handles better when they are dry

28. Accidental poisoning of children can occur when
    A. Harmful products are kept in their original containers
    B. Harmful substances are labeled and stored in high, locked areas
    C. Drugs are carried in purses, backpacks, and briefcases
    D. Safety latches are used on kitchen, bathroom, garage, basement, and workshop cabinets

29. Poison warning stickers should be placed on common poisons such as
    A. Foods
    B. Bottled waters and sodas
    C. Fruits and vegetables
    D. Harmful substances

30. Children are at risk for lead poisoning between the ages of
    A. Birth and 3 months
    B. 6 months and 6 years
    C. 6 years and 9 years
    D. 12 years and 18 years

31. How can you prevent exposure to lead-based plumbing?
    A. Use only bottled water.
    B. Run the water until it is hot before drinking.
    C. Boil all water used in cooking.
    D. Let cold water run 1 to 2 minutes before using it for cooking or coffee.

32. A gas that can cause suffocation is
    A. Oxygen   C. Carbon monoxide
    B. Carbon dioxide   D. Nitrogen

33. All of these are sources of carbon monoxide *except*
    A. Furnaces
    B. Automobiles, especially if one is running in a garage
    C. Gas stoves or space heaters
    D. Electric appliances

34. A choking hazard for older persons can be
    A. Loose dentures that fit poorly
    B. Sitting up in a wheelchair to eat
    C. Food that is cut into small, bite-sized pieces
    D. Making sure the person is positioned properly in bed

35. Which of these would prevent choking in children?
    A. Position infants on their stomachs for sleep.
    B. Use Mylar balloons instead of latex ones.
    C. Give the child food such as hot dogs, peanuts, or popcorn.
    D. Place an infant on a soft pillow or comforter to sleep.

36. The universal sign of choking is when the
    A. Person begins to cough forcefully
    B. Conscious person clutches at the throat
    C. Person tells you he is choking
    D. Person becomes unconscious

37. Abdominal thrusts given for choking can be used on
    A. Pregnant women
    B. Obese people
    C. Infants
    D. Other adults or children over 1 year of age

38. When giving abdominal thrusts, the correct procedure is to
    A. Make a fist, place the thumb side against the abdomen, and quickly thrust upward
    B. Press your fist against the abdomen and slowly push straight down
    C. Gently thrust upward with the fist
    D. Lay the hands flat on the abdomen and push down

39. If you see a foreign object in the mouth of an unconscious person, you should
    A. Turn the head to one side
    B. Leave the object in place
    C. Grasp and remove the object if it is within reach
    D. Ask the person to cough out the object

40. If an infant is choking, you should
    A. Take the infant to the emergency room
    B. Give abdominal thrusts
    C. Hold the infant face down over your forearm and give 5 forceful back slaps between the shoulder blades
    D. Reach in the mouth and try to retrieve the object

41. If a choking person becomes unresponsive, you should
    A. Make sure EMS or RRT was called
    B. Begin abdominal thrusts
    C. Begin chest thrusts
    D. Do a finger sweep for foreign objects in the mouth

42. If you find a piece of equipment that is damaged, take it to the
    A. Nurse
    B. Maintenance department
    C. Fire department
    D. Director of nursing

43. When using electrical items, you
    A. Should always use a three-pronged plug
    B. May touch the equipment even if you are wet
    C. Should unplug the equipment before turning it off
    D. May use water to put out an electrical fire

44. An electrical shock is especially dangerous because it can
    A. Start a fire
    B. Damage equipment
    C. Affect the heart and cause death
    D. Violate OBRA regulations

45. If you are shocked by electrical equipment, you should
    A. Report the shock at once
    B. Try to see what is wrong with the equipment
    C. Make sure it has a ground prong
    D. Test the equipment in a different outlet

46. _____ requires that health care employees understand the risks of hazardous substances and how to handle them safely.
    A. Omnibus Budget Reconciliation of 1987 (OBRA)
    B. Occupational Safety and Health Administration (OSHA)
    C. Joint Commission on Accreditation of Healthcare Organization (JCAHO)
    D. Safety data sheet (SDS)

47. Warning labels may include all of these *except*
    A. Physical hazards and health hazards
    B. What protective equipment to wear
    C. The phone number of the local emergency system
    D. Storage and disposal information

48. Where would you find the safety data sheets (SDSs) for hazardous materials?
    A. Attached to the substance
    B. In the administrator's office
    C. In a place on your nursing unit
    D. On the Internet

49. All of these things are needed for a fire *except*
    A. Spark or flame
    B. Electrical equipment
    C. Materials that will burn
    D. Oxygen

50. When a person is receiving oxygen, which of these is allowed in the room?
    A. Visitors may smoke but the person receiving oxygen may not
    B. Wool blankets and fabrics that cause static electricity
    C. Electrical items that are in good working order
    D. Oil, grease, alcohol, and nail polish remover

51. If a fire occurs, what should you do first?
    A. Rescue people in immediate danger.
    B. Sound the nearest fire alarm and call the switchboard operator.
    C. Close doors and windows to confine the fire.
    D. Use a fire extinguisher on a small fire that has not spread to a larger area.

52. If evacuation is necessary, persons who are
    A. Closest to the outside door are rescued first
    B. Able to walk are rescued last
    C. Closest to the fire are evacuated first
    D. Helpless are rescued last

53. If a space heater is used in a home, a safety practice is to
    A. Place the heater in doorways or on stairs
    B. Keep the heater 3 feet away from curtains, drapes, and furniture
    C. Store fuel near the heater
    D. Fill the heater when it is hot or running

54. If there is a disaster, you
    A. Are expected to go to your agency immediately
    B. May be called into work if you are off duty
    C. Should stay away or leave to get out of the way
    D. May go home to check on your family

55. Nurses and nursing assistants are at risk for workplace violence for these reasons *except*
    A. Patients may be persons who are arrested or convicted of crimes
    B. Acutely disturbed and violent persons are often patients
    C. Agency pharmacies are a source of drugs and therefore a target for robberies
    D. They are not allowed to defend themselves if attacked

56. Which of these would *not* be effective to prevent or control workplace violence?
    A. Stand away from the person.
    B. Know where to find panic buttons, call bells, and alarms.
    C. Sit quietly with the person in his room. Hold his hand to calm him.
    D. Tell the person you will get a nurse to speak to her.

57. You can help prevent workplace violence by doing all of these *except*
    A. Wearing long hair up and off the collar
    B. Making sure shoes have good soles that do not slip
    C. Wearing necklaces, bracelets, and earrings
    D. Wearing uniforms that fit well

58. If you are uncomfortable or threatened in a home setting, you should
    A. Tell the nurse
    B. Stay at the home and try to resolve the matter
    C. Confront the person who is making you uncomfortable
    D. Ignore the situation and continue to give care

59. A yellow color-coded wristband may indicate that the person
    A. Has allergies
    B. Has a "Do Not Resuscitate" order
    C. Has a restricted diet
    D. Is at risk for falling

Matching

Match each safety measure to the risk it prevents.

A. Burns
B. Poisoning
C. Suffocation
D. Equipment accident
E. Hazardous substances
F. Fire

60. _____ Do not allow person to sleep with a heating pad.

61. _____ Supervise persons who smoke.

62. _____ Keep child-resistant caps on all harmful products.

63. _____ Wear PPE to clean spills and leaks.

64. _____ Report loose teeth or dentures to the nurse.

65. _____ Do not touch a person who is experiencing an electrical shock.

66. _____ Open doors and windows if you notice gas odors.

67. _____ Have water heaters set at 120°F or less.

68. _____ Never call drugs or vitamins "candy."

69. _____ Store fuel and flammable liquids in locked cabinets.

Fill in the Blank

70. Write out the meaning of the abbreviations.

    A. AED _Automated external defibrillator_

    B. CDC _Centers for Disease Control and_

    C. CO _Carbon monoxide_

    D. CPR _Cardiopulmonary resuscitation_

    E. EMS _Emergency Medical Service_

    F. FBAO _Foreign-body airway obstruc_

    G. HCS _Hazard Communication Standard_

    H. OSHA _Occupational Safety and H. Admin_

    I. PASS _Pull the safety pin, aim low,_

    J. RACE _Rescue, alarm, confine, extinguish_

    K. RRT _Rapid Response Team_

    L. SDS _Safety data sheet_

71. As part of the team, you can help provide a safe setting by correcting something that is unsafe. What could you do if

    A. You see a water spill _____

    B. You see a person sliding out of a wheelchair

    _____

    C. A person is having problems holding a cup of coffee _____

    D. Food is left unattended in a microwave

    _____

    E. A grab bar is loose in the bathroom

    _____

72. A person who is agitated or aggressive may be at risk for injuries. What can cause these behaviors?

    A. _____

    B. _____

    C. _____

    D. _____

73. What health hazards can be caused by hazardous chemicals?

    A. _____

    B. _____

    C. _____

    D. _____

74. When a fire occurs, what action is taken for each of these steps?

    A. R _____

    B. A _____

    C. C _____

    D. E _____

75. The word PASS is used to remember how to use a

    _____

    What action is taken for each of these steps?

    A. P _____

    B. A _____

    C. S _____

    D. S _____

76. If a disaster occurs, the agency usually has a plan that generally provides for

    A. _____

    B. _____

    C. _____

    D. _____

    E. _____

Use the FOCUS ON PRIDE section to complete these statements.

77. If you make a mistake, you show personal and professional responsibility when you

    A. _____

    B. _____

    C. _____

78. You work as a team when you ensure the safety of all staff arriving and leaving the agency by

    A. _____

    B. _____

    C. _____

    D. _____

    E. _____

Optional Learning Exercises

What safety measure to prevent burns is being followed in each example? (Box 13-1)

79. Smoke alarm batteries are checked in spring and fall.

    _____

80. A child is placed in the playpen nearby while you are cooking. _____

81. A heating pad is removed from the bed for the night.

    _____

82. A wet pot-holder is replaced with a dry one.

    _____

83. You place Mr. Smith's cigarettes in a designated area of the nurses' station. _____

84. You keep matches on the top shelf of the cupboard.

_____

85. When you get ready to cook, you take off your bulky sweater. _____

86. The nursing assistant sits with the confused person while he smokes. _____

Read the following examples and write the related safety measure. (Boxes 13-2 and 13-3)

87. You check the labels on harmful products in your home. _____

88. You ask a visitor to your home to put her purse on a shelf. _____

89. Use your glazed pottery for decoration only.

_____

90. You discard a can of food when you notice it was canned in Mexico. _____

Read the following examples and write the related safety measure. (Box 13-7)

91. The nursing assistant tells the person his shower will be delayed until the storm passes.

_____

92. The nursing assistant tells the nurse she has never used the portable foot bath before.

_____

93. The nursing assistant dries her hands carefully before plugging in a razor. _____

94. An electric fan will not work and the staff member follows the correct procedure to have it repaired.

_____

_____

95. The nursing assistant moves an electrical cord that is lying across a heat vent. _____

_____

What should you do in these situations related to hazardous chemicals? (Box 13-8)

96. When cleaning up a hazardous chemical, how do you know what equipment to wear?

_____

97. When a spill occurs, what is the correct way to wipe it up? _____

_____

98. The nurse tells the nursing assistant the person is having an x-ray done in her room.

_____

99. The nurse tells you to open the windows in a room where you are cleaning up a hazardous chemical.

_____

What fire prevention measure is being practiced in each example? (Box 13-9)

100. The person is taken to the smoking area in his wheelchair. _____

101. When cleaning a smoking area, the staff uses a metal can partially filled with sand.

_____

What measures to prevent or control workplace violence are being used or should be used in these examples? (Box 13-10)

102. What types of jewelry can serve as a weapon?

_____

_____

103. Why is long hair worn up? _____

104. Why are pictures, vases, and other items removed from certain areas?

_____

105. What type of glass protects nurses' stations, reception areas, and admitting areas?

_____

106. What clothing items should be worn by staff to assist the ability to run?

_____

List personal safety practices that apply in these situations. (Box 13-11)

107. What safety practices should be used when parking your car in a parking garage?

_____

_____

108. What items should you keep in the car for safety?

_____

_____

109. Why is a "dry run" important?

_____

_____

110. If you think someone is following you, what should you do? _____

_____

111. How can you use your car keys as a weapon?

_____

_____

112. How can you use your thumbs as a weapon?

_____

_____

113. What part of the body can you attack on either a man or a woman? _____

_____

Fill in the Blank: Key Terms

Bed rail   Gait belt   Transfer belt

1. A device used to support a person who is unsteady or disabled is a _____.

2. A _____ is a device that serves as a guard or barrier along the side of the bed.

3. Another name for a transfer belt is a

   _____.

Circle the Best Answer

4. Most falls occur in
   A. Hallways
   B. Resident rooms and bathrooms
   C. Outside areas
   D. Dining areas

5. In nursing centers the most common causes of falling are
   A. Confusion and dementia
   B. Weakness and walking problems
   C. Throw rugs and clutter on the floor
   D. Loose or missing hand rails and grab bars

6. Which of these would help to prevent falls?
   A. Answer call light promptly.
   B. Take the person to the bathroom once per shift.
   C. Always keep side rails up.
   D. Have the person wear socks to walk in the room.

7. A safety measure that can help prevent falls would be
   A. Have the person wear reading glasses when walking
   B. Assist the person to the bathroom or provide the bedpan, urinal, or commode
   C. Re-arrange the furniture in the room often
   D. Turn off lights and night-lights at night

8. A bed or chair alarm
   A. Prevents the person from getting out of bed or the chair
   B. Can be turned off by the person
   C. Makes a sound or has a recorded message that alerts the staff that the person is getting up unassisted
   D. Is considered a restraint

9. Bed rails
   A. Are used for all older persons
   B. Must be in the person's best interest
   C. Prevent falls
   D. Are never used when giving care

10. Information about whether to raise bed rails for a particular person can be found in the
    A. Care plan   C. Agency policies
    B. Doctor's orders   D. Procedure book

11. When giving bedside care, the bed wheels are
    A. Unlocked
    B. Locked
    C. Unlocked on the side of the bed where you are working
    D. Locked when moving the bed

12. A transfer belt is
    A. Applied over clothing
    B. Applied with the buckle in the front
    C. Applied very loosely
    D. Always applied next to the skin

13. Check with the nurse before using a transfer belt when a person
    A. Is unsteady when moving from a chair to the bed
    B. Needs help to walk
    C. Has an abdominal wound, incision, or drainage tube
    D. Needs help to stand up

14. If a person begins to fall, you should
    A. Try to prevent the fall
    B. Call for help and hold the person up
    C. Ease the person to the floor
    D. Stand back and let the person fall

15. If a bariatric person starts to fall, you should
    A. Try to prevent the fall
    B. Ease the person to the floor
    C. Quickly move any items that could cause injury out of the way
    D. Call for help and hold the person up

Fill in the Blank

16. Write out the meaning of these abbreviations.
    A. CDC _____
    B. CMS _____

17. You may calm an agitated person by giving the person
    a _____, _____,
    or a _____.

18. Tubs and showers may be made safer if they have
    _____ surfaces.

19. Bed rails are used according to the _____ and
    _____.

20. You raise the bed to give care. If the person uses bed rails and you are working alone, what do you do with the side rails?
    A. _____
    B. _____

21. After you are done giving care, how is the bed positioned? _____
    _____.

22. When using bed or chair alarms safely, you should
    A. _____
    B. _____
    C. _____
23. Hand rails in hallways and stairways give support to persons who are _____
24. Bed wheels are locked when
    A. _____
    B. _____
25. When a transfer belt is applied, you should be able to slide _____ under the belt.
26. Check with the nurse before using a transfer belt if the person has
    A. _____
    B. _____
    C. _____
    D. _____
    E. _____
    F. _____
    G. _____
27. When a person starts to fall, you can protect the person's _____ as you ease the person to the floor.
28. If you must manually lift a person who falls, you should protect yourself from _____.

Use the FOCUS ON PRIDE section to complete these statements.

29. To show personal and professional responsibility, you do not take short cuts and take time to
    A. _____
    B. _____
    C. _____
    D. _____
    E. _____
30. You support the person's right to safety and security when you promote comfort using good
    _____
31. When assisting a co-worker with a transfer, what information do you need?
    A. _____
    B. _____
    C. _____
    D. _____
    E. _____
    F. _____

Optional Learning Exercises

32. Why are falls more likely to happen during shift changes? Staff _____
    _____. Confusion
    _____.
33. What kinds of equipment and safety measures help to make bathrooms and showers safer?
    A. _____
    B. _____
    C. _____
    D. _____
    E. _____
    F. _____
34. Why should floor coverings be one color in areas where older persons are living? _____
    _____
35. Why are falls prevented when the person's phone, lamp, and personal belongings are at the bedside?
    _____
36. What kind of footwear and clothing will help to prevent falls?
    A. Footwear
    _____
    _____
    B. Clothing
    _____
    _____
37. Why is it important to answer call lights promptly?
    _____
    _____
38. If a person needs bed rails, keep them up at all times except _____.
39. For a person who uses bed rails, always raise the far bed rail if you _____.
40. If a person does not use bed rails and you are giving care, how do you protect him or her from falling?
    _____
    _____
41. Wheels are locked at all times except when
    _____
42. If a person starts to fall, you _____. This lets you control _____.
43. If a bariatric person starts to fall, you should
    A. _____
    B. _____
    C. _____
    D. _____
    E. _____

15 Restraint Alternatives and Safe Restraint Use

Fill in the Blank: Key Terms

Chemical restraint   Discipline
Convenience   Enabler

Freedom of movement   Physical restraint
Medical symptom   Remove easily

1. Any action taken to control or manage a person's behavior that requires less effort by the staff is a

_____.

2. Any manual method or physical or mechanical device, material, or equipment attached to or near the person's body that he or she cannot remove easily is a

_____.

3. _____ is a term used when a manual method device, material, or equipment can be removed intentionally by the person in the same manner it was applied by the staff.

4. A device that limits freedom of movement but is used to promote independence is an

_____.

5. Any change in place or position for the body that the person is physically able to control is called

_____.

6. An indication or characteristic of a physical or psychological condition is a

_____.

7. A _____ is any drug used for discipline or convenience and not required to treat medical symptoms.

8. Any action taken by the agency to punish or penalize a patient or resident is _____.

Circle the Best Answer

9. Restraints are used
   A. Whenever the nurse feels they are necessary
   B. Only to treat a medical symptom or for the immediate physical safety of the person or others
   C. To make sure the person does not fall
   D. To decrease work for the staff

10. Research shows that restraints
    A. Prevent falls
    B. Cause falls
    C. Are used whenever the nurse decides
    D. Are not effective

11. A person's harmful behaviors may be caused by all of these except
    A. Being afraid of a new setting
    B. Being too hot or too cold
    C. Being hungry or thirsty
    D. Being uncooperative with staff

12. Guidelines about using restraints are part of the resident rights in
    A. CDC regulations
    B. OSHA rules
    C. OBRA, FDA, CMS, and TJC regulations
    D. The nurse practice act

13. Restraints are *not* used to
    A. Prevent harm to the person
    B. Control the person's behaviors
    C. Prevent a person from pulling at a wound or dressing
    D. Keep an IV from being pulled out

14. Which of these is a type of restraint?
    A. A soft chair with a footstool to elevate the feet
    B. A bed without bed rails
    C. A chair with a tray that prevents the person from rising
    D. A drug that helps a person function at his or her highest level

15. The most serious risk from restraints is
    A. Cuts, bruises, and fractures
    B. Death from strangulation
    C. Falls
    D. Depression, anger, and agitation

16. Using a restraint requires informed consent. This consent is obtained by
    A. The person's legal representative
    B. The doctor or nurse
    C. The person
    D. The nursing assistant

17. All of these are legal aspects of restraint use except
    A. Unnecessary restraint use is false imprisonment
    B. Nurses can decide when to use restraints, what type of restraints to use, and how long to use the restraints
    C. The least restrictive method is used
    D. Restraints must protect the person

18. Restraints may increase
    A. Rest and sleep
    B. Confusion and agitation
    C. Calmness and alertness
    D. Cooperation with care and procedures

19. If you do not know how to apply a restraint, you should
    A. Read the directions before applying the restraint and then apply the restraint
    B. Ask the nurse to observe you applying the restraint
    C. Watch someone else apply it to a person
    D. Apply it to the person independently

20. Which of these is a physical restraint?
    A. Vest
    B. Bed rail
    C. Wedge cushion
    D. Pillow

21. When restraining a combative and agitated person, it should be done
    A. Slowly by only one person
    B. Only after explaining to the person what will be done
    C. With enough staff to complete the task safely and quickly
    D. In a public area so the person is distracted

22. The person who is restrained must be observed every
    A. 5 minutes
    B. 15 minutes
    C. Hour
    D. 2 hours

23. When a person is restrained, at least every 2 hours you should
    A. Check the person
    B. Remove the restraints, re-position the person, and meet basic needs
    C. Make sure the restraints are secure
    D. Remove the restraints until the next shift

24. Wrist restraints are used when a person
    A. Tries to get out of bed
    B. Moves his or her wheelchair without permission
    C. Pulls at tubes used in medical treatments
    D. Slides out of a chair easily

25. A roll belt restraint
    A. Is more restrictive than other restraints
    B. Allows the person to turn from side to side
    C. Must be released by the staff
    D. Can be used only in a chair

26. The straps of vest and jacket restraints
    A. Always cross in the front
    B. Are applied next to the skin under clothing
    C. Must be secured very tightly to be safe
    D. May cross in the back

27. Elbow restraints are used
    A. To prevent older persons from pulling at tubes
    B. For children to limit movements and prevent scratching and touching incisions
    C. On only one arm at a time
    D. To prevent injury to the staff by a confused person

28. When applying wrist restraints
    A. Tie the straps to the bed rail
    B. Tie firm knots in the straps
    C. Place the restraints over clothing
    D. Place the soft or foam part toward the skin

29. If you are using padded mitt restraints, you should
    A. Give the person a hand roll to hold
    B. Pad the mitt with soft material
    C. Make sure the person's hands are clean and dry
    D. Tie the straps to the bed rails

30. A belt restraint should be
    A. Used only when the person is in a chair or wheelchair
    B. Secured tightly with no slack in the straps
    C. Checked to make sure the person is comfortable and in good body alignment
    D. Applied next to the skin

31. When using a vest restraint in bed
    A. The ties are secured to the bed frame out of the person's reach
    B. The ties are secured to the bed rail
    C. The vest crosses in the back
    D. The person can turn over

32. When you check a person in vest, jacket, or belt restraint, report at once if
    A. The skin is slightly reddened under the restraint
    B. The person needs to urinate
    C. The person is not breathing or is having difficulty breathing
    D. You need to re-position the person

Matching

Match the laws and safety guidelines with the correct example.
A. Restraints must protect the person
B. Restraints require a written doctor's order.
C. The least restrictive method of restraint is used
D. Restraints are used only after other methods fail to protect the person.
E. Unnecessary restraint is false imprisonment.
F. Informed consent is required for restraint use.
G. The manufacturer's instructions are followed.
H. Restraints are applied with enough help to protect the person and staff from injury.
I. Restraints can increase a person's confusion and agitation.
J. Quality of life must be protected.
K. The person is observed at least every 15 minutes or more often as required by the care plan.
L. The restraint is removed, the person repositioned, and basic needs met at least every 2 hours.

33. _____ Injuries and deaths have occurred from improper restraint and poor observation.

34. _____ A restraint is used only when it is the best safety precaution for the person.

35. _____ You are provided the manufacturer's instructions for applying and securing restraints.

36. _____ Restrained persons need repeated explanations and reassurance.

37. _____ The doctor gives the reason for the restraint, what to use, and how long to use the restraint.

38. _____ Persons in immediate danger of harming themselves or others are restrained quickly.

39. _____ Passive physical restraints are the least restrictive so should be used when possible.

40. _____ Restraints are used for as short a time as possible and needs are met with as little restraint as possible.

41. _____ If told to apply a restraint, you must clearly understand the need for restraints and the risks.

42. _____ Restraint is removed. Person is ambulated or range-of-motion exercises are performed.

43. _____ The care plan must include measures to protect the person and to prevent the person from harming others.

44. _____ The person must understand the reason for the restraints.

Fill in the Blank

45. Write out the abbreviations.

A. CMS _____

B. FDA _____

C. ID _____

D. OBRA _____

E. ROM _____

F. TJC _____

46. When using restraints, what information is reported and recorded?

A. _____

B. _____

C. _____

D. _____

E. _____

F. _____

G. _____

H. _____

I. _____

J. _____

K. _____

L. _____

M. Complaints to report at once:

   i. _____

   ii. _____

   iii. _____

   iv. _____

47. When you check a mitt, wrist, or ankle restraint every 15 minutes, tell the nurse at once if you observe these signs or symptoms.

A. _____

B. _____

C. _____

D. _____

48. When you remove the restraints every 2 hours, what are the basic needs that should be met?

A. _____

B. _____

C. _____

D. _____

E. _____

F. _____

G. _____

49. Persons restrained in a supine position must be monitored constantly because they are at great risk for _____.

50. You should carry scissors with you because in an emergency _____
_____

51. When you are delegated to apply restraints, what information do you need from the nurse and the care plan?

A. _____

B. _____

C. _____

D. _____

E. _____

F. _____

G. _____

H. _____

I. _____

J. _____

K. _____

L. _____

M. _____

N. _____

Use the FOCUS ON PRIDE section to complete these statements.

52. When a person has restraints in place, your professional responsibilities mean you must

A. _____

B. _____

C. _____

D. _____

E. _____

F. _____

53. When you practice ethical behavior, you would treat a person like _____ with
_____.

Optional Learning Exercises

54. Drugs or drug dosages are restraints if they

A. _____

B. _____

55. How can a geriatric chair be an enabler instead of a restraint?

_____
_____

56. What life-long habits and routines could be included in the nursing care plan as alternatives to restraints?

_____
_____

57. Why would a person in restraints be at risk for dehydration?

_____

58. What is the purpose of padded hip protectors and floor cushions?

_____

16 Preventing Infection

Fill in the Blank: Key Terms

Antibiotic
Antisepsis
Asepsis
Biohazardous waste
Carrier
Clean technique
Communicable disease
Contagious disease
Contamination

Cross-contamination
Disinfectant
Disinfection
Healthcare-associated infection (HAI)
Immunity
Infection
Infection control
Medical asepsis

Microbe
Microorganism
Non-pathogen
Normal flora
Pathogen
Reservoir
Spore
Sterile
Sterile field

Sterile technique
Sterilization
Surgical asepsis
Vaccination
Vaccine
Vector
Vehicle

1. _____ is passing microbes from 1 person to another by contaminated hands, equipment, or supplies.

2. A carrier (animal, insect) that transmits disease is a _____.

3. A _____ is a small living plant or animal seen only with a microscope; a microbe.

4. A human or animal that is a reservoir for microbes but does not have signs and symptoms of infection is a _____.

5. Protection against a certain disease is _____.

6. A preparation containing dead or weakened microbes is a _____.

7. A work area free of all pathogens and non-pathogens is a _____.

8. _____ are items contaminated with blood, body fluids, secretions, and excretions that may be harmful to others.

9. _____ are the practices used to remove or destroy pathogens and to prevent their spread from one person or place to another person or place; clean technique.

10. A communicable disease is also called a _____.

11. An _____ is a disease state resulting from the invasion and growth of microorganisms in the body.

12. _____ is the practices that keep equipment and supplies free of all microbes; sterile technique.

13. A _____ is a disease caused by pathogens that spread easily; contagious disease.

14. The process of destroying pathogens is _____.

15. The processes, procedures, and chemical treatments that kill microbes or prevent them from causing an infection are _____.

16. A _____ is an infection that develops in a person cared for in any setting where health care is given.

17. _____ is being free of disease-producing microbes.

18. Another name for a microorganism is a _____.

19. The environment in which microbes live and grow is a _____.

20. Medical asepsis is also called _____.

21. The process of becoming unclean is _____.

22. The absence of all microbes is _____.

23. Surgical asepsis is also called _____.

24. A bacterium protected by a hard shell is a _____.

25. _____ are microbes that usually live and grow in a certain area.

26. A microbe that does not usually cause an infection is a _____.

27. _____ is the process of destroying all microbes.

28. A microbe that is harmful and can cause an infection is a _____.

29. The administration of a vaccine to produce immunity against an infectious disease is _____.

30. Practices and procedures that prevent the spread of disease are _____.

31. An _____ is a drug that kills microbes that cause infections.

32. Any substance that transmits microbes is a _____.

33. A _____ is a liquid chemical that can kill many or all pathogens except spores.

Circle the Best Answer

34. Which type of microbe can cause an infection in any body system?
    A. Protozoa
    B. Fungi
    C. Viruses
    D. Bacteria

35. Rickettsiae are transmitted to humans by
    A. Plants
    B. Other humans
    C. Insect bites
    D. One-celled animals

36. In order to live and grow, all microbes require
    A. Oxygen
    B. A reservoir
    C. A hot environment
    D. Plenty of light

37. Normal flora
    A. Are always pathogens
    B. Are always non-pathogens
    C. Become pathogens when transmitted from their natural site to another site
    D. Cause signs and symptoms of an infection

38. Multidrug-resistant organisms are organisms that
    A. Can be destroyed by certain antibiotics
    B. Can resist the effects of antibiotics
    C. Are viruses that cause influenza and colds
    D. Are spread by insects

39. Which of these is *not* a sign or symptom of infection?
    A. Rash
    B. Fatigue and loss of energy
    C. Constipation
    D. Sores on mucous membranes

40. An older person is at higher risk for infection because of changes in
    A. Diet
    B. The immune system
    C. Mobility
    D. Independence

41. The source of infection is
    A. A break in the skin
    B. A human or animal
    C. Nutritional status
    D. A pathogen

42. In the chain of infection, a portal of exit can be
    A. Blood
    B. Humans and animals
    C. General health
    D. A carrier

43. Healthcare-associated infections often occur when
    A. Insects are present
    B. Hand-washing is poor
    C. Medical asepsis is used correctly
    D. A person is in isolation

44. The practice that keeps equipment and supplies free of *all* microbes is
    A. Medical asepsis
    B. Clean technique
    C. Contamination
    D. Surgical asepsis

45. To prevent the spread of microbes
    A. Sterilize all equipment
    B. Use only disposable equipment
    C. Keep all residents in isolation
    D. Wash your hands

46. When washing hands, you should
    A. Use hot water
    B. Keep hands lower than the elbows
    C. Turn off faucets after lathering
    D. Keep hands higher than the elbows

47. Clean under the fingernails by rubbing your fingers against your palms
    A. Each time you wash your hands
    B. If you have long nails
    C. Only for the first hand-washing of the day
    D. For at least 10 seconds

48. To avoid contaminating your hands, turn off the faucets
    A. After soap is applied
    B. Before drying hands
    C. With clean paper towels
    D. With your elbows

49. An alcohol-based hand rub may be used to decontaminate your hands
    A. When the hands are visibly dirty or soiled with blood, body fluids, or secretions and excretions
    B. After using the restroom
    C. After contact with the intact skin
    D. Before eating

50. You can prevent the spread of microbes in the home by
    A. Thawing frozen foods at room temperature
    B. Using a disinfectant to clean surfaces in the bathroom
    C. Refreezing food items that have partially thawed
    D. Wiping cutting boards with a dry paper towel after use

51. Older persons with dementia rely on others to protect them from infection because they
    A. Do not understand aseptic practices
    B. Are more resistant to infection
    C. Resist hand-washing and other aseptic practices
    D. Never learned good hygiene practices

52. When cleaning contaminated equipment
    A. Wear personal protective equipment (PPE)
    B. Rinse it in hot water first
    C. Use the clean utility room
    D. Remove any organic materials with a paper towel

53. Organic material is removed from re-usable items with
    A. Soap and hot water
    B. An autoclave
    C. A rinse in cold water
    D. A disinfectant

54. A good, cheap disinfectant to use in the home is
    A. Chlorine bleach
    B. Ammonia
    C. White vinegar solution
    D. Soap and water

55. If you use boiling water to sterilize items in the home, you should
    A. Pour the water over the items in a sink
    B. Boil the items for at least 10 minutes depending on elevation
    C. Boil the items for 30 to 45 minutes
    D. Place the items in the water, bring the water to a boil, and turn it off

56. Isolation precautions are used for
    A. All persons
    B. Any person who has had surgery
    C. All older persons
    D. As a method to prevent spreading communicable diseases

57. Standard Precautions are used
    A. For a person with a respiratory infection
    B. For a person with a wound infection
    C. For a person with tuberculosis
    D. For all persons whenever care is given

58. Gloves worn in Standard Precautions
    A. Do not need to be changed when performing several tasks for the same person
    B. Can be worn until they tear or are punctured
    C. Are changed before caring for another person
    D. Are worn only if the person has an infection

59. When you are working in a room with isolation precautions, you use paper towels to
    A. Handle clean items
    B. Turn faucets on and off
    C. Give the person personal care
    D. Wipe up spills on the floor

60. Practice hand hygiene
    A. After removing gloves
    B. Only when you leave the isolation area
    C. Only when moving between residents
    D. Only if gloves were not worn

61. If you are allergic to latex gloves, you should
    A. Wash your hands each time you remove the gloves
    B. Make sure the gloves have powder inside
    C. Wear latex-free gloves
    D. Never wear any gloves

62. When you wear a gown for isolation precautions, the contaminated areas are
    A. The ties at the neck and waist
    B. The gown front and sleeves
    C. The gown back and sleeves
    D. Only the areas that touch the patient

63. When you remove gown and gloves worn for isolation precautions, what step is done first?
    A. Untie the neck and waist strings.
    B. Remove and discard your gloves.
    C. Turn the gown inside out as it is removed.
    D. Pull the gown down from each shoulder toward the same hand.

64. Personal protective equipment is worn when entering a room
    A. Isolated for airborne precautions
    B. Isolated for droplet precautions
    C. Isolated for Standard Precautions
    D. Depending on what tasks, procedures, and care measures you will do

65. Which of these statements about wearing gloves is *true?*
    A. The inside of the glove is contaminated.
    B. Slightly used gloves can be saved and re-used.
    C. You may need more than 1 pair of gloves for a task.
    D. Gloves are easier to put on when hands are damp.

66. When removing gloves
    A. Make sure that glove touches only glove
    B. Pull the gloves off by the fingers
    C. Reach inside the glove with the gloved hand to pull it off
    D. Hold the discarded gloves tightly in your ungloved hand

67. When removing a mask, only the ties or elastic bands are touched because
    A. The front of the mask is contaminated
    B. The front of the mask is sterile
    C. Your gloves are contaminated
    D. Your hands are contaminated

68. When donning a gown, which of these is done *first?*
    A. Tie the strings at the back of the neck.
    B. Tie the waist strings at the back.
    C. Put on the gloves.
    D. It doesn't matter.

69. When removing personal protective equipment, which of these is done *first?*
    A. Remove the face mask.
    B. Remove and discard the gloves.
    C. Remove the gown.
    D. Untie the waist strings of the gown.

70. If you wear re-usable eyewear and it is contaminated
    A. It should be discarded
    B. It should be autoclaved
    C. Follow agency policy
    D. Rinse it in cool running water

71. How are contaminated items identified when sent to the laundry or trash collection?
    A. Bags are transparent so materials are visible.
    B. Labeled as "contaminated."
    C. Always are double-bagged.
    D. Labeled with BIOHAZARD symbol.

72. How are specimens collected in a contaminated room handled?
    A. Place specimen container in a biohazard specimen bag.
    B. It depends on center policy.
    C. Testing must be done in the room.
    D. Special containers are needed.

73. If a resident in Transmission-Based Precautions must be transported to another area, all of these would be done *except*
    A. The person wears a mask as required by the Transmission-Based Precautions used
    B. The staff wear gown, mask, and gloves as required
    C. The staff in the receiving area are alerted so they can wear protective equipment as needed
    D. The wheelchair or stretcher is disinfected after use

74. When a person is in isolation, you can help to meet love, belonging, and self-esteem needs when you
    A. Restrict all visitors
    B. Keep the door open so the person can see others in the hallway
    C. Say "hello" from the doorway often
    D. Avoid going into the room

75. When a child is in isolation, it may be helpful if
    A. Favorite toys or blankets are brought from home
    B. Personal protective equipment is put on before entering the room
    C. The child is given a mask, eyewear, and a gown to touch and play with
    D. You avoid the room so you do not upset the child

76. You can help a person with poor vision, confusion, or dementia to tolerate isolation by
    A. Putting on personal protective equipment outside the room
    B. Keeping the door open so they can see people in the hall
    C. Letting the person see your face before putting on personal protective equipment
    D. Not wearing a mask when in the room

77. A person with measles, chicken pox, or tuberculosis would be isolated with
    A. Contact precautions
    B. Bloodborne Pathogen Standard
    C. Droplet precautions
    D. Airborne precautions

78. When the person has airborne precautions, you do not need to wear a mask when
    A. The person no longer has skin lesions
    B. You are transporting the person
    C. The person is not sneezing or coughing
    D. The skin lesions are covered

79. When contact precautions are being used, gloves are worn when
    A. Entering the room or care setting
    B. The skin has open lesions
    C. You have direct contact with the person
    D. It is likely you will have contact with surfaces or equipment near the person

80. What viruses are bloodborne pathogens?
    A. Influenza and pneumococcus
    B. Measles and chicken pox
    C. Human immunodeficiency virus (HIV) and hepatitis B virus (HBV)
    D. Staphylococcus and streptococcus

81. All of these can transmit bloodborne pathogens *except*
    A. Body fluid that is visibly contaminated with blood
    B. Dressings soaked with body fluids
    C. Used needles and suction equipment
    D. Sweat

82. How do staff members know what to do if exposed to a bloodborne pathogen?
    A. Free training is provided upon employment and yearly by employers.
    B. Information is provided on the Internet.
    C. They may attend classes offered at colleges or hospitals.
    D. The nurse tells them what they need to know.

83. The hepatitis B virus (HBV) vaccine
    A. Requires only 1 vaccination
    B. Must be given every year
    C. Involves 3 injections
    D. Is required by law

84. Which of these is *not* a correct work practice control to reduce exposure risks?
    A. Discard contaminated needles and sharp instruments in containers that are closable, puncture-resistant, and leak-proof.
    B. Do not store food or drinks where blood or potential infectious materials are kept.
    C. Break contaminated needles before discarding them.
    D. Wash hands after removing gloves.

85. Personal protective equipment
    A. Is free to staff
    B. Is purchased by staff members
    C. Must be worn by all employees instead of regular uniforms
    D. Is paid for by deducting the cost from the employee's paycheck

86. Broken glass is cleaned up by
    A. Picking it up carefully with gloved hands
    B. Using a brush and dustpan or tongs
    C. A person specially trained to remove biohazardous materials
    D. Wiping it up with wet paper towels

87. When discarding regulated waste, the containers are
    A. Plastic bags that are specially labeled
    B. Labeled as "BIOHAZARD" in red letters
    C. Melt-away bags
    D. Closable, puncture-resistant, leak-proof and labeled with the BIOHAZARD symbol

88. If you are working in a home and need to dispose of sharps, you may need to
    A. Place needles, syringes, and other sharp items into hard plastic containers
    B. Take them with you at the end of each shift
    C. Place them in a plastic bag labeled with the BIOHAZARD symbol
    D. Discard them with the regular trash each day

89. If an exposure incident occurs
    A. Report it at once
    B. Wash your hands thoroughly with soap and water
    C. Discard any contaminated clothing
    D. Observe yourself for any symptoms of the disease

90. If a sterile item touches a clean item, the sterile item
    A. Can still be used
    B. Is contaminated
    C. Should be handled with sterile gloves
    D. Can be placed on the sterile field

91. When working with a sterile field, you should
    A. Always wear a mask
    B. Keep items within your vision and above your waist
    C. Keep the door open
    D. Wear clean gloves

92. When arranging the inner package of sterile gloves
    A. Have the right glove on the left and the left glove on the right
    B. Have the fingers pointing toward you
    C. Have the right glove on the right and the left glove on the left
    D. Straighten the gloves to remove the cuff

93. When picking up the first glove
    A. Pick it by the cuff and touch only the inside
    B. Reach under the cuff with your fingers
    C. Grasp the edge of the glove with your hand
    D. Unfold the cuff

Matching

Match the kind of asepsis being used with each example.
    A. Medical asepsis (clean technique)
    B. Surgical asepsis (sterile technique)

94. _____ An item is placed in an autoclave.

95. _____ Each person has his or her own toothbrush, towel, washcloth, and other personal care items.

96. _____ Hands are washed before preparing food.

97. _____ Contaminated items are boiled in water for at least 10 minutes.

98. _____ Disposable supplies and equipment reduce the spread of infection.

99. _____ Liquid or gas chemicals are used to destroy microbes.

100. _____ Hands are washed every time you use the bathroom.

Match the aseptic measures used to control the related chain of infection with the step in the chain.
    A. Reservoir (host)   D. Portal of entry
    B. Portal of exit   E. Susceptible host
    C. Transmission

101. _____ Provide the person with tissues to use when coughing or sneezing.

102. _____ Make sure linens are dry and wrinkle-free to protect the skin.

103. _____ Use leak-proof plastic bags for soiled tissues, linens, and other materials.

104. _____ Wear personal protective equipment.

105. _____ Hold equipment and linens away from your uniform.

106. _____ Assist with cleaning or clean the genital area after elimination.

107. _____ Clean from cleanest area to the dirtiest.

108. _____ Label bottles with the person's name and the date it was opened.

109. _____ Follow the care plan to meet the person's nutritional and fluid needs.

110. _____ Make sure drainage tubes are properly connected.

111. _____ Do not use items that are on the floor.

112. _____ Assist the person with cough and deep-breathing exercises as directed.

113. _____ Do not sit on a person's bed. You will pick up microorganisms and transfer them.

Match the practices with the correct principles for surgical asepsis.
    A. A sterile item can only touch another sterile item.
    B. Sterile items or a sterile field is always kept within your vision and above your waist.
    C. Airborne microbes can contaminate sterile items or a sterile field.
    D. Fluid flows down, in the direction of gravity.
    E. The sterile field is kept dry, unless the area below it is sterile.
    F. The edges of a sterile field are contaminated.
    G. Honesty is essential to sterile technique.

114. _____ Consider any item as contaminated if it touches a clean item.

115. _____ Wear a mask if you need to talk during the procedure.

116. _____ Place all sterile items inside the 1-inch margin of the sterile field.

117. _____ Do not turn your back on a sterile field.

118. _____ Prevent drafts by closing the door and avoiding extra movements.

119. _____ Avoid spilling and splashing when pouring sterile fluids into sterile containers.

120. _____ If you cannot see an item, it is contaminated.

121. _____ You report to the nurse that you contaminated an item or a field.

122. _____ Hold wet items down.

Fill in the Blank

123. Write out the meaning of the abbreviations.
    A. AIDS _____
    B. CDC _____
    C. cm _____
    D. EPA _____
    E. GI _____
    F. HAI _____
    G. HBV _____
    H. HIV _____
    I. MDRO _____
    J. MRSA _____
    K. OPIM _____
    L. OSHA _____
    M. PPE _____
    N. TB _____
    O. VRE _____

Use the FOCUS ON PRIDE section to complete these statements.

124. You show personal and professional responsibility when you prevent infections by

    A. Practicing good hand hygiene _____

    and _____ giving care

    B. Removing items that become

    _____

    C. Not using a _____

    D. Being honest with _____

125. If delegated care of a person at increased risk for infection, you must

    A. _____

    B. _____

    C. _____

    D. _____

    E. _____

    F. _____

    G. _____

    H. _____

    I. _____

    J. _____

Labeling

126. The figure shows how to remove gloves. List the steps of the procedure shown in each drawing.

    A.

    i. _____

    ii. _____

    B.

    i. _____

    C.

    i. _____

    ii. _____

    D.

    i. _____

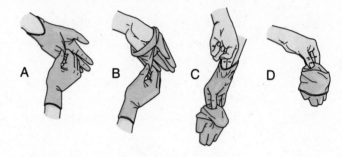

CROSSWORD

Fill in the crossword by answering the clues below with the words from this list:

Asepsis	HBV	*Parenteral*	Sharps
Autoclave	HIV	PPE	Sterilize
Bacteria	Isolation	Protozoa	Viruses
Fungi	OPIM	Rickettsiae	

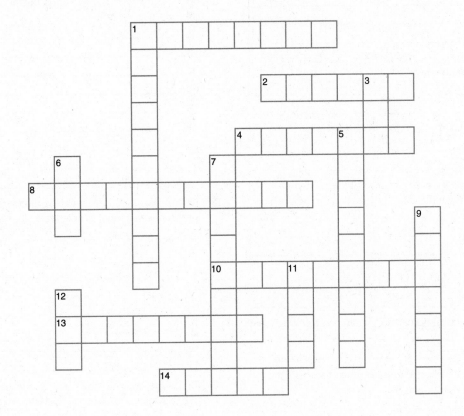

Across
1. One-celled animals; can infect the blood, brain, intestines, and other body areas
2. Any object, such as needles, scalpels, broken glass, and broken capillary tubes, that can penetrate the skin
4. Grows in living cells; causes many diseases such as the common cold, herpes, and hepatitis
8. Found in fleas, lice, ticks, and other insects; spread to humans by insect bites
10. A pressure-steam sterilizer
13. Plant life that multiplies rapidly; a type of microbe
14. Plants that live on other plants or animals; can infect the mouth, vagina, skin, feet, and other body areas

Down
1. Piercing mucous membranes or the skin barrier through such events as needle-sticks, human bites, cuts, and abrasions
3. Clothing or equipment worn by an employee for protection against a hazard
5. The use of physical or chemical procedure designed to destroy all microbial life, including highly resistant bacterial spores
6. Human immunodeficiency virus
7. Barriers that prevent the escape of pathogens to other areas; usually this area is the person's room
9. Being free of disease-producing microbes
11. Other potentially infectious materials; human body fluids, any tissue or organ from a human, HIV-containing cell or tissue cultures
12. Hepatitis B virus

Optional Learning Exercises

127. Compare medical asepsis to surgical asepsis.

    A. Medical asepsis is _____

    _____

    _____

    B. Surgical asepsis is _____

    _____

    _____

    _____

128. Why are hands and forearms kept lower than elbows in hand-washing?

    _____

    _____

129. Why is lotion applied after hand-washing?

    _____

    _____

130. When are the following worn when practicing Standard Precautions?

    A. Gloves

    _____

    _____

    B. Masks, eye protection, and face shields

    _____

    _____

131. If a person has measles and you are susceptible, what should you do?

    _____

132. If a person in airborne precautions must leave the room, the person must wear a

    _____

133. When you wear gloves, you protect yourself and the person.

    A. They protect you from _____

    _____

    B. They protect the person from _____.

134. Why is a gown turned inside out as you remove it?

    _____

    _____

135. Why is a moist mask or gown changed?

    _____

    _____

136. What basic needs may not be met when a person is in isolation?

    _____

137. What information is included in training about bloodborne pathogens?

    A. _____

    B. _____

    C. _____

    D. _____

    E. _____

    F. _____

    G. _____

    H. _____

    I. _____

138. OSHA requires these measures for safely handling and using personal protective equipment.

    A. _____

    B. _____

    C. _____

    D. _____

    E. _____

    F. _____

    G. _____

    H. _____

139. If you are asked to assist with a sterile procedure, what information do you need before beginning?

    A. _____

    B. _____

    C. _____

    D. _____

    E. _____

    F. _____

17 Body Mechanics

Fill in the Blank: Key Terms

Base of support
Body alignment
Body mechanics
Dorsal recumbent position

Ergonomics
Fowler's position
Lateral position
Posture

Prone position
Semi-prone side position
Side-lying position
Sims' position

Supine position
Work-related musculo-skeletal disorders

1. Another name for the lateral position is
_____.

2. The way in which the head, trunk, arms, and legs are aligned with one another is _____ or posture.

3. The _____ is also called the side-lying position.

4. The _____ is the same as the back-lying or supine position.

5. The area on which an object rests is the
_____.

6. _____ are injuries and disorders of the muscles, tendons, ligaments, joints, and cartilage; they are caused or made worse by the work setting.

7. _____ is a left side-lying position in which the upper leg is sharply flexed so that it is not on the lower leg and the lower arm is behind the person.

8. A semi-sitting position with the head of the bed elevated 45 to 60 degrees is _____.

9. Lying on the abdomen with the head turned to one side is _____.

10. _____ is using the body in an efficient and careful way.

11. The back-lying or dorsal recumbent position is also called the _____.

12. _____ or body alignment is the way in which body parts are aligned with one another.

13. _____ is the science of designing the job to fit the worker.

14. Another name for the Sims' position is
_____.

Circle the Best Answer

15. Using good body mechanics will
    A. Prevent good posture
    B. Cause back injuries
    C. Reduce the risk of injury
    D. Cause muscle injury

16. For a wider base of support and balance
    A. Keep your feet close together
    B. The head, trunk, arms, and legs are aligned with one another
    C. Stand with your feet apart
    D. Make sure you are in good physical condition

17. When you bend your knees and squat to lift a heavy object, you are
    A. Using good body alignment
    B. In danger of injury
    C. Likely to strain your back
    D. Using good body mechanics

18. If you need to move a heavy object, you should *not*
    A. Push, slide, or pull the object
    B. Get help from a co-worker
    C. Bend your hips and knees to lift from the floor
    D. Work alone so you can control how to move the object

19. Work-related musculo-skeletal disorders (MSDs) are a risk
    A. When the worker does not exercise regularly
    B. When the worker is small and weak
    C. When force or repeating action is used when moving persons
    D. Only when the staff member is using poor body mechanics

20. If you have pain when standing or rising from a seated position, you
    A. May have a back injury
    B. Are using poor body mechanics
    C. Have worked too many hours
    D. Should exercise more

21. According to the Occupational Safety and Health Administration (OSHA), which of these is *not* a factor that can lead to back disorders?
    A. Reaching while lifting
    B. Getting help when lifting or moving heavy objects
    C. Bending while lifting
    D. Lifting with forceful movement

22. Which of these activities will help to prevent back injury?
    A. Reach across the bed to give care.
    B. Bend at the waist to pick up an object from the floor.
    C. Lift an object above your shoulder.
    D. Keep objects close to your body when you lift, move, or carry.

23. Regular position changes and good alignment
    A. Cause pressure ulcers and contractures
    B. Promote comfort and well-being
    C. Interrupt rest and sleep
    D. Decrease circulation

24. A resident who depends on the nursing team for position changes needs to be positioned
    A. At least every 2 hours   C. Every 15 minutes
    B. Once an hour   D. Once a shift

25. Linens need to be clean, dry, and wrinkle-free to help prevent
    A. Pressure ulcers
    B. Contractures
    C. Breathing problems
    D. Frequent repositioning

26. Persons with heart and respiratory disorders usually can breathe more easily in the
    A. Fowler's position
    B. Semi-Fowler's position
    C. Supine position
    D. Prone position

27. Most older persons have limited range of motion in their necks and so do not tolerate
    A. Lateral position
    B. Semi-Fowler's position
    C. Fowler's position
    D. Prone position

28. When positioning a person in the supine position, the nurse may ask you to place a pillow under the person's lower legs to
    A. Improve the circulation
    B. Assist the person to breathe easier
    C. Prevent the heels from rubbing on the sheets
    D. Prevent swelling of the legs and feet

29. A small pillow is positioned against the person's back in the
    A. Lateral position   C. Supine position
    B. Prone position   D. Semi-Fowler's position

30. When a person cannot keep his or her upper body erect in a chair
    A. A vest restraint may be used
    B. Postural supports help keep him or her in good alignment
    C. A geriatric chair with a tray will be used
    D. A belt restraint can be applied

31. In the chair position, a pillow is not used
    A. To position paralyzed arms
    B. To support the feet
    C. Under the upper arm and hand
    D. Behind the back if restraints are used

Fill in the Blank

32. Write out the abbreviations.
    A. MSD _____
    B. OSHA _____

33. Where are strong, large muscles that are used to lift and move heavy objects located?
    A. _____
    B. _____
    C. _____
    D. _____

34. Back injuries are a major risk when lifting. For good body mechanics you should
    A. _____
    B. _____

35. Describe these risk factors for musculo-skeletal disorders (MSDs) in nursing centers.
    A. Force _____
    B. Repeating action _____
    C. Awkward postures _____
    D. Heavy lifting _____

36. Early signs and symptoms of MSDs are _____
    _____.

37. What nursing tasks are known to be high risk for MSDs?
    A. _____
    B. _____
    C. _____
    D. _____
    E. _____
    F. _____
    G. _____
    H. _____
    I. _____
    J. _____
    K. _____
    L. _____
    M. _____
    N. _____
    O. _____
    P. _____
    Q. _____

38. Instructions to re-position a person are received from the _____ and the
    _____.

39. If you are delegated the task of positioning the person, what information do you need?
    A. _____
    B. _____
    C. _____
    D. _____
    E. _____
    F. _____
    G. _____
    H. _____
    I. _____
    J. _____
    K. _____

In the following questions, list the measures needed for good alignment in each position.

40. What measures are needed for good alignment when the person is in Fowler's position?

    A. _____

    B. _____

    C. _____

41. For supine position?

    A. _____

    B. _____

    C. _____

42. For prone position?

    A. _____

    B. _____

    C. _____

43. For lateral position?

    A. _____

    B. _____

    C. _____

    D. _____

    E. _____

    F. _____

44. For Sims' position?

    A. _____

    B. _____

    C. _____

    D. _____

45. For chair position?

    A. _____

    B. _____

    C. _____

Use the FOCUS ON PRIDE section to complete these statements.

46. You take responsibility for protecting yourself from harm when moving patients. What decisions do you make about protecting yourself?

    A. _____

    B. _____

    C. _____

    D. _____

    E. _____

47. How can you promote comfort, independence, and social interaction for a person you are caring for?

    A. _____

    B. _____

    C. _____

    D. _____

Labeling

48. Label the positions in each of the drawings.

A. _____

B. _____

C. _____

D. _____

E. _____

F. _____

Optional Learning Exercises

49. According to OSHA, certain activities can lead to back injuries. Read the examples and list the activity that could cause a back injury in each one *(listed in textbook)*.

   A. The nursing assistant does not raise the level of the bed when changing linens. _____

   B. While you are walking with Mr. Smith, he slips and starts to fall. _____

   C. Mrs. Tippett slides down in bed and looks uncomfortable. _____
   _____

   D. You assist Mrs. Miller to use the toilet in her small bathroom. _____

   E. Mr. Thomas is confused and often hits you when being moved. _____

   F. You lean across the bed to hold the person while the nurse washes his back. _____
   _____

50. Regular position changes and good alignment promote

   A. _____

   B. _____

   C. _____

   D. _____

   It prevents

   E. _____

   F. _____

51. When you properly position and re-position a person, you help prevent a lack of joint or mobility or

   _____.

Fill in the Blank: Key Terms

Bed mobility   Logrolling
Friction   Shearing
Functional status   Weight-bearing

1. _____ is to put weight on one's legs.

2. _____ occurs when skin sticks to a surface and muscles slide in the direction the body is moving.

3. How a person moves to and from a lying position, turns from side to side, and re-positions in bed or other furniture is _____.

4. The rubbing of one surface against another is

_____.

5. Turning the person as a unit, in alignment, with one motion is _____.

6. _____ is the person's ability to perform the activities of daily living.

Circle the Best Answer

7. To prevent injuries when moving older persons
   A. Move the person without help
   B. Grab the person under the arms
   C. Allow the person to move himself or herself
   D. Provide for comfort and avoid causing pain

8. When moving a person up in bed, prevent hitting the head-board with the head by
   A. Keeping the person in good body alignment
   B. Placing the pillow upright against the head-board
   C. Placing your hand on the person's head
   D. Asking the person to bend his or her neck forward

9. When moving residents, it is best if you move the person
   A. By yourself
   B. With at least 2 staff members
   C. Using a mechanical lift
   D. Only with staff members who you like

10. To prevent work-related injuries, OSHA recommends that
    A. Manual lifting be minimized or eliminated when possible
    B. Manual lifting be used at all times
    C. You never lift any person or object alone
    D. You always use mechanical lifts for any lifting

11. When the person needs help to turn, re-position, sit up, and move in bed, you know that the person's level of dependence is
    A. Level 4
    B. Level 3
    C. Level 2
    D. Level 1

12. Why are beds raised to move persons in bed?
    A. It prevents the person from falling out of bed.
    B. It reduces friction and shearing.
    C. It prevents pulling on drainage tubes.
    D. It reduces bending and reaching for staff members.

13. How can you reduce friction and shearing?
    A. Raise the head of the bed to a sitting position before moving the person.
    B. Roll or lift the person to re-position.
    C. Pull the person up in bed by grasping under the arms.
    D. Massage the skin.

14. If a person with dementia resists being moved, you should
    A. Move the person by yourself
    B. Proceed slowly and use a calm voice
    C. Let the person alone and do not re-position him or her
    D. Tell the person firmly that he or she must cooperate to be moved

15. When you are delegated to move a person in bed, you need to know all of these *except*
    A. What equipment is needed
    B. Whether the person is awake
    C. The number of staff needed to move the person safely
    D. Any limits in the person's ability to move or be re-positioned

16. When raising a person's head and shoulders
    A. It is best to have help with an older person to prevent pain and injury
    B. A mechanical lift should be used
    C. You can always do this alone
    D. A transfer belt will be needed

17. To correctly raise the head and shoulders
    A. Both of your hands are placed under the person's back
    B. The person puts his or her near arm under your near arm and behind your shoulder
    C. Use a lift sheet to raise the person up
    D. Your free arm rests on the edge of the bed

18. You may move a person up in bed alone if the
    A. Person can assist using a trapeze
    B. Rest of the staff is busy and cannot help
    C. Nurse tells you to use a lift sheet or slide sheet
    D. Nurse tells you to move the person alone

19. What is the position of the bed when you are moving a person up in bed?
    A. Fowler's
    B. Flat
    C. As flat as possible for the person's condition
    D. Semi-Fowler's

20. The person is moved
    A. On the "count of 3"
    B. On the "count of 2"
    C. When the person says he or she is ready
    D. As soon as the workers are all in position

21. An assist device such as a lift sheet is used for
    A. A person who can use the trapeze to help
    B. All patients regardless of size or functional status
    C. A person with a functional status of Level 4: Total Dependence
    D. Moving a person when you are working alone

22. Where is the lift sheet positioned?
    A. Under the head and shoulders
    B. Under the buttocks
    C. From the head to above the knees or lower
    D. From the hips to below the knees

23. When using a lift sheet as an assist device, the workers should
    A. Roll the sheet up close to the person near the shoulders and hips
    B. Grasp the sheet at the edges
    C. Move one side of the sheet at a time
    D. Grasp the sheet only at the top edge

24. A person is moved to the side of the bed before turning because
    A. Otherwise, after turning, the person lies on the side of the bed
    B. It makes it easier to turn the person
    C. It prevents injury to the person
    D. It prevents friction and shearing

25. When you move a person in segments, which of these is *incorrect*?
    A. Place your arm under the person's neck and shoulders and grasp the far shoulder.
    B. First move the hips and legs.
    C. Move the center part of the body by placing one arm under the waist and one under the thighs.
    D. Rock backward and shift your weight to your rear leg when moving the upper part of the body.

26. When using a drawsheet to move a person to the side of the bed, support the person's
    A. Back
    B. Knees
    C. Head
    D. Hips

27. After the person is turned
    A. Give the person good personal care
    B. Position him or her in good body alignment
    C. Elevate the head of the bed
    D. Elevate the bed to its highest position

28. When delegated to turn a person, you need all of this information from the nurse and care plan *except*
    A. How much help the person needs
    B. Which procedure to use
    C. Whether the doctor has ordered turning
    D. What supportive devices are needed for positioning

29. When a person is turned, musculo-skeletal injuries, skin breakdown, and pressure ulcers could occur if a person is not in
    A. A special bed
    B. Good body alignment
    C. Good body mechanics
    D. The middle of the bed

30. How do you decide whether to turn the person toward you or away from you?
    A. Check the doctor's order.
    B. It depends on the person's condition and the situation.
    C. Use the method you like best.
    D. Ask the person which way is best.

31. Why do you need 2 or 3 staff members to logroll a person?
    A. A person who is being logrolled is usually in pain.
    B. It is important to keep the spine straight and in alignment.
    C. The person is probably at Level 4: Total Dependence and needs extra help.
    D. No assist devices are used when you logroll.

32. When preparing to logroll a person, place a pillow
    A. At the head of the bed
    B. Between the knees
    C. Under the head
    D. Under the shoulders

33. What information do you need before dangling a person?
    A. The person's diagnosis
    B. When the person ate last
    C. The person's functional status
    D. Whether the person likes to dangle

34. What should you do if a person who is dangling becomes faint or dizzy?
    A. Lay the person down and tell the nurse.
    B. Report this at the end of the shift.
    C. Tell the person to take deep breaths.
    D. Have the person move his or her legs back and forth in circles.

35. When preparing to dangle a person, the head of the bed should be
    A. Flat
    B. Slightly raised
    C. In a sitting position
    D. At a comfortable height for the person

36. All of these are important reasons to re-position a person sitting in a chair or wheelchair *except*
    A. The person needs to be in good body alignment
    B. The back and buttocks need to be against the back of the chair
    C. Some persons cannot move and re-position themselves
    D. The person gets bored sitting in the same position all day

Fill in the Blank

37. To prevent injuries in older persons with fragile bones and joints, what safety measures need to be used?
    A. _____
    B. _____
    C. _____
    D. _____
    E. _____
    F. _____

38. To promote mental comfort when handling, moving, or transferring the person, you should

    A. _____

    B. _____

39. To promote physical comfort when handling, moving, or transferring the person, you should

    A. _____

    B. _____

    C. _____

    D. _____

40. To prevent work-related injuries when moving a person, the nurse and health team determine

    A. _____

    B. _____

    C. _____

    D. _____

41. Explain how a person is moved for each functional status level.

    A. Level 4: Total Dependence

    _____

    _____

    B. Level 3: Extensive Assistance

    _____

    _____

    C. Level 2: Limited Assistance

    _____

    _____

    D. Level 1: Supervision

    _____

    _____

    E. Level 0: Independent

    _____

    _____

42. When you move a person in bed, report and record

    A. _____

    B. _____

    C. _____

    D. _____

    E. _____

43. Friction and shearing can be reduced when moving a person in bed by

    A. _____

    B. _____

44. When moving a person up in bed and the person can assist, ask the person to

    A. Grasp the _____

    B. Flex _____

    C. Move on the count of _____

45. What assist devices, other than mechanical lifts, are used to move persons to the side of the bed?

    _____

    _____

    _____

46. Why are assist devices used when moving a person to the side of the bed?

    A. Prevent _____ and _____ damage

    B. Prevent injury to the _____

47. Before turning and re-positioning a person, what information do you need from the nurse and care plan?

    A. _____

    B. _____

    C. _____

    D. _____

    E. _____

    F. _____

    G. _____

    H. _____

    I. _____

        i. _____

        ii. _____

        iii. _____

        iv. _____

        v. _____

    J. _____

    K. _____

48. After turning and re-positioning a person, it is common to place a small pillow under the

    _____.

49. When a person is logrolled, the spine is

    _____.

50. Logrolling is used to turn these persons.

    A. _____

    B. _____

    C. _____

    D. _____

51. When a person is dangling, the circulation can be stimulated by having the person move

    _____.

52. What observations should be reported and recorded after dangling a person?

    A. _____

    B. _____

    C. _____

    D. _____

    E. _____

    F. _____

    G. _____

    H. _____

    I. _____

    J. _____

53. While a person is dangling, check the person's condition by

    A. Asking _____

    B. Checking _____

    C. Checking _____

    D. Noting _____

54. When re-positioning a person in a chair or wheelchair, you *do not* _____
    _____ .

Use the FOCUS ON PRIDE section to complete these statements.

55. What information is provided to staff that will help them reduce risk to themselves and patients?

    A. _____

    B. _____

    C. _____

56. When moving a person, you promote pride and independence when you

    A. _____

    B. _____

    C. _____

    D. _____

Optional Learning Exercises

57. When planning to move a person, why is it important to know the person's height and weight, functional status, physical abilities, and medical condition?

    _____

    _____

58. If you need to move a person with dementia, he or she may resist because he or she may not _____ . What measures in the care plan will help you give safe care?

    A. _____

    B. _____

    C. _____

59. It is safe to move a person up in bed alone only if

    A. _____

    B. _____

    C. _____

    D. _____

    E. _____

    F. _____

    G. _____

60. What types of pads are not strong enough to be used during a lift? _____
    _____ For a safe lift, the under-pad must

    A. _____

    B. _____

    C. _____

61. How does moving a person to the side of the bed avoid work-related injuries for you?

    _____

62. When you are delegated to turn a person, how will you know whether to turn them alone, with help, or by using logrolling? _____

63. When you turn a person and re-position them, what must be done to the bed level before you leave the room? _____
    _____

64. When two staff members are logrolling a person without a turning sheet, where does each person place the hands? (See Figure 18-11.)

    A. Staff at head _____

    B. Staff at legs _____

65. Why should a person dangle for 1 to 5 minutes before walking or transferring?

    _____

66. What simple hygiene measures can be performed while the person is dangling? _____
    _____

    In addition to refreshing the person, what is another benefit this activity will provide? _____
    _____

Fill in the Blank: Key Terms

Lateral transfer   Transfer
Pivot

1. _____ is how a person moves to and from surfaces such as bed, chair, wheelchair, toilet, or standing position.

2. When a person moves between 2 horizontal surfaces, it is a _____.

3. To turn one's body from a set standing position is to _____.

Circle the Best Answer

4. If an agency has a lift team, they will
   A. Perform all lifts in the agency
   B. Only do manual lifts
   C. Carry out scheduled lifts
   D. Only assist when you ask

5. When preparing to transfer a person, you should
   A. Arrange the room so there is enough space for a safe transfer
   B. Keep furniture in the position the resident likes
   C. Remove all furniture from the room
   D. Ask the person how to arrange the furniture

6. The person being transferred should wear non-skid footwear to
   A. Protect the person from falls
   B. Allow the person to bend the feet more easily
   C. Promote comfort for the person
   D. Keep the feet warm

7. Lock the bed, wheelchair, or assist device wheels when transferring to
   A. Help the staff use good body mechanics
   B. Prevent damage to the equipment being used
   C. Prevent the bed and the device from moving during the transfer
   D. Make sure the person is kept in good body alignment

8. When a person is transferring to a chair or wheelchair, help the person out of bed on
   A. The right side of the bed
   B. His or her strong side
   C. His or her weak side
   D. The side of the bed that is most convenient for the staff

9. If not using a mechanical lift, which of these is the preferred method for chair or wheelchair transfers?
   A. Use a gait/transfer belt.
   B. Have the person put his or her arms around your neck.
   C. Put your arms around the person and grasp the shoulder blades.
   D. Have the person use a trapeze.

10. When a person is seated in a wheelchair, you can increase the person's comfort by
    A. Placing pillows around the person
    B. Making sure nothing covers the vinyl seat and back
    C. Covering the back and seat with a folded bath blanket
    D. Removing any cushions or positioning devices

11. When you transfer a person, the nurse may ask you to take and report the _____ before and after the transfer.
    A. Blood pressure   C. Respirations
    B. Pulse rate   D. Temperature

12. When using a transfer belt, you can prevent the person from sliding or falling by
    A. Bracing your knees against the person's knees
    B. Holding the person close to your body
    C. Having another staff member hold the person's feet in place
    D. Grasping the belt in the back to give you better balance

13. A transfer belt must be used for a transfer unless
    A. The doctor has written an order that states no belt is needed
    B. You are directed by the nurse and care plan to transfer without a belt
    C. The person asks you not to use the belt
    D. You feel safer moving the person without the belt

14. When you are transferring a person back to bed from a chair or wheelchair, the person should be positioned
    A. With the weak side near the bed
    B. With the strong side near the bed
    C. With the chair in the same position as it was when the person got out of bed
    D. Where you have the most space to work

15. When moving a person from a bed to a stretcher, it is most important that you prevent
    A. The person from becoming chilled
    B. Friction and shearing injuries
    C. The person from assisting with the move
    D. Using too many linens

16. When moving a person to a stretcher, you should
    A. Always use a mechanical lift
    B. Use the bed linens as a lift sheet
    C. Raise or lower the stretcher so it is ½ inch lower than the bed
    D. Raise or lower the stretcher so it is ½ inch higher than the bed

17. A mechanical lift is used
    A. For all persons regardless of functional status
    B. For persons who are too heavy for the staff to move
    C. When staff members prefer to use them instead of lifting manually
    D. Only when ordered by the doctor

18. When you are delegated to use a mechanical lift, you need to know all of this information *except*
    A. The person's functional status
    B. What sling to use
    C. How many staff members are needed to perform the task safely
    D. Whether the person wants you to use the lift

19. As a person is lifted in the sling of the mechanical lift, the person
    A. May hold the swivel bar
    B. May hold the straps or chains
    C. Crosses the arms across the chest
    D. Should keep the legs outstretched

20. When transferring a person from a wheelchair to the toilet
    A. The toilet should have a raised seat
    B. The toilet seat should be removed
    C. Always position the wheelchair next to the toilet
    D. Unlock the wheelchair to allow movement during the transfer

21. A slide board may be used to transfer a person from a wheelchair to a toilet if
    A. The person can stand and pivot
    B. There is enough room to position the wheelchair next to the toilet
    C. The staff member does not want to use a transfer belt
    D. The person has lower body strength

22. When moving a person who weighs more than 200 pounds to a stretcher
    A. Use a lateral sliding aid and 2 staff members
    B. Use a mechanical ceiling lift or a mechanical lateral transfer device
    C. Use a lateral sliding aid or a friction-reducing device and 2 staff members
    D. Use a drawsheet, turning pad, or large re-usable waterproof under-pad

Fill in the Blank

23. A person can transfer from the bed to the chair with a stand and pivot transfer if
    A. _____
    B. _____
    C. _____

24. During a chair or wheelchair transfer, the person must not put his or her arms around your neck because
    _____ .

25. Locked wheelchairs may be considered restraints if the person _____
    _____ .

26. When using a transfer belt to transfer a person to a chair or wheelchair, grasp the belt at _____ and from
    _____

27. If you transfer a person to a chair without a transfer belt, place your hands _____
    and around the person's _____ .

28. For what reasons would you use the slings listed?
    A. Standard full sling _____
    B. Extended length sling _____
    C. Bathing sling _____
    D. Toileting sling _____
    E. Amputee sling _____
    F. Bariatric sling _____

29. What information do you need when you are delegated to use a mechanical lift?
    A. _____
    B. _____
    C. _____
    D. _____
    E. _____
    F. _____
    G. _____

30. To promote mental comfort when using a mechanical lift you should explain _____ and show the person
    _____ .

Use the FOCUS ON PRIDE section to complete these statements.

31. When transferring a person, you respect the person's privacy when you
    A. _____
    B. _____
    C. _____

32. Your speech and tone must convey
    _____. When giving directions
    A. _____
    B. _____
    C. _____
    D. _____
    E. _____
    F. _____
    G. _____

Optional Learning Exercises

33. When transferring a person to and from the toilet, why should the person have a raised toilet seat?
    _____

34. What safety measures are important when transferring a bariatric person to and from the toilet?
    A. _____
    B. _____
    C. _____

35. When moving a person to a stretcher, you know that for a safe transfer

 A. A _____ device is used

 B. At least _____ staff are needed

 C. If the person weighs less than 200 pounds, a

 _____

 device or _____ is used

36. When moving a person to a stretcher, if a person weighs more than 200 pounds, what are 3 devices that may be used?

 A. _____

 B. _____

 C. _____

37. After you are finished using a mechanical lift, what should you do with it that will help teamwork and time management?

 A. Return _____

 B. Do not leave _____

 C. Follow _____ to charge or

 _____

38. Stand-assist lifts are used for persons who can

 A. _____

 B. _____

 C. _____

 D. _____

39. Why should you know the person's weight before using a mechanical lift? _____

 _____

40. What should you do if the mechanical lift available is different than one you have used before?

 _____

 _____

Fill in the Blank: Key Terms

Entrapment
Fowler's position
Full visual privacy

High-Fowler's
 position
Hospital bed system

Person's unit
Reverse Trendelenburg's
 position

Semi-Fowler's position
Trendelenburg's position

1. The personal space, furniture, and equipment provided for the person by the agency is the

   _____.

2. In _____,
   the head of the bed is raised 30 degrees and the knee portion is raised 15 degrees; or the head of the bed is raised 30 degrees.

3. _____ is a semi-sitting position; the head of the bed is raised 45 to 60 degrees.

4. The head of the bed is raised and the foot of the bed is lowered in _____

5. Getting caught, trapped, or entangled in spaces created by the bed rails, the mattress, the bed frame, the head-board, or the foot-board is _____.

6. In _____, the head of the bed is lowered and the foot of the bed is raised.

7. The person has the means to be completely free from public view while in bed when they have

   _____

8. _____ is a semi-sitting position with the head of the bed raised 60 to 90 degrees.

9. The _____ is the bed frame and its parts; the parts include the mattress, bed rails, head- and foot-boards, and bed attachments.

Circle the Best Answer

10. When people share a room
    A. You may re-arrange items and furniture in the room as needed
    B. A resident cannot take or use another person's space
    C. They may use each other's belongings
    D. They generally share furniture such as a dresser

11. OBRA and CMS require that nursing centers maintain a temperature range of
    A. 68°F to 74°F
    B. 61°F to 71°F
    C. 71°F to 81°F
    D. 78°F to 85°F

12. Older persons or those who are ill may
    A. Need cooler room temperatures
    B. Need higher room temperatures
    C. Be insensitive to room temperature changes
    D. Need a warmer room at night

13. The nursing staff cannot control which factor that affects comfort?
    A. Illness   C. Noise
    B. Temperature   D. Odors

14. You may best protect a person who is sensitive to drafts by
    A. Putting the person to bed
    B. Giving the person a hot shower or bath
    C. Offering a lap robe or making sure the person is wearing enough clothing
    D. Pulling the privacy curtain around the person

15. Older persons are sensitive to cold because they
    A. Have poor circulation and a loss of fatty tissue
    B. Are often confused about their surroundings
    C. Are more active
    D. Are used to wearing heavier clothes

16. If unpleasant odors occur, do all of these *except*
    A. Use spray deodorizers wherever odors are present
    B. Provide good personal hygiene for persons
    C. Change and dispose of soiled linens and clothing
    D. Empty and clean bedpans, commodes, urinals, and kidney basins promptly

17. Noises in a health care agency may keep a person from meeting the need for
    A. Love and belonging   C. Rest
    B. Self-esteem   D. Safety and security

18. Which of these measures will *not* reduce noises in a health care agency?
    A. Having drapes in rooms
    B. Using metal equipment
    C. Answering telephones promptly
    D. Keeping equipment in good working order

19. Bright lighting is helpful for all of these *except*
    A. Persons with poor vision
    B. Helping the staff to perform procedures
    C. Making the room more cheerful
    D. Helping persons to rest and relax

20. Beds are kept at the lowest horizontal position to
    A. Give care
    B. Let the person get out of bed with ease
    C. Transfer the person to a stretcher
    D. Maintain good body alignment

21. Cranks on manual beds are kept down when not in use to
    A. Prevent persons from operating the bed
    B. Prevent anyone walking past the crank from bumping into it
    C. Keep the bed in the correct position
    D. Make sure they are ready to use at all times

22. How can the staff prevent a person from adjusting an electric bed to unsafe positions?
    A. Lock the bed into a position.
    B. Unplug the bed.
    C. Put the person in a bed that cannot be re-positioned.
    D. Keep reminding the person not to change the position.

23. What bed position raises the head of the bed and the knee portion?
    A. Fowler's
    B. Semi-Fowler's
    C. Trendelenburg's
    D. Reverse Trendelenburg's

24. The bed wheels are locked
    A. Only when giving care
    B. When the person is not using bed rails
    C. At all times except when moving the bed
    D. When the person requests it

25. Hospital bed entrapment can occur with persons who are
    A. Alert and oriented
    B. Able to move easily in bed independently
    C. Older, frail, and confused
    D. Large in size

26. A person who weighs 600 pounds will need
    A. An electric bed   C. A bariatric bed
    B. A manual bed   D. Bed rails

27. Hospital bed entrapment zone 4 is between
    A. The top of the compressed mattress and the bottom of the bed rail and at the end of the bed rail
    B. The split bed rails
    C. The top of the compressed mattress and the bottom of the bed rail and between the rail supports
    D. The bed rail and the mattress

28. A child can become entrapped in a crib if the
    A. Mattress is larger than the crib
    B. Mattress is smaller than the crib
    C. Mattress is too soft
    D. Bumper pad does not fit correctly

29. What items are never placed on the over-bed table?
    A. Meals
    B. Personal care items
    C. Writing and reading materials
    D. Bedpans, urinals, and soiled linens

30. Where are the bedpan and urinal kept in the bedside stand?
    A. Wherever the person wants
    B. On the top shelf
    C. On the bottom shelf or in the lower drawer
    D. In the top drawer

31. Privacy curtains
    A. Are sometimes used in rooms with more than 1 bed
    B. Are always pulled completely around the bed when giving care
    C. Can block sounds and conversations
    D. May be open when giving personal care

32. Full visual privacy as required by OBRA and CMS can be achieved by all of these except
    A. Closing a privacy curtain
    B. Placing a movable screen around the person
    C. Closing the door in a private room
    D. Making other persons in the room go to another area

33. Personal care items
    A. May be supplied by the agency
    B. Must be supplied by the person
    C. Are supplied when ordered by the doctor
    D. Cannot be brought into the agency by the person

34. When the person is weak on the left side, the call light is
    A. Placed on the left side
    B. Removed from the room
    C. Placed on the right side
    D. Replaced by an intercom

35. If a confused person cannot use a call light
    A. Explain often how to use the call light
    B. Use an intercom instead
    C. Remove the call light
    D. Check the person often to make sure needs are met

36. When a person turns on a call light, who should answer it?
    A. Only the person assigned to give care to the person.
    B. Any nursing team member who is available should answer and assist the person as needed.
    C. The charge nurse.
    D. Another team member may answer but is not expected to give any care.

37. Elevated toilet seats
    A. Help persons with joint problems
    B. Make wheelchair transfers more difficult
    C. Help if you transfer the person with a mechanical lift
    D. Are used if the person is very tall

38. When a person uses a bathroom call light
    A. It flashes red above the room door and at the nurses' station.
    B. It makes the same sound as the room call light
    C. It activates the intercom
    D. It flashes the same color as the room call light

39. Closet and drawer space
    A. Is shared by persons in a room with more than 1 person
    B. Can be cleaned out by a staff member
    C. Can be searched without the person's permission
    D. Must give the person free access to the closet and drawers

40. Which of these is not a responsibility when maintaining the person's unit?
    A. Throw away extra papers and other items that may clutter the room.
    B. Arrange personal items as the person prefers.
    C. Empty the wastebasket as least once a day.
    D. Explain the causes of strange noises.

Fill in the Blank

41. Write out the abbreviations.

    A. CMS _____

    B. CNA _____

    C. F _____

    D. IV _____

    E. OBRA _____

42. If you smoke, before giving care you should

    A. _____

    B. _____

    C. _____

43. According to the CMS, a "comfortable" sound level

    A. _____

    B. _____

    C. _____

44. According to CMS, comfortable lighting

    A. _____

    B. _____

    C. _____

45. Describe each hospital bed system entrapment zone

    A. Zone 1 _____

    B. Zone 2 _____

    C. Zone 3 _____

    D. Zone 4 _____

    E. Zone 5 _____

    F. Zone 6 _____

    G. Zone 7 _____

Use the FOCUS ON PRIDE section to complete these statements.

46. You help to protect the rights of the person and respect the person when you allow personal choice when arranging items. Make sure the person's choices

    A. _____

    B. _____

    C. _____

47. The location of items in the person's unit can prevent injuries when you help the person to

    A. _____

    B. _____

    C. _____

Labeling

48. In this figure

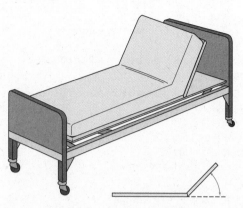

    A. What is the bed position called?

    _____

    B. What is the angle of the head of the bed?

    _____

49. In this figure

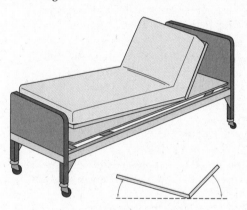

    A. What is the bed position called?

    _____

    B. What is the angle of the head of the bed?

    _____

    C. What is the angle of the foot of the bed?

    _____

50. In this figure

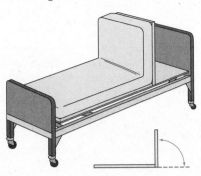

    A. What is the bed position called?

    _____

    B. What is the angle of the head of the bed?

    _____

51. In this figure

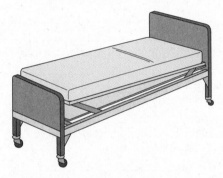

    A. What is the bed position called?

    _____

    B. What is the position of the head of the bed and the foot of the bed?

    _____

    C. Who decides this position is to be used?

    _____

52. In this figure

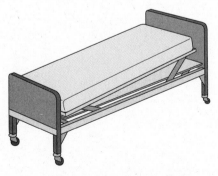

    A. What is the bed position called?

    _____

    B. What is the position of the head of the bed and the foot of the bed?

    _____

    C. Who decides this position is to be used?

    _____

Optional Learning Exercises

53. Comfort is affected by three factors that cannot be controlled. These factors are

    A. _____

    B. _____

    C. _____

54. What factors can be controlled that affect comfort?

    A. _____

    B. _____

    C. _____

    D. _____

    E. _____

55. In these situations, how would you protect a person from drafts?
    A. The person is dressing for the day.

    _____

    B. The person is sitting in a wheelchair.

    _____

    C. You are assisting a person who is going to bed for the night. _____

    _____

    D. You are giving personal care to the person.

    _____

56. How can you help to eliminate odors in these situations?
    A. You are caring for a person who is frequently incontinent. _____

    _____

    B. The person is vomiting and has wound drainage.

    _____

    C. The person changes his own ostomy drainage bag in his bathroom. _____

    D. The person keeps a urinal at his bedside and uses it himself during the day. _____

57. When the staff talks loudly and laughs in hallways, some persons may think that

    _____

58. How can the staff reduce noises and increase the person's comfort?
    A. Control _____

    B. Handle _____

    C. Keep _____

    D. Answer _____

59. What are 2 times when bright lights are helpful for a person with poor vision?
    A. _____
    B. _____
60. What does OBRA require for the furniture and equipment listed?
    A. Closet space _____
    B. Bedding _____
    C. Chair _____
    D. Temperature _____
    E. Toilet seat _____
    F. Number of persons in a room _____
    G. Windows _____
    H. Call system _____
    I. Lighting _____
       _____
    J. Hand rails _____
61. The bed in the flat position is used when sleeping and
    A. After _____
    B. For _____
62. Semi-Fowler's has 2 different definitions. They are
    A. _____
    B. _____
63. How do you know which of the ways to position the bed when semi-Fowler's position is ordered? _____

64. What 2 methods are used to raise the foot of the bed with Trendelenburg's position?
    A. _____
    B. _____
65. How can you place a person in Fowler's or semi-Fowler's position if the person has a regular bed?
    _____
66. When the nursing team uses the over-bed table as a work area, what are the only items that can be placed on it? _____
67. What are your responsibilities in these situations regarding the call light?
    A. The person is sitting in a chair next to the bed.
       _____
    B. The person is weak on the right side.
       _____
    C. The person calls out instead of using the call light.
       _____
    D. The person is embarrassed because she soiled the bed after calling for assistance.
       _____
    E. The call light in a bathroom rings while you are busy in another room.
       _____

21 Bedmaking

Fill in the Blank: Key Terms

Cotton drawsheet   Drawsheet
Padded waterproof drawsheet

1. A drawsheet placed between the bottom sheet and cotton drawsheet to keep the mattress and bottom linens clean and dry is a

   _____.

2. A _____ is a small sheet placed over the middle of the bottom sheet.

3. A drawsheet made of cotton that helps keep the mattress and bottom linens clean is a

   _____.

Circle the Best Answer

4. In nursing centers, a complete linen change is usually done
   - A. Only when the linens are wet or soiled
   - B. Every day
   - C. On the person's bath or shower day
   - D. Only once a week

5. Beds are made
   - A. When the person requests it
   - B. Once a week
   - C. To promote comfort and prevent skin breakdown
   - D. Only when linens are soiled or wet

6. A closed bed is
   - A. Not in use
   - B. Made with the top linens fan-folded back to make it easier for the person to get into bed
   - C. Made with the person in it
   - D. Made to transfer a person from a stretcher to the bed

7. An open bed is
   - A. Made with the person in it
   - B. In use; the top linens are folded back so that the person can get into bed
   - C. Not in use until bedtime; the top linens are not folded back
   - D. Made to transfer a person from a stretcher to the bed

8. When making a bed, medical asepsis is practiced by
   - A. Putting clean or used linens on the floor
   - B. Shaking the linens as you place them on the bed
   - C. Raising the bed to a comfortable height to prevent injury to the nursing assistant
   - D. Holding the linens away from your uniform

9. If extra clean linens are brought to a person's room, you should
   - A. Return the un-used linens to the linen room
   - B. Use the linens for the person's roommate
   - C. Put the un-used linens in the laundry because they are contaminated
   - D. Use the linens for a person in the next room

10. Which of these linens will be collected first when making a bed?
    - A. Bath towel
    - B. Bath blanket
    - C. Mattress pad (if needed)
    - D. Top sheet

11. When you remove used linens, which of these actions is *incorrect*?
    - A. Gather all used linens in 1 large roll.
    - B. Roll each piece away from you.
    - C. Top and bottom sheets, drawsheets, and pillowcases are always changed.
    - D. The blanket and bedspread may be re-used for the same person.

12. You allow the person the right of personal choice when you
    - A. Allow the person to choose the time when you make the bed
    - B. Decide which linens will look best in the room
    - C. Tell the person you will make the bed at 9 AM
    - D. Choose the pillows and blanket the person needs for comfort

13. When caring for a person in the home, the linens are usually changed
    - A. Once a day
    - B. Twice a week
    - C. Only if the person gives you permission
    - D. Weekly or more often if the person asks you to do so

14. A padded waterproof drawsheet
    - A. Protects against skin breakdown
    - B. Can easily be kept tight and wrinkle-free
    - C. Protects the mattress and bottom linens from dampness and soiling
    - D. Is always disposable

15. When caring for a person at home, the mattress and linens may be protected with all of these *except*
    - A. A flat sheet folded in half
    - B. A plastic trash bag
    - C. A cotton drawsheet
    - D. A plastic mattress protector

16. When you are delegated to make a bed, why do you need to know the person's schedule for treatments, therapies, and activities?
    - A. You need to make sure the bed is flat.
    - B. It is best to change linens after the treatment or when the person is out of the room.
    - C. You need to unlock beds that have been locked in a certain position.
    - D. You will know what type of bed to make.

17. When making a bed in the home, you should
    - A. Always follow the person's wishes
    - B. Make the bed only as stated in the care plan
    - C. Follow the person's wishes unless he or she asks you to do something unsafe
    - D. Use your own methods to make the bed

18. When making a bed, you are using good body mechanics when you
    A. Bend from the waist to remove and replace linens
    B. Stretch across the bed to smooth linens
    C. Raise the bed to a comfortable height to work
    D. Lock the wheels

19. When a person is discharged, what is done in addition to changing the bed?
    A. New pillows are placed on the bed.
    B. The bed system is cleaned and disinfected.
    C. The bed is sterilized.
    D. The bedspread and blanket may be re-used.

20. When making a bed, position the bottom flat sheet with
    A. The lower edge even with the top of the mattress
    B. The hem stitching facing outward, away from the person
    C. The large hem at the bottom and the small hem at the top
    D. The crease cross-wise on the bed.

21. When the top sheet, blanket, and bedspread are in place on the bed
    A. Each one is tucked under the mattress separately
    B. The sheet and blanket are tucked together and the bedspread is allowed to hang loose over them
    C. All top linens are tucked together under the foot of the bed and the corners are mitered
    D. All three are allowed to hang loose over the foot of the bed

22. The pillow is placed on the bed
    A. So the open end is away from the door
    B. So the seam of the pillowcase is toward the foot of the bed
    C. Leaning against the head of the bed
    D. So the open end is toward the door

23. An open bed is made
    A. With the linens fan-folded to one side
    B. The same as a closed bed with the top linens fan-folded to the foot of the bed
    C. With the person in the bed
    D. When the room is unoccupied

24. When you change the linens for a comatose person, it is important to
    A. Keep the bed in the low position
    B. Unlock the wheels
    C. Use special linens
    D. Explain each step of the procedure to the person before it is done

25. When making an occupied bed, a bath blanket is used to
    A. Protect the person while he is being bathed
    B. Cover the person for warmth and privacy
    C. Protect the bed linens
    D. Protect the person from used linens

26. When making an occupied bed for a person who does not use bed rails, you should
    A. Have a co-worker work on the other side of the bed
    B. Push the bed against the wall
    C. Always keep 1 hand on the person while you are making the bed
    D. Change linens only when the person is out of the bed for tests or therapies

27. When making an occupied bed
    A. Remove all used linens from the bed first
    B. Have the person roll from side to side for each piece of the bottom linens
    C. Tuck the used bottom linens and the clean bottom linens under the person
    D. Ask the person to raise his or her hips so you can push the linens under the buttocks

28. Which of these steps is *not* done when making a surgical bed?
    A. Tuck all top linens under the mattress together and make mitered corners.
    B. Remove all linens from the bed.
    C. Put the mattress pad on the mattress.
    D. Place the bottom flat sheet with the lower edge even with the bottom of the mattress.

Fill in the Blank

29. Number this list from 1 to 13 in the order you would collect the linens to make a bed.
    _____ Pillowcase(s)
    _____ Top sheet
    _____ Gown
    _____ Bottom sheet (flat or fitted)
    _____ Mattress pad (if needed)
    _____ Bedspread
    _____ Plastic drawsheet, waterproof drawsheet, or waterproof under-pad (if needed)
    _____ Bath blanket
    _____ Hand towel
    _____ Cotton drawsheet (if needed)
    _____ Bath towel(s)
    _____ Blanket
    _____ Washcloth

30. Beds are made every day to
    A. Promote _____
    B. Prevent _____
    C. Prevent _____

31. When doing home care, what guidelines should you follow when doing laundry?
    A. _____
    B. _____
    C. _____
    D. _____

32. How will you be able to tell the difference between a closed bed and an open bed?
    _____
    _____

33. When you make a surgical bed, fan-fold linens
    _____
    _____.

Use the FOCUS ON PRIDE section to complete these statements.

34. When handling used linens, it is important as a team member that you

    A. Do not _____

    B. Linens must not _____

       If you see a full cart, _____

    C. If you fill a cart, _____

       If you place an item in a cart that will cause an

       odor, _____

    D. Place used linens _____

    E. Follow agency policy for _____

Optional Learning Exercises

35. Compare how often linen changes are made in a hospital and nursing center.

    A. How often is a complete linen change made in a

       nursing center? _____

       _____

    B. How often are linens changed in a hospital?

       _____

36. Even when a complete linen change is not scheduled, you should do the following to keep beds neat and clean.

    A. _____

    B. _____

    C. _____

    D. _____

    E. _____

37. The mattress pad, waterproof drawsheet, blanket, and bedspread are re-used when making a bed unless they

    are _____.

38. If you were making a bed in a home, how would you

    use a twin sheet for a drawsheet? _____

    _____

39. When giving care in a home, what should you tell a family member who suggests using a plastic trash bag to protect the linens and mattress?

    A. _____

    B. _____

    C. _____

Fill in the Blank: Key Terms

AM care
Aspiration
Circumcised

Denture
Diaphoresis
Early morning care

Evening care
Morning care
Oral hygiene

Pericare
Perineal care
Plaque

PM care
Tartar
Uncircumcised

1. The person is _____ when he has a foreskin covering the head of the penis.

2. Care given at bedtime or PM care is

   _____

3. _____ is cleaning the genital and anal areas; pericare.

4. Sometimes evening care is called

   _____

5. Sometimes early morning care is called

   _____

6. _____ is mouth care.

7. Hardened plaque on teeth is

   _____

8. _____ occurs when breathing fluid, food, vomitus, or an object into the lungs.

9. Care given after breakfast is called

   _____

   Hygiene measures are more thorough at this time.

10. Another name for perineal care is

    _____

11. _____ is a thin film that sticks to the teeth. It contains saliva, microbes, and other substances.

12. Another name for AM care is

    _____

13. An artificial tooth or a set of artificial teeth is a

    _____

14. Profuse sweating is _____.

15. When the foreskin covering the glans of the penis was surgically removed, the man is _____.

Circle the Best Answer

16. If a person needs help with personal hygiene, you can find out what needs they have by
    A. Following the nurse's directions and the care plan
    B. Asking the family
    C. Asking other staff members
    D. Making your own decisions

17. You should assist a person with personal hygiene
    A. Only when the person asks
    B. Only in the morning
    C. Whenever help is needed
    D. Only when it is your assignment

18. When giving personal hygiene, you need to remember to protect the person's right to
    A. Privacy and personal choice
    B. Care and security of personal possessions
    C. Activities
    D. Environment

19. Which of these hygiene measures is *not* done before breakfast?
    A. Assisting with elimination
    B. Straightening resident units, including making beds
    C. Assisting with activity by providing range-of-motion exercises
    D. Assisting with oral hygiene

20. Which of these is done every time you assist with hygiene measures throughout the day?
    A. Assist with dressing and hair care
    B. Face and hand washing and oral hygiene
    C. Assist with activity
    D. Helping the person change into sleepwear

21. If good oral hygiene is not done regularly, the person may develop tartar, which will lead to
    A. A dry mouth
    B. Periodontal disease
    C. A bad taste in the mouth
    D. Plaque

22. All of these health team members may assess the person's need for mouth care *except* the
    A. Speech-language pathologist
    B. Physical therapist
    C. Nurse
    D. Dietitian

23. Teeth are flossed
    A. When teeth cannot be brushed
    B. Once or twice a week
    C. To help prevent periodontal disease
    D. Every time oral care is offered

24. Sponge swabs are used for
    A. Persons with sore, tender mouths and for unconscious persons
    B. Cleaning dentures
    C. Oral care on children
    D. Oral care on all residents

25. You follow Standard Precautions and the Bloodborne Pathogen Standard when giving oral hygiene because
    A. You will not spread bacteria to the person
    B. It will help you avoid bad breath odors from the person
    C. Gums may bleed during mouth care
    D. You will avoid any loose teeth or rough dentures

26. When the person is able to perform oral hygiene in bed, you arrange the items on
    A. The over-bed table
    B. The bedside table
    C. The sink counter
    D. The bed

27. When you are brushing the person's teeth, which of these steps would be *incorrect*?
    A. Let the person rinse the mouth with water.
    B. Use only a sponge swab to clean the teeth.
    C. Brush the person's tongue gently, if needed.
    D. Floss the person's teeth.

28. Which of these steps is *incorrect* to do when flossing the teeth?
    A. Start at the lower back tooth on the right side.
    B. Hold the floss between the middle fingers.
    C. Move the floss gently up and down between the teeth.
    D. Move to a new section of floss after every second tooth.

29. When providing mouth care for an unconscious person, position the person on 1 side with the head turned well to the side to
    A. Make it easier to brush the teeth
    B. Make the person more comfortable
    C. Prevent or reduce the risk of aspiration
    D. Make it easier for the person to breathe

30. When giving oral hygiene to an unconscious person who wears dentures, you should
    A. Remove the dentures, clean them, and replace them in the mouth
    B. Dentures are not worn when the person is unconscious
    C. Clean the dentures in the mouth without removing them
    D. Place a padded tongue blade in the mouth to prevent biting

31. Mouth care is given to an unconscious person
    A. After each meal
    B. When AM and PM care is given
    C. At least every 2 hours
    D. Once a day

32. A padded tongue blade is used when giving oral hygiene to an unconscious person to
    A. Keep the mouth open
    B. Clean the teeth
    C. Clean the tongue
    D. Prevent aspiration

33. When cleaning dentures at a sink, line the sink with a towel to
    A. Prevent infections
    B. Prevent damage to the dentures if they fall in the sink
    C. Dry the dentures
    D. Clean the dentures

34. If dentures are not worn after cleaning, store them in
    A. Cool water
    B. Hot water
    C. A soft towel
    D. Soft tissues or a napkin

35. If the person cannot remove the dentures, you can use _____ to get a good grip on the slippery dentures.
    A. Gloves
    B. Washcloth
    C. Gauze squares
    D. Bare hands

36. Older persons usually need a complete bath or shower only twice a week because
    A. They are less active
    B. They are often ill
    C. They have increased perspiration
    D. Dry skin often occurs with aging

37. If a person has dry skin, which of these will help keep it soft?
    A. Soaps
    B. Creams, lotions, and oils
    C. Powders
    D. Deodorants and antiperspirants

38. If a person with dementia resists bathing, you may
    A. Hurry through the bath
    B. Speak firmly in a loud voice
    C. Try giving the bath during a time of day when the person is calmer
    D. Use restraints so the person will not harm you

39. When choosing skin care products for bathing, you should use
    A. Soap
    B. Products the person prefers whenever possible
    C. Bath oils
    D. Creams and lotions

40. The water temperature for a complete bed bath is usually between 110°F and 115°F (43.3°C to 46.1°C) for adults. For older persons, the temperature
    A. Should be between 110°F and 115°F (43.3°C to 46.1°C)
    B. May need to be lower
    C. Should be whatever you feel is comfortable
    D. May need to be warmer

41. When applying powder
    A. Shake or sprinkle the powder directly on the person
    B. Sprinkle a small amount of powder onto your hands or a cloth
    C. Apply a thick layer of powder
    D. You should never use powder on any older person

42. When helping a bariatric person with hygiene, it is important to
    A. Use only water to prevent dry skin
    B. Dry under skin folds to prevent skin breakdown
    C. Work alone to protect the person's privacy
    D. Apply a thick layer of powder in skin folds

43. A complete bed bath is given to persons who
    A. Ask for a complete bath
    B. Are being cared for at home
    C. Are weak from illness or surgery
    D. Are newly admitted to a facility

44. When you are giving a complete bed bath, the bed is made
    A. Only if needed
    B. Before the bath begins
    C. After the bath is completed
    D. After the person gets out of bed

45. Offering the bedpan, urinal, commode, or bathroom is
    A. Done before the bath begins
    B. Done after the bath ends
    C. Not important in giving a bath
    D. Not needed at all during the bath procedure

46. During the bed bath, the bath blanket is placed
    A. Over the person after the top linens are removed
    B. Under the top linens
    C. Over the person before top linens are removed
    D. Under the person

47. Do not use soap when washing
    A. The face, ears, and neck
    B. Around the eyes
    C. The abdomen
    D. The perineal area

48. How do you avoid exposing the person when washing the chest?
    A. Keep the bath blanket over the area.
    B. Keep the top linens over the chest.
    C. Place a towel over the chest cross-wise.
    D. Make sure the curtains are closed.

49. Bath water is changed
    A. Every 5 minutes during the bath
    B. When it becomes cool and soapy
    C. Only once during the bath
    D. After washing the face, ears, and neck

50. A person _____ may respond well to a towel bath.
    A. With dementia
    B. Who has been incontinent
    C. With breaks in the skin
    D. Who needs a partial bath

51. A partial bath involves bathing
    A. The entire body
    B. The face, hands, axillae (underarms), back, buttocks, and perineal area
    C. The arms, legs, and feet
    D. The chest, abdomen, and underarms

52. When giving any type of bath, you should
    A. Wash from the dirtiest to the cleanest areas
    B. Allow the skin to air dry to avoid rubbing
    C. Provide for privacy
    D. Decide what is best for the person

53. A tub bath should not last longer than
    A. 10 minutes
    B. 15 minutes
    C. 20 minutes
    D. 30 minutes

54. If a person is weak or unsteady, a _____ should be used when the person showers.
    A. Shower chair, shower trolley, or shower stall
    B. Transfer belt
    C. Wheelchair
    D. Stretcher

55. Which of these would be good time management when giving a tub bath or shower?
    A. Take the person to the shower room and then collect your equipment.
    B. Ask a co-worker to give the shower for you.
    C. Ask a co-worker to make the person's bed while you give the bath.
    D. Clean and disinfect the tub or shower before returning the person to his or her room.

56. When assisting with a tub bath or shower, which of these steps is first?
    A. Help the person undress and remove footwear.
    B. Assist or transport the person to the tub or shower room.
    C. Put the occupied sign on the door.
    D. Place a rubber bath mat in the tub or on the shower floor.

57. When cleaning the perineal area
    A. You do not need to wear gloves
    B. Work from the anal area to the urethral area (back to front, bottom to top)
    C. Work from the urethral area to the anal area (front to back, top to bottom)
    D. Work from the dirtiest area to the cleanest area

58. When gathering equipment for perineal care, you will need
    A. 1 washcloth
    B. 2 washcloths
    C. At least 3 washcloths
    D. At least 4 washcloths

59. When giving perineal care to a male, you
    A. Retract the foreskin if he is uncircumcised
    B. Wash from the scrotum to the tip of the penis
    C. Use 1 washcloth for the entire procedure
    D. Leave the foreskin retracted after finishing the care

Matching

Match the skin care product with the benefit or the problem that may occur if you use the product.

A. Soaps
B. Bath oils
C. Creams and lotions
D. Powders
E. Deodorants and antiperspirants

60. _____ Absorbs moisture and prevents friction

61. _____ Makes showers and tubs slippery

62. _____ Protects skin from the drying effect of air and evaporation

63. _____ Excessive amounts can cause caking and crusts that can irritate the skin

64. _____ Masks and controls body odors or reduces perspiration

65. _____ Tends to dry and irritate skin

66. _____ Keeps skin soft and prevents drying of skin

67. _____ Removes dirt, dead skin, skin oil, some microbes, and perspiration

Fill in the Blank

68. Write out the abbreviations.

A. ADA _____

B. C _____

C. F _____

D. ID _____

69. The _____ and the _____ of the mouth, genital area, and anus must be intact to prevent microbes from entering the body and causing an _____

70. The religion of East Indian Hindus requires at least _____ a day.

71. Some Hindus believe that bathing is _____ after a meal.

72. When should you give or offer oral hygiene to a person?

A. _____

B. _____

C. _____

D. _____

73. When you are delegated to give oral hygiene, what observations should you report?

A. _____

B. _____

C. _____

D. _____

E. _____

F. _____

74. If flossing is done only once a day, the best time to floss is at _____.

75. When giving oral care to an unconscious person, explain what you are doing because you always assume _____ _____

76. When following the rules for bathing in Box 22-2, you protect the skin by following these rules:

A. Rinse _____

B. Pat _____

C. Dry _____

D. Bathe _____

77. What methods can be used to measure the water temperature for a bed bath?

A. _____

B. _____

78. When you place a person's hand in the basin during the bed bath, you may have the person _____ the hands and fingers.

79. When assisting with partial baths, most people need help with washing the _____.

80. A tub bath can cause a person to feel _____, especially if the person has been on bedrest.

81. When the shower room has more than 1 stall or cabinet, you must protect the person's right to _____

What can you do to protect this right?

A. _____

B. _____

82. When giving a tub bath or shower, you use safety measures to protect the person from _____, _____, and _____

83. When you are assisting a person with perineal care, what terms may help the person understand what you are going to do? _____ _____

84. What observations made while assisting with hygiene should be reported at once?

A. _____

B. _____

C. _____

D. _____

E. _____

Use the FOCUS ON PRIDE section to complete these statements.

85. You show personal and professional responsibility when you focus on the quality of life steps before performing procedures. They are:

   A. _____

   B. _____

   C. _____

   D. _____

   E. _____

   F. _____

86. You can promote independence and social interaction when you allow

   A. Personal choice of _____

   B. Encourage the person to _____

Labeling

87. Look at the figure and answer these questions.

   A. Why is the person positioned on his side?

   _____

   B. What is the purpose of the padded tongue blade?

   _____

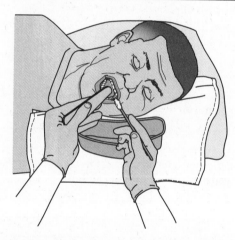

88. In this figure, what is the staff member using to remove the upper denture?

   _____

   Why? _____

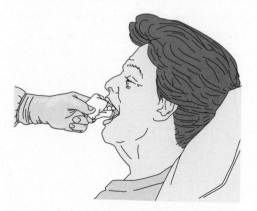

89. In this figure, explain what the staff member is doing.

   _____

   Why is the towel positioned vertically on the person?

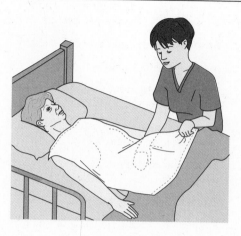

Optional Learning Exercises

90. Hygiene promotes comfort, safety, and health. Answer these questions about hygiene.

   A. What does intact skin prevent? _____

   B. What other areas must be clean to maintain intact skin? _____

   _____

   C. Besides cleansing, what are the other benefits of good hygiene?

   i. Prevents _____ and _____

   ii. It is _____

   iii. Increases _____

91. What factors cause mouth dryness for an unconscious person?

   A. _____

   B. _____

   C. _____

92. The factors listed above cause crusting on the

   _____ and

   _____.

93. Oral hygiene (mouth care) does the following:

   A. _____.

   B. _____

   C. _____.

   D. _____

   E. _____

94. What are the benefits of bathing?
    A. Cleans _____
    B. Also cleans _____
    C. Removes _____
    D. Bath is _____ and

    _____
    E. Stimulates _____
    F. Exercises _____
    G. You can make _____
    H. You have time _____

95. When you are bathing a person with dementia, what measures are important to help the person through the bath?
    A. Comfort
       i. Provide for _____
       ii. Provide good _____
       iii. Play _____
    B. Safety
       i. Use a hand-held _____
       ii. Have the person use a shower _____
       iii. Do not _____
       iv. Do not leave _____
    C. Tell the person _____
    D. Try a partial _____
    E. Try a bath _____

96. You are delegated to give Mrs. Johnson a bath. Before beginning, what information do you need?
    A. _____
    B. _____
    C. _____
    D. _____
    E. _____
    F. _____
    G. _____
    H. _____

97. As you are bathing Mrs. Johnson, what observations should you make to report and record?
    A. _____
    B. _____
    C. _____
    D. _____
    E. _____
    F. _____
    G. _____
    H. _____
    I. _____
    J. _____
    K. _____
    L. _____

98. You are preparing to give perineal care to Mrs. Johnson. How many washcloths should you gather?
    _____ Why?
    _____
    _____
    _____

Fill in the Blank: Key Terms

Alopecia	Hirsutism	Mite	Pediculosis corporis
Anticoagulant	Infestation	Pediculosis	Pediculosis pubis
Dandruff	Lice	Pediculosis capitis	Scabies

1. Being in or on a host in an _____.

2. The infestation with lice is _____.

3. A very small spider-like organism is a

   _____.

4. _____ is an excessive amount of dry, white flakes from the scalp.

5. The infestation of the body with lice is

   _____.

6. Hair loss is _____.

7. _____ is the infestation of the pubic hair with lice.

8. Excessive body hair is _____.

9. The infestation of the scalp with wingless insects is

   _____.

10. Another description of pediculosis is

    _____.

11. A drug that prevents or slows down blood clotting is an

    _____.

12. _____ is a skin disorder caused by the female mite.

Circle the Best Answer

13. Hair care, shaving, and nail and foot care are important to many people because these measures affect
    A. Safety and security needs
    B. Love, belonging, and self-esteem needs
    C. Physical needs
    D. Self-actualization needs

14. If you see any signs of lice, you should report it to the nurse because
    A. Lice bites can cause severe infections
    B. Lice are easily spread to other persons through clothing, furniture, bed linens, and sexual contact
    C. Lice can cause the person's hair to fall out
    D. The lice will cause the hair to mat and tangle

15. If a person has scabies, what signs or symptoms may be present?
    A. You may see lice that are small and tan to grayish white in color.
    B. The person has a rash and intense itching between the fingers, around the wrists, and in other areas.
    C. You may see eggs (nits) attached to the hair shaft.
    D. The person has an excessive amount of dry, white flakes on the scalp.

16. Who chooses how you will brush, comb, and style a person's hair?
    A. The person
    B. You decide
    C. The nurse tells you
    D. It is written in the care plan

17. If long hair becomes matted or tangled, you should
    A. Braid the hair
    B. Cut the hair to remove the tangles and matting
    C. Tell the nurse and ask for directions
    D. Get the family's permission to change the hairstyle

18. If hair is curly, coarse, and dry, which of these would *not* be done?
    A. Braid or cut the hair
    B. Use a wide-toothed comb
    C. Work upward, lifting and fluffing hair outward
    D. Apply a conditioner or petroleum jelly to make combing easier

19. When shampooing the person who has small braids
    A. Undo the hair and re-braid it each time it is shampooed
    B. The braids are left intact for shampooing
    C. Undo the braids only at night
    D. Comb out the braids once a week

20. If a woman's hair is done by the beautician in long-term care
    A. Wash her hair only once a week
    B. Shampoo her hair on the day she goes to the beautician
    C. Have her wear a shower cap during the tub bath or shower
    D. Wash her hair each time she gets a shower or tub bath

21. If a person has limited range of motion in the neck, he or she is not shampooed
    A. At the sink or on a stretcher
    B. In the shower
    C. During a tub bath
    D. In bed

22. Which of these is *not* an observation that is made when shampooing?
    A. Scalp sores
    B. The presence of nits or lice
    C. The amount of hair on the head
    D. Matted or tangled hair

23. If a person receives anticoagulants and needs shaving
    A. Use an electric razor
    B. Use disposable safety razors
    C. It must be done by the nurse or barber
    D. It should be done only during the shower or bath

24. When using safety razors (blade razors)
    A. The same razor can be used for several persons until it becomes dull
    B. Use the resident's own razor as many times as possible
    C. Discard the disposable razor or razor blade in the sharps container
    D. Be careful when shaving a person who takes anticoagulants

25. Why is an electric razor used when shaving a person with dementia?
    A. The person usually bleeds easily.
    B. The person may not understand what you are doing and resist care or move suddenly.
    C. It is faster than using a safety razor.
    D. The skin is tender and sensitive.

26. When shaving a person with a safety razor, wear gloves
    A. To protect the person from infections
    B. To prevent contact with blood
    C. When applying shaving cream
    D. To maintain sterile technique

27. When caring for a mustache and beard, all of these are done *except*
    A. Wash the mustache or beard daily
    B. Comb the mustache or beard daily
    C. Ask the person how to groom his beard or mustache
    D. Trim a beard or mustache when you notice it is too long

28. The nursing assistant can cut or trim toenails
    A. Whenever he or she has time
    B. On all persons
    C. If agency policy allows them to trim toenails
    D. If the person agrees to the care

29. When caring for the fingernails or toenails, which of these is *wrong*?
    A. Cut the nails with small scissors.
    B. Clean under the nails with an orangewood stick.
    C. Clip the nails straight across with nail clippers.
    D. Shape the nails with an emery board or nail file.

30. When changing clothing, remove the clothing from
    A. The weak side first
    B. The lower limbs first
    C. The right side last
    D. The strong or "good" side first

31. When you are undressing a person, it is usually done
    A. In the bed in the supine position
    B. With the person sitting in a chair
    C. By having the person stand at the bedside
    D. In the bathroom

32. When you are undressing a person, you use good body mechanics when you
    A. Lower the bed rail on the person's weak side
    B. Position the person in a supine position
    C. Raise the bed to a good working level
    D. Turn the person away from you

33. To provide warmth and privacy when changing clothes, you
    A. Keep the top sheets in place
    B. Cover the person with a bath blanket
    C. Close the curtains
    D. Close the door

34. When changing the gown of a person with an IV
    A. Turn off the IV
    B. Lay the IV bag on the bed and remove the gown
    C. Slide the gathered sleeve over the tubing, hand, arm, and IV site
    D. Disconnect the IV

35. When you have finished changing the gown of a person with an IV, you should
    A. Restart the pump
    B. Reconnect the IV
    C. Ask the nurse to check the flow rate
    D. Check the flow rate

Fill in the Blank

36. Write out the abbreviations.
    A. C _____
    B. F _____
    C. ID _____
    D. IV _____

37. When you brush and comb the hair, you should report and record
    A. _____
    B. _____
    C. _____
    D. _____
    E. _____
    F. _____
    G. _____
    H. _____

38. If you give hair care to a person in bed after a linen change, collect falling hair by _____

39. It may help to prevent tangled and matted hair when you brush and comb small sections of the hair, starting at the _____.

40. If hair is curly, coarse, and dry, special measures are needed. You should
    A. Use a _____
    B. Start at _____
    C. Work _____,
       lift and _____
    D. Wet _____
       or apply _____

41. You can protect the person's eyes during shampooing by asking the person to hold a _____

    _____

42. What delegation guidelines do you need when shaving a person?

    A. _____

    B. _____

    C. _____

    D. _____

    E. _____

    F. _____

    G. _____

    H. _____

43. What should be reported *at once* when you are shaving a person?

    A. _____

    B. _____

    C. _____

    D. _____

44. When you are shaving the face and underarms with a safety razor, shave in the direction of the

    _____.

45. When shaving legs with a safety razor, shave

    _____

46. When using an electric shaver, shave

    _____

47. When you are delegated to give nail and foot care, report and record

    A. _____

    B. _____

    C. _____

    D. _____

    E. _____

    F. _____

48. Foot care for persons with diabetes or poor circulation is provided by _____

    or _____

49. When undressing the person who cannot raise the head and shoulders

    A. _____

    B. _____

    C. _____

    D. _____

    E. _____

50. When dressing the person who cannot raise the hips and buttocks off the bed

    A. _____

    B. _____

    C. _____

    D. _____

    E. _____

51. Before changing a person's hospital gown, what information do you need from the nurse and the care plan?

    A. _____

    B. _____

Use the FOCUS ON PRIDE section to complete these statements.

52. When a person has clean _____,

    _____, and _____,

    it helps mental well-being.

53. It is important for you to be _____ and have a professional _____ because others may question the quality of care you provide if you are not groomed well.

54. When you respect the person's choice of hairstyles and personal care products, it shows you respect the person's right to _____.

55. When a person allows family members to assist with giving personal care, this promotes

    _____.

56. If you cut a person's hair or shave a mustache or beard without permission, you have violated the person's right to be free from

    _____.

Optional Learning Exercises

57. You are caring for a person who is receiving cancer treatments. What effect could this treatment have on the person's hair? _____

    _____

58. Dandruff not only occurs on the scalp, but also may involve the _____.

59. Brushing the hair increases _____ to the scalp. It also brings _____ along the hair shaft.

60. Why do older persons usually have dry hair?

    _____

61. What water temperature is usually used when shampooing the hair?

_____

62. How can the beard be softened before shaving?

_____

_____

63. After shaving, why do some people apply after-shave or lotion?

    A. Lotion _____

    B. After-shave _____

64. Injuries to the feet of a person with poor circulation are serious because poor circulation prolongs

_____

65. When changing clothing or hospital gowns, what rules should be followed?

    A. _____

    B. _____

    C. _____

    D. _____

    E. _____

    F. _____

    G. _____

    H. _____

Fill in the Blank: Key Terms

Dysuria
Functional incontinence
Hematuria
Micturition
Mixed incontinence

Nocturia
Oliguria
Over-active bladder
Over-flow incontinence
Polyuria

Reflex incontinence
Stress incontinence
Transient incontinence
Urge incontinence
Urinary frequency

Urinary incontinence
Urinary retention
Urinary urgency
Urination
Voiding

1. Another name for urge incontinence is
   _____

2. The production of abnormally large amounts of urine is _____

3. _____ is the combination of stress incontinence and urge incontinence.

4. _____ is the loss of bladder control.

5. Frequent urination at night is
   _____

6. The loss of small amounts of urine that leak from a bladder that is always full is
   _____

7. Another name for urination or voiding is
   _____

8. _____ occurs when the person has bladder control but cannot use the toilet in time.

9. The process of emptying urine from the bladder is micturition, voiding, or _____

10. Blood in the urine is _____.

11. Voiding at frequent intervals is _____.

12. When urine leaks during exercise and certain movements that cause pressure on the bladder, it is called _____.

13. Another word for urination or micturition is
    _____

14. _____ is the need to void at once.

15. The loss of urine in response to a sudden, urgent need to void is _____.

16. Painful or difficult urination is
    _____

17. The loss of urine at predictable intervals when the bladder is full is _____

18. A scant amount of urine, usually less than 500 mL in 24 hours, is _____.

19. _____ is temporary or occasional incontinence that is reversed when the cause is treated.

20. The inability to void is _____.

Circle the Best Answer

21. Solid wastes are removed from the body by the
    A. Digestive system   C. Blood
    B. Urinary system   D. Integumentary system

22. A healthy adult excretes about _____1500_____ of urine a day.
    A. 500 mL
    B. 1000 mL
    C. 1500 mL
    D. 2000 mL

23. All of these will provide privacy when the person is voiding *except*
    A. Pull drapes or window shades
    B. Always stay in the room to give assistance
    C. Pull the curtain around the bed
    D. Close room and bathroom doors

24. If the person has difficulty starting the urine stream, it may help to
    A. Play music on the TV
    B. Provide perineal care
    C. Use a stainless steel bedpan
    D. Run water in a nearby sink

25. The urine may be bright yellow if the person eats
    A. Asparagus
    B. Carrots or sweet potatoes
    C. Beets or blackberries
    D. Rhubarb

26. If you are caring for an infant, which of these observations should be reported to the nurse at once?
    A. The infant has had a wet diaper 4 times in 3 hours.
    B. The infant has not had a wet diaper for several hours.
    C. The urine in the diaper is pale yellow.
    D. The urine in the diaper has a faint odor.

27. When you are getting ready to give a person the bedpan, you should
    A. Raise the head of the bed slightly for the person's comfort
    B. Position the person in the Fowler's position
    C. Wash the person's hands
    D. Place the bed in a flat position

28. Urinals are usually placed at the bedside on
    A. Bed rails
    B. Over-bed tables
    C. Bedside stands
    D. The floor

29. If a man is unable to stand and place a urinal to void, you should
    A. Tell the nurse
    B. Ask a male co-worker to help the man
    C. Place and hold the urinal for him
    D. Pad the bed with incontinence pads

30. A commode chair is used when
    A. The person is unable to stand and pivot
    B. The person is not allowed to get out of bed
    C. The person needs to be in the normal position for elimination
    D. The bathroom is being used by another person

31. When you place a commode over the toilet
    A. Use restraints on the person
    B. Stay in the room with the person
    C. Lock the wheels
    D. Make sure the container is in place

32. When you do not answer call lights quickly or do not position the call light within the person's reach, it can cause
    A. Over-flow incontinence
    B. Mixed incontinence
    C. Reflex incontinence
    D. Functional incontinence

33. You are caring for an incontinent person who often wets right after you have changed the clothes and bedding. It would be correct if you
    A. Wait 15 to 30 minutes before changing the person each time
    B. Re-use some of the linens that are only slightly damp
    C. Talk to the nurse at once if you find yourself becoming impatient
    D. Tell the person that you can change him or her only once a shift

34. When a person has dementia, what measures may help keep the person clean and dry?
    A. Tell the person to use the call light when he or she needs to void.
    B. Increase fluid intake at bedtime.
    C. Observe for signs that the person may need to void, such as pulling at the clothing.
    D. Remove any incontinence garments and seat the person on a commode at all times.

35. When discussing incontinence products, it may lower a person's self-esteem if the products are called
    A. Incontinence briefs
    B. Underwear
    C. Adult diapers
    D. By the brand name

36. When applying an incontinence product, you should
    A. Apply a new one only when the old one is very wet
    B. Weigh the old product to determine the urine output
    C. Mark the date, time, and your initials on the new product
    D. Clean the skin by rubbing hard with dry paper towels

37. The goal of bladder training is
    A. To keep the person dry and clean
    B. Control of urination
    C. Prevention of skin breakdown
    D. Prevention of infection

38. When you are assisting the person with habit training to have normal elimination
    A. Help the person to the bathroom every 15 or 20 minutes
    B. Voiding is scheduled at regular times to match the person's voiding habits
    C. Make sure the person drinks at least 1000 mL each shift
    D. Tell the person he or she can void only once a shift

39. When you assist with bladder training for a person with an indwelling catheter
    A. Empty the drainage bag every hour
    B. At first, clamp the catheter for 1 hour
    C. At first, clamp the catheter for 3 to 4 hours
    D. Give the person 15 to 20 minutes to start voiding

Fill in the Blank

40. Write out the abbreviations.
    A. BM _____
    B. mL _____
    C. UTI _____

41. What substances increase urine production?
    A. _____
    B. _____
    C. _____
    D. _____

42. A normal position for voiding for women is _____.
    For men, a normal position is _____.

43. What can you do to mask urination sounds?
    A. _____
    B. _____
    C. _____

44. Fracture pans are used for persons
    A. _____
    B. _____
    C. _____
    D. _____
    E. _____
    F. _____
    G. _____

45. A bariatric bedpan is placed with the _____ end under the buttocks.

46. When a person voids in a bedpan or urinal, what observations about the urine are important?
    A. _____
    B. _____
    C. _____
    D. _____
    E. _____

47. You should report complaints of _____, _____, or _____ when the person is voiding.

48. When you are handling bedpans, urinals, and commodes and their contents, you should follow
    _____
    and _____.

49. When you are delegated to provide a urinal, what guidelines should you follow?
    A. _____
    B. _____
    C. _____
    D. _____
    E. _____
    F. _____
    G. _____
    H. _____

50. When you transfer a person to a commode from bed, you must practice safe transfer procedures and use a
    _____
    and _____ the wheels.

51. Name risk factors and causes of incontinence related to
    A. Women _____
    B. Men _____
    C. Age _____
    D. Over-weight _____
    E. Smoking _____
    F. Diabetes _____

52. How are these related to transient incontinence?
    A. Alcohol _____
    B. Bladder irritation caused by _____
    C. Caffeine _____
    D. Constipation or fecal impaction _____
    E. Increased fluid intake _____
    F. Urinary tract infection _____

53. When you are delegated to apply incontinence products, you need this information from the nurse and care plan.
    A. _____
    B. _____
    C. _____
    D. _____
    E. _____
    F. _____

54. What observations should you report and record when you are delegated to apply incontinence products?
    A. _____
    B. _____
    C. _____
    D. _____
    E. _____
    F. _____
    G. _____

55. When you provide perineal care after a person is incontinent, remember to
    A. _____
    B. _____
    C. _____
    D. _____
    E. _____
    F. _____

56. The catheter is clamped for 1 hour at first and, over time, for 3 to 4 hours when _____ is being done.

Use the FOCUS ON PRIDE section to complete these statements.

57. If you notice a person is uncomfortable talking about urinary elimination, what ways can you put the person at ease?
    A. Pay attention _____
    B. Modify _____
    C. Always be _____
    D. Speak with _____

58. Urine-filled devices in the person's room do not respect the person's right to
    _____

Crossword

Fill in the crossword by answering the clues below with words from this list:

Dysuria	Hematuria	Nocturia	Polyuria
Frequency	Incontinence	Oliguria	Urgency

Across

6. Scant amount of urine, usually less than 500 mL in 24 hours
8. Inability to control loss of urine from bladder

Down

1. Production of abnormally large amount of urine
2. Painful or difficult urination
3. Blood in the urine
4. Voiding at frequent intervals
5. Frequent urination at night
7. Need to void immediately

Optional Learning Exercises

59. When a person eats a diet high in salt, it causes the body to _____.
When this happens, how does it affect urine output?

_____

60. You would ask the nurse to observe urine that looks

or _____.
The nurse uses the information for the

_____

61. A fracture pan can be used with older persons who have _____

or _____.

62. Covering the lap and legs of a person using a commode provides _____ and promotes

_____

63. If you are caring for an incontinent person and you become short-tempered and impatient,

_____

What right are you protecting when you do this?

_____

64. When using incontinence products, it is important to use the correct size. If the product is too large,

_____

If it is too small, the product will cause

_____

65. When bladder training is being done, the person needs to

A. _____

B. _____

C. _____

25 Urinary Catheters

Fill in the Blank: Key Terms

Catheter   Condom catheter   Indwelling catheter   Straight catheter
Catheterization   Foley catheter   Retention catheter

1. A soft sheath that slides over the penis and is used to drain urine is a _____.

2. A Foley or indwelling catheter is also called a _____

3. The process of inserting a catheter is _____

4. A catheter left in the bladder so urine drains constantly into a drainage bag is called a retention, Foley, or _____

5. A _____ is a tube used to drain or inject fluid through a body opening.

6. A catheter that drains the bladder and then is removed is a _____

7. An indwelling or retention catheter is also called a _____

Circle the Best Answer

8. A catheter is used for all of these *except*
   A. To keep the bladder empty before, during, and after surgery
   B. When a person is dying
   C. For all persons with incontinence
   D. To protect wounds and pressure ulcers from contact with urine

9. When securing the drainage tubing, you should
   A. Pin the tubing to the person's gown
   B. Pin the tubing so that it is stretched tight and straight
   C. Pin the tubing to the bottom linens
   D. Attach the tubing to the bed rails

10. When cleaning a catheter, you should
    A. Wipe 4 inches up the catheter to the meatus
    B. Disconnect the tubing from the drainage bag
    C. Clean the catheter from the meatus down the catheter about 4 inches
    D. Wash and rinse the catheter by washing up and down the tubing

11. The drainage bag from a catheter should *not* be attached to the
    A. Bed frame   C. Wheelchair
    B. Back of a chair   D. Bed rail

12. If a catheter is accidentally disconnected from the drainage bag, you should tell the nurse at once and then
    A. Quickly reconnect the drainage system
    B. Clamp the catheter to prevent leakage
    C. Wipe the end of the tube with an antiseptic wipe and the end of the catheter with another antiseptic wipe
    D. Discard the drainage bag and get a new bag

13. If a person uses a leg drainage bag, it
    A. Is switched to a drainage bag when the person is in bed
    B. Is attached to the clothing with tape or safety pins
    C. Is attached to the bed rail when the person is in bed
    D. Can be worn 24 hours a day

14. A leg bag needs to be emptied more often than a drainage bag because
    A. It holds less than 1000 mL and the drainage bag holds about 2000 mL
    B. It is more likely to leak than the drainage bag
    C. It holds about 250 mL and the drainage bag holds 1000 mL
    D. It interferes with walking if it is full

15. When you empty a drainage bag, you
    A. Disconnect the bag from the tubing
    B. Clamp the catheter to prevent leakage
    C. Open the clamp on the drain and let urine drain into a graduate
    D. Take the bag into the bathroom to empty it

16. When removing an indwelling catheter, a syringe is needed to
    A. Remove water in the balloon
    B. Insert water into the balloon
    C. Flush the catheter with water
    D. Clean the perineal area after removing the catheter

17. A condom catheter is changed
    A. Daily after perineal care
    B. Once or twice a week on bath days
    C. Only when the adhesive becomes loose and the catheter leaks
    D. When the drainage system is changed from a leg bag to a large drainage bag

18. When applying a condom catheter
    A. Apply elastic tape in a spiral around the penis
    B. Make sure the catheter tip is touching the head of the penis
    C. Apply adhesive tape securely in a circle entirely around the penis
    D. Remove and reapply every shift

Fill in the Blank

19. When a catheter is inserted after a person voids and then removed, it is used to measure the

_____.

20. A catheter is secured to the inner thigh or the man's abdomen to prevent

_____.

21. When a person has a catheter, what observations should you report and record?

A. _____

B. _____

C. _____

D. _____

E. _____

F. _____

G. _____

H. _____

22. When you give catheter care, clean the catheter about _____ inches. Clean _____ from the meatus with _____ stroke.

23. Is the urinary drainage system sterile or non-sterile?

_____

24. What happens if a drainage bag is higher than the bladder? _____ This can cause

_____.

25. If a drainage system is disconnected accidentally, what should you do?

A. Tell _____

B. Do not _____

C. Practice _____ Put _____

D. Wipe _____

E. Wipe _____

F. Do not _____

G. Connect _____

H. Discard _____

I. Remove _____

26. When you are allowed to remove a catheter, what information is needed from the nurse?

A. _____

B. _____

C. _____

D. _____

E. _____

F. _____

27. Do not apply a condom catheter if the penis is

_____, _____,

or shows signs of _____.

Labeling

28. Mark the places you would secure the catheter and drainage bag.

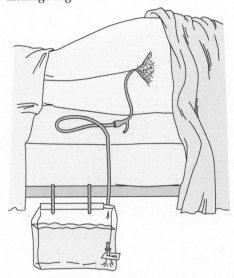

29. Mark the places you would secure the catheter.

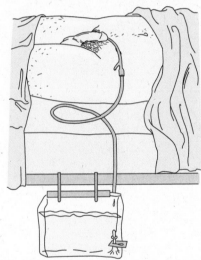

30. Why is it important to secure the catheters and drainage tubing as shown in the drawings?

_____

_____

Use the FOCUS ON PRIDE section to complete these statements.

31. When you are careful handling and caring for catheters, you decrease the risk of _____ for the person.

32. When you need to move a drainage bag to the other side of the bed, you must

A. _____

B. _____

C. _____

D. _____

Optional Learning Exercises

33. Even though catheters create a risk of urinary tract infections, they are used to

    A. _____

    B. _____

    C. _____

    D. _____

    E. _____

    F. _____

34. What can happen if microbes enter a closed drainage system? _____

35. How can you make a person with a catheter feel less embarrassed and more comfortable when visitors are coming?

    A. _____

    B. _____

36. What type of tape is used to apply a condom catheter?
    _____ Why?

    What can happen if you use the wrong tape?
    _____

37. Even though catheters are a last resort for incontinent persons, they may be used with weak, disabled, or dying persons to

    A. Promote _____

    B. Prevent _____

    C. Protect _____

       and _____

26 Bowel Elimination

Fill in the Blank: Key Terms

Colostomy   Diarrhea   Feces   Ostomy   Stool
Constipation   Enema   Flatulence   Peristalsis   Suppository
Defecation   Fecal impaction   Flatus   Stoma
Dehydration   Fecal incontinence   Ileostomy

1. A surgically created opening is a stoma or
_____

2. The process of excreting feces from the rectum through the anus is a bowel movement or
_____

3. The excessive formation of gas in the stomach and intestines is _____

4. A _____ is a cone-shaped solid drug that is inserted into a body opening.

5. The frequent passage of liquid stools is
_____

6. _____ is the prolonged retention and buildup of feces in the rectum.

7. _____ is the excessive loss of water from tissues.

8. Gas or air passed through the anus is
_____

9. The introduction of fluid into the rectum and lower colon is an _____

10. Excreted feces is _____

11. An artificial opening between the colon and abdominal wall is a _____

12. _____ is the alternating contraction and relaxation of intestinal muscles.

13. The passage of a hard, dry stool is
_____

14. _____ is the inability to control the passage of feces and gas through the anus.

15. A surgically created opening is an ostomy or
_____

16. The semi-solid mass of waste products in the colon is
_____

17. An artificial opening between the ileum and the abdominal wall is an _____

Circle the Best Answer

18. People normally have a bowel movement
    A. Every day
    B. Every 2 to 3 days
    C. 2 or 3 times a day
    D. All of these can be normal

19. Bleeding in the stomach and small intestines causes stool to be
    A. Brown   C. Red
    B. Black   D. Clay-colored

20. The characteristic odor of stool is caused by
    A. Poor personal hygiene
    B. Poor nutrition
    C. Bacterial action in the intestines
    D. Adequate fluid intake

21. When you observe stool that is abnormal
    A. Ask the nurse to observe the stool
    B. Report your observation and discard the stool
    C. Ask the person if the stool is normal for him or her
    D. Record your observations when you finish giving care

22. Which of these could interfere with defecation?
    A. Being able to relax by reading a book or newspaper
    B. Eating a diet with high-fiber foods
    C. Having others present in a semi-private room
    D. Drinking 6 to 8 glasses of water daily

23. A person who must stay in bed most of the time may have irregular elimination and constipation because of
    A. Poor diet   C. Inactivity
    B. Poor fluid intake   D. Lack of privacy

24. Which of these would provide safety for the person during bowel elimination?
    A. Make sure the bedpan is warm.
    B. Place the call light and toilet tissue within the person's reach.
    C. Provide perineal care.
    D. Allow enough time for defecation.

25. Constipation can be relieved by
    A. Giving the person a low-fiber diet
    B. Increasing activity
    C. Decreasing fluids
    D. Ignoring the urge to defecate

26. A person tries several times to have a bowel movement and cannot. Liquid feces seep from the anus. This may mean he has
    A. Diarrhea   C. A fecal impaction
    B. Constipation   D. Fecal incontinence

27. When a fecal impaction is present, it is relieved by
    A. Changing the person's diet
    B. Giving more fluids
    C. Removing the fecal mass with a gloved finger
    D. Increasing the activity of the person

28. When checking and removing a fecal impaction, all of these are true *except*
    A. All nursing assistants do these procedures as part of routine care
    B. The procedures must be in your job description
    C. Your state must allow you to perform this procedure
    D. You must have the necessary education and training
29. Good skin care is important when a person has diarrhea because
    A. This prevents odors
    B. Skin breakdown and pressure ulcers are risks
    C. It prevents the spread of microbes
    D. It prevents fluid loss
30. Why is diarrhea very serious in older persons?
    A. It causes skin breakdown.
    B. It causes odors.
    C. It can cause dehydration and death.
    D. It increases activity.
31. If a person with diarrhea has *C. difficile*, you should
    A. Wear sterile gloves and gown
    B. Practice Standard Precautions and contact precautions
    C. Restrict all visitors from visiting the person
    D. Use alcohol hand rubs to clean your hands
32. When fecal incontinence occurs, the person may need all of these *except*
    A. Increased fluid intake
    B. Bowel training
    C. Help with elimination after meals and every 2 to 3 hours
    D. Incontinence products to keep garments and linens clean
33. If flatus is not expelled, the person may complain of
    A. Abdominal cramping or pain
    B. Diarrhea
    C. Fecal incontinence
    D. Nausea
34. Which of these is *not* a goal of bowel training?
    A. To give laxatives daily to maintain regular bowel movements
    B. To gain control of bowel movements
    C. To develop a regular pattern of elimination
    D. To prevent fecal impaction, constipation, and fecal incontinence
35. When bowel training is planned, which of these is included in the care plan?
    A. The amount of stool the person expels
    B. How many bowel movements the person has each day
    C. The usual time of day the person has a bowel movement
    D. The foods that cause flatus
36. When the nurse delegates you to prepare a soapsuds enema for an adult, mix
    A. 2 teaspoons of salt in 1000 mL of tap water
    B. 3 to 5 mL of castile soap in 500 to 1000 mL of tap water
    C. 2 mL of castile soap in 200 mL of tap water
    D. Mineral oil with sterile water

37. When you give a cleansing enema, it should be given to the person
    A. Within 5 minutes
    B. Over about 30 minutes
    C. Over about 10 to 15 minutes
    D. Over about 20 minutes
38. The person receiving an enema is usually placed in a
    A. Supine position
    B. Prone position
    C. Semi-Fowler's position
    D. Left side-lying or Sims' position
39. When you prepare and give an enema to an adult, you will do all of these *except*
    A. Prepare the solution at 110°F
    B. Insert the tubing 2 to 4 inches into the rectum
    C. Hold the solution container about 12 inches above the bed
    D. Lubricate the enema tip before inserting it into the rectum
40. When the doctor orders enemas until clear
    A. Give 1 enema
    B. Give as many enemas as necessary to return a clear fluid
    C. Ask the nurse how many enemas to give
    D. Give only tap water enemas
41. If you are giving an enema and the person complains of cramping
    A. Tell the person that is normal and continue to give the enema
    B. Clamp the tube until the cramping subsides
    C. Discontinue the enema immediately and tell the nurse
    D. Lower the bag below the level of the bed
42. If you are giving a cleansing enema to a child, which of the following is correct?
    A. Mix 3 mL of castile soap with 500 mL of tap water.
    B. A saline enema is used when giving a cleansing enema to a child.
    C. Use only a small-volume enema.
    D. Use room temperature tap water for the solution.
43. When giving a small-volume enema, do not release pressure on the bottle because
    A. It will cause cramping if pressure is released
    B. The fluid will leak from the rectum
    C. Solution will be drawn back into the bottle
    D. It will cause flatulence
44. When giving a small-volume enema
    A. Place the person in the prone position
    B. Insert the enema tip 2 inches into the rectum
    C. Heat the solution to 105°F
    D. Clamp the tubing if cramping occurs
45. An oil-retention enema is given to
    A. Cleanse the bowel to prepare for surgery
    B. Regulate the person who is receiving bowel training
    C. Relieve flatulence
    D. Soften the feces and lubricate the rectum

46. If you feel resistance when you are giving an enema
    A. Lubricate the tube more thoroughly
    B. Push more firmly to insert the tube
    C. Stop tube insertion
    D. Ask the person to take a deep breath and relax

47. When you are caring for a person with an ostomy, you know
    A. All of the stools are solid and formed
    B. The stoma does not have sensation and touching it does not cause pain
    C. An ostomy is always temporary and is reconnected after healing
    D. A pouch is worn to protect the stoma

48. Which of these statements about an ileostomy is *true?*
    A. The stool is solid and formed.
    B. The stoma is an opening into the colon.
    C. The pouch is changed daily.
    D. The skin around the ileostomy can be irritated by the digestive juices in the stool.

49. When caring for a person with an ostomy, the pouch is
    A. Changed daily
    B. Changed every 2 to 7 days and when it leaks
    C. Worn only when the person thinks he or she will have a bowel movement
    D. Changed every time the person has a bowel movement

50. The best time to change the ostomy bag is before breakfast because
    A. The stoma is less likely to expel feces at this time
    B. The person has more time in the morning
    C. It should be changed before morning care
    D. The person tolerates the procedure better before eating

51. When cleaning the skin around the stoma, you use
    A. Sterile water and sterile gauze pads
    B. Alcohol and sterile cotton
    C. Gauze pads or washcloths and water and soap or cleansing agents as delegated by the nurse
    D. Adhesive remover and sterile cotton balls

Fill in the Blank

52. Write out the abbreviations
    A. BM _____
    B. CMS _____
    C. GI _____
    D. ID _____
    E. IV _____
    F. mL _____
    G. oz _____
    H. SSE _____

53. When observing stool, what should be reported to the nurse?
    A. _____
    B. _____
    C. _____
    D. _____
    E. _____
    F. _____
    G. _____
    H. _____
    I. _____

54. What 3 food groups are high in fiber?
    A. _____
    B. _____
    C. _____

55. Name 6 gas-forming foods.
    A. _____
    B. _____
    C. _____
    D. _____
    E. _____
    F. _____

56. Drinking warm fluids such as coffee, tea, hot cider, and warm water will increase _____.

57. If you are delegated to remove a fecal impaction, what observations should you report and record?
    A. _____
    B. _____
    C. _____
    D. _____

58. When checking and removing impactions, the vagus nerve may be stimulated. Why is this dangerous?
    _____

59. How will dehydration affect these?
    A. Skin is _____.
    B. Urine is _____.
    C. Blood pressure is _____.
    D. Pulse and respirations are _____.

60. Flatulence may be caused when a tense or anxious person _____ while eating and drinking.

61. When a nurse inserts a suppository, how soon would you expect the person to defecate?
    _____

62. Before giving an enema, make sure that
    A. Your state _____
    B. The procedure _____
    C. You have _____
    D. You review _____
    E. A nurse _____

63. After giving an enema, what should be reported and recorded?
    A. _____
    B. _____
    C. _____
    D. _____
    E. _____
    F. _____
    G. _____

64. Because it is likely you will have contact with stool while giving an enema, you should follow

    _____ and

    _____.

65. How can cramping be prevented during an enema?
    A. _____
    B. _____

66. How long does it usually take for a tap water, saline, or soapsuds enema to take effect?

    _____

67. A small-volume enema contains _____ of solution.

68. A person should retain a small-volume enema

    _____.

69. When you start to insert the tube to give an enema, ask the person to _____

70. What can you place in the ostomy pouch to prevent odors? _____

71. Showers and baths are delayed 1 or 2 hours after applying a new pouch to allow

    _____

Use the FOCUS ON PRIDE section to complete these statements.

72. If your state allows a nursing assistant to insert suppositories, you may be allowed to insert them in

    persons who _____.
    You are not allowed to give a suppository for

    _____.

73. When the person needs to have a bowel elimination, you can provide comfort and privacy when you
    A. _____
    B. _____
    C. _____
    D. _____
    E. _____
    F. _____
    G. _____

Labeling
Answer questions 74-77 using these figures.

74. Name the four colostomies shown.
    A. _____
    B. _____
    C. _____
    D. _____

75. Which colostomy will have the most solid and formed stool? _____

76. Which colostomy will have the most liquid stool?

    _____

77. Which colostomy is a temporary colostomy?

    _____

Answer questions 78-80 using this figure.

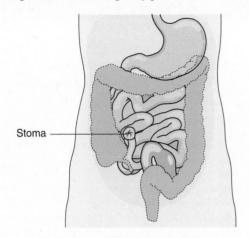

Stoma

78. What type of ostomy is shown?

_____

79. What part of the bowel has been removed?

_____

80. Will the stool from the ostomy be liquid or formed?

_____

Optional Learning Exercises

81. You are caring for Mr. Evans, who is in a semi-private room. His roommate has a large family and many visitors. Mr. Evans has not had a bowel movement in 3 days, even though he is eating well and taking medications to assist elimination. What could be a reason he has not had a bowel movement?

_____

_____

_____

82. Mrs. Weller usually has a bowel movement after breakfast. What are some activities that may assist her to defecate more easily?

_____

_____

83. The nurse tells you to make sure Mr. Johnson eats the high-fiber foods in his diet to assist in his elimination. What foods are high in fiber?

_____

_____

84. Mrs. Shaffer tells you she cannot digest fruits and vegetables and she refuses to eat them. What may be added to her cereal and prune juice to provide fiber?

_____

85. You offer Mr. Murphy _____ of water each day to promote normal bowel elimination.

86. Mr. Hernandez has been taking an antibiotic to treat his pneumonia and he has developed diarrhea. You think he may have diarrhea because

_____

87. You are caring for 83-year-old Mrs. Chen and you helped her to the bathroom 30 minutes ago where she had a bowel movement. When you enter her room to make her bed, she tells you she needs to use the bathroom for a bowel movement. You know that older

people _____

_____

_____

88. Why can tap water enemas be dangerous? _____

_____

How many tap water enemas can be given? _____
Why? _____

_____

89. Compare small-volume enemas and oil-retention enemas.

A. Small-volume enemas _____
the rectum. This causes _____.
Oil-retention enemas are given to

_____

B. Small-volume enemas take effect in about
_____ minutes.
Oil-retention enemas should be retained for at

least _____ minutes.

27 Nutrition and Fluids

Fill in the Blank: Key Terms

Anorexia	Cholesterol	Edema	Intake	Nutrition
Aspiration	Dehydration	Graduate	Nutrient	Output
Calorie	Dysphagia	Hydration		

1. Having an adequate amount of water in body tissues is _____.

2. _____ is the amount of fluid taken in.

3. The loss of appetite is

   _____.

4. The amount of fluid lost is

   _____.

5. A substance that is ingested, digested, absorbed, and used by the body is a

   _____.

6. _____ is difficulty or discomfort in swallowing.

7. The breathing of fluid, food, vomitus, or an object into the lungs is _____.

8. The many processes involved in the ingestion, digestion, absorption, and use of food and fluids by the body is _____.

9. The amount of energy produced from the burning of food by the body is a _____.

10. A decrease in the amount of water in body tissues is

    _____.

11. A _____ is a calibrated container used to measure fluid.

12. _____ is the swelling of body tissues with water.

13. A soft, waxy substance found in the bloodstream and all body cells is _____.

Circle the Best Answer

14. Which of these occur when the person has a poor diet and poor eating habits?
    A. Decreased risk for infection and chronic diseases
    B. Wounds heal well
    C. Increased risk for accidents and injuries
    D. Decreased risk of acute and chronic infections

15. Body fuel for energy is found in
    A. Vitamins
    B. Minerals
    C. Fats, proteins, and carbohydrates
    D. Water

16. All of these food choices are included in MyPlate *except*
    A. Eating high-fat foods
    B. Making half of your plate fruits and vegetables
    C. Avoiding over-sized portions
    D. Drinking water instead of sugary drinks

17. The amount needed from each food group in MyPlate depends on
    A. The ethnic background of the person
    B. The age, sex, and physical activity of the person
    C. The likes and dislikes of the person
    D. The budget available to the person

18. Whole grains in the grain group include
    A. Bulgur, oatmeal, and brown rice
    B. White flour and white rice
    C. Black beans, lentils, and split peas
    D. Potatoes, green bananas, and water chestnuts

19. When choosing from the protein food group, foods that may have a higher risk for heart disease are those
    A. Lower in calories
    B. Higher in iron, zinc, and magnesium
    C. That are lean or low-fat meats and poultry
    D. That are high in fat and cholesterol

20. All of these are food group in MyPlate *except*
    A. Grains   C. Fruits
    B. Vegetables   D. Oils

21. An example of moderate physical activity in MyPlate is
    A. Bicycling at less than 10 miles per hour
    B. Freestyle swimming laps
    C. Chopping wood
    D. Running and jogging at 5 miles per hour

22. Which nutrient is needed for tissue growth and repair?
    A. Carbohydrates   C. Vitamins
    B. Fats   D. Protein

23. Which vitamin is needed for the formation of substances that hold tissue together?
    A. Vitamin K
    B. Vitamin C
    C. Vitamin A
    D. Vitamin B_{12}

24. Food labels have all of this information *except*
    A. The serving size
    B. All vitamins and minerals in the food
    C. Total amount of fat and amount of saturated and trans fats
    D. Amount of cholesterol and sodium

25. A cultural group that eats a diet high in sodium is in
    A. The Philippines
    B. China
    C. Poland
    D. Mexico

26. All pork and pork products are forbidden by
    A. Seventh Day Adventists
    B. Muslims or Islam
    C. The Church of Jesus Christ of Latter-Day Saints
    D. Roman Catholics

27. People with limited incomes often buy
    A. More protein foods
    B. Carbohydrate foods
    C. Foods high in vitamins and minerals
    D. Fatty foods

28. When people buy cheaper foods, the diet may lack
    A. Fats
    B. Starch
    C. Protein and certain vitamins and minerals
    D. Sugars

29. Appetite can be stimulated by
    A. Illness and medications
    B. Decreased senses of taste and smell
    C. Aromas and thoughts of food
    D. Anxiety, pain, and depression

30. During illness
    A. Appetite increases
    B. Fewer nutrients are needed
    C. Nutritional needs increase to fight infection and heal tissue
    D. The person will prefer protein foods

31. All of these may occur with aging *except*
    A. Increases in taste and smell
    B. Decrease in secretion of digestive juices
    C. Difficulty in chewing
    D. A need for fewer calories than younger people

32. Requirements for food served in nursing centers are made by
    A. The FDA
    B. OBRA
    C. The nursing center
    D. The public health department

33. All of these are requirements for food served in long-term care centers *except*
    A. The center provides needed adaptive equipment and utensils
    B. The person's diet is well balanced, nourishing, and tastes good
    C. All food is served at room temperature
    D. Each person must receive at least 3 meals a day and be offered a bedtime snack

34. A general diet
    A. Is ordered for a person with difficulty swallowing
    B. Has no dietary limits or restrictions
    C. May have restricted amounts of sodium
    D. Increases the amount of sugar in the diet

35. The body needs no more than _____ of sodium each day.
    A. 2300 mg
    B. 3000 mg
    C. 5000 mg
    D. 1000 mg

36. When the body tissues swell with water, what organ has to work harder?
    A. Kidneys
    B. Liver
    C. Heart
    D. Lungs

37. When you are caring for a person with diabetes, you should do all of these *except*
    A. Serve the person's meals and snacks on time
    B. Tell the nurse what the person did and did not eat
    C. Give the person extra food and snacks whenever it is requested
    D. Provide between-meal nourishment if all of the food was not eaten

38. A person may be given a mechanical soft diet because
    A. The person is over-weight
    B. The person has chewing problems
    C. The person has been advanced from a clear-liquid diet
    D. The person has constipation

39. If you are serving a meal to a person on a fiber- and residue-restricted diet, the meal would *not* include
    A. Raw fruits and vegetables
    B. Strained fruit juices
    C. Canned or cooked fruit without skin or seeds
    D. Plain pasta

40. A person who has serious burns would receive a
    A. Sodium-controlled diet
    B. Fat-controlled diet
    C. High-calorie diet
    D. High-protein diet

41. When a person has dysphagia, the thickness of the food served is chosen by the
    A. Person
    B. Nursing assistant
    C. Family
    D. Speech-language pathologist, occupational therapist, dietitian, and doctor or nurse

42. All of these may be a sign of a swallowing problem (dysphagia) *except*
    A. Person complains that food will not go down or that food is stuck
    B. Foods that need chewing are avoided
    C. There is excessive drooling of saliva
    D. Person is able to eat a regular diet without problems

43. When assisting a person who is on aspiration precautions, you can help to prevent aspiration while the person is eating by placing him or her in
    A. Semi-Fowler's position
    B. As upright a position as the nurse and care plan direct
    C. The side-lying position
    D. The supine position

44. If fluid intake exceeds fluid output, the person will
    A. Have edema (swelling) in the tissues
    B. Be dehydrated
    C. Have vomiting and diarrhea
    D. Have increased urinary output

45. How much fluid is needed every day for normal fluid balance?
    A. 1500 mL
    B. 1000 to 1500 mL
    C. 2000 to 2500 mL
    D. 3000 to 4000 mL

46. If the person you are caring for has an order for restricted fluids, which of these should you do?
    A. Offer a variety of liquids.
    B. Thicken all fluids.
    C. Remove the water mug or keep it out of sight.
    D. Do not allow the person to swallow any liquids during oral hygiene.

47. When you are keeping I&O records, you should measure all of these as intake *except*
    A. Milk, water, coffee, and tea
    B. Mashed potatoes and creamed vegetables
    C. Soups and gelatin
    D. Ice cream, custard, and pudding

48. When you are measuring I&O, you need to know that 1 ounce equals
    A. 10 mL
    B. 500 mL
    C. 100 mL
    D. 30 mL

49. When you are using the graduate to measure output, you read the amount by
    A. Holding the graduate at waist level and reading the amount
    B. Looking at the graduate while it is held above eye level
    C. Placing the graduate at eye level to read it
    D. Setting the graduate on the floor and reading it

50. When I&O is ordered, which of the following is *not* included in the measurement?
    A. Urine
    B. Solid stool
    C. Drainage from suction
    D. Vomitus

51. When residents are served meals in a family dining program
    A. They serve themselves as at home
    B. The person can eat any time the buffet is open
    C. Meal time distractions are prevented
    D. Food is served as in a restaurant

52. Which of the following needs to be done before the person is served a meal?
    A. Give complete personal care.
    B. Change all linens.
    C. Check the person's position.
    D. Make sure the person has been shaved or has make-up applied.

53. You can provide comfort during meals by doing all of these *except*
    A. Making sure unpleasant sights, sounds, and odors are removed
    B. Making sure dentures, eyeglasses, or hearing aids are in place
    C. Giving the person good oral care before and after meals
    D. Giving complete personal hygiene and a linen change

54. What should you do if a food tray has not been served within 15 minutes?
    A. Re-check the food temperatures.
    B. Serve the tray immediately.
    C. Throw the food away.
    D. Serve only the cold items on the tray.

55. How can you make sure the food tray is complete?
    A. Ask the person being served.
    B. Ask the nurse.
    C. Call the dietary department.
    D. Check items on the tray with the dietary card.

56. If you become impatient while feeding a resident with dementia, you should
    A. Refuse to continue caring for the person
    B. Return the person to his or her room
    C. Talk to the nurse
    D. Make the person eat his or her food

57. When you are feeding a person, you should
    A. Not allow the person to assist
    B. Give the person a fork and knife to assist with cutting the food
    C. Feed the person in a private area to maintain confidentiality
    D. Use a teaspoon because it is less likely to cause injury

58. When feeding a person, liquids are given
    A. Only at the start of feeding
    B. During the meal, alternating with solid foods
    C. At the end of the meal when all solids have been eaten
    D. Only if the person has difficulty swallowing

59. When delegated to provide drinking water, what information do you need from the nurse and the care plan?
    A. Whether a person likes water
    B. If a person can have ice
    C. Whether a person can pour water himself or herself
    D. How often to refill the mug

60. When re-heating cooked foods, it should be heated
    A. To room temperature
    B. According to agency policy
    C. To 212°F
    D. To the temperature the person requests

61. A safe temperature for hot foods is
    A. 40°F or below
    B. 212°F or higher
    C. 140°F or higher
    D. Room temperature for up to 4 hours

Fill in the Blank

62. Write out the abbreviations.

A. F _____

B. FDA _____

C. GI _____

D. ID _____

E. I&O _____

F. mg _____

G. mL _____

H. NPO _____

I. OBRA _____

J. oz _____

K. USDA _____

63. How many calories are in each of these?

A. 1 gram of fat _____

B. 1 gram of protein _____

C. 1 gram of carbohydrate _____

Use the Dietary Guidelines for Americans, 2010 to answer questions 64-67.

64. The *Dietary Guidelines for Americans* are for persons

A. _____

B. _____

65. Certain diseases are linked to poor diet and lack of physical activity. They are

A. _____

B. _____

C. _____

D. _____

E. _____

F. _____

66. The *Dietary Guidelines* help people

A. _____

B. _____

C. _____

67. The *Dietary Guidelines* focus on

A. _____

B. _____

C. _____

Questions 68-71 relate to MyPlate.

68. What are the 5 food groups in MyPlate?

A. _____

B. _____

C. _____

D. _____

E. _____

69. When using MyPlate, calories are balanced by

A. _____

B. _____

70. When making food choices, which foods are increased in the diet?

A. _____

B. _____

C. _____

71. Which food group or groups has the following health benefits?

A. Builds and maintains bone mass throughout life

_____

B. Provide B vitamins and vitamin E

_____

C. May prevent constipation

_____

D. May reduce risk of kidney stones _____ or

E. May prevent birth defects

_____

F. May help lower calorie intake _____

or _____

G. Provides nutrients needed for health and body maintenance _____

72. What is the most important nutrient?

_____

73. If dietary fat is not needed by the body, it is stored as

_____.

74. What is the function of each of these nutrients?

A. Protein _____

B. Carbohydrates _____

C. Fats _____

D. Vitamins _____

E. Minerals _____

F. Water _____

75. Which vitamins can be stored by the body?

_____

76. Which vitamins must be ingested daily?

_____

77. What vitamin is important for these functions? *Formation of substances that hold tissues together; healthy blood vessels, skin, gums, bones, and teeth; wound healing; prevention of bleeding; resistance to infection*

_____

78. Milk and milk products, liver, green leafy vegetables, eggs, breads, and cereals are good sources of which vitamin? _____

79. What mineral allows red blood cells to carry oxygen?

_____

80. When the diet does not have enough

_____, it may affect nerve function, muscle contraction, and heart function.

81. Calcium is needed for _____

_____.

82. What information is found on food labels?

    A. _____

    B. _____

    C. _____

83. Those who practice _____ as their religion eat only fish with scales and fins.

84. Alcohol and coffee are avoided or not allowed by these religious groups.

    A. _____

    B. _____

    C. _____

85. What religious group may have members that fast from meats on certain Fridays of the year?

    _____

86. Nutritional needs increase during illness when the body must _____

    _____.

87. Older persons need _____ calories than younger people do.

88. Why do the diets of some older people lack protein?

    _____

89. What OBRA requirement relates to the temperature of foods served in long-term care centers?

    _____

    _____

90. What foods are included in a clear-liquid diet?

    _____

    _____

    _____

    _____

91. When the person receives a full-liquid diet, it will include all of the foods on the clear-liquid diet as well as these foods. _____

    _____

92. If a person has poorly fitted dentures and has chewing problems, the doctor may order a

    _____ diet.

93. A person who is constipated and has other GI disorders may receive a _____ diet. The foods in this diet increase the

    _____

    to stimulate _____.

94. If a person is receiving a high-calorie diet, the calorie intake is _____ daily.

95. What vegetable juices are high in sodium?

    _____

96. When a person is receiving a diabetic diet, the same amount of _____ are eaten each day.

97. If you are feeding a person a dysphagia diet, what observations should be reported to the nurse immediately?

    A. _____, _____, or _____ during or after meal

    B. _____ or _____

98. Why is it important to offer water often to older persons? _____

    _____

99. When you give oral hygiene to a person who is receiving nothing by mouth, the person must not _____.

100. List the amount of milliliters in the following.

    A. 1 ounce equals _____ mL

    B. 1 pint equals about _____ mL

    C. 1 quart equals about _____ mL

101. What information do you need when you are delegated to measure intake and output?

    A. _____

    B. _____

    C. _____

    D. _____

    E. _____

102. What 2 types of dining programs may be used with persons who are quietly confused?

    _____

103. What can be done to promote comfort when preparing residents for meals?

    A. _____

    B. _____

    C. _____

    D. _____

    E. _____

    F. _____

104. If a food tray is not served within 15 minutes, what should be checked? _____

105. When you are delegated to serve meal trays, what information do you need from the nurse or care plan?

    A. _____

    B. _____

    C. _____

    D. _____

    E. _____

    F. _____

    G. _____

106. When you are serving meal trays, you make sure the right person gets the right tray by

    A. _____

    B. _____

107. When you are feeding a person, the spoon should be filled _____.

108. Why is it important to sit facing the person when you feed him or her?

   A. _____

   B. _____

   C. _____

109. What should be reported after you have fed a person?

   A. _____

   B. _____

   C. _____

   D. _____

110. Explain each of the concepts below that are recommended by the USDA to keep food safe.

   A. Clean _____

   _____

   B. Separate _____

   _____

   C. Cook _____

   _____

   D. Chill _____

   _____

111. The safe temperature to keep foods at are

   A. Cold foods _____

   B. Hot foods _____

   C. The danger zone for foods is

   _____ for more than

   _____ hours or

   _____ hour if temperature is warmer than 90°F

   D. Keep the refrigerator at _____ or below. Keep the freezer at _____ or below.

Use the FOCUS ON PRIDE section to complete these statements.

112. When a nursing center uses 24-hour catering or mobile food carts, it allows the residents to have freedom and _____.

113. When you respect the person's likes and dislikes of food or complaints about the food, it meets the right to _____.

114. When family members bring food to a resident, it is important that you tell _____. The food must not interfere with the _____.

Labeling

115. Enter the information below on the Intake and Output record. Total amounts for the 8-hour and 24-hour periods. Amounts in () indicate how much the person ate or drank. (Use 2400–0800, 0800–1600, and 1600–2400 as 8-hour periods.)

OSF℠ ST. JOSEPH MEDICAL CENTER

Bloomington, Illinois

DATE _____

FLUID BALANCE CHART

Water Glass	250cc	Ice Cream	120cc	
Styrofoam Cup	180cc	Ice Chips	1/2 amt. of cc's in cup	
Cup (coffee)	250cc			
Milk Carton	240cc	Pitcher		
Pop (1 can)	360cc	(Yellow)	1000cc	
Broth-Soup	175cc			
Juice Carton	120cc			
Juice Glass	120cc			
Jello	120cc			

TIME	ORAL	Parenteral	Amt. cc Absbd.	URINE Method Collected	URINE Amt. (cc)	OTHER Method Collected	OTHER Amt. (cc)	CONT. IRRIGATION In	CONT. IRRIGATION Out
2400-0100		cc from previous shift							
0100-0200									
0200-0300									
0300-0400									
0400-0500									
0500-0600									
0600-0700									
0700-0800									
		8 - hour Sub-total		8-hr T		8-hr T			
0800-0900		cc from previous shift							
0900-1000									
1000-1100									
1100-1200									
1200-1300									
1300-1400									
1400-1500									
1500-1600									
		8 - hour Sub-total		8-hr T		8-hr T			
1600-1700		cc from previous shift							
1700-1800									
1800-1900									
1900-2000									
2000-2100									
2100-2200									
2200-2300									
2300-2400									
		8 - hour Sub-total		8-hr T		8-hr T			
		24 - hour Sub-total		24-hr T		24-hr T			

Source Key:

URINE

V - Voided
C - Catheter
INC - Incontinent
U.C. - Ureteral Catheter

Source Key:

OTHER

G.I.T. - Gastric Intestinal Tube
T.T. - T. Tube
Vom. - Vomitus
Liq S. - Liquid Stool
H.V. - Hemovac

310' Marie Mills

Form No. MF36722 (Rev. 5/97) *MFI*

Modified from OSF St. Joseph Medical Center, Bloomington, Ill.

0200	Voided	300 mL	1530	Vomited	50 mL
0600	Voided	500 mL	1545	1 can of soda	(whole can)
0730	**Breakfast**		1730	**Dinner**	
	Orange juice	(whole glass)		Soup	(whole bowl)
	Milk	(½ carton)		Tea	(1 cup)
	Coffee	(1 cup)		Juice	(whole glass)
0700	Voided	300 mL		Ice cream	(all)
1000	Water pitcher filled		1730	Voided	250 mL
1130	**Lunch**		1830	Vomited	100 mL
	Soup	(whole bowl)	1915	Voided	500 mL
	Milk	(½ carton)	2000	Milk	(1 carton)
	Tea	(1 cup)	2015	Voided	300 mL
	Jello	(1 serving)	2330	Voided	200 mL
1330	Voided	450 mL			
1430	Water pitcher (refilled)	500 mL			

116. Label the plate in the figure with numbers so that you can describe the location of food to a blind person. What would you tell a visually impaired person who asks you where to find these food items on the plate?

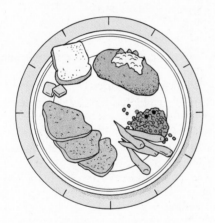

A. Bread _____

B. Baked potato _____

C. Vegetables _____

D. Meat _____

Optional Learning Exercises

117. This is a person's food intake for one day. Place the foods in the correct food groups on MyPlate.

BREAKFAST
¾ cup Orange juice
1 cup Oatmeal
2 slices Toast
¼ cup Milk
2 cups Black coffee

LUNCH
1 cup Tomato soup
Grilled cheese sandwich
½ cup Applesauce
Can of regular soda
Candy bar

DINNER
2–4 oz. Pork chops
Baked potato/butter
¼ cup Green beans
2 Brownies
2 cups Black coffee

SNACKS
1 Apple
1 4-ounce bag Potato chips
⅓ cup Nuts
Can of regular soda
½ cup Ice cream

A. Grains _____

_____

B. Vegetables _____

_____

C. Fruits _____

_____

D. Dairy _____

_____

E. Proteins _____

F. Oils _____

_____

G. Other _____

_____

Fill in the Blank: Key Terms

Aspiration	Gavage	Naso-enteral tube	Percutaneous endoscopic
Enteral nutrition	Intravenous (IV) therapy	Naso-gastric (NG) tube	gastrostomy (PEG) tube
Flow rate	Jejunostomy tube	Parenteral nutrition	Regurgitation
Gastrostomy tube			

1. Giving nutrients into the gastro-intestinal (GI) tract through a feeding tube is

   _____.

2. A _____ is a tube inserted through a surgically created opening in the stomach.

3. _____ is the backward flow of stomach contents into the mouth.

4. A _____ is a feeding tube inserted into a surgically created opening in the jejunum of the small intestine.

5. The process of giving a tube feeding is called

   _____.

6. The _____ is the number of drops per minute.

7. _____ is breathing fluid, food, vomitus, or an object into the lungs.

8. Giving nutrients through a catheter inserted into a vein is _____.

9. _____ is giving fluids through a needle or catheter inserted into a vein.

10. A feeding tube inserted through the nose into the stomach is a _____.

11. A _____ is a feeding tube inserted into the stomach through a small incision made through the skin.

12. A feeding tube inserted through the nose into the small bowel is a _____.

Circle the Best Answer

13. The doctor may order nutritional support for a person who
    A. Cannot eat enough to meet his or her nutritional needs
    B. Has a problem swallowing
    C. Refuses to eat or drink
    D. All of the above

14. Which of these tubes are used for short-term nutritional support?
    A. Naso-gastric tubes
    B. Gastrostomy tubes
    C. Jejunostomy tubes
    D. PEG tubes

15. Opened formula for a tube feeding can remain at room temperature for
    A. 1 hour
    B. About 8 hours
    C. About 4 hours
    D. Overnight

16. If a person is receiving intermittent (scheduled) feedings, the nurse will
    A. Attach the feeding to a pump
    B. Give feeding 4 or more times each day
    C. Give the feedings over a 24-hour period
    D. Give the feeding directly from the refrigerator

17. A major risk with tube feedings is
    A. Nausea
    B. Complaints of flatulence
    C. Aspiration
    D. Elevated temperature

18. If a person is receiving a tube feeding, you should report at once
    A. Elevated blood pressure
    B. Signs and symptoms of respiratory distress
    C. A normal pulse rate
    D. That the person is sleeping

19. You can help to prevent regurgitation when a person is receiving gavage when you
    A. Position the person in a left side-lying position
    B. Maintain Fowler's or semi-Fowler's position after the feeding
    C. Position the person in a supine position
    D. Position the person in prone position

20. When a person is receiving nutrition through a tube, frequent mouth care is needed because
    A. It stimulates peristalsis to aid digestion
    B. It prevents discomfort from dry mouth, dry lips, and sore throat
    C. It provides additional fluid intake
    D. It provides additional nutrition

21. Which of these are *never* done by nursing assistants?
    A. Insert a feeding tube or check it for placement.
    B. Remove a feeding tube.
    C. Give tube feedings.
    D. Clean area around a feeding tube.

22. When a person is receiving TPN, the nursing assistant would assist by
    A. Removing the tube
    B. Inserting the tube
    C. Providing frequent oral hygiene and other basic needs
    D. Giving the feedings

23. When caring for a person receiving IV therapy, the nursing assistant can
    A. Adjust the flow rate if it is too fast or too slow
    B. Tell the nurse at once if no fluid is dripping
    C. Disconnect the IV to give basic care
    D. Change the IV bag when it is empty

24. You may change a dressing on a peripheral IV if
    A. The nurse asks you to do this
    B. You observe that it is loose and soiled
    C. Your state and agency allows nursing assistants to perform the procedure
    D. You think you know how to do this procedure

Fill in the Blank

25. Write out the abbreviations.
    A. GI _____
    B. gtt _____
    C. gtt/min _____
    D. IV _____
    E. mL _____
    F. mL/hr _____
    G. NG _____
    H. NPO _____
    I. oz _____
    J. PEG _____
    K. TPN _____

26. Naso-gastric and naso-enteral tubes are in place for short-term nutritional support, usually for less than _____.

27. Gastrostomy, jejunostomy, and PEG tubes are used for long-term support, usually longer than _____.

28. Formula is given through a feeding tube at room temperature because cold fluids cause _____.

29. It shows good teamwork when you warm a container of formula by placing it _____.

30. Coughing, sneezing, vomiting, suctioning, and poor positioning can move a tube out of place and are common causes of _____.

31. What can the nursing assistant do to assist the nurse in preventing regurgitation and aspiration?
    A. _____
    B. _____
    C. _____

32. What comfort measures will help a person with a feeding tube who has a dry mouth?
    A. _____
    B. _____
    C. _____

33. The nose and nostrils are cleaned every 4 to 8 hours because a feeding tube can _____ and _____.

34. If you are delegated to give a tube feeding, the nurse should
    A. Check _____ and residual _____
    B. Tell you what feeding method to use _____ , _____ , or _____
    C. Tell you how to position the person _____ or _____

35. How much flushing solution is used before giving a tube feeding to an adult? _____

36. Parenteral nutrition solution given intravenously contains _____.

37. When caring for a person receiving IV therapy, what signs and symptoms of complications may occur at the IV site?
    A. _____
    B. _____
    C. _____
    D. _____
    E. _____
    F. _____

Use the FOCUS ON PRIDE section to complete these statements.

38. You have a responsibility when a person has an IV. You follow the ethics and laws.
    A. When you hear an alarm, _____
    B. If the battery is low, _____.
    C. You DO NOT adjust _____ on IV pumps or _____ on IV tubing.

Optional Learning Exercises

39. What type of feeding tube would each of these persons probably have in place?
    A. The nurse tells you Mr. S is expected to have a feeding tube to his stomach for 2 to 3 weeks. _____
    B. Mrs. G. has had a feeding tube inserted into her stomach for 9 months. _____ or _____
    C. The nurse tells you to observe Mr. H. for irritation of his nose and nostrils when you give care. _____ or _____
    D. The nurse tells you that Mrs. K. is at great risk for regurgitation from her feeding tube. _____ or _____

40. When you are assisting with tube feedings, why do you turn the lights on in a dark room before beginning?

    _____

    _____

41. You are caring for a person receiving a continuous tube feeding. You note that the formula was hung 7¾ hours ago, so you tell the nurse. Why did you report this to the nurse?

    _____

    _____

42. Why are older persons more at risk for regurgitation and aspiration?
    A. _____
    B. _____

43. What would you do if a person with a feeding tube asks you for something to eat or drink?

    _____ Why?

    _____

    _____

44. Mrs. H. has a feeding tube in her nose. Answer these questions about caring for her nose and nostrils.
    A. How often should the nose and nostrils be cleaned?

       _____

    B. How is the tube secured to the nose?

       _____

    C. Why is the tube secured to the person's garment at the shoulder?

       _____

       _____

    D. What are 2 ways the tube can be secured at the shoulder?
       i. _____
       ii. _____

45. If a person is receiving TPN, how will you assist the nurse?
    A. _____
    B. _____
    C. _____

46. How can you check the flow rate of an IV?

    _____

47. What would you tell the RN at once when you check the flow rate?
    A. _____
    B. _____
    C. _____
    D. _____

29 Measuring Vital Signs

Fill in the Blank: Key Terms

Afebrile	Diastolic pressure	Pulse deficit	Systolic pressure
Apical-radial pulse	Febrile	Pulse rate	Tachycardia
Blood pressure	Fever	Respiration	Thermometer
Body temperature	Hypertension	Sphygmomanometer	Vital signs
Bradycardia	Hypotension	Stethoscope	
Diastole	Pulse	Systole	

1. _____ means with a fever.

2. A rapid heart rate is _____.
   The heart rate is over 100 beats per minute.

3. The _____ is taking the apical and radial pulse at the same time.

4. An instrument used to listen to the sounds produced by the heart, lungs, and other body organs is a _____.

5. When the systolic blood pressure is below 90 mm Hg and the diastolic pressure is below 60 mm Hg it is called _____.

6. The _____ is the number of heartbeats or pulses felt in 1 minute.

7. The amount of heat in the body that is a balance between the amount of heat produced and amount lost by the body is the _____.

8. _____ is the period of heart muscle contraction.

9. _____ is when the blood pressure measurements remain above a systolic pressure of 140 mm Hg or a diastolic pressure of 90 mm Hg.

10. The cuff and measuring device used to measure blood pressure is a _____.

11. The beat of the heart felt at an artery as a wave of blood passes through the artery is the _____.

12. Without a fever is _____.

13. Temperature, pulse, respirations, and blood pressure are _____.

14. _____ is a slow heart rate; the rate is less than 60 beats per minute.

15. The amount of force it takes to pump blood out of the heart into the arterial circulation is the _____.

16. The period of heart muscle relaxation is _____.

17. The difference between the apical and radial pulse rates is the _____.

18. _____ is the amount of force exerted against the walls of an artery by the blood.

19. Breathing air into and out of the lungs is _____.

20. _____ is the pressure in the arteries when the heart is at rest.

21. Elevated body temperature is _____.

22. A _____ is a device used to measure temperature.

Circle the Best Answer

23. Persons in nursing centers usually have vital signs measured
    A. Once a shift
    B. Every 4 hours
    C. Once a month
    D. Weekly

24. Unless otherwise ordered, take vital signs when the person
    A. Is lying or sitting
    B. Has been walking or exercising
    C. Has just finished eating
    D. Is getting ready to take a shower or tub bath

25. Body temperature is lower in the
    A. Afternoon
    B. Morning
    C. Evening
    D. Night

26. If you are taking vital signs on a person with dementia, it may be better if
    A. You have a co-worker hold the person so he or she does not move
    B. The vital signs are taken when the person is asleep
    C. You take the pulse and respirations at one time, and the temperature and blood pressure at another time
    D. You ask the nurse to take the vital signs

27. What should you do if a person asks for their vital sign measurements?
    A. You can tell the person the measurements if center policy allows.
    B. Tell the nurse that the person wants to know the measurements.
    C. Tell the person you cannot tell them this information.
    D. This information is private and cannot be shared.

28. If you take a rectal temperature, the normal range of the temperature would be
    A. 96.6 °F to 98.6 °F (35.9 °C to 37.0 °C)
    B. 97.6 °F to 99.6 °F (36.5 °C to 37.5 °C)
    C. 98.6 °F to 100.6 °F (37.0 °C to 38.1 °C)
    D. 98.6 °F (37 °C)

29. If you are taking the temperature of an older person, you would expect the temperature to be
    A. Lower than the normal range
    B. Higher than the normal range
    C. About in the middle of the normal range
    D. The same as in a younger adult

30. A glass rectal thermometer has
    A. A stubby tip color-coded in red
    B. A long or slender tip
    C. A pear-shaped tip
    D. A blue color-coded end

31. To read a glass thermometer you should hold it at the
    A. Stem above eye level and look up to read it
    B. Bulb end and bring it to eye level to read it
    C. Stem and bring it to eye level to read it
    D. Bulb at waist level and look down to read it

32. If you are preparing to take an oral temperature, ask the person not to
    A. Eat, drink, smoke, or chew gum for at least 15 to 20 minutes
    B. Shower or bathe right before the temperature is taken
    C. Exercise for 30 minutes before
    D. Eat, drink, or smoke for at least 5 to 10 minutes

33. An electronic thermometer is inserted into the rectum
    A. 1 inch
    B. 2 inches
    C. ½ inch
    D. 3 inches

34. When taking a temperature for persons who are confused and resist care, the best choice would be to
    A. Take a rectal temperature
    B. Use a glass oral thermometer
    C. Take an axillary temperature
    D. Use a tympanic or temporal artery thermometer

35. Which pulse is most commonly used?
    A. Carotid
    B. Brachial
    C. Radial
    D. Popliteal

36. A _____ pulse is taken during cardiopulmonary resuscitation (CPR).
    A. Carotid
    B. Temporal
    C. Femoral
    D. Radial

37. When using a stethoscope, you can help to prevent infection by
    A. Warming the diaphragm in your hand
    B. Wiping the ear-pieces and diaphragm with antiseptic wipes before and after use
    C. Placing the diaphragm over the artery
    D. Placing the ear-pieces in your ears so the bend of the tips point forward

38. When a pulse rate is 120 beats per minute, you
    A. Report that the person has bradycardia
    B. Know that this is a normal pulse rate
    C. Report that the person has tachycardia
    D. Report that the pulse is irregular

39. The pulse rate is the number of heartbeats or pulses felt in
    A. 30 seconds
    B. 15 seconds
    C. 1 minute
    D. 5 minutes

40. You need to feel the pulse to determine the
    A. Force
    B. Rate
    C. Rhythm (whether it is regular or irregular)
    D. Blood pressure

41. When taking the radial pulse, place
    A. The thumb over the pulse site
    B. Two or three fingers on the middle of the wrist
    C. Two or three fingers on the thumb side of the wrist over the radial artery
    D. The stethoscope on the chest wall

42. You may count the radial pulse for 30 seconds and multiple by 2 if
    A. The pulse is irregular
    B. You lose count after 30 seconds
    C. The pulse is regular
    D. The doctor's order permits counting for 30 seconds

43. The apical pulse is taken
    A. For a full minute
    B. At least once a day for all persons
    C. On persons who have a regular heartbeat
    D. For 30 seconds and multiplied by 2

44. An apical pulse of 72 is recorded as
    A. Pulse 72
    B. 72 – Apical pulse
    C. 72Ap
    D. P 72

45. An apical-radial pulse is taken by
    A. Taking the radial pulse for 1 minute and then taking the apical pulse for 1 minute
    B. Subtracting the apical pulse from the radial pulse
    C. Having one staff member take the apical pulse and a second staff member take the radial pulse at the same time
    D. Having 2 persons take the apical pulse at the same time

46. A pedal pulse is found
    A. By listening to the heart with a stethoscope
    B. Over a foot bone
    C. On the thumb side of the wrist
    D. At the apex of the heart, just below the left nipple

47. When counting respirations, the best way is to
    A. Place your hand on the person's chest and watch the chest rise and fall
    B. Keep your fingers or stethoscope over the pulse site so the person thinks you are still counting the pulse
    C. Tell the person to breathe normally so you can count the respirations
    D. Use the stethoscope to hear the respirations clearly and count for 1 full minute

48. Each respiration involves
    A. 1 inhalation
    B. 1 exhalation
    C. 1 inhalation and 1 exhalation
    D. Counting for 30 seconds and multiplying by 2

49. The blood pressure may be higher in older persons because
    A. They have orthostatic hypotension
    B. Their diet is higher in sodium
    C. Blood pressure increases with age
    D. They are usually over-weight

50. The blood pressure may not be taken
    A. On an arm that has a dialysis access site
    B. If the person is sleeping
    C. If the person is very obese
    D. When the person is sitting in a chair

51. You will find out the size of blood pressure cuff needed
    A. By asking the nurse
    B. By measuring the person's arm
    C. In the doctor's orders
    D. By asking the person

52. When taking the blood pressure, you place the stethoscope diaphragm
    A. Over the radial artery on the thumb side of the wrist
    B. Over the brachial artery at the inner aspect of the elbow
    C. Lightly against the skin
    D. Over the apical pulse site

53. When getting ready to take the blood pressure, position the person's arm
    A. Above the level of the heart
    B. Level with the heart
    C. Below the level of the heart
    D. Abducted from the body

54. The blood pressure cuff is inflated _____ beyond the point where you last felt the radial pulse.
    A. 10 mm Hg   C. 30 mm Hg
    B. 20 mm Hg   D. 40 mm Hg

Fill in the Blank

55. Write out the abbreviations.
    A. BP _____
    B. C _____
    C. DUS _____
    D. F _____
    E. Hg _____
    F. ID _____
    G. IV _____
    H. mm _____
    I. mm Hg _____
    J. TPR _____

56. Vital signs are taken when the person takes drugs that affect _____

57. When vital signs are taken, report to the nurse at once if
    A. _____
    B. _____

58. Sites for measuring temperature are the
    A. _____
    B. _____
    C. _____
    D. _____
    E. _____

59. Which site has the highest normal range temperature?
    _____

60. Which site has the lowest baseline temperature?
    _____

61. If a glass thermometer breaks, _____ at once because it may contain _____, which is a _____.

62. When you read a Fahrenheit thermometer, the short lines mean _____.

63. List how long the glass thermometer remains in place for these sites.
    A. Oral _____ or as required by center policy
    B. Rectal _____ or as required by center policy
    C. Axillary _____ or as required by center policy

64. When taking an oral temperature, place the bulb end of the thermometer
    _____

65. When taking an axillary temperature, the axilla must be _____.

66. Tympanic membrane and temporal artery thermometers are used for confused persons because they are _____.

67. When using an electronic thermometer, what does the color of the probe mean?
    A. Blue _____
    B. Red _____

68. When you take a rectal temperature, you _____ the tip of the thermometer or the end of the covered probe before inserting it into the rectum.

69. When taking a tympanic membrane temperature on an adult, pull up and back on the ear to
    _____

70. The adult pulse rate is between
    _____ beats per minute.

71. List words used to describe:
    A. Forceful pulse _____
    B. Hard-to-feel pulse _____

72. If a pulse is irregular, count the pulse for
    _____

73. When you take a pulse, what observations should be reported and recorded?
    A. _____
    B. _____
    C. _____
    D. _____
    E. _____

74. Do not use your thumb to take a pulse because _____.

75. When taking an apical pulse, each *lub-dub* sound is counted as _____.

76. The apical pulse rate is never less than the _____.

77. The nurse may mark the skin with an X where the _____ is found.

78. A healthy adult has _____ respirations per minutes.

79. What observations should be reported and recorded when counting respirations?
    A. _____
    B. _____
    C. _____
    D. _____
    E. _____
    F. _____

80. One respiration is counted for each _____.

81. Respirations are counted for _____ if they are abnormal or irregular.

82. Blood pressure is controlled by
    A. _____
    B. _____
    C. _____

83. Report blood pressures that have these readings.
    A. Systolic over _____;
       systolic below _____
    B. Diastolic over _____;
       diastolic below _____

84. Let the person rest for _____ before taking the blood pressure.

85. When you are taking a blood pressure, the person should be in a _____ or _____ position. Sometimes the doctor orders blood pressure in the _____ position.

86. When listening to the blood pressure, the first sound you hear is the _____ pressure and the point where the sound disappears is the _____ pressure.

Use the FOCUS ON PRIDE section to complete these statements.

87. Measurements of the vital signs is important because they help the nurse _____ and _____ the person's care.

88. You are responsible for
    A. Knowing _____
    B. Reporting _____

89. You allow the person to have _____ when you use the arm for blood pressure or pulse that the person prefers.

90. If you cannot feel a pulse or hear a blood pressure, you should never _____.

Labeling

91. Identify the type of thermometers shown
    A. _____
    B. _____
    C. _____
    D. An axillary or oral temperature can be taken with _____ thermometers.
    E. A rectal temperature is taken with a _____ thermometer.

92. Fill in the drawings so that the thermometers read correctly.
    A   95.8° F
    B   98.4° F
    C   100.2° F
    D   35.5° C
    E   36.5° C
    F   37° C

93. Name the pulse sites shown.

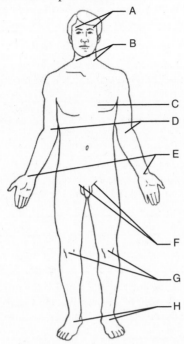

A. _____

B. _____

C. _____

D. _____

E. _____

F. _____

G. _____

H. _____

I. Which pulse is used during cardiopulmonary resuscitation (CPR)?

_____

J. Which pulse is most commonly taken?

_____

K. Which pulse is used when placing the stethoscope to take the blood pressure?

_____

L. Which pulse is found with a stethoscope?

_____

94. Fill in the drawings so that the dials show the correct blood pressures.

A   168/102

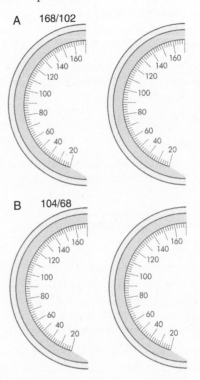

B   104/68

95. Fill in the drawings so that the mercury columns show the correct blood pressures.

A   152/86

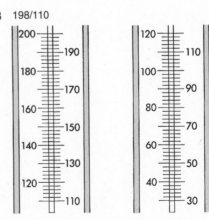

B   198/110

Optional Learning Exercises

Taking Temperatures

96. You prepare to take Mr. Harrison's temperature with a glass thermometer. When you take the thermometer from the container, it reads 97.8 °F. What should you do? _____

97. If the thermometer registers between 2 short lines, record the temperature to the

_____

Taking Pulses and Respirations

98. You are assigned to take Mrs. Sanchez's pulse and respirations. You note that the pulse rate and respirations are regular, so you take each

one for _____. When you complete counting the pulse, you keep

your _____ and count

_____. This is done so that

Mrs. Sanchez will _____.

99. When you finish counting Mrs. Sanchez's pulse and respirations, your numbers are pulse 36 and respirations 9. What numbers should be recorded?

Pulse _____ Respirations _____

Why? _____

100. The nurse tells you to take an apical-radial pulse on Mrs. Hellman. Why do you ask a co-worker to help

you? _____

101. How long is an apical-radial pulse counted?

_____ After you have taken the apical-radial pulse, how do you find the pulse deficit?

_____

_____

Taking Blood Pressures

102. You are assigned to take Mr. Hardaway's blood pressure. You know that he goes for dialysis 3 times a week. What do you need to know before you take his

blood pressure? _____

_____

Why? _____

_____

103. When you inflate the cuff, you cannot feel the pulse after you pump the cuff to 130 mm Hg. How high will you inflate the cuff to take his blood pressure?

_____

104. You should deflate the cuff at an even rate of

_____ per second.

30 Exercise and Activity

Fill in the Blank: Key Terms

Abduction	Deconditioning	Footdrop	Orthotic device	Rotation
Adduction	Dorsiflexion	Hyperextension	Plantar flexion	Supination
Ambulation	Extension	Internal rotation	Postural hypotension	Syncope
Atrophy	External rotation	Opposition	Pronation	
Contracture	Flexion	Orthostatic hypotension	Range of motion (ROM)	

1. Touching the opposite finger with the thumb is
   _____.

2. The foot is bent down at the ankle when
   _____ is present.

3. A brief loss of consciousness or fainting is
   _____.

4. Bending a body part is
   _____.

5. Moving a body part away from the mid-line of the
   body is _____.

6. _____ is
   the movement of a joint to the extent possible without
   causing pain.

7. Turning the joint outward is
   _____.

8. A drop in blood pressure when the person suddenly
   stands up is postural hypotension or
   _____.

9. _____ occurs when
   moving a body part toward the mid-line of the body.

10. Turning the joint upward is called
    _____.

11. Bending the toes and foot up at the ankle is
    _____.

12. Excessive straightening of a body part is
    _____.

13. A decrease in size or a wasting away of tissue is
    _____.

14. Turning the joint is
    _____.

15. _____ is straightening
    of a body part.

16. _____ is another name
    for orthostatic hypotension.

17. _____ is permanent
    plantar flexion; the foot falls down at the ankle.

18. The act of walking is
    _____.

19. _____ is turning the
    joint downward.

20. The loss of muscle strength from inactivity is
    _____.

21. _____ is turning
    the joint inward.

22. The lack of joint mobility caused by abnormal
    shortening of a muscle is a
    _____.

23. A device used to support a muscle, promote a certain
    motion, or correct a deformity is an
    _____.

Circle the Best Answer

24. If a person is on bedrest, he or she
    A. May be allowed to perform some activities of daily
       living (ADL)
    B. Can use the bedside commode for elimination needs
    C. May not perform any ADL
    D. Can use the bathroom for elimination needs

25. Complications of bedrest include all of these *except*
    A. Contractures in fingers, wrists, knees, and hips
    B. Muscle atrophy
    C. Increased appetite and improved muscle strength
    D. Orthostatic hypotension and syncope

26. If a contracture develops
    A. It will require extra range-of-motion exercises to
       correct it
    B. You need to position the person in good body
       alignment
    C. The contracted muscle is fixed into position, is
       deformed, and cannot stretch
    D. It will be relieved as soon as the person is able to
       walk and exercise

27. When you are caring for a person who has orthostatic
    hypotension, you should
    A. Raise the head of the bed slowly to Fowler's
       position
    B. Have the person get out of bed quickly to prevent
       weakness
    C. Keep the bed flat when getting the person out of bed
    D. Have the person walk around to decrease
       weakness and dizziness

28. Nursing care that prevents complications from bedrest include all of these *except*
    A. Positioning in good body alignment
    B. Range-of-motion exercises
    C. Frequent position changes
    D. Deconditioning

29. If a person sitting on the edge of the bed complains of weakness, dizziness, or spots before the eyes, you should
    A. Assist the person to stand
    B. Help the person to sit in a chair or walk around
    C. Have the person sit on the side of the bed for a short while
    D. Tell the person that is a normal response and continue to get the person up

30. Bed-boards are used to
    A. Keep the person in alignment by preventing the mattress from sagging
    B. Prevent plantar flexion that can lead to footdrop
    C. Keep the hips abducted
    D. Keep the weight of top linens off the feet

31. Plantar flexion must be prevented to
    A. Keep the feet from bending down at the ankle (footdrop)
    B. Keep the hips from rotating outward
    C. Keep the wrist, thumb, and fingers in normal position
    D. Maintain good body alignment

32. To prevent the hips and legs from turning outward, you can use
    A. Bed cradles   C. Trochanter rolls
    B. Hip abduction wedges   D. Splints

33. You help the person to exercise when you
    A. Perform all activities of daily living (ADL) for the person
    B. Turn and move the person in bed without the person helping
    C. Encourage the person to use a trapeze to lift the trunk off the bed
    D. Allow the person to remain in bed all day

34. When another person moves the joints through their range of motion, it is called
    A. Active range-of-motion
    B. Activities of daily living
    C. Active-assistive range-of-motion
    D. Passive range-of-motion

35. A nursing assistant can perform range-of-motion exercises on the _____ only if allowed by center policy.
    A. Shoulder   C. Hip
    B. Neck   D. Knee

36. Depending on activity limits, it is best if exercise for children is
    A. Only passive ROM exercises
    B. Active-assistive ROM exercises
    C. Play activities that promote active ROM exercises
    D. Delayed until they are able to get out of bed

37. When exercising the wrist, you will perform all of these motions *except*
    A. Abduction   C. Flexion
    B. Hyperextension   D. Extension

38. Which of these joints can be adducted and abducted?
    A. Neck   C. Forearm
    B. Hip   D. Knee

39. When you help a person who is weak and unsteady to walk, you should
    A. Apply a gait (transfer) belt
    B. Help the person lean on furniture to walk around the room
    C. Put soft socks on the feet without shoes
    D. Let the person walk without any help

40. When the person is walking with crutches, the person should wear
    A. Soft slippers on the feet   C. Clothes that are loose
    B. Clothes that fit well   D. A gait belt

41. When walking with a cane, it is held
    A. On the strong side of the body
    B. On the weak side of the body
    C. In the right hand
    D. On the left side of the body

42. When a person is using a walker, it is
    A. Picked up and moved 3 to 4 inches in front of the person
    B. Moved forward with a rocking motion
    C. Moved first on the left side and then on the right
    D. Pushed and moved 6 to 8 inches in front of the person's feet

43. When you are caring for a person who wears a brace, it is important to report at once
    A. How far the person walks
    B. What care the person can do alone
    C. The amount of mobility in joints when doing range-of-motion exercises
    D. Any redness or signs of skin breakdown when you remove a brace

Fill in the Blank

44. Write out the abbreviations.
    A. ADL _____
    B. CMS _____
    C. ID _____
    D. OBRA _____
    E. ROM _____

45. You assist the nurse in promoting _____ and _____ in all persons to the extent possible.

46. Bedrest is ordered to
    A. _____
    B. _____
    C. _____
    D. _____
    E. _____

47. The nurse tells you the resident is on bedrest, but can use the bathroom for elimination. This type of bedrest is _____.

48. When a person is moved from lying or sitting to a standing position, the blood pressure may _____. This is called _____.

49. Supportive devices such as bed-boards are used to _____ and _____ the person in a certain position.

50. When you use a foot-board, the soles of the feet are _____ against it to prevent _____.

51. A trochanter roll is placed along the body to prevent the hips and legs from _____.

52. Hand rolls or grips prevent _____ of the thumb, fingers, and wrists.

53. A splint is used to keep these joints in their normal positions.
    A. _____
    B. _____
    C. _____
    D. _____
    E. _____
    F. _____

54. Bed cradles are used because the weight of top linens can cause _____ and _____.

55. A trapeze bar allows the person to lift the _____ off the bed. It also allows the person to _____ and _____ in bed.

56. When a person does exercises with some help, they are doing _____ range-of-motion exercises.

57. When range-of-motion exercises are done, what should be reported or recorded?
    A. _____
    B. _____
    C. _____
    D. _____
    E. _____
    F. _____

58. When performing range-of-motion exercises, each movement should be repeated _____ times or the _____.

59. List the safety measures to follow when performing range-of-motion exercises.
    A. _____
    B. _____
    C. _____
    D. _____
    E. _____
    F. _____
    G. _____
    H. _____
    I. _____

60. When you help a person to walk, you should walk to the _____ and _____ the person. Provide support with the _____.

61. Many people prefer a walker because it gives more support than a _____.

Use the FOCUS ON PRIDE section to complete these statements.

62. You can promote activity, exercise, and well-being when you
    A. _____
    B. _____
    C. _____
    D. _____
    E. _____

63. OBRA requires _____ programs for nursing center residents. These programs are important for _____ and _____ well-being.

64. Activities in nursing centers must meet the interests and needs of each resident. These needs are
    A. _____
    B. _____
    C. _____

Labeling

65. ROM exercises for the _____ joint are shown in these drawings. Name the movements shown in each drawing.

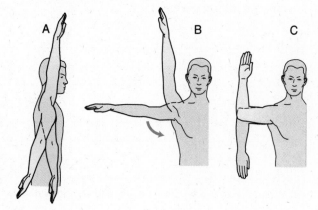

A. _____
B. _____
C. _____

66. ROM exercises for the _____ are shown in these drawings. Name the movements shown in each drawing.

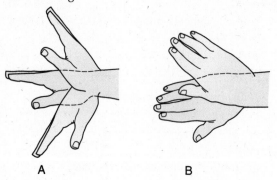

A. _____
B. _____

67. ROM exercises for the _____ are shown in these drawings. Name the movements shown in each drawing.

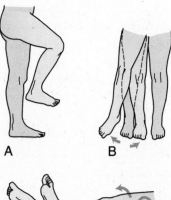

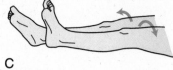

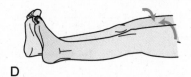

A. _____
B. _____
C. _____
D. _____

Crossword

Fill in the crossword by answering the clues below with the words from this list:

Abduction	Flexion	Rotation	External rotation	Pronation
Adduction	Hyperextension	Internal rotation	Plantar flexion	Supination
Extension	Dorsiflexion			

Across

5. Turning the joint upward
7. Turning the joint inward
10. Straightening a body part
11. Bending the toes and foot up at the ankle
12. Turning the joint downward

Down

1. Bending a body part
2. Bending the foot down at the ankle
3. Turning the joint outward
4. Excessive straightening of a body part
6. Turning the joint
8. Moving a body part away from the midline of the body
9. Moving a body part toward the midline of the body

Optional Learning Exercises

68. What kind of range of motion would be used with each of these residents?

    A. The resident needs complete care for bathing, grooming, and feeding.

    _____

    B. The resident takes part in many activities in the center. She walks to most activities independently.

    _____

    C. The resident has weakness on his left side. He is able to feed himself but needs help with bathing and dressing.

    _____

69. As you plan to help a person out of bed, you are concerned about orthostatic hypotension. To make sure the person is able to stand and get up safely, you plan to take the blood pressure, pulse, and respirations several times. When would you take the blood pressure?

    A. _____

    B. _____

    C. _____

    D. _____

    E. _____

70. When doing range-of-motion exercises, you should ask the person if he or she

    A. _____

    B. _____

    C. _____

71. When you are going to assist a person to ambulate, you can promote comfort and reduce fears when you explain

    A. _____

    B. _____

    C. _____

    D. _____

    E. _____

72. When you help a person to walk, what observations are reported and recorded?

    A. _____

    B. _____

    C. _____

    D. _____

    E. _____

73. When using a cane, the person walks as follows:

    A. Step A: _____

    B. Step B: _____

    C. Step C: _____

74. Why does the nurse assess the skin under braces every shift? _____

    _____

31 Comfort, Rest, and Sleep

Fill in the Blank: Key Terms

Acute pain	Discomfort	Insomnia	Phantom pain	Rest
Chronic pain	Distraction	NREM sleep	Radiating pain	Sleep
Circadian rhythm	Enuresis	Pain	Relaxation	Sleep deprivation
Comfort	Guided imagery	Persistent pain	REM sleep	Sleepwalking

1. The amount and quality of sleep are reduced in
   _____.

2. Another name for discomfort is _____.

3. _____ is pain that is felt suddenly from injury, disease, trauma, or surgery.

4. _____ is a way to change a person's center of attention.

5. A state of unconsciousness, reduced voluntary muscle activity, and lowered metabolism is _____.

6. Pain lasting longer than 6 months is _____. It is constant or occurs off and on.

7. _____ is to be free from mental or physical stress.

8. _____ is a state of well-being. The person has no physical or emotional pain and is calm and at peace.

9. To be calm, at ease, and relaxed is to _____. The person is free of anxiety and stress.

10. Creating and focusing on an image is
    _____.

11. The stage of sleep when there is rapid eye movement is
    _____.

12. _____ is a chronic condition in which the person cannot sleep or stay asleep all night.

13. The day-night cycle or body rhythm is also called
    _____. This daily rhythm is based on a 24-hour cycle.

14. _____ is pain felt at the site of tissue damage and in nearby areas.

15. To ache, hurt, or be sore is _____. It is also called pain.

16. _____ is the phase of deep sleep when there is no rapid eye movement.

17. Pain felt in a body part that is no longer there is
    _____.

18. Urinary incontinence in bed at night is
    _____.

19. Another name for chronic pain is
    _____.

20. When the person leaves the bed and walks about, it is
    _____.

Circle the Best Answer

21. Rest and sleep are needed to
    A. Restore well-being and energy
    B. Decrease function and quality of life
    C. Increase muscle strength
    D. Relieve pain

22. OBRA and CMS requirements related to comfort, rest, and sleep include
    A. Only 2 people in a room
    B. Bright lighting in all areas
    C. Room temperature between 65°F and 71°F
    D. Adequate ventilation and room humidity

23. When a person complains of pain or discomfort
    A. The person has pain or discomfort
    B. It must be carefully measured to see if the person really has pain
    C. You can easily measure to find out how much pain is present
    D. You can tell if the person really has pain by the way he or she acts

24. When a person complains of pain that is nearby an area of tissue damage, this is _____ pain.
    A. Acute
    B. Chronic
    C. Radiating
    D. Phantom

25. If pain is ignored or denied, it may be because the person thinks pain is a sign of weakness. Which factor that affects pain would this be?
    A. Attention
    B. Past experience
    C. Value or meaning of pain
    D. Support from others

26. A person from Mexico may react to pain by
    A. Showing a strong emotional response
    B. Appearing very stoic
    C. Accepting pain quietly
    D. Viewing it as the will of God

27. When a person has anxiety, the person
    A. May feel increased pain
    B. Will usually feel less pain
    C. May deny having pain
    D. May be stoic and show no reaction to pain

28. When you ask a person, "Where is the pain?" you are asking the person to
    A. Describe the pain
    B. Explain the intensity of the pain
    C. Tell you the onset and duration of the pain
    D. Tell you the location of the pain

29. A child may deal with pain by
    A. Restricting play or school activities
    B. Describing pain to an adult
    C. Asking for pain medications
    D. Concentrating on reading, watching TV, or playing quietly

30. Older persons may ignore new pain because they
    A. Cannot verbally communicate pain
    B. May think it is related to a known health problem
    C. Have increased anxiety
    D. Are used to being in pain

31. When a person tells you he or she has pain when coughing or deep breathing, this is
    A. A factor causing pain
    B. A measurement of the onset of pain
    C. Words used to describe the pain
    D. The location of the pain

32. A distraction measure to promote comfort and relieve pain may be
    A. Asking the person to focus on an image
    B. Learning to breathe deeply and slowly
    C. Listening to music or playing games
    D. Contracting and relaxing muscle groups

33. If the nurse has given a person pain medication, it is best if you
    A. Give the person a bath
    B. Walk the person according to the care plan
    C. Wait 30 minutes before giving care
    D. Give care before the medication makes the person sleepy

34. You may help to promote comfort and relieve pain by doing all of these *except*
    A. Allowing family members and friends at the bedside as requested by the person
    B. Keeping the room brightly lit and play loud music
    C. Providing blankets for warmth and to prevent chilling
    D. Using touch to provide comfort

35. You can promote comfort and help relieve pain when you
    A. Perform passive range-of-motion exercises
    B. Give a back massage
    C. Make sure the person ambulates every 2 hours
    D. Keep the person in the supine position

36. Lotion is used for back massage because it
    A. Stimulates circulation
    B. Heals any skin breakdown
    C. Reduces friction during the massage
    D. Cools the skin

37. Back massages are dangerous for persons with all of these disorders *except*
    A. Certain heart diseases
    B. Lung disorders
    C. Arthritis
    D. Back injuries or surgeries

38. The best position for a back massage is
    A. Prone position
    B. Supine position
    C. Semi-Fowler's position
    D. Fowler's position

39. When giving a back massage, the strokes
    A. Start at the shoulders and go down to the lower back
    B. Should be light and gentle
    C. Start at the lower back and go up to the shoulders
    D. Are continued for at least 10 minutes

40. You can help to promote rest by doing all of these *except*
    A. Meeting physical needs such as thirst, hunger, and elimination needs
    B. Making sure the person feels safe
    C. Allowing the person to practice rituals or routines before resting
    D. Giving care at a time most convenient to you

41. When caring for an ill or injured person, you know the person may need more rest. You can help the person to get rest by making sure you
    A. Provide plenty of exercise to prevent weakness
    B. Provide rest periods during or after a procedure
    C. Give complete hygiene and grooming measures quickly
    D. Spend time talking with the person to distract him or her

42. Which of these does *not* occur during sleep?
    A. The person is unaware of the environment.
    B. Metabolism is reduced during sleep.
    C. Vital signs are higher.
    D. There are no voluntary arm or leg movements.

43. Some people function better in the morning because of
    A. The circadian rhythm
    B. Getting enough sleep
    C. Interference with the body rhythm
    D. Changes in the work schedule

44. During REM sleep the person
    A. Is hard to arouse
    B. Has a gradual fall in vital signs
    C. Is easily aroused
    D. Has tension in voluntary muscles

45. Which stage of sleep is usually *not* repeated during the cycles of sleep?
    A. REM
    B. Stage 1: NREM
    C. Stage 2: NREM
    D. Stage 3: NREM

46. Which age-group requires the least amount of sleep?
    A. Newborns
    B. Pre-schoolers
    C. Teenagers
    D. Adults, including the elderly

47. Which of these factors increases the need for sleep?
    A. Illness
    B. Weight loss
    C. Emotional problems
    D. Drugs and other substances

48. When a person takes sleeping pills, sleep may not restore the person mentally because
    A. Caffeine prevents sleep
    B. Some have difficulty falling asleep
    C. The length of REM sleep is reduced
    D. It upsets the usual sleep routines

49. Exercise should be avoided for 2 hours before sleep because
    A. It requires energy
    B. People usually feel good after exercise
    C. It causes the release of substances in the bloodstream that stimulate the body
    D. The person tires after exercise

50. Persons who are ill, in pain, or receiving hospital care are at risk for
    A. Sleep deprivation
    B. Sleepwalking
    C. Insomnia
    D. Increased sleep times

51. If a person has decreased reasoning; red, puffy eyes; and coordination problems, report this to the nurse because the person
    A. Is having a reaction to sleeping medications
    B. Has signs and symptoms of sleep disorders
    C. Needs more exercise before bedtime
    D. May need an increase in sleeping pills

52. Which of these measures *would not* help to promote sleep?
    A. Provide blankets or socks for those who tend to be cold.
    B. Have the person void or make sure incontinent persons are clean and dry.
    C. Follow bedtime rituals.
    D. Offer the person a cup of coffee or tea at bedtime.

53. When a person with Alzheimer's disease wanders at night, you can assist her by
    A. Giving her a cup of coffee or tea
    B. Turning on the TV in the room to distract her
    C. Quietly and calmly directing her to her room
    D. Explaining to her that it is night and she needs to go to bed

Fill in the Blank

54. Write out the abbreviations.
    A. CMS _____
    B. NREM _____
    C. OBRA _____
    D. REM _____

55. OBRA and CMS have requirements about the person's room. List the requirements that relate to each of these.
    A. Suspended curtain _____
    B. Linens _____
    C. Bed _____
    D. Room temperature _____
    E. Persons in room _____

56. Name the type of pain described.
    A. A person with an amputated leg may still sense leg pain. _____
    B. There is tissue damage. The pain decreases with healing. _____
    C. Pain from a heart attack is often felt in the left chest, left jaw, left shoulder, and left arm.
    _____
    D. The pain remains long after healing. Common causes are arthritis and cancer.
    _____

57. What is the reason that persons from the Philippines may appear stoic in reaction to pain?
    _____
    _____

58. Older persons may ignore or deny new pain because
    A. _____
    B. _____

59. In persons with dementia, pain may be signalled by changes
    _____

60. When gathering information about a person in pain, you can use a scale of 1 to 10. Which end of the scale is the most severe pain? _____

61. What happens to vital signs when the person has acute pain? _____

62. What happens to vital signs when the person has chronic pain? _____

63. When the person uses words such as *aching, knifelike,* or *sore* to describe pain, what do you report to the nurse? _____
    _____

64. What body responses that you can see or measure (objective signs) may mean the person has pain?
    A. _____
    B. _____
    C. _____
    D. _____

65. What changes in these behaviors may be symptoms of pain?
    A. Speech _____
    B. Affected body part _____
    C. Body position _____

66. List nursing measures to promote comfort and relieve pain related to these clues.
    A. Position of the person _____
    B. Linens _____
    C. Blankets _____
    D. Pain medications _____
    E. Family members _____

67. If a person is receiving strong pain medication or sedatives, what safety measures are important?

    A. _____

    B. _____

    C. _____

    D. _____

68. When giving a back massage, what is the effect of

    A. Fast movements _____

    B. Slow movements _____

69. When you are delegated to give a back massage, what observations should you report and record?

    A. _____

    B. _____

    C. _____

    D. _____

70. When you explain the procedure before performing it, you may help a person to rest better because you met the need for _____.

71. A clean, neat, and uncluttered room can promote rest by meeting _____ needs.

72. The mind and body rest, the body saves energy, and body functions slow during _____.

73. Mental restoration occurs during a phase of sleep called _____.

74. The deepest stage of sleep occurs during

    _____

75. If work hours change, it can affect the normal _____ cycle or _____ rhythm.

76. Alcohol tends to cause drowsiness and sleep but it interferes with _____.

77. Insomnia may be caused by

    A. Fear of _____

    B. Fear of not _____

    C. Fear of not being able _____

    D. Physical and emotional _____

78. When a person has dementia and wanders at night, the best approach for some persons is to allow

    _____

Use the FOCUS ON PRIDE section to complete these statements.

79. When you are caring for persons who have pain, what is your responsibility?

    A. Report _____ and _____.

    B. Report what the person _____ and what _____.

80. It is important to report signs and symptoms of pain because the nurse uses this information to _____.

81. Take pride in providing care that focuses on the person as a _____.

82. You can affect the person's well-being by meeting these needs.

    A. _____

    B. _____

    C. _____

Optional Learning Exercises

83. You are caring for 2 residents who both have arthritis. Mr. Forman tells you this is the first time he has had any health problems. Mrs. Wegman tells you she has had several surgeries and has had 3 children. Who is likely to be more anxious about the pain and to be unable to handle the pain well, Mr. or Mrs. Forman?

    _____ Why? _____

84. Mr. Forman tells you his pain seems much worse at night. What could be the reason for this reaction?

    _____

    _____

85. You are caring for Mrs. Reynolds. She tells you she misses her children who have moved to another state. Today, Mrs. Reynolds is complaining of pain in her abdomen. In spite of providing nursing comfort measures, she still rates her pain at a 7. What is a possible reason that Mrs. Reynolds is not getting relief of her pain? _____

    _____

86. When a person is ill, how do these affect sleep?

    A. Treatments and therapies _____

    B. Care devices such as traction or a cast

    _____

    C. Emotions that affect sleep include

    _____

87. Certain foods affect sleep. Tell how these foods affect sleep and list foods that contain the substances.

    A. Caffeine _____ sleep. It is found in

    _____

    B. Trytophan _____ sleep. It is found in _____

Fill in the Blank: Key Terms

Admission   Discharge   Transfer

1. _____ is moving a person from one room or nursing unit to another.

2. The official entry of a person into a nursing agency is

_____.

3. _____ occurs with the official departure of a person from a nursing agency.

Circle the Best Answer

4. Admission to a hospital or nursing center may include all of these *except*
   A. Anxiety and fear
   B. Concerns about who gives care, how care is given, and if the correct care is given
   C. Being separated from family and friends
   D. Excitement about having a new experience and meeting new friends

5. Usually, _____ is a happy time.
   A. Admission   C. Transfer
   B. Discharge   D. Home care

6. The admissions process starts with the
   A. Doctor
   B. Nurse on the nursing unit
   C. Admitting office
   D. Activities director

7. When a person with dementia is admitted to a nursing center, the person
   A. Is usually depressed
   B. May have an increase in confusion
   C. May have a decrease in confusion
   D. Usually feels safer in the new setting

8. Persons being admitted
   A. Are always admitted by the RN
   B. Are usually admitted by the nursing assistant
   C. May be admitted by the nursing assistant if the person has no discomfort or distress
   D. Are never admitted by the nursing assistant

9. If a person being admitted is arriving by stretcher, you should
   A. Raise the bed to the level of the stretcher
   B. Leave the bed closed
   C. Raise the head of the bed to Fowler's position
   D. Lower the bed to its lowest level

10. When admitting a person, identify him or her by
    A. Asking the person his or her name
    B. Checking the information on the admission form and the ID bracelet
    C. Asking the family the person's name
    D. Asking the nurse to identify the person

11. When weighing a resident, have the person
    A. Wear socks and shoes and a bathrobe
    B. Remove regular clothes and wear a gown or pajamas
    C. Wear regular street clothes
    D. Remove clothing after weighing and then weigh the clothes

12. A chair scale is used when a person
    A. Cannot transfer from a wheelchair
    B. Cannot stand
    C. Can stand and walk independently
    D. Is in the supine position

13. When a person cannot stand on the scale to have his or her height measured
    A. Ask the person or the family the height of the person
    B. Have the person sit in a chair and use a tape measure from head to toe to measure the person
    C. Position the person in supine position if the position is allowed and measure with a tape measure
    D. Estimate the height of the person by observing him or her

14. When a person is being moved to a new room, who is told about the transfer?
    A. The doctor
    B. The social worker
    C. The family and the business office
    D. The person's roommate

15. When you are transferring a person, you should do all of these *except*
    A. Identify the person by checking the ID bracelet with the transfer slip
    B. Explain the reasons for the transfer
    C. Collect the person's personal belongings and bedside equipment
    D. Report to the receiving nurse

16. If a person wishes to leave the center without the doctor's permission, you should
    A. Tell the person this is not allowed
    B. Prevent the person from leaving
    C. Tell the nurse at once
    D. Try to convince the person to stay

17. When you are assisting a person who is being discharged, you should do all of these *except*
    A. Check all drawers and closets
    B. Check off the clothing list and personal belongings list
    C. Help the person dress as needed
    D. Provide discharge instructions

Fill in the Blank

18. Write out the abbreviations.

    A. ft _____

    B. ID _____

    C. in _____

    D. lb _____

19. OBRA and CMS have standards for transfers and discharges. List the ways these standards affect the person's rights.

    A. Reasons for _____ or

    _____ are

    part of the person's _____.

    B. The _____ and

    _____ are told of transfer or discharge plans.

    C. A procedure is followed if the person

    _____

    D. An _____ often works with the person and family to protect

    _____

20. When you are delegated to assist with admissions, transfers, or discharges, what information do you need from the nurse?

    A. _____

    B. _____

    C. _____

    D. _____

    E. _____

    F. _____

    G. _____

    H. _____

    I. _____

    J. _____

21. When a person is being admitted, what identifying information is obtained?

    A. _____

    B. _____

    C. _____

22. During admission, what is the person given to allow the staff to identify the person?

    _____ and

    _____

23. The person may also have a _____ ID taken.

24. When you are asked to admit a person, what can you do to make a good first impression?

    A. _____

    B. _____

    C. _____

    D. _____

    E. _____

25. Why is it important to have a person void before being weighed? _____

26. What is done to the balance scale before having the person step on it?

    A. _____

    B. _____

    C. _____

27. When measuring a person in the supine position, the ruler is placed _____.

28. When you transfer or discharge a person, tell the nurse when the person is ready, so that the nurse can

    A. _____

    B. _____

    C. _____

    D. _____

29. When you assist with a discharge, you should report and record

    A. _____

    B. _____

    C. _____

    D. _____

    E. _____

    F. _____

Use the FOCUS ON PRIDE section to complete these statements.

30. When you admit, transfer, or discharge a person, it is your responsibility to help the person adjust by

    A. _____

    B. _____

    C. _____

    D. _____

    E. _____

31. If a person tells you he or she does not want certain people to visit, you should tell _____. The staff must _____ the person's wishes.

Optional Learning Exercises

Answer the questions about the following person and situation:
Rosa Romirez, 65, had a stroke (CVA) last week and is being
admitted to a rehabilitation unit in the nursing care center
where you work.

32. Since you know Mrs. Romirez is arriving by
    wheelchair, you leave the bed _____ and
    _____ the bed to its _____.

33. The nurse instructs you to collect the needed
    equipment to admit a new person. You collect

    A. _____

    B. _____

    C. _____

    D. _____

    E. _____

    F. _____

    G. _____

    H. _____

    I. _____

    J. _____

34. When Mrs. Romirez arrives with her husband, it may
    help them feel more comfortable if you offer them

    _____.

35. You greet Mrs. Romirez by name and ask her if a

    certain _____

36. Mrs. Romirez has some weakness on her left side and
    cannot stand alone, but can safely transfer from the
    wheelchair to chairs or the bed. The nurse tells you to

    weigh Mrs. Romirez with the _____ scale.

When you arrive at work one day, you are told Mrs. Romirez is
being transferred to another nursing unit and you are asked to
assist. Answer these questions about transferring her.

37. When you transport Mrs. Romirez in a wheelchair, she

    is covered with a _____.

38. What items are taken with Mrs. Romirez to the new
    unit?

    _____

39. What information is recorded and reported about the
    transfer?

    A. _____

    B. _____

    C. _____

    D. _____

    E. _____

    F. _____

    G. _____

Several weeks later, you are sent to the nursing unit where
Mrs. Romirez is living and find she is going home. Answer these
questions about her discharge.

40. Mrs. Romirez tells you she and her family have been

    taught about her _____, _____,

    _____, _____,

    and _____.

41. Good communication skills should be used when
    assisting with the discharge. When Mrs. Romirez and
    her family leave, you should

    _____.

Fill in the Blank: Key Terms

Dorsal recumbent position
Genupectoral position
Horizontal recumbent position

Knee-chest position
Laryngeal mirror
Lithotomy position

Nasal speculum
Ophthalmoscope
Otoscope

Percussion hammer
Tuning fork
Vaginal speculum

1. An instrument vibrated to test hearing is a

_____

2. In the _____, the woman lies on her back with her hips at the edge of the exam table, her knees are flexed, her hips are externally rotated, and her feet are in stirrups.

3. The supine position with the legs together is called the

_____

4. An _____ is a lighted instrument used to examine the external ear and the eardrum (tympanic membrane).

5. A _____ is an instrument used to open the vagina so it and the cervix can be examined.

6. When a person kneels and rests the body on the knees and chest, the head is turned to one side, the arms are above the head or flexed at the elbows, the back is straight, and the body is flexed about 90 degrees at the hip, the person is in the _____.

7. A _____ is an instrument used to tap body parts to test reflexes.

8. An instrument used to examine the mouth, teeth, and throat is called a _____.

9. An instrument used to examine the inside of the nose is a _____.

10. The dorsal recumbent position is also called the

_____

11. An _____ is a lighted instrument used to examine the internal structures of the eye.

12. Another name for knee-chest position is

_____

Circle the Best Answer

13. In nursing centers, residents have a physical examination
    A. Only when the person is admitted
    B. Once a month
    C. At least once a year
    D. Only when the person is ill

14. If a person is having a physical examination, you may be asked to do all of these *except*
    A. Measure vital signs, height, and weight
    B. Have the person void
    C. Explain why the examination is being done and what to expect
    D. Position and drape the person

15. When the doctor is examining the person's mouth, teeth, and throat, you may be asked to hand him or her the
    A. Ophthalmoscope
    B. Percussion hammer
    C. Tuning fork
    D. Laryngeal mirror

16. Which of these would provide for privacy for a person having a physical examination?
    A. Having the person urinate before the examination begins
    B. Telling the person who will do the exam and when it will be done
    C. Screening the person and closing the room door
    D. Allowing a family member to decide who will be in the room during the exam

17. When a child is examined, all of the following are true *except*
    A. All clothing is removed
    B. Parents are allowed to be present
    C. Underpants are worn by toddlers, pre-school children, and school-age children
    D. Protect the child from chilling

18. It is important to have a person empty the bladder before an examination because
    A. An empty bladder allows the examiner to feel the abdominal organs
    B. A full bladder may cause the person to be incontinent
    C. A urine specimen is always collected before an examination
    D. A full bladder will cause the person to have intense pain

19. Which of these steps *would not* promote safety and comfort during an exam?
    A. The procedure is not explained to the person.
    B. Have an extra bath blanket nearby.
    C. Prevent drafts to protect the person from chilling.
    D. Do not leave the person unattended.

20. After you have taken the person to the exam room and placed the person in position, you should
    A. Put on the call light for the examiner
    B. Leave the room
    C. Go to the examiner to report that the person is ready
    D. Open the door so that the examiner knows you are ready

21. When the abdomen, chest, and breasts are to be examined, you will place the person in the
    A. Lithotomy position
    B. Sims' position
    C. Dorsal recumbent (horizontal recumbent) position
    D. Knee-chest position

22. If a person is asked to stand on the floor during an exam, you should
    A. Assist the person to put on shoes or slippers
    B. Place paper or paper towels on the floor
    C. Place a sheet on the floor
    D. Wipe the floor carefully with an antiseptic cleaner before the person stands on it

Fill in the Blank

23. Physical exams are done to:
    A. _____
    B. _____
    C. _____

24. List the equipment you need to collect when the ears are being examined.
    A. _____
    B. _____

25. What equipment is needed to examine the eyes?
    A. _____
    B. _____

26. When the nose, mouth, and throat are being examined, you should collect
    A. _____
    B. _____
    C. _____
    D. _____

27. What are concerns the person may have when a physical examination is done?
    A. _____
    B. _____
    C. _____

28. When the examiner is a man and the person being examined is female, who else should be in the examination room? _____
    Why? _____

29. After the examination is completed, you make sure the exam room _____
    _____.

Use the FOCUS ON PRIDE section to complete these statements.

30. Fears about the exam affect the person's well-being. Common fears are
    A. _____
    B. _____
    C. _____
    D. _____

31. You violate the Health Insurance Portability and Accountability Act of 1996 (HIPAA) when you
    _____.

32. Failure to follow HIPAA can result in
    _____.

Labeling

Look at the instruments and answer the questions.

33. Name the instruments.

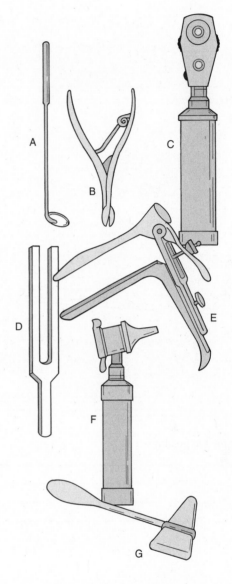

    A. _____
    B. _____
    C. _____
    D. _____
    E. _____
    F. _____
    G. _____

34. Which instrument is used to examine the nose?
    _____

35. When the eye is examined, the examiner uses the
    _____.

36. If a person has a sore throat, the examiner will look at the throat with the _____.

37. The reflexes are examined by using the

    _____.

Look at the positions and answer these questions.

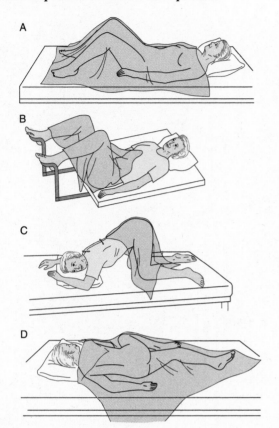

A

B

C

D

38. Name the positions.
    A. _____
    B. _____
    C. _____
    D. _____

39. Which positions may be used when a rectal examination is done?
    A. _____
    B. _____

40. When the abdomen, chest, and breasts are examined, the person is placed in _____.

41. The _____
    position is used for a vaginal exam.

Optional Learning Exercises

42. When you are delegated the job of preparing a person for an exam, why do you need the following information?

    A. What time is the examination? _____
    _____

    B. What are 2 reasons it would be helpful to know which examinations will be done?
    _____
    _____

    C. What equipment will you need if you are assigned to take vital signs? _____
    _____
    _____

43. You are a female nursing assistant assisting a male examiner with an examination of a female resident. The nurse tells you to stay in the exam room during the entire procedure. Why is this important to the examiner and to the woman? _____
    _____

34 Collecting and Testing Specimens

Fill in the Blank: Key Terms

Acetone
Glucometer
Glucosuria

Glycosuria
Hematoma
Hematuria

Hemoptysis
Ketone
Ketone body

Melena
Sputum

1. Bloody sputum is _____.

2. Ketone or acetone is also called

   _____.

3. A black, tarry stool is

   _____.

4. _____ is glucosuria or sugar in the urine.

5. _____ is mucus from the respiratory system that is expectorated through the mouth.

6. _____ is a substance that appears in urine from the rapid breakdown of fat for energy.

7. Another name for ketone or ketone body is

   _____.

8. Sugar in the urine is called glycosuria or

   _____.

9. _____ is blood in the urine.

10. A swelling that contains blood is a

    _____.

11. A device for measuring blood glucose is a

    _____.

Circle the Best Answer

12. Specimens are collected and tested for all of these reasons *except*
    A. To measure the specimen
    B. To prevent diseases
    C. To detect diseases
    D. To treat diseases

13. When you are collecting a specimen, which of these is *incorrect?*
    A. Use a clean container for each specimen.
    B. Gloves are not needed.
    C. Do not touch the inside of the container or lid.
    D. Place the specimen container in a *BIOHAZARD* plastic bag.

14. When collecting a urine specimen from an older child or teenager, the specimen may be placed in a paper bag to
    A. Prevent embarrassing the person
    B. Protect the specimen from light
    C. Follow Standard Precautions
    D. Keep the specimen sterile

15. A random urine specimen is collected
    A. First thing in the morning
    B. After meals
    C. At any time
    D. At bedtime

16. When a person is collecting a random urine specimen, remind the person to put the toilet tissue in
    A. The wastebasket or toilet
    B. The specimen container
    C. The specimen pan
    D. Any of the above

17. When obtaining a midstream specimen, the perineal area is cleaned to
    A. Remove all microbes from the area
    B. Reduce the number of microbes in the urethral area
    C. Follow Standard Precautions and the Bloodborne Pathogen Standard
    D. Reduce infection during specimen collection

18. When collecting a midstream specimen, which of these is *correct?*
    A. Collect the entire amount of urine voided.
    B. Collect about 4 oz (120 mL) of urine.
    C. Have the person start to void, then stop. A sterile specimen container is positioned to catch urine as the person begins to void again.
    D. Collect several specimens and mix them together.

19. When collecting a 24-hour urine specimen, the urine is kept
    A. Chilled on ice or refrigerated during the entire time
    B. At room temperature
    C. In a sterile container at the nurses' station
    D. In a drainage collection bag at the bedside

20. A 24-hour urine specimen collection is started
    A. At the beginning of a shift
    B. After a meal
    C. At night
    D. After the person voids and that urine is discarded

21. At the end of 24-hour specimen collection
    A. The person voids and that urine is saved
    B. Write down any missed or spilled urine
    C. Record the amount of urine collected
    D. The person voids and that urine is discarded

22. When a urine specimen is needed from infants or very young children, it is obtained by
    A. Inserting a straight catheter
    B. Using a collection bag applied over the urethra
    C. Having the parent hold the child on a potty chair until the child voids
    D. Applying a diaper and then squeezing the urine out of the diaper

23. A child may be able to void for a specimen if you give the child fluids
    A. 5 to 10 minutes before the test
    B. 30 minutes before the test
    C. 1 hour before the test
    D. While you are obtaining the specimen

24. When you test urine with a reagent strip, it is important that you
    A. Follow the manufacturer's instructions
    B. Use a sterile urine specimen
    C. Wear sterile gloves
    D. Make sure the urine is cold

25. When you are assigned to strain a person's urine, you
    A. Have the person void directly into the strainer
    B. Send all urine to the lab
    C. Have the person void into the voiding device and then pour the urine through the strainer
    D. Discard the strainer if it contains any stones

26. If a warm stool specimen is required, it is
    A. Placed in an insulated container
    B. Stored on the nursing unit until the end of the shift
    C. Tested at once on the nursing unit
    D. Taken at once to the laboratory or the storage area

27. When collecting a stool specimen, ask the person to
    A. Void and have a bowel movement in a bedpan
    B. Use only a bedpan or commode to collect the specimen
    C. Urinate into the toilet and collect the stool in the specimen pan
    D. Place the toilet tissue in the bedpan, commode, or specimen pan with the stool

28. When collecting the stool specimen
    A. Pour it into the specimen container
    B. Use your gloved hand to obtain a specimen to place in the container
    C. Use a tongue blade to take about 2 tablespoons of stool from the middle of the formed stool
    D. Use a tongue blade to place the entire stool specimen in the container

29. When you test a stool specimen
    A. It must be sent to the laboratory
    B. The specimen must be sterile
    C. You will need to test the entire stool specimen
    D. Use a tongue blade to smear a small amount of stool on the test paper

30. A sputum specimen is more easily collected
    A. Upon awakening   C. At bedtime
    B. After eating   D. After activity

31. Before obtaining a sputum specimen, ask the person to
    A. Rinse the mouth with clear water
    B. Brush the teeth and use mouthwash
    C. Cough and discard the first sputum expectorated
    D. Sit in an upright position to loosen secretions

32. Postural drainage is used when collecting a sputum specimen to
    A. Collect sterile specimens
    B. Make the sputum specimen more liquid
    C. Stimulate coughing
    D. Help secretions drain by gravity

33. If a sputum specimen is needed from an infant or small child, you may assist the nurse by
    A. Positioning the child for postural drainage
    B. Holding the child's head and arms still
    C. Positioning the sputum specimen cup near the child's mouth
    D. Explaining the procedure to the child

34. If you are delegated to do blood glucose testing, the most common site for testing is
    A. The earlobe
    B. A fingertip
    C. The forearm
    D. The abdomen

35. It is important to do glucose testing at correct times because
    A. The nurse uses the results to make decisions about administering drugs for the person
    B. It must be done before meals
    C. It must be done after meals
    D. It must be done at a time when the person is not sleeping

Fill in the Blank

36. Write out the abbreviations.
    A. BM _____
    B. ID _____
    C. I&O _____
    D. mL _____
    E. oz _____
    F. SDS _____
    G. U/A _____

37. When collecting urine specimens, what observations are reported and recorded?
    A. _____
    B. _____
    C. _____
    D. _____
    E. _____
    F. _____

38. How much urine is collected for a random urine specimen? _____

39. When collecting a midstream urine specimen, the person may not be able to stop voiding. If so, you will pass _____

40. When you are obtaining a midstream specimen from a female, spread the labia with your thumb and index finger with your _____ hand.

41. When cleaning the female perineum for a midstream specimen, clean from _____

42. When cleaning the male perineum for a midstream specimen, clean the penis starting

_____

43. What information is marked on the room and bathroom container labels for a 24-hour urine collection?

_____

44. Urine ph measures if the urine is _____

    or _____.

45. When you use reagent strips, you read the strip by comparing it to the _____.

46. When you strain urine, you are looking for stones that can develop in the _____.

47. The strainer is placed in the specimen container if any _____ appear.

48. Stool specimens are studied and checked for

    A. _____

    B. _____

    C. _____

    D. _____

    E. _____

49. After collecting a stool specimen, place the container in a _____

    _____.

50. When you are delegated to collect a stool specimen, what observations are reported and recorded?

    A. _____

    B. _____

    C. _____

    D. _____

    E. _____

51. When stools are black and tarry, there is bleeding in the _____.

52. Blood in the stool that is hidden is called

    _____

53. Mouthwash is not used before a sputum specimen is collected because it _____.

54. When you are delegated to collect a sputum specimen, report and record

    A. _____

    B. _____

    C. _____

    D. _____

    E. _____

    F. _____

    G. _____

    H. _____

    I. _____

55. When you are assisting a person to collect a sputum specimen, ask the person to take 2 or 3

    _____ and

    _____ the sputum.

56. Why do you avoid swollen, bruised, cyanotic, or calloused sites when testing for blood glucose?

    _____

57. Why do you avoid the center, fleshy part of the fingertip when you make a skin puncture? _____

    _____

58. When you test for blood glucose, what should you report and record?

    A. _____

    B. _____

    C. _____

    D. _____

    E. _____

    F. _____

    G. _____

    H. _____

Use the FOCUS ON PRIDE section to complete these statements.

59. When collecting a specimen, you are responsible to correctly _____ the person.

60. What information may you need to place on the specimen container?

    A. _____

    B. _____

    C. _____

61. When collecting specimens, you respect the person's right to privacy when you

    A. _____

    B. _____

    C. _____

    D. _____

62. If you did not collect a specimen correctly, why is it important to report this to the nurse?

    _____

    _____

Crossword

Fill in the crossword by answering the clues below with the words from this list:

Calculi	Expectorated	Midstream	Postural	Specimens
Dysuria	Labia	Occult	Random	Suctioning

Across

1. Samples
3. Urine specimen that can be collected at any time
6. Hidden, as in blood in stool
8. Position with head lower than body used to cause fluid to flow downward
9. Folds of tissue on each side of the vagina
10. Pain when urinating

Down

2. Expelled, as in sputum through the mouth
4. Urine specimen that is collected after the person starts to void
5. Stones that develop in kidneys, ureters, or bladder
7. Removal of sputum from the trachea with a machine

Optional Learning Exercises

63. If you are collecting a midstream specimen, what should you do if it is hard for the person to stop the stream of urine? _____

_____

64. You are caring for a person who is having a 24-hour urine specimen test. He tells you he forgot to save a specimen an hour ago. What should you do and why?

_____

_____

65. What is normal pH for urine? _____
What can cause changes in the normal pH?

_____

66. When the body cannot use sugar for energy, it uses fat. When this happens _____ appear in the urine.

67. Why is privacy important when collecting a sputum specimen? _____

_____

35 The Person Having Surgery

Fill in the Blank: Key Terms

Anesthesia
Elective surgery
Embolus

Emergency surgery
General anesthesia
Local anesthesia

Postoperative
Preoperative
Regional anesthesia

Sedation
Thrombus
Urgent surgery

1. The loss of consciousness and all feeling or sensation is
   _____.

2. _____ is surgery done by choice to improve the person's life or well-being.

3. A blood clot is called a _____.

4. _____ is the loss of feeling or sensation produced by a drug.

5. An _____ is a blood clot that travels through the vascular system until it lodges in a blood vessel.

6. _____ is before surgery.

7. _____ is surgery needed for the person's health. It is done soon to prevent further damage or disease.

8. _____ is after surgery.

9. The loss of feeling or sensation in a large area of the body is _____
   _____.

10. Surgery done immediately to save life or function is
    _____.

11. _____ is the loss of feeling or sensation in a small area.

12. A state of quiet, calmness, or sleep produced by a drug is _____

Circle the Best Answer

13. A surgery that can be delayed for a few days is
    A. Emergency surgery
    B. Elective surgery
    C. Urgent surgery
    D. Out-patient surgery

14. When an accident occurs, the person often requires
    A. Elective surgery   C. General anesthesia
    B. Emergency surgery   D. Urgent surgery

15. When a person tells you about fears and concerns before surgery, you should
    A. Explain that the surgeon is very skilled
    B. Tell the person not to worry
    C. Respect the person's fears by showing warmth, sensitivity, and caring
    D. Change the subject and talk about something else

16. When a patient asks you about test results or the diagnosis
    A. Answer the questions honestly
    B. Tell the person you will get the nurse
    C. Tell the person that information is not available
    D. Explain that you do not know but will find out

17. Which of these is *not* part of your role when caring for a surgical patient?
    A. Explain the care you will give.
    B. Provide care with skill and ease.
    C. Tell the person about your own experience with the same surgery.
    D. Report a request to see a member of the clergy to the nurse.

18. The nurse will tell the patient that deep-breathing and coughing exercises will be done after surgery
    A. Once a shift
    B. Every 1 or 2 hours when the person is awake
    C. Every 4 hours
    D. Every 2 hours for the first 48 hours after surgery

19. How is a child prepared for surgery?
    A. The parents are responsible for explaining the surgery to the child.
    B. A doll may be used to show the site of the surgery.
    C. Children are not told about the surgery as it may frighten them.
    D. A child does not need an explanation as the idea of surgery is too difficult for the child to understand.

20. If blood loss is expected during surgery, what test is done preoperatively?
    A. Type and crossmatch   C. Urinalysis
    B. Complete blood count   D. Electrocardiogram

21. A person is NPO for 6 to 8 hours before surgery to reduce
    A. Breathing problems after surgery
    B. Pain post-operatively
    C. Diarrhea
    D. Vomiting and aspiration during and after surgery

22. Cleansing enemas may be ordered before surgery to
    A. Prevent contamination of the abdominal cavity during surgery
    B. Prevent incontinence after surgery
    C. Prevent diarrhea after surgery
    D. Prevent pain

23. The person being prepared for surgery needs to void
    A. Right before leaving the room
    B. The morning of surgery
    C. Before the nurse gives the pre-operative drugs
    D. Before an enema is given

24. Make-up, nail polish, and fake nails are removed before surgery because
    A. This reduces wound infection
    B. It reduces the number of microbes on the body
    C. The skin, lips, and nail beds are observed for color during and after surgery
    D. It makes the person more comfortable after surgery

25. When preparing a child for surgery, it is important to report
    A. A dry mouth
    B. Any loose teeth
    C. Any missing teeth
    D. That you removed hair clips from the hair

26. If a person is allowed to wear a wedding ring during surgery, you should
    A. Record this information on the chart
    B. Secure it in place with gauze and tape
    C. Make sure it fits well and will not come off
    D. Put a clean glove on the person's hand

27. If you are assigned to do a skin preparation with a razor pre-operatively, you should be careful
    A. Not to cut, scratch, or nick the skin
    B. To shave against the direction of hair growth
    C. To shave the entire body
    D. Not to shave too closely to the skin

28. The surgery consent
    A. Is signed by the person and sometimes the nearest relative
    B. Is signed by the person's attorney
    C. May be obtained by the nursing assistant
    D. Is not needed for emergency surgery

29. Pre-operative medications are given
    A. To prevent pain
    B. Before the person is transported to the operating room
    C. Immediately before surgery
    D. In the operating room

30. When you are delegated to assist with the pre-operative checklist, it must be completed
    A. Before the nurse gives the pre-operative drugs
    B. Before the patient falls asleep after receiving the pre-operative drugs
    C. Before the patient leaves the unit for surgery
    D. The night before the surgery

31. When a child is transported to the operating room, the parents
    A. Must stay in the child's room
    B. May stay in the OR until the anesthesia is given and the child is asleep
    C. Are allowed to go with the child as far as the OR entrance
    D. May stay with the child during surgery

32. A person stays in the PACU for 1 to 2 hours after surgery or until
    A. Vital signs need to be taken only every 4 hours
    B. All IVs are removed
    C. The person can respond and call for needed help
    D. The person is completely awake

33. When you prepare a room for a person to return from surgery
    A. You make a closed bed
    B. The bed is in the lowest position
    C. The bed is raised for a transfer from a stretcher
    D. You make an open bed

34. You may be assigned to take the vital signs after surgery. They are usually measured
    A. Once a shift
    B. Every 15 minutes until the person is stable
    C. Every 2 hours
    D. Every 5 minutes for the first hour

35. Post-operatively, the person is positioned
    A. In supine position
    B. To allow for easy and comfortable breathing
    C. In Fowler's position
    D. In reverse Trendelenburg position

36. Coughing and deep-breathing exercises are done after surgery to
    A. Make the person more comfortable
    B. Prevent complications such as pneumonia and atelectasis
    C. Decrease pain and discomfort
    D. Prevent nausea and vomiting

37. Leg exercises are important to prevent
    A. Pneumonia and atelectasis
    B. Thrombus and embolus (blood clots) from forming
    C. Pain at the surgical site
    D. Low blood pressure

38. Leg exercises are done
    A. At least every 1 to 2 hours while the person is awake
    B. Once a shift
    C. When the person is able to do them independently
    D. After the person begins to ambulate

39. Elastic stockings are used to
    A. Prevent swelling in the legs
    B. Prevent orthostatic hypotension
    C. Promote venous blood return to the heart and prevent blood clots
    D. Increase blood pressure

40. When applying elastic stockings, you should have the person
    A. Lie in a supine position
    B. Sit in a chair
    C. In Fowler's position
    D. First walk around the room for few minutes

41. When applying elastic bandages
    A. Start at the proximal part of the extremity
    B. Completely cover the fingers or toes
    C. Apply the bandages very loosely
    D. Expose the fingers and toes if possible

42. When you assist a person to walk after surgery, you first measure
    A. The person's temperature
    B. The blood pressure and pulse
    C. The distance from the bed to the door
    D. The person's weight

43. If a person is NPO after surgery, important personal hygiene is
    A. Frequent oral hygiene
    B. Giving ice chips frequently
    C. Offering sips of cool water
    D. Giving a complete bed bath

44. It is important to report the time and amount of the first voiding after surgery because the person must void
    A. Within 2 hours after surgery
    B. During the first 24 hours after surgery
    C. Within 8 hours after surgery
    D. At least 1000 mL within the first 4 hours after surgery

Fill in the Blank

45. Write out the abbreviations.
    A. AE _____
    B. CBC _____
    C. ECG _____
    D. EKG _____
    E. ID _____
    F. IV _____
    G. NG _____
    H. NPO _____
    I. OR _____
    J. PACU _____
    K. Pre-op _____
    L. Post-op _____
    M. SCD _____
    N. TED _____

46. If a person has out-patient, 1-day, or ambulatory surgery, the person is admitted in the morning and _____.

47. Before surgery, special personal care is done. Describe the care given and the reasons it is important.
    A. Baths _____
    B. Removing make-up, nail polish, and fake nails _____
    C. Hair care _____
    D. Oral hygiene _____

48. Some people do not like being seen without their dentures. How can you promote dignity and self-esteem when dentures must be removed before surgery? _____

49. When you are delegated a skin preparation, what is reported and recorded?
    A. _____
    B. _____
    C. _____
    D. _____

50. What vital signs are recorded on the pre-operative checklist? _____

51. After the pre-operative drugs are given, the person is not allowed _____.

52. When a person returns to the room after surgery, how often are vital signs usually measured?
    A. _____
    B. _____
    C. _____
    D. _____

53. What post-operative observations of the vital signs should be reported to the nurse?
    A. Temperature _____
    B. Pulse
        i. _____
        ii. _____
        iii. _____
        iv. _____
    C. Respirations
        i. _____
        ii. _____
        iii. _____
        iv. _____
        v. _____
        vi. _____
        vii. _____
    D. Blood pressure _____

54. You may be able to turn a person who has had surgery by yourself when the person's condition _____.

55. Why are older persons at risk for respiratory complications?
    A. _____
    B. _____
    C. _____

56. Leg exercises are done at least every _____.
    These exercises are done _____ times.

57. Leg exercises are

    A. _____

    B. _____

    C. _____

    D. _____

58. When you apply elastic stockings, you avoid twists because they can _____. Creases and wrinkles can cause _____.

59. When you apply elastic bandages, what observations are reported and recorded?

    A. _____

    B. _____

    C. _____

    D. _____

    E. _____

    F. _____

    G. _____

    H. _____

60. Early ambulation prevents

    A. _____

    B. _____

    C. _____

    D. _____

    E. _____

Use the FOCUS ON PRIDE section to complete these statements.

61. How can you ease a person's fears and concerns when he or she has surgery?

    A. _____

    B. _____

    C. _____

    D. _____

62. What questions can you answer when caring for a person having surgery? _____

    _____

63. When you are delegated to take post-operative vital signs, what should you report at once to the nurse?

    A. _____

    B. _____

    C. _____

Labeling

64. Color in the area on the figure that needs a skin preparation for the surgery listed.

A. Breast surgery

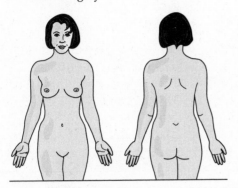

B. Cervical spine surgery

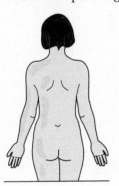

C. Knee surgery

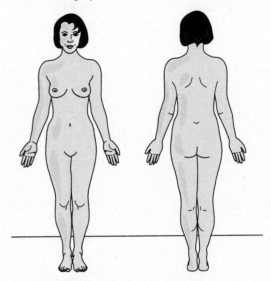

D. Abdominal and leg surgery

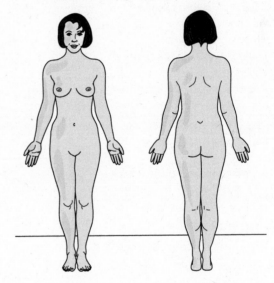

65. A pre-operative checklist is completed before a person
    is sent to surgery. Mark the steps that a nursing
    assistant can do and report to the nurse.

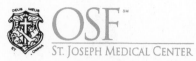

OSF ℠
ST. JOSEPH MEDICAL CENTER

2200 E. Washington Street, Bloomington, Illinois 61701
Phone (309) 662-3311

PRE-OPERATIVE CHECKLIST

DATE OF SURGERY: _____

CHART PREPARATION	ADEQUATE INITIAL HERE	NOT ADEQUATE INITIAL HERE AND EXPLAIN
1. HISTORY AND PHYSICAL ON CHART HT. _____ WT. _____		
2. SURGICAL CONSENT ON CHART, SIGNED		
3. CONSENT FOR ADM BLOOD/BLOOD PROD.		
4. PREGNANCY TEST OBTAINED WHEN INDICATED		
5. URINALYSIS REPORT ON CHART		
6. BLOOD WORK TYPE _____		
7. TYPE AND CROSSMATCH		
8. CHEST X-RAY REPORT ON CHART		
9. EKG REPORT ON CHART READ _____		
10. KNOWN ALLERGIES AND SENSITIVITIES NOTED ON CHART		
11. KNOWN EXPOSURE AND/OR ALLERGY TO **LATEX** NOTED ON CHART		

PATIENT PREPARATION	ADEQUATE INITIAL HERE	NOT ADEQUATE INITIAL HERE AND EXPLAIN
12. FAMILY NOTIFIED OF SURGERY NAME _____ DATE/TIME _____		
13. PATIENT IDENTIFICATION ON WRIST		
14. ALL PROSTHESIS REMOVED (INCLUDING DENTURES, WIGS, HAIRPINS, CONTACT LENSES, COSMETICS, NAIL POLISH, ARTIFICIAL EYES, LIMBS, ETC.)		
15. ALL JEWELRY REMOVED		
16. CLOTHING REMOVED EXCEPT HOSPITAL GOWN WITH TIES		
17. SURGICAL PREP DONE		
18. TIME OF LAST MEAL OR FLUIDS _____ TIME		
19. PRE-OP TPR AND BP: T_____ P_____ R_____ BP_____		
20. VOIDED TIME _____ OR FOLEY		
21. PRE-OP IV AND/OR ANTIBIOTIC: TIME:		

	DRUG	DOSAGE	ROUTE
PREOPERATIVE MEDICATION GIVEN,	_____	_____	_____

TIME _____ GIVEN BY _____

☐ SIDE RAILS UP

READY FOR O.R.   DATE _____ TIME _____   SIGNATURE _____

PATIENT IDENTIFIED BY TRANSPORTER AND STAFF NURSE   TIME _____

FLOOR NURSE
SIGNATURE _____

OR TRANSPORTER
SIGNATURE _____

OR NURSE
SIGNATURE _____

IDENTIFICATION OF INITIALS			
INITIALS	SIGNATURE	INITIALS	SIGNATURE

Optional Learning Exercises

Mr. Shafer is an 82-year-old man admitted for knee replacement surgery. Answer the questions about Mr. Shafer and his pre-operative care.

66. This surgery is done by choice and is an

    _____ surgery.

67. When you are in the room, you listen quietly while Mr. Shafer talks about his fears and concerns. By sitting quietly and showing concern for his feelings, you can assist in Mr. Shafer's

    _____ care.

68. The nurse comes to Mr. Shafer's room. What kind of pre-operative teaching will be given to him?

    A. _____
    B. _____
    C. _____
    D. _____
    E. _____
    F. _____
    G. _____
    H. _____
    I. _____
    J. _____

69. The nurse tells you she will give Mr. Shafer his pre-operative drugs in 10 minutes. What should you do? _____

Mrs. Johnson is a 70-year-old woman who is scheduled for abdominal surgery. Answer these questions about her care.

70. The nurse tells you she is busy and asks you to have Mrs. Johnson sign the surgery consent. What should

    you do? _____

    _____

71. Mrs. Johnson returns to her room 2 hours after the surgery is completed. You know she is transported to her room when

    A. _____
    B. _____
    C. _____

72. How is the room prepared for Mrs. Johnson's return?

    A. _____
    B. _____
    C. _____

73. When Mrs. Johnson returns to her room, she has sequential compression devices (SCDs) on her legs. What is the purpose of an SCD?

    _____

    _____

74. You are caring for Mrs. Johnson 3 days after her surgery. She tells you she has not had a bowel movement since before surgery. You know that one reason for constipation can be drugs given for

    _____.

Fill in the Blank: Key Terms

Abrasion
Arterial ulcer
Chronic wound
Circulatory ulcer
Clean-contaminated
  wound
Clean wound
Closed wound
Contaminated wound
Contusion
Dehiscence

Diabetic foot ulcer
Dirty wound
Edema
Evisceration
Excoriation
Full-thickness wound
Gangrene
Hematoma
Hemorrhage
Incision
Infected wound

Intentional wound
Laceration
Open wound
Partial-thickness wound
Penetrating wound
Phlebitis
Puncture wound
Purulent drainage
Sanguineous drainage
Serosanguineous drainage
Serous drainage

Shock
Skin tear
Stasis ulcer
Trauma
Ulcer
Unintentional wound
Vascular ulcer
Venous ulcer
Wound

1. A _____ is a break or rip in the skin that separates the epidermis from underlying tissues.

2. An open wound with clean, straight edges, usually intentional from a sharp instrument, is an

   _____

3. A shallow or deep crater-like sore of the skin or mucous membrane is an

   _____

4. When tissues are injured but the skin is not broken, it is a _____.

5. _____ is thick green, yellow, or brown drainage.

6. When the dermis and epidermis of the skin are broken, it is called a

   _____

7. A _____ is a break in the skin or mucous membrane.

8. A wound that is not infected and that microbes have not entered is a

   _____

9. An _____ is a partial-thickness wound caused by the scraping away or rubbing of the skin.

10. A _____ is an open wound on the foot caused by complications from diabetes.

11. Thin, watery drainage that is blood-tinged is called

    _____

12. An _____ is a wound containing large amounts of bacteria and that shows signs of infection; dirty wound.

13. An open sore on the lower legs or feet caused by decreased blood flow through arteries or veins is a

    _____

14. A swelling that contains blood is a

    _____

15. _____ is an inflammation of a vein.

16. A wound with a high risk of infection is a

    _____

17. A condition in which there is death of tissue is

    _____

18. A _____ is an open wound with torn tissues and jagged edges.

19. A wound resulting from trauma is an

    _____

20. An _____ is an open wound on the lower legs and feet caused by poor arterial blood flow.

21. Clear, watery fluid is _____

22. The excessive loss of blood in a short time is

    _____

23. An infected wound is a

    _____

24. A wound that occurs from surgical entry of the urinary, reproductive, respiratory, or gastro-intestinal system is a _____.

25. A _____ is a wound that does not heal easily.

26. An open sore on the lower legs or feet caused by poor blood flow through the veins is a

    _____; stasis ulcer.

27. An open wound made by a sharp object is a

    _____

    The entry of the skin and underlying tissues may be intentional or unintentional.

28. A wound created for therapy is an

_____.

29. A _____ is an open wound that breaks the skin and enters a body area, organ, or cavity.

30. _____ is the separation of wound layers.

31. A circulatory ulcer is also called a

_____.

32. Swelling that is caused by fluid collecting in tissues is

33. A _____ occurs when the dermis, epidermis, and subcutaneous tissue are penetrated. Muscle and bone may be involved.

34. An accident or violent act that injuries the skin, mucous membranes, bones, and internal organs is called _____.

35. The separation of the wound along with the protrusion of abdominal organs is

_____.

36. A _____ is another name for a venous ulcer.

37. Bloody drainage is called

_____.

38. A closed wound caused by a blow to the body is a

_____.

39. An _____ occurs when the skin or mucous membrane is broken.

40. _____ results when tissues do not get enough oxygen.

41. _____ is the loss of epidermis caused by scratching or when skin rubs against skin, clothing, or other materials.

Circle the Best Answer

42. When you inspect a resident's elbow, you find some of the skin is rubbed away. You would report this to the nurse as
    A. A laceration
    B. An abrasion
    C. A contusion
    D. An incision

43. When you look at a resident's arm that caught on the wheelchair, the tissue is torn with jagged edges. You know this is a
    A. Puncture wound
    B. Abrasion
    C. Penetrating wound
    D. Laceration

44. Which of these *would not* place a person at risk for skin tears?
    A. The person is obese.
    B. The person requires total help in moving.
    C. The person has poor nutrition.
    D. The person has altered mental awareness.

45. Applying lotion will help to prevent skin breakdown or skin tears because it may prevent
    A. Loss of fatty layer under the skin
    B. General thinning of the skin
    C. Dryness of the skin by keeping the skin moisturized
    D. Moisture in areas of the body where perspiration occurs

46. Ulcers of the feet and legs are caused by
    A. Poorly fitted shoes
    B. Decreased blood flow through arteries or veins
    C. Increased activity
    D. Increased fluid intake

47. A measure to prevent venous (stasis) ulcers is
    A. Use elastic or rubber band–type garters to hold the person's socks in place
    B. Remind the person not to sit with the legs crossed
    C. Cut the toenails to keep them short
    D. Massage the legs and feet

48. Common causes of arterial ulcers are
    A. Poor blood flow through the veins
    B. Leg or foot surgery
    C. High blood pressure, diabetes, and injuries
    D. Surgery on bones and joints

49. It is important to check the feet of a diabetic every day because
    A. The person may not feel a cut, blister, burn, or other trauma to the foot
    B. Toenails grow quickly
    C. Injuries heal well
    D. It relieves pain when you inspect and massage the feet

50. A person with diabetes should
    A. Go barefoot as much as possible
    B. Place feet near heat or use heating pads to stimulate circulation
    C. Break in new shoes slowly
    D. Soak feet in water to keep skin moisturized

51. During wound healing, what phase is happening when the wound is about 1 year old?
    A. Initial phase
    B. Inflammatory phase
    C. Maturation phase
    D. Proliferative phase

52. A surgical wound that is closed with sutures, staples, clips, special glue, or adhesive strips is an example of wound healing by
    A. Delayed intention
    B. First intention
    C. Second intention
    D. Third intention

53. A sign of internal hemorrhage is
    A. Dressings that are soaked with blood
    B. Bloody drainage
    C. An increase in the blood pressure
    D. A hematoma

54. If you observe signs of shock or hemorrhage, you should
    A. Report it to the nurse at once
    B. Re-position the person into a more comfortable position
    C. Make a note of your observations on the flow sheet
    D. Report the observations at the end of your shift

55. The nurse tells you to make sure Mrs. Reynolds supports her abdominal wound when she coughs. The nurse wants this done to protect against
    A. Secondary intention healing
    B. Infection
    C. Scarring
    D. Dehiscence

56. When you are caring for Mrs. Reynolds, you notice thin, watery drainage that is blood-tinged. When you report your observations, you would tell the nurse that the wound has _____ drainage.
    A. Purulent   C. Serous
    B. Serosanguineous   D. Sanguineous

57. A wet dressing will
    A. Provide a moist environment for wound healing
    B. Be kept moist at all times
    C. Allow air to reach the wound but prevent fluids and bacteria from doing so
    D. Stick to the wound

58. Plastic and paper tape may be used to secure a dressing
    A. Because they allow movement of the body part
    B. When the dressing must be changed frequently
    C. If the person is allergic to adhesive tape
    D. Because they stick well to the skin

59. If you care for a person who has Montgomery ties to secure a dressing, you should
    A. Replace the cloth ties when you give care
    B. Tell the nurse if the adhesive strips are soiled and need to be replaced
    C. Replace the adhesive strips each time you give care
    D. Re-tie the cloth ties when you re-position the person

60. If you are assigned to change a dressing, which of these is important information to have?
    A. What kind of medication the person receives
    B. The person's diagnosis
    C. When pain medication was given and how long until it takes effect
    D. When the dressing was last changed

61. You can make the person more comfortable when changing a dressing by doing all of the following *except*
    A. Control your nonverbal communication when looking at the wound
    B. Remove tape by pulling it toward the wound
    C. Encourage the person to look at the wound
    D. Make sure the person does not see the old dressing when it is removed

62. When you are assigned to change dressings, you should
    A. Change gloves after removing old dressing
    B. Use sterile technique
    C. Only wear gloves to remove old dressings
    D. Use 1 pair of gloves throughout the dressing change

63. A binder promotes healing because it will
    A. Prevent infection
    B. Reduce drainage
    C. Reduce swelling, promote comfort, and prevent injury
    D. Stop bleeding

64. A binder should be applied
    A. With firm, even pressure over the area
    B. And secured with safety pins positioned where they are easy to reach
    C. Very loosely to prevent interfering with movement
    D. Only once a day and removed only during AM care

65. Which of these measures *will not* be helpful when a person has a wound?
    A. Tell the person the wound looks fine and he or she shouldn't be upset.
    B. Encourage the person to eat well so that the body can heal better.
    C. Remove any soiled dressings from the room as soon as possible.
    D. Allow pain medications to take effect before giving wound care.

Fill in the Blank

66. Write out the abbreviations.
    A. GI _____
    B. PPE _____

67. What are common causes of skin tears?
    A. _____
    B. _____
    C. _____
    D. _____
    E. _____
    F. _____
    G. _____
    H. _____

68. List ways to prevent skin tears in the following:
    A. Keep the person hydrated by _____
       _____.
    B. What kind of clothing would be helpful? _____
       _____.
    C. Nail care of the person _____
       _____.
    D. Lift and turn the person with an _____
       _____.
    E. Support the arms and legs _____
       _____.
    F. Pad _____.
    G. Keep your fingernails _____
       and _____. Do not wear rings with
       _____.

69. Skin tears are portals _____.

70. When the person has circulatory ulcers, report any

_____.

71. You are caring for a person with a disease that affects venous circulation. You notice her toenails are long and sharp. You should _____

_____.

72. What 2 diseases are common causes of arterial ulcers?

_____

73. When a person has diabetes, what complications can occur with the following?
A. Nerves—person does not feel

_____. Can develop

_____.

B. Blood vessels—blood flow _____.
What can occur? _____

74. Explain what can happen if a person with diabetes has these foot problems.
A. Athlete's foot _____
B. Ingrown toenails _____
C. Hammer toes _____
D. Dry and cracked skin _____

75. With primary intention healing, the wound edges are

held together with _____.

76. Secondary intention healing is used for _____ wounds. Because healing

takes longer, the threat of _____
is great.

77. If you suspect a person has external hemorrhage, where would you check for drainage?

_____

78. What should you do if you find a person's wound has

dehiscence or evisceration? _____

_____

79. What observations would you make about wound appearance?
A. _____
B. _____
C. _____
D. _____
E. _____

80. When you are delegated to change a dressing, what should you do if the old dressings stick to the wound?

_____

81. If the person has drainage from a wound, how is it measured?
A. _____
B. _____
C. _____

82. What are purposes of a transparent adhesive film dressing?
A. _____
B. _____
C. _____
D. _____

83. When large amounts of drainage are expected, the

doctor inserts a _____
into the wound.

84. What drainage systems prevent microbes from

entering a wound? _____

85. When taping a dressing in place, the tape should not

encircle the entire body part because _____

_____.

86. When delegated to apply dressings, list what observations should be reported and recorded.
A. _____
B. _____
C. _____
D. _____
E. _____
F. _____
G. _____
H. _____
I. _____
J. _____
K. _____
L. _____

Use the FOCUS ON PRIDE section to complete these statements.

87. When you are giving care, you are responsible to protect the person's safety and well-being. What are your responsibilities regarding wound care in these situations?
A. If you are careless during a transfer, you can cause

a _____.
B. If you rush during a bath, you may not notice a

_____ between skin folds on a bariatric
person.
C. If you do not apply shoes properly on a diabetic

person, _____ can develop.

88. To promote comfort and interaction with family and friends for a person with a wound, you may
A. _____
B. _____
C. _____
D. _____
E. _____

Optional Learning Exercises

You are assigned to care for Mrs. Stevens. She is 87 years old and has diabetes and high blood pressure. She walks with difficulty and spends most of her day sitting in her chair. She is somewhat over-weight and tells you she had a knee replacement 5 years ago and had phlebitis after surgery. The nurse tells you to watch carefully for signs of circulatory ulcers.

89. What risk factors does Mrs. Stevens have that place her at risk for venous ulcers?

    A. _____

    B. _____

    C. _____

    D. _____

    E. _____

90. What risk factors does Mrs. Stevens have that place her at risk for arterial ulcers?

    A. _____

    B. _____

Mr. Hawkins, age 74, was in an automobile accident and has a wound on his leg that is large and open. It has become infected and he is being treated with antibiotics. When you are talking with him, he tells you he has smoked for 55 years and has poor circulation in his legs. He lives alone and generally eats takeout foods or eats cereal when he is at home.

91. Why is he receiving antibiotics?

    _____

    _____

92. What side effect of the antibiotics can cause a problem that could interfere with healing? _____

    _____

93. What factors would increase Mr. Hawkins' risk for complications?

    A. _____

    B. _____

    C. _____

    D. _____

94. What is missing in Mr. Hawkins' diet that is needed to help in healing the wound? _____

You are assisting the nurse with wound care. She is changing dressings for 2 different persons. Mrs. Henderson has a wound that has a large amount of drainage. Mr. Wendel has a drain in his wound that is attached to suction.

95. Why does the nurse weigh Mrs. Henderson's new dressings before applying them to the wound and the old dressings when they are removed?

    _____

    _____

96. How does she find out the amount of drainage from Mr. Wendel's wound? _____

    _____

97. What other ways can be used to measure drainage in old dressings?

    A. _____

    B. _____

    C. _____

    D. _____

    E. _____

    F. _____

98. When you are changing a nonsterile dressing, why do you need 2 pairs of gloves? _____

    _____

99. When a wound is infected and has poor circulation, the wound may be left open at first and then closed later. This type of wound healing is called healing through _____. This type of healing combines _____ and _____ intention healing.

37 Pressure Ulcers

Fill in the Blank: Key Terms

Avoidable pressure ulcer
Bedfast
Bony prominence
Chairfast

Colonized
Epidermal stripping
Eschar
Friction

Intact skin
Pressure point
Pressure ulcer
Shear

Skin breakdown
Slough
Unavoidable pressure
ulcer

1. Normal skin and skin layers without damage or breaks is _____.

2. _____ is the presence of bacteria on the wound surface or in wound tissue; the person does not have signs and symptoms of an infection.

3. Dead tissue that is shed from the skin is _____

4. A pressure ulcer that develops from the improper use of the nursing process is an _____.

5. A _____ is an area where the bone sticks out or projects from the flat surface of the body.

6. Thick, leathery dead tissue that may be loose or adhered to the skin is _____

7. Another name for bony prominence is _____.

8. _____ occurs when layers of the skin rub against each other; when the skin remains in place and underlying tissues move and stretch and tear underlying capillaries and blood vessels causing tissue damage.

9. _____ means confined to bed.

10. The rubbing of one surface against another is _____.

11. An _____ is a pressure ulcer that occurs despite efforts to prevent one through proper use of the nursing process.

12. A localized injury to the skin and/or underlying tissue, usually over a bony prominence, resulting from pressure or pressure in combination with shear is a _____

13. _____ means confined to a chair.

14. Removing the epidermis as tape is removed from the skin is _____.

15. Changes or damage to intact skin is _____

Circle the Best Answer

16. A pressure ulcer occurs because
    A. The person re-positions himself or herself in the bed or chair
    B. The person drinks too many fluids
    C. Skin and underlying tissue is damaged by pressure or pressure in combination with shear and/or friction
    D. The person is re-positioned too frequently

17. Older and disabled persons are at great risk for pressure ulcers because of
    A. Acute illnesses
    B. Increased activity
    C. Thin and fragile skin
    D. Good nutrition

18. Risk factors for pressure ulcers are *all* of the following *except*
    A. Sitting in one position for 4 hours
    B. Pulling a person up in a bed or chair and causing shearing
    C. Helping the person to drink plenty of liquids
    D. Having skin that is irritated by urine or feces

19. The first sign of a pressure ulcer in an area may be
    A. Reddened skin over a bony prominence
    B. Swelling in the area
    C. A break in the skin
    D. Exposed tissue and some drainage from the area

20. Mrs. Greene keeps sliding down in bed. The nurse tells you to raise the head of the bed no more than 30 degrees. This position will prevent tissue damage caused by
    A. Pressure over hard surfaces
    B. Shearing
    C. Poor body mechanics
    D. Poor fluid balance

21. In children and infants, pressure ulcers commonly occur
    A. Over bony areas such as the hips
    B. Underneath the breasts
    C. Between abdominal folds
    D. On the back of the head

22. A Kennedy terminal ulcer occurs
    A. Because of poor nursing care
    B. Over a bony prominence 2 to 3 days before death
    C. Because of poor hydration
    D. In patients who are incontinent

23. A Stage 3 pressure ulcer would have
    A. Intact skin with redness or different skin coloring over a bony prominence
    B. Exposed subcutaneous fat and slough
    C. Full-thickness tissue loss with muscle, tendon, and bone exposure
    D. A blister or shallow ulcer

24. The most common site for a pressure ulcer is the
    A. Elbow   C. Thighs
    B. Sacrum   D. Ears

25. When following a re-positioning schedule, the person should be re-positioned
    A. According to the person's re-positioning schedule
    B. Every 2 hours
    C. Every 15 minutes
    D. As often as you have time

26. One way to prevent friction in the bed is to
    A. Use soap when cleansing the skin
    B. Rub or massage reddened areas
    C. Use pillows and blankets to prevent skin from being in contact with skin
    D. Powder sheets lightly

27. Bed cradles are used to
    A. Position the person in good body alignment
    B. Prevent pressure on the legs, feet, and toes
    C. Keep the heels off the bed
    D. Distribute body weight evenly

28. When the person is using some special beds, it allows
    A. The person to move around easily
    B. Re-positioning without moving the person
    C. 1 staff member to move the person every 2 hours
    D. The head of the bed to be elevated

Fill in the Blank

29. Write out the abbreviations.
    A. CMS _____
    B. NPUAP _____
    C. TJC _____

30. Name the stage of pressure ulcer described in each of these.
    A. The skin is gone and subcutaneous fat may be exposed. _____
    B. In a person with dark skin, skin color may differ from surrounding areas. _____
    C. Muscle, tendon, and bone are exposed and damaged. Eschar may be present. _____
    D. The wound may involve an abrasion, blister, or shallow crater. _____

31. You can help prevent shearing by raising the head of the bed only _____. The care plan tells you
    A. _____
    B. _____
    C. _____

32. Explain how the following conditions place a person at risk for pressure ulcers.
    A. Urinary or fecal incontinence _____
       _____
    B. Poor nutrition _____
       _____
    C. Limited mental awareness _____
       _____
    D. Circulatory problems _____
       _____
    E. Have weight loss or are very thin _____
       _____

33. Explain how these protective devices help prevent pressure ulcers.
    A. Bed cradle prevents pressure on
       _____.
    B. Heel and elbow protectors promote
       _____
       and reduce _____
       and _____.
    C. Heel and foot elevators raise
       _____.
    D. Gel or fluid-filled pads have
       _____
    E. Special beds distribute
       _____. There is little
       pressure on _____.

34. Describe dressings used to treat pressure ulcers.
    A. Wet dressings must be _____.
       If too moist, the dressing can _____.
    B. Dressing may absorb _____.
       When the dressing is removed, the _____
       is removed.

35. According to the CMS, infection is present in Stages _____ of pressure ulcers.

Use the FOCUS ON PRIDE section to complete these statements.

36. When you observe and report skin problems to the nurse, it can prevent _____

37. When you speak up for your patients and residents, this is called being an _____.

Labeling

Answer questions 38 and 39 using the following illustration.

38. Name this position.

_____

39. Place an "X" on each of the 5 pressure points. Name the bony point for each one.

    A. _____

    B. _____

    C. _____

    D. _____

    E. _____

Answer questions 40 and 41 using the following illustration.

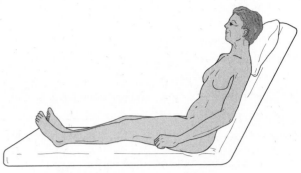

Answer questions 44 and 45 using the following illustration.

40. Name this position. _____

41. Place an "X" on each of the 10 pressure points. Name the bony point for each one.

    A. _____

    B. _____

    C. _____

    D. _____

    E. _____

    F. _____

    G. _____

    H. _____

    I. _____

    J. _____

Answer questions 42 and 43 using the following illustration.

44. Name this position. _____

45. Place an "X" on each of the 6 pressure points. Name the bony point for each one.

    A. _____

    B. _____

    C. _____

    D. _____

    E. _____

    F. _____

Answer questions 46 and 47 using the following illustration.

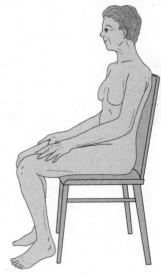

42. Name this position. _____

43. Place an "X" on each of the 10 pressure points. Name the bony point for each one.

    A. _____

    B. _____

    C. _____

    D. _____

    E. _____

    F. _____

    G. _____

    H. _____

    I. _____

    J. _____

46. Name this position. _____

47. Place an "X" on each of the 5 pressure points. Name the bony point for each one.

    A. _____

    B. _____

    C. _____

    D. _____

    E. _____

Optional Learning Exercises

48. After admission to a nursing center, many pressure ulcers develop within the first _____ after admission.

49. How quickly can a person develop a pressure ulcer after the onset of pressure? _____

50. When handling, moving, and positioning a person, it is important to follow the _____ _____ in the person's care plan.
   A. How often should a bedfast person be re-positioned? _____
   B. How often should a chairfast person be re-positioned? _____
   C. Why would a person be re-positioned more frequently (as often as every 15 minutes)?
   _____

51. What are 2 ways pressure ulcers can occur on the ears?
   A. _____
   B. _____

52. If you are interviewed by the CMS staff about pressure ulcers, what questions may be asked?
   A. _____
   B. _____
   C. _____
   D. _____
   E. _____

38 Heat and Cold Applications

Fill in the Blank: Key Terms

Compress   Cyanosis   Hyperthermia   Pack

Constrict   Dilate   Hypothermia

1. A body temperature that is much higher than the person's normal range is

   _____.

2. _____ means to narrow.

3. A treatment that involves wrapping a body part with a wet or dry application is a

   _____

4. A _____ is a soft pad applied over a body area.

5. _____ means to expand or open wider.

6. _____ occurs when the body temperature is very low.

7. A bluish color is _____.

Circle the Best Answer

8. Heat applications can be applied
   A. Only to extremities
   B. To areas with metal implants
   C. To almost any body part
   D. To persons who have difficulty sensing heat or pain

9. When heat is applied to the skin
   A. Blood vessels in the area dilate
   B. Tissues have less oxygen
   C. Blood flow decreases
   D. Blood vessels constrict

10. When heat is applied for too long, a complication that occurs is
    A. Blood vessels dilate
    B. Blood flow increases
    C. Blood vessels constrict
    D. More nutrients reach the area

11. Moist heat applications have cooler temperatures than dry heat applications because
    A. Dry heat penetrates more deeply
    B. Dry heat cannot cause burns
    C. Heat penetrates deeper with a moist application
    D. Moist heat has a slower effect than dry heat

12. When heat is applied to an area, which of these is an expected response?
    A. The skin is red and warm.
    B. The skin is pale, white, or gray.
    C. The person begins to shiver.
    D. The area is excessively red.

13. The care plan states that the person receives a heat application of 110 °F. As a nursing assistant you know that you should
    A. Measure the temperature carefully before applying heat to the person
    B. Not apply an application that is above 106 °F
    C. Ask the person if the application is too warm
    D. Apply the application and remind the person not to remove it

14. Heat and cold applications are applied for no longer than
    A. 1 hour   C. 15 to 20 minutes
    B. 30 minutes   D. 4 hours

15. When a hot or cold application is in place, you should check the area
    A. Every 15 to 20 minutes
    B. Every 5 minutes
    C. About every 30 minutes
    D. Once an hour

16. When hot compresses are in place, you may apply an aquathermia pad over the compress
    A. To keep the compress wet
    B. To protect the area from injury
    C. To measure the temperature of the compress
    D. To maintain the correct temperature of the compress

17. A hot soak is applied
    A. By putting the body part into water
    B. By applying a soft pad to a body part
    C. And is covered with plastic wrap
    D. Only until the water temperature cools down

18. When giving a sitz bath
    A. Check the person often to assess for weakness, fainting, or fatigue
    B. Keep the door open so you can see the person from the hallway
    C. Give the person privacy by closing the door and leaving the person alone for the entire time
    D. Make sure the water temperature is hot

19. When you use an aquathermia pad
    A. The pad temperature will cool off after about 20 to 30 minutes
    B. The temperature is maintained by the flow of water through the pad
    C. It is a form of moist heat
    D. You do not need to check the person as often as with other heat applications

20. When a cold application is applied, the numbing effect helps to
  A. Reduce or relieve pain in the part
  B. Constrict blood vessels
  C. Decrease blood flow
  D. Cool the body part

21. Which of these cold applications is moist?
  A. Ice bag   C. Ice glove
  B. Ice collar   D. Cold compress

22. You should remove the heat or cold application if
  A. The skin is red and warm with a heat application
  B. The person tells you the cold application has numbed the area and relieved some pain
  C. The skin appears pale, white, gray, or bluish in color
  D. The person is slightly chilled and asks for another blanket

23. When a person has hyperthermia, ice packs are applied to all of these areas *except*
  A. The abdomen   C. The underarms
  B. The head   D. The groin

Fill in the Blank

24. Write out the abbreviations.
  A. F _____
  B. C _____

25. What are the effects of heat applications?
  A. _____
  B. _____
  C. _____
  D. _____
  E. _____

26. When you are caring for a confused person and heat or cold is applied, how can you know if the person is in pain? _____

27. What are the advantages of dry heat applications?
  A. _____
  B. _____

28. Give 2 examples of dry heat applications.
  _____

29. When the nurse delegates you to prepare a warm soak, what is the correct temperature range?
  _____

30. When you are giving a sitz bath, what observations should be reported to the nurse?
  _____

31. When using an aquathermia pad, you should make sure the hoses do not have kinks or air bubbles to allow the water to _____

32. Name the uses for cold applications.
  A. _____
  B. _____
  C. _____
  D. _____
  E. _____

33. When you prepare an ice bag, ice collar, or ice glove remove the excess air by _____
  _____.

34. When a cooling blanket is being used, _____ are checked often.

35. How can you manage your time to stay in or near the person's room during a heat or cold application?
  A. _____
  B. _____
  C. _____
  D. _____
  E. _____
  F. _____

Use the FOCUS ON PRIDE section to complete these statements.

36. When applying heat or cold, you must allow time for
  A. _____
  B. _____
  C. _____
  D. _____
  E. _____

37. When applying heat and cold, harm and legal action can result if you
  A. _____
  B. _____
  C. _____
  D. _____
  E. _____
  F. _____
  G. _____

Optional Learning Exercises

Situation: The nurse instructs you to apply a cold pack to a resident who has twisted her ankle. Use the information you learned in this chapter to answer these questions about carrying out this treatment.

38. What is the purpose of the cold application for this injury? _____
  _____

39. What can you use to make a cool dry application to the ankle if no commercial packs are available?
  _____

40. Why do you squeeze the application tightly after filling it with ice? _____

41. How will you protect the person's skin?

_____

42. How often do you check the application?

_____

43. When you check the area where the cold pack was applied, what signs and symptoms should be reported?

 A. _____
 B. _____
 C. _____
 D. _____
 E. _____
 F. _____
 G. _____

44. What should you do if any of these signs or symptoms are present? _____

45. How long should you leave the application in place?

_____

46. What happens if you leave the cold pack in place for too long? _____

39 Oxygen Needs

Fill in the Blank: Key Terms

Allergy
Apnea
Atelectasis
Biot's respirations
Bradypnea
Cheyne-Stokes respirations

Cyanosis
Dyspnea
Hemoptysis
Hyperventilation
Hypoventilation
Hypoxemia

Hypoxia
Kussmaul respirations
Orthopnea
Orthopneic position
Oxygen concentration
Pollutant

Pulse oximetry
Respiratory arrest
Respiratory depression
Sputum
Tachypnea

1. _____ are respirations that are rapid and deep followed by 10 to 30 seconds of apnea.

2. Bloody sputum is called

   _____

3. Rapid breathing where respirations are usually greater than 20 per minute is called

   _____

4. An _____ is a sensitivity to a substance that causes the body to react with signs and symptoms.

5. Difficult, labored, or painful breathing is

   _____

6. Mucus from the respiratory system that is expectorated through the mouth is

   _____

7. Being able to breathe deeply and comfortably only while sitting is _____

8. Respirations that are less than 12 per minute is slow breathing or _____

9. A reduced amount of oxygen in the blood is

   _____

10. _____ describes slow, weak respirations that occur at a rate of fewer than 12 per minute.

11. The lack or absence of breathing is

    _____

12. _____ is a pattern of respirations that is rapid and deeper than normal.

13. A harmful chemical or substance in the air or water is a _____

14. _____ are respirations that gradually increase in rate and depth and then become shallow and slow. Breathing may stop for 10 to 20 seconds.

15. The _____ is sitting up and leaning over a table to breathe.

16. When breathing stops, it is _____

17. Very deep and rapid respirations are

    _____

18. _____ is the amount of hemoglobin containing oxygen.

19. When cells do not have enough oxygen, it is called

    _____

20. Respirations that are slow, shallow, and sometimes irregular is _____

21. The collapse of a portion of the lung is

    _____

22. _____ is a bluish color to the skin, lips, mucous membrane, and nail beds.

23. _____ measures the oxygen concentration in arterial blood.

Circle the Best Answer

24. The _____ brings O_2 into the lungs and removes CO_2.
    A. Respiratory system
    B. Circulatory system
    C. Nervous system
    D. Red blood cells

25. Oxygen needs increase when
    A. The person is aging
    B. Drugs are taken
    C. The person has fever or pain
    D. The person is well nourished

26. Respiratory depression or arrest can occur when
    A. The person exercises
    B. Allergies are present
    C. Narcotic drugs are taken in large doses
    D. The person smokes

27. Restlessness is one of the early signs of
    A. Hypoxia
    B. Apnea
    C. Hyperventilation
    D. Bradypnea

28. Which of these would *not* be a sign of hypoxia?
    A. Disorientation and confusion
    B. Decrease in pulse rate and respirations
    C. Apprehension and anxiety
    D. Cyanosis of the skin, mucous membranes, and nail beds

29. If a pulse oximeter is being used on a person with tremors or poor circulation, which of these sites would be best to use?
    A. A toe on a foot that is swollen
    B. A finger that has nail polish on the nail
    C. A toe with an open wound
    D. An earlobe

30. When you are delegated to place a pulse oximeter on a person, report to the nurse if
    A. The person is sleeping
    B. The pulse rate is above or below the alarm limit
    C. You remove nail polish on the nail before attaching the pulse oximeter
    D. You tape the oximeter in place

31. When a person has breathing difficulties, it is usually easier for the person to breathe
    A. In the supine position
    B. Lying on one side for long periods
    C. In the semi-Fowler's or Fowler's position
    D. In the prone position

32. Deep-breathing and coughing exercises
    A. Help prevent pneumonia and atelectasis
    B. Decrease pain after surgery or injury
    C. Are done once a day
    D. Cause mucus to form in the lungs

33. When assisting with coughing and deep breathing, you ask the person to
    A. Inhale through the mouth
    B. Hold the breath for 30 seconds
    C. Exhale slowly through pursed lips
    D. Repeat the exercise 1 or 2 times

34. The goal when using an incentive spirometer is to
    A. Encourage the person to take shallow breaths
    B. Increase the number of respirations
    C. Improve lung function and prevent complications
    D. Have the person exhale quickly

35. If a person is receiving oxygen, you may
    A. Set the flow rate
    B. Apply the oxygen device to the person
    C. Set up the system
    D. Turn on the oxygen

36. If you are caring for a person with oxygen therapy, you may *not*
    A. Start and maintain oxygen therapy
    B. Maintain adequate water level in the humidifier
    C. Tell the nurse if the rate is too high or too low
    D. Check for irritation from the device

37. When oxygen is in use, you do all of these *except*
    A. Place no smoking signs in the room and on the room door
    B. Turn off electrical items before unplugging them
    C. Do not use wool or synthetic fabrics in the room
    D. Turn off all electrical equipment

38. If a person receives oxygen through a nasal cannula, it is important to look for irritation
    A. On the nose, ears, and cheekbones
    B. Under the mask
    C. In the throat
    D. In the oral cavity

39. If you are delegated to set up for oxygen administration, you will do all of these *except*
    A. Collect the device with connecting tubing
    B. Attach the flowmeter to the wall outlet or tank
    C. Apply the oxygen device to the person
    D. Fill the humidifier with distilled water

40. If you are near a person receiving oxygen, which of these should you report?
    A. The humidifier is bubbling.
    B. The humidifier has enough water.
    C. The humidifier is not bubbling.
    D. The person is in a semi-Fowler's position.

Fill in the Blank

41. Write out the meaning of the abbreviations.
    A. CO_2 _____
    B. ID _____
    C. L/min _____
    D. O_2 _____
    E. RBC _____
    F. SpO_2 _____

42. As a person ages, what factors affect the person's oxygen needs?
    A. Respiratory muscles _____
    B. Lung tissue _____
    C. Strength for coughing _____
    D. Risk increases for developing _____

43. Three diseases are caused by or are a risk factor related to smoking. They are
    A. _____
    B. _____
    C. _____

44. How does alcohol increase the risk of aspiration?
    It depresses the _____, reduces the
    _____, and increases
    _____.

45. What terms can be used to describe sputum when reporting and recording?
    A. Color: _____
    B. Odor: _____
    C. Consistency: _____
    D. Hemoptysis: _____

46. The normal range for oxygen concentration is

_____.

47. If you are caring for a person with a pulse oximeter, what observations should be reported and recorded?

A. _____

B. _____

C. _____

D. _____

E. _____

F. _____

48. If a pulse oximeter is in place, what should be reported at once to the nurse?

A. SpO$_2$ _____

B. Pulse rate _____

C. Signs and symptoms of _____ and

_____

49. If a person has difficulty breathing, he or she may prefer a position where the person is sitting

_____.

This position is called _____

50. If a person has a productive cough, what respiratory hygiene and cough etiquette should be taught?

A. Cover _____

B. Use _____

C. Dispose of tissues _____

D. Wash _____

51. If a person is using an incentive spirometer, how long is the breath held to keep the balls floating?

_____

52. What observations should be reported after a person uses an incentive spirometer?

A. _____

B. _____

C. _____

D. _____

53. When a person wears a mask to receive oxygen, what should you do when the person needs to eat?

_____

How will the person receive oxygen during the meal?

_____

54. Oxygen is humidified because otherwise it will

_____.

Use the FOCUS ON PRIDE section to complete these statements.

55. When you remind the person or visitors not to smoke when NO SMOKING signs are used, you are protecting the person's right to a

_____.

56. You do not adjust the oxygen flow rate unless allowed by your _____ and

_____ and instructed _____.

Crossword

Fill in the crossword by answering the clues below with the words from this list:

Apnea   Bradypnea   Dyspnea   Hypoventilation   Orthopnea
Biot's   Cheyne-Stokes   Hyperventilation Kussmaul   Tachypnea

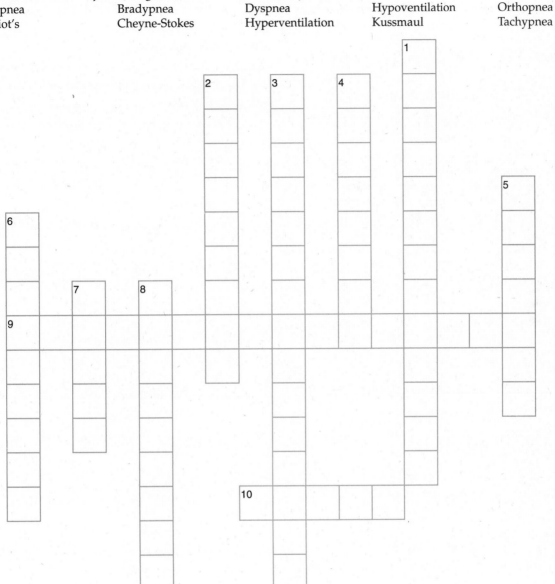

Across
9. Respirations are rapid and deeper than normal
10. Rapid and deep respirations followed by 10 to 30 seconds of apnea; occur with nervous disorders

Down
1. Respirations gradually increase in rate and depth; common when death is near
2. Respirations are 20 or more per minute
3. Respirations are slow, shallow, and sometimes irregular
4. Very deep and rapid respirations; signal diabetic coma
5. Difficult, labored, or painful breathing
6. Breathing deeply and comfortably only when sitting
7. Lack or absence of breathing
8. Respirations are fewer than 12 per minute

Optional Learning Exercises

Situation: You are caring for Mr. R., age 84, who has chronic obstructive pulmonary disease. Answer questions 57 and 58 about caring for Mr. R.

57. What position would make it easier for Mr. R. to breathe when he is in bed? _____

_____

58. How can you increase his comfort when he is sitting up? _____

_____ What is this

position called? _____

Situation: Mrs. F. is receiving oxygen through a nasal cannula at 2 L/min. Her respirations are unlabored at 16 per minute unless she is walking about or doing personal care. Then her respirations are 28 and dyspneic. Answer questions 59 to 62 about her care.

59. Why is there no humidifier with the oxygen setup for Mrs. F.? _____

_____

60. Where should you check for signs of irritation from the cannula? _____

_____

61. You should make sure there are _____ in the tubing and that Mrs. F. does not

_____ of the tubing.

62. What are the abnormal respirations that Mrs. F. has with activity called? _____

40 Respiratory Support and Therapies

Fill in the Blank: Key Terms

Hemothorax   Mechanical ventilation   Pleural effusion   Suction
Intubation   Patent   Pneumothorax   Tracheostomy

1. The escape and collection of fluid in the pleural space is _____.

2. _____ is blood in the pleural space.

3. A _____ is a surgically created opening into the trachea.

4. _____ is the process of withdrawing or sucking up fluid.

5. Inserting an artificial airway is _____.

6. _____ is air in the pleural space.

7. _____ is using a machine to move air into and out of the lungs.

8. _____ is open or unblocked.

Circle the Best Answer

9. When caring for a person with an artificial airway, you should tell the nurse at once if
   A. The vital signs remain stable
   B. Frequent oral hygiene is done
   C. The airway comes out or is dislodged
   D. The person feels as if he or she is gagging

10. Because a person with an endotracheal tube (ET) cannot speak, it is important to
    A. Never ask questions
    B. Avoid talking to the person
    C. Always keep the call light within reach
    D. Avoid explaining what you are going to do

11. The person with an ET can communicate by
    A. Whispering or speaking softly
    B. Using paper and pencil, Magic Slates, or communication boards
    C. Having a family member ask and answer questions
    D. Covering the tube opening

12. If you are caring for a person with an artificial airway, your care should always include
    A. Removing the device to clean it
    B. Comforting and re-assuring the person that the airway helps breathing
    C. Suctioning to maintain the airway
    D. Making sure the person never takes a tub bath

13. The stoma or tube must be
    A. Covered when shaving
    B. Covered with plastic when outdoors
    C. Covered with a loose gauze dressing when bathing
    D. Uncovered when the person is out of doors

14. If you are assisting with tracheostomy care, you may be delegated to
    A. Use clean technique when handling the equipment
    B. Provide care every 2 to 4 hours
    C. Clean a re-usable cannula with a cleaning agent that the nurse tells you to use
    D. Remove the inner and outer cannulas to clean them

15. When suctioning is done, the nurse
    A. Follows Standard Precautions and the Bloodborne Pathogen Standard
    B. Makes sure a suction cycle is not more than 20 to 30 seconds
    C. Waits about 5 seconds between each suction cycle
    D. Suctions as many times as needed to clear the airway

16. If you are caring for a person who needs suctioning, you know that suctioning is done
    A. On a regular schedule
    B. When signs and symptoms of respiratory distress are observed
    C. When the nurse directs you to do the suctioning
    D. When the person asks for suctioning

17. When the alarm sounds on a machine used for mechanical ventilation, you should first
    A. Report to the nurse at once
    B. Re-set the alarms
    C. Re-assure the person that the alarm is normal
    D. Check to see if the person's tube is attached to the ventilator

18. When caring for a person with chest tubes, tell the nurse at once if
    A. Vital signs are unchanged since last assessment
    B. There is a small amount of drainage in the chest tube
    C. The bubbling in the drainage system has increased
    D. The person tells you he or she has no pain

19. Petrolatum gauze is kept at the bedside of a person with chest tubes to
    A. Cover the insertion site if the chest tube comes out
    B. Lubricate the site of the chest tube
    C. Cleanse the skin around the chest tube
    D. Cover the site of the chest tube insertion to prevent drainage

Fill in the Blank

20. Write out the meaning of the abbreviations.

    A. CO_2 _____

    B. ET _____

    C. O_2 _____

    D. RT _____

21. When assisting with suctioning, tell the nurse if there is

    A. A decrease in _____ to

      less than _____

    B. Irregular _____ rhythm

    C. An increase or decrease in _____

    D. Signs of _____

    E. Decrease in oxygen _____

22. What are the 3 parts of a tracheostomy tube?

    A. _____

    B. _____

    C. _____

23. Which part of the tracheostomy tube is removed for cleaning and mucus removal? _____

24. Which part of the tracheostomy tube is not removed?

_____

25. If a person with a tracheostomy is outdoors, what is used to cover the tracheostomy? _____

_____

26. A suction cycle takes no more than _____ seconds. The cycle involves

    A. _____

    B. _____

    C. _____

27. Before, during, and after suctioning, what is checked and observed?

    A. _____

    B. _____

    C. _____

    D. _____

28. When a person has mechanical ventilation, what should you do when you enter the room? _____

_____

29. What should you do each time you leave the room of a person with mechanical ventilation? _____

_____

30. If chest tubes are in place, what should be reported to the nurse at once?

    A. _____

    B. _____

    C. _____

    D. _____

    E. _____

    F. _____

Use the FOCUS ON PRIDE section to complete these statements.

31. It is important to report signs and symptoms that a person needs suctioning because the airway must be clear for _____.

32. When a person has an ET tube, you show dignity and respect when providing care by

    A. _____

    B. _____

    C. _____

    D. _____

    E. _____

Optional Learning Exercises

33. If you are caring for a person with a tracheostomy, why is the tracheostomy covered when the person is outdoors? _____

_____

34. What is done to protect the stoma in the following situations?

    A. Showers _____

    B. Shaving _____

    C. Shampooing _____

35. The stoma is never covered with _____

_____.

    Why? _____

_____

36. What do you need to check before using an Ambu bag attached to oxygen? _____

    Why? _____

_____

37. If a person has mechanical ventilation, where do you find a plan for communication? _____

    Why is it important for everyone to use the same signals for communication? _____

_____

38. If a person has chest tubes, why is it important to prevent kinks in the tubing? _____

_____

41 Rehabilitation and Restorative Nursing Care

Fill in the Blank: Key Terms

Activities of daily living   Rehabilitation
Disability   Restorative aide
Prosthesis   Restorative nursing care

1. A nursing assistant with special training in restorative nursing and rehabilitation skills is a

   _____

2. _____ are activities usually done during a normal day in a person's life.

3. An artificial replacement for a missing body part is a

   _____

4. Care that helps persons regain their health, strength, and independence is _____.

5. A _____ is any lost, absent, or impaired physical or mental function.

6. The process of restoring the disabled person to the highest possible level of physical, psychological, social, and economic functioning is

   _____

Circle the Best Answer

7. One of the goals of rehabilitation is to
   A. Improve abilities
   B. Restore function to normal
   C. Help the person regain health and strength
   D. Prevent injury

8. Restorative nursing programs include measures that promote all of these *except*
   A. Self-care, elimination, and positioning
   B. Mobility, communication, and cognitive function
   C. Maintaining the highest level of function
   D. Restoration of all abilities to normal

9. If you are a restorative aide, it means you have
   A. Special training in restorative nursing and rehabilitation skills
   B. Taken required classes for restorative aides
   C. Passed a special test to show you can perform these duties
   D. The most seniority at the facility

10. When assisting with rehabilitation and restorative care, it is important to
    A. Give complete care to prevent exertion by the person
    B. Make sure you do everything for the person
    C. Encourage the person to perform ADL to the extent possible
    D. Complete care quickly

11. Which of these would be most helpful for a person receiving rehabilitative care?
    A. Give the person pity or sympathy when tasks are difficult.
    B. Remind the person not to try new skills or those that are difficult.
    C. Give praise when even a little progress is made.
    D. Encourage the person to perform ADL quickly.

12. Complications can be prevented by
    A. Doing all ADL for the person
    B. Allowing the person to decide if he or she wants to move or exercise
    C. Making sure the person is in good alignment, is turned and re-positioned, and has range-of-motion exercises
    D. Making sure rehabilitation is fast-paced

13. Rehabilitation begins
    A. After the person has recovered
    B. When the person first seeks health care
    C. When the person asks for help
    D. When a discharge date has been set

14. Self-help devices help to meet the goal of
    A. Recovery of all normal abilities
    B. Self-care
    C. Living alone
    D. Dependence on others

15. Rehabilitation includes ways to help the person adjust to
    A. Only physical care needs
    B. Only ambulation needs
    C. Physical, psychological, social, and economic needs
    D. Only psychological and social needs

16. The rehabilitation team meets to evaluate the person's progress
    A. Every 90 days
    B. Often, to discuss the person and make needed changes
    C. Every week
    D. Only when requested by the family or person

17. A person who has had a joint replacement would receive
    A. Spinal cord rehabilitation
    B. Amputee rehabilitation
    C. Orthopedic rehabilitation
    D. Stroke rehabilitation

18. OBRA requires that nursing centers
    A. Have a full-time physical therapist
    B. Provide rehabilitation services
    C. Provide physical care only
    D. Employ full-time occupational and speech therapists

19. When a home is assessed for a rehabilitation patient, scalding is prevented by
    A. Telling the caregiver to use only a hand-held shower nozzle
    B. Making sure the person can get in and out of the shower or bathtub easily
    C. Making faucets easy to use
    D. Regulating the water temperature

Fill in the Blank

20. Write out the meaning of the abbreviations.
    A. ADL _____
    B. ROM _____

21. The goals of rehabilitation are to
    A. _____
    B. _____
    C. _____

22. In long-term care, residents may have progressive illnesses. Goals for them are to
    A. _____
    B. _____

23. A person with health problems or a disability needs to adjust in these areas.
    A. _____
    B. _____
    C. _____
    D. _____

24. Rehabilitation takes longer in which age-group?
    _____ What are reasons for this?
    A. Changes affect _____.
    B. Chronic _____.
    C. Risk for _____.

25. What are some self-help devices that will assist in self-feeding?
    A. _____
    B. _____
    C. _____

26. The goal for a prosthesis is for the device to _____
    _____.

27. When you are assisting with rehabilitation and restorative care, why should you practice the task that the person must perform? _____
    _____

28. When assisting with rehabilitation and restorative care, what complications can be prevented if you report early signs and symptoms? _____
    _____

29. The key team member of the rehabilitation team is the
    _____. Other members are
    A. _____
    B. _____
    C. _____
    D. _____

30. What rehabilitation program would help a person with
    A. Severe vision problems _____
    B. Chronic obstructive pulmonary disease _____
    C. Severe burns _____
    D. Traumatic brain injury _____
    E. A fractured leg _____

31. What can you do to promote the person's quality of life?
    A. _____
    B. _____
    C. _____
    D. _____
    E. _____
    F. _____
    G. _____

Use the FOCUS ON PRIDE section to complete these statements.

32. If a nursing assistant is being considered for promotion to a restorative aide position, what qualities are considered first?
    A. _____
    B. _____
    C. _____

33. To promote independence when a person is receiving rehabilitation and restorative care, you can
    A. _____
    B. _____
    C. _____
    D. _____
    E. _____
    F. _____
    G. _____

Optional Learning Exercises

Mrs. Mercer is 82 years old. She is a resident in a rehabilitation unit because she had a stroke that has caused weakness on her left side. Although she is right-handed, she needs to learn to use several self-help devices as she re-learns ways to carry out ADLs. She often becomes angry or depressed. Answer the following questions about Mrs. Mercer and her care.
NOTE: Some of these questions will require information contained in other chapters.

34. Mrs. Mercer is having difficulty with controlling urinary and bowel elimination. What would be the goal of her care for these problems?

    _____

    _____ Her plan of care would

    include programs for _____.

35. What should you do to prepare Mrs. Mercer's food at meal time so she can feed herself? *(Ch. 27, Nutrition and Fluids)* _____

    _____

36. Mrs. Mercer can brush her teeth but needs help getting prepared. What should you do to get her ready to brush her teeth? *(Ch. 22, Personal Hygiene)*

    _____

37. Why does she need help at meal time and to brush her teeth? *(Ch 22, 27)* _____

    _____

38. Mrs. Mercer needs help to get in and out of bed. When helping her to transfer, you remember to position the

    chair on her _____

    side. *(Ch 19, Safely Transferring the Person)*

39. When Mrs. Mercer becomes discouraged because progress is slow, how can you help her? You can stress

    _____ and focus on

    _____.

Fill in the Blank: Key Terms

Aphasia   Cerumen   Hearing loss   Receptive aphasia
Blindness   Deafness   Low vision   Tinnitus
Braille   Expressive aphasia   Mixed aphasia   Vertigo
Broca's aphasia   Global aphasia   Motor aphasia   Wernicke's aphasia

1. _____ is a touch reading and writing system that uses raised dots for each letter of the alphabet.

2. Another name for receptive aphasia is
   _____.

3. Another name for earwax is _____.

4. _____ is dizziness.

5. A ringing, roaring, hissing, or buzzing sound in the ears is _____.

6. The total or partial loss of the ability to use or understand language is _____.

7. _____ is not being able to hear the normal range of sounds associated with normal hearing.

8. _____ is difficulty expressing or sending out thoughts through speech or writing; motor aphasia, Broca's aphasia.

9. Eyesight that cannot be corrected with eyeglasses, contact lenses, medicine, or surgery is
   _____.

10. _____ is also called expressive aphasia.

11. A hearing loss in which it is impossible for the person to understand speech through hearing alone is
    _____.

12. Another name for expressive aphasia is
    _____.

13. _____ is difficulty expressing or sending out thoughts and difficulty understanding language; mixed aphasia.

14. The absence of sight is
    _____.

15. Another name for global aphasia is
    _____.

16. Difficulty understanding language is
    _____;
    also called Wernicke's aphasia.

Circle the Best Answer

17. If a person has chronic otitis media, the person may develop
    A. Vertigo
    B. Permanent hearing loss
    C. Diarrhea
    D. Nausea and vomiting

18. If a young child has otitis media, you may observe all of these problems *except*
    A. The child has a problem with balance
    B. Fluid draining out of the ear
    C. The child does not respond to quiet sounds
    D. The child turns and cups the better ear toward the speaker

19. How would you know a person with dementia has otitis media?
    A. The person would tell you he or she has pain.
    B. The person would speak softly.
    C. You might notice the person tugging or pulling at one or both ears.
    D. The person would have tinnitus.

20. If you are caring for a person who has Meniere's disease, it is important to
    A. Assist with walking
    B. Assist the person to move quickly
    C. Keep the lights in the room very bright
    D. Encourage the person to be active

21. Which of these is preventable cause of hearing loss?
    A. Aging
    B. Heredity
    C. Exposure to very loud sounds and noises
    D. Birth defects

22. When you are caring for a person with a hearing loss, which of these would *not* help communication?
    A. Gain the person's attention by lightly touching his or her arm.
    B. Speak as loudly as possible.
    C. Face the person when you are speaking.
    D. Use gestures and facial expressions to give useful clues.

23. A child with normal hearing begins to babble in a speech-like way at
    A. Birth to 3 months
    B. 7 months to 1 year
    C. 4 to 6 months
    D. 1 to 2 years

24. A person with a hearing loss
    A. Is able to understand others if he or she listens carefully
    B. Still is able to speak clearly
    C. Is often senile
    D. May deny he or she has a hearing loss

25. When you are caring for a person with a hearing aid, report to the nurse
    A. When turning the hearing aid off at night
    B. If a new battery is inserted
    C. If the hearing aid is lost or damaged
    D. When removing the battery at night

26. If a person has expressive aphasia, he or she
    A. Would not understand simple language
    B. Would speak in complete sentences
    C. Would have difficulty hearing what was said
    D. Might speak in single words or put words in the wrong order

27. An effective measure to use when caring for a speech-impaired person is to
    A. Speak in a child-like way
    B. Ask the person questions to which you know the answer
    C. Use long, involved sentences
    D. Make sure the TV and radio is loud

28. Cataracts most commonly are caused by
    A. Aging
    B. Injury
    C. Increased pressure in the eye
    D. Surgery

29. When a person has had eye surgery for cataracts, the care includes
    A. Removing the eye shield or patch for naps and at night
    B. Having the person cover both eyes during a shower or shampoo
    C. Reminding the person not to rub or press on the affected eye
    D. Placing the over-bed table on the operative side

30. After cataract surgery, report to the nurse at once if
    A. The person complains of eye pain or has eye drainage
    B. Glasses need to be cleaned
    C. The person asks for equipment to clean contact lenses
    D. The person asks for help with basic needs

31. If a person has advanced age-related macular degeneration (AMD)
    A. It can be treated with surgery
    B. The person will need to use eye drops for the rest of his or her life
    C. The person will eventually be blind
    D. The person will need to wear corrective glasses to see clearly

32. Which of these measures can reduce the risk of AMD?
    A. Exposing the eyes to sunlight
    B. Eating a healthy diet high in green leafy vegetables and fish
    C. Eating a diet high in red meats
    D. Decreasing the amount of exercise

33. Diabetic retinopathy is the result of
    A. High blood pressure
    B. Tiny blood vessels in the retina being damaged as a complication of diabetes
    C. A clouding of the lens
    D. Increased pressure in the eye

34. When a person has glaucoma, he or she may have difficulty seeing objects
    A. That are far away
    B. To the right side or left side of the person
    C. Directly in front of the person
    D. That are bright colors

35. Which of these groups of persons are at risk for glaucoma?
    A. Everyone over 60 years of age
    B. Caucasians and Asians over 40 years of age
    C. Those with diabetes
    D. Those who need corrective glasses to see clearly

36. A person who is legally blind
    A. Is totally unable to see anything
    B. May sense some light but have no usable vision
    C. May have some usable vision but cannot read newsprint
    D. All of the above may be true

37. When you enter the room of a blind person, you should first
    A. Touch the person to let him or her know you are there
    B. Speak loudly to make sure the person knows you are there
    C. Make sure the lights are bright
    D. Identify yourself and give your name, title, and reason for being there

38. When a person is blind, you should not
    A. Re-arrange furniture and equipment
    B. Use words such as "see," "look," or "read"
    C. Let the person move about
    D. Let the person perform self-care

39. When you assist a blind person to walk, it is best if you
    A. Walk slightly behind the person and link your arm with the person's arm
    B. Walk slightly ahead of the person and allow the person to hold on to your arm just above the elbow
    C. Grasp the person's arm firmly to guide him or her
    D. Walk very slowly to allow the person to take small steps

40. If a blind person uses a cane, you can assist by
    A. Grasping the person by the arm holding the cane
    B. Coming up behind the person and grasping his or her elbow
    C. Giving the person verbal cues to avoid objects in the way
    D. Asking if you can assist before trying to help

41. If a blind person uses a guide dog, it is correct to
    A. Take the person by the arm on the side opposite from the dog
    B. Avoid distracting a guide dog by petting or feeding the dog
    C. Give the dog commands to avoid danger
    D. Greet the dog and pet it

42. Eyeglasses should be cleaned with
    A. Special cleaning solution or warm water
    B. Boiling water
    C. Detergent
    D. Dry cleansing tissues

43. When cleaning an ocular prosthesis, you should
    A. Wash the artificial eye with mild soap and warm water
    B. Wash the eyelid and eyelashes with sterile water
    C. Dry the artificial eye before inserting it in the socket
    D. Use sterile technique throughout the entire procedure

Fill in the Blank

44. Write out the abbreviations.
    A. AMD _____
    B. ASL _____
    C. TRS _____

45. Otitis media often begins with _____ _____.

46. If a person has chronic otitis media, it can cause permanent _____.

47. When a person has Meniere's disease, safety practices include
    A. _____
    B. _____
    C. _____
    D. _____
    E. _____

48. What are examples of noises that can cause hearing loss?
    A. _____
    B. _____
    C. _____
    D. _____

49. What problems occur with a hearing loss?
    A. _____
    B. _____
    C. _____
    D. _____

50. Symptoms of hearing loss include
    A. _____
    B. _____
    C. _____
    D. _____
    E. _____
    F. _____
    G. _____
    H. _____
    I. _____

51. If a woman is speaking to a hearing-impaired person, why should she adjust the pitch of her voice?
    _____
    _____

52. Why is it important for a person with a hearing loss to see your face when you are speaking to the person?
    _____

53. What are common causes of speech disorders?
    A. _____
    B. _____
    C. _____

54. If a person has apraxia, the brain _____.

55. Measures you can use to communicate with a speech-impaired person are
    A. Listen, and give _____.
    B. Repeat _____.
    C. Write down _____.
    D. Allow the person _____.
    E. Watch _____.

56. When a person has expressive aphasia, the person knows what _____.

57. When a person has receptive aphasia, the person has trouble _____.

58. Symptoms of glaucoma include
    A. Peripheral _____
    B. Blurred _____
    C. Halos _____

59. Drugs and surgery are used with glaucoma to _____.

60. Most cataracts are caused by _____.
    Other risk factors are
    A. _____
    B. _____
    C. _____
    D. _____
    E. _____

61. When you are caring for a person after cataract surgery, an eye shield is worn as directed, and is worn for _____.

62. When assisting a blind or visually impaired person, what can be done to provide a consistent meal-time setting?

    A. _____

    B. _____

    C. _____

    D. _____

    E. _____

    F. _____

    G. _____

63. A person with age-related macular degeneration (AMD) would develop a blind spot

    _____.

64. Everyone with diabetes is at risk for

    _____.

65. How can a person with low vision use a computer as an adaptive device?

    A. _____

    B. _____

66. The legally blind person sees at 20 feet what a person with normal vision sees at

    _____.

67. When you orient a person to the room, why do you let the person move about the room?

    _____

Use the FOCUS ON PRIDE section to complete these statements.

68. When you are referring to a person who has speech, hearing, or vision problems, he or she should be referred to by _____, not by the

    _____

69. Braille signs for areas with public access are required by the _____.

Optional Learning Exercises

Mr. Herman is an 85-year-old man with a hearing loss that has developed as he has gotten older. Answer these questions about his care.

70. Two nursing assistants, a male and a female, are caring for Mr. Herman. They notice that he answers questions asked by the male nursing assistant more quickly. What is the likely reason for this?

    _____

71. The nursing assistants have found that Mr. Herman is alert and oriented. They are surprised when Joan, another nursing assistant, tells them he is "senile." Why would Joan make this statement?

    _____

72. Mr. Herman says he is too tired to go to the game room for a party. He says no one likes him. What are some reasons for his actions and statements?

    A. Tired because

    _____

    B. No one likes him

    _____

73. When giving care, the nursing assistant turns off the TV and radio in Mr. Herman's room. Why is this done? _____

You are caring for Mrs. Sanchez, who is legally blind because of glaucoma. Answer the questions about her care.

74. When you enter the room, you notice that Mrs. Sanchez is looking at her mail with a magnifying glass. How is this possible since you thought she was blind? _____

    _____

75. When you enter the room, Mrs. Sanchez asks you to adjust the blinds. Why? _____

76. When you are helping Mrs. Sanchez to move about the room, you are careful to tell her where furniture is located. Why? _____

    _____

Fill in the Blank: Key Terms

Benign tumor   Malignant tumor   Mole   Tumor
Cancer   Metastasis   Stomatitis

1. A _____ is a tumor that invades and destroys nearby tissue and can spread to other body parts.

2. Inflammation of the mouth is _____.

3. A tumor that does not spread to other body parts is a _____.

4. A new growth of abnormal cells that may be benign or malignant is a _____.

5. The spread of cancer to other body parts is _____.

6. Another name for a malignant tumor is _____.

7. A _____ is a brown, tan, or black spot on the skin that is flat or raised and round or oval.

Circle the Best Answer

8. Benign tumors
   A. Do not spread to other body parts
   B. Invade healthy tissue
   C. Are always very small
   D. Divide in an orderly and controlled way

9. When cancer occurs in children, it
   A. Is usually fatal
   B. Has a high cure rate
   C. Is treated very easily
   D. Is very rare

10. Risk factors that increase cancer include all of the following *except*
   A. Exposure to sun and tanning booths
   B. Smoking
   C. A diet high in fresh fruits and vegetables
   D. Close relatives with certain types of cancer

11. When surgery is done to treat cancer
   A. It cures or controls the cancer
   B. The cancer cells are killed
   C. The tumor shrinks
   D. It prevents metastasis

12. When you care for a person receiving radiation therapy, you might expect the person to
   A. Have pain related to the therapy
   B. Need extra rest related to fatigue
   C. Be at risk for bleeding and infections
   D. Complain of flu-like symptoms such as chills, fever, and muscle aches

13. Chemotherapy involves
   A. X-ray beams aimed at the tumor
   B. Giving drugs that prevent the production of certain hormones
   C. Therapy to help the immune system
   D. Giving drugs that kill cells

14. While caring for a person receiving chemotherapy, she tells you she is upset because her hair is falling out. You know that
   A. The hair often falls out when a person receives chemotherapy
   B. This is a symptom of her disease
   C. You should report this to the nurse at once
   D. You should change the subject so she will not be so upset

15. When hormone therapy is used to treat cancer, a woman may experience
   A. Stomatitis
   B. Flu-like symptoms
   C. Weight gain, hot flashes, and fluid retention
   D. Burns and skin breakdown

16. Complementary and alternative medicine treatment includes
   A. Chemotherapy
   B. Massage therapy, herbal products, and spiritual healing
   C. Implanting of radiation implants
   D. Giving blood-forming stem cells

17. A person with cancer may complain of constipation because of
   A. The side effects of pain-relief drugs
   B. Pain
   C. The side effects of cancer treatments
   D. Fluid and nutrition intake

18. When a person has cancer and expresses anger, fear, and depression, you can help most by
   A. Telling the person not to worry or get upset
   B. Giving the person privacy and time alone
   C. Being there when needed and listening to the person
   D. Changing the subject to distract the person

19. Treatment for autoimmune disorders is aimed at
   A. Curing the illness
   B. Suppressing the immune system
   C. Removing the affected organs
   D. Preventing metastasis

20. HIV is *not* spread by
    A. Blood
    B. Semen
    C. Sneezing or coughing
    D. Breast-milk

21. To protect yourself from HIV and AIDS, you should
    A. Avoid all body fluids when giving care
    B. Refuse to give care to persons diagnosed with these diseases
    C. Follow Standard Precautions and the Bloodborne Pathogen Standard when giving care
    D. Always use the sterile technique when giving any care

22. Shingles is caused by the same virus that causes
    A. HIV
    B. Measles
    C. Chicken pox
    D. Mumps

Fill in the Blank

23. Write out the abbreviations.
    A. AIDS _____
    B. CDC _____
    C. HIV _____
    D. STD _____
    E. TB _____

24. Cancer is the _____ most common cause of death in the United States.

25. The goals of cancer treatment are
    A. _____
    B. _____
    C. _____

26. The general signs and symptoms of cancer are
    A. _____
    B. _____
    C. _____
    D. _____
    E. _____
    F. _____
    G. _____
    H. _____
    I. _____
    J. _____
    K. _____
    L. _____
    M. _____
    N. _____
    O. _____
    P. _____

27. When radiation therapy is used, _____ cells and _____ cells are both destroyed.

28. With radiation therapy, skin care measures are needed at the treatment site because these can occur.
    A. _____
    B. _____
    C. _____
    D. _____
    E. _____
    F. _____

29. When chemotherapy is used, it affects _____ cells and _____ cells.

30. When a person is receiving chemotherapy, what side effects might occur?
    A. _____
    B. _____
    C. _____
    D. _____
    E. _____

31. Biological therapy treats cancer by
    A. _____
    B. _____

32. Complementary and alternative medicine (CAM) is sometimes used with standard cancer treatment. Treatments include
    A. _____
    B. _____
    C. _____
    D. _____
    E. _____
    F. _____

33. When a person has an autoimmune disorder, it means the _____ system attacks the _____.

34. Autoimmune disorder treatment is aimed at
    A. _____
    B. _____
    C. _____

35. Acquired immunodeficiency syndrome (AIDS) is caused by a _____ that attacks the _____.

36. How is human immunodeficiency virus (HIV) mainly transmitted?

    A. _____

    B. _____

37. When caring for a person with HIV, the main threat to health care workers is from

    _____

38. Those at risk for developing shingles are

    A. _____

    B. _____

    C. _____

Use the FOCUS ON PRIDE section to complete these statements.

39. If you work on an oncology unit, staff and patients value a person who is _____,

    _____, _____,

    and _____

40. When you work closely with oncology patients and families, you must protect the person's privacy and rights and avoid crossing _____.

Optional Learning Exercises

Mrs. Myers is a 62 year old who is having chemotherapy to treat cancer. She has not been eating well and complains of feeling very tired. When you assist her with personal care, you notice a large amount of hair on her pillow. Answer these questions about Mrs. Myers and her care.

41. Mrs. Myers may not be eating well because the chemotherapy _____ the gastro-intestinal tract and causes _____,

    _____, _____, and

    _____.

42. She may also have _____,

    which is called stomatitis. You can help to relieve the discomfort from this side effect when

    you provide _____.

43. What is causing Mrs. Myers to lose her hair?

    _____

    This condition is called _____.

44 Nervous System and Musculo-Skeletal Disorders

Fill in the Blank: Key Terms

Amputation	Closed fracture	Gangrene	Paralysis	Simple fracture
Arthritis	Compound fracture	Hemiplegia	Paraplegia	Tetraplegia
Arthroplasty	Fracture	Open fracture	Quadriplegia	

1. An open fracture is also called a

_____.

2. Another name for quadriplegia is

_____.

3. The removal of all or part of an extremity is

_____.

4. A _____ is when the bone is broken but the skin is intact.

5. _____ is paralysis and loss of sensory function in the arms, legs, and trunk. It can also be called tetraplegia.

6. Paralysis on one side of the body is

_____.

7. Joint inflammation is

_____.

8. A closed fracture can also be called

_____.

9. A _____ is a broken bone.

10. An _____ occurs when the broken bone has come through the skin. It is also called a compound fracture.

11. An _____ is the surgical replacement of a joint.

12. Paralysis and loss of sensory function in the legs is

_____.

13. A condition in which there is death of tissue is

_____.

14. _____ is loss of motor function, loss of sensation, or both.

Circle the Best Answer

15. The leading cause of disability in the United States is
    A. Heart disease
    B. Cancer
    C. Stroke
    D. Diabetes

16. If a person has stroke-like symptoms that last a few minutes, it means that
    A. The person has had a transient ischemic attack (TIA)
    B. It is not a dangerous situation since it was temporary
    C. The person needs to lie down at once
    D. No further treatment is needed

17. Which of these is *not* a risk factor for stroke?
    A. High blood pressure
    B. Cigarette smoking
    C. Regular physical activity
    D. Diabetes

18. When a person has "neglect" after a stroke, it means that
    A. There is paralysis on 1 side of the body
    B. The person may forget about or ignore the weaker side
    C. The person is incontinent
    D. The speech is slowed or slurred

19. When you are caring for a person who has had a stroke, the call light
    A. Should be removed from the room
    B. Is placed on the weak side of the body
    C. Is placed on the strong side of the body
    D. Is given to a family member to use for the person

20. A safety concern for a person with Parkinson's disease would be
    A. Changes in speech
    B. Swallowing and chewing problems
    C. A mask-like expression
    D. Emotional changes

21. Multiple sclerosis (MS) is a disease that
    A. Is an acute illness from which the person recovers completely
    B. Always follows the same course with the same symptoms
    C. Has remissions and flare-ups, with more symptoms with each flare-up
    D. Is easily treated with medications

22. As amyotrophic lateral sclerosis (ALS) progresses, the person is
    A. Confused and disoriented
    B. Able to walk with assistance even as the disease progresses
    C. Incontinent of bladder and bowel functions
    D. Unable to move the arms, legs, and body

23. If a person is in a vegetative state after traumatic brain injury, he or she
    A. Is unconscious, unaware, and cannot be aroused
    B. Is unconscious; has sleep-wake cycles; and may open the eyes, make sounds, or move
    C. Is unresponsive but can be aroused briefly
    D. Has a complete loss of brain function

24. A person who has a spinal cord injury in the lumbar region will likely have
    A. Quadriplegia
    B. Paraplegia
    C. Hemiplegia
    D. Tetraplegia

25. When caring for a person with paralysis, it is important to
    A. Keep the bed in semi-Fowler's position
    B. Check bath water, heat applications, and food for proper temperature
    C. Apply elastic stockings to prevent thrombi in the legs
    D. Place objects on the unaffected side

26. Autonomic hyperreflexia occurs in a person who has paralysis
    A. Of any kind
    B. Above the mid-thoracic level
    C. In the lumbar region
    D. That is incomplete

27. If you are caring for a person with autonomic hyperreflexia, report to the nurse at once if
    A. The person is sweating
    B. The blood pressure is low
    C. The person complains of pain below the level of the injury
    D. The person has sweating below the level of the injury

28. If a person is at risk for autonomic hyperreflexia, it is best if only the nurse
    A. Gives basic care
    B. Makes sure the catheter is draining properly
    C. Checks for fecal impactions or gives an enema
    D. Re-positions the person at least every 2 hours

29. Osteoarthritis differs from rheumatoid arthritis because osteoarthritis
    A. Is an inflammatory disease
    B. Occurs when cartilage covering the ends of the bone wears away
    C. Means that the person does not feel well
    D. Occurs on both sides of the body

30. When you are caring for a person with arthritis, which of these would be most helpful to the person?
    A. Allow the person to stay in bed as much as desired.
    B. Keep the room cool at all times.
    C. Help the person use good body mechanics and good posture and get regular rest.
    D. Tell the person not to exercise, as the exercise will prevent healing.

31. When caring for a person who has had a total hip replacement, which of these measures should *not* be done?
    A. Have a high, firm chair for the person to use when out of bed.
    B. Remove the pillow between the legs when the person is sleeping.
    C. Remind the person not to cross his or her legs.
    D. Make sure the person has a raised toilet seat.

32. Which of these will help to strengthen bones in a person at risk for osteoporosis?
    A. Bedrest
    B. Decrease calcium intake
    C. Exercise weight-bearing joints
    D. Increase alcohol and caffeine intake

33. Which of these is not a sign or symptom of a fracture?
    A. Full range of motion in the affected limb
    B. Bruising and color change in the skin of the affected area
    C. Pain
    D. Swelling

34. When a closed reduction is done, the person has
    A. A fracture with no bone exposed
    B. Surgery to allow the bone to be moved into alignment
    C. Devices to keep the bones in place such as pins, screws, or wires
    D. The bone exposed so it can be moved into alignment

35. When a person has a newly applied plaster cast, it will dry in
    A. 2 to 4 hours   C. 24 to 48 hours
    B. 3 to 4 days   D. 12 to 24 hours

36. You can prevent flat spots on a cast by
    A. Positioning the cast on a hard, flat surface
    B. Supporting the entire cast with pillows
    C. Using your fingertips to lift the cast
    D. Covering the cast with a blanket

37. If a person complains of numbness in a part that is in a cast, you should
    A. Tell the person to move the limb a little to relieve the numbness
    B. Re-position the person to help the numbness
    C. Gently rub the exposed toes or fingers
    D. Tell the nurse at once

38. When giving care to a person in traction, you should
    A. Put bottom linens on the bed from the top down
    B. Remove the weights while you are giving care
    C. Turn the person from side to side to change the bed and to give care
    D. Assist the person to use the commode chair when needed

39. After surgery to repair a hip fracture, the operated leg should be
    A. Abducted at all times
    B. Adducted at all times
    C. Exercised with range-of-motion exercises every 4 hours
    D. Positioned to keep the leg in external rotation

40. When you assist a person to get up in a chair after hip surgery
    A. Place the chair on the affected side
    B. Place the chair on the unaffected side
    C. Have a low, soft chair for the person to use
    D. Remind the person to cross the legs

41. If a person complains of pain in the amputated part
    A. Report this to the nurse at once
    B. Assume that the person is confused or disoriented
    C. Re-assure the person that this is a normal reaction
    D. Tell the person that this a temporary sensation that will go away shortly

Fill in the Blank

42. Write out the abbreviations.
    A. ADL _____
    B. ALS _____
    C. CVA _____
    D. JRA _____
    E. MS _____
    F. RA _____
    G. ROM _____
    H. TBI _____
    I. TIA _____

43. What are the warning signs of stroke?
    A. _____
    B. _____
    C. _____
    D. _____
    E. _____

44. What are signs and symptoms of Parkinson's disease?
    A. _____
    B. _____
    C. _____
    D. _____

45. A person with Parkinson's disease will receive
    A. Drugs to control _____
    B. Exercise and physical therapy to help _____
    C. Therapy for speech and _____
    D. Safety measures to prevent _____

46. Multiple sclerosis (MS) may present in many ways.
    A. When symptoms disappear, the person is in _____
    B. When symptoms flare up, the person is in a _____

47. What effect does amyotrophic lateral sclerosis have on
    A. Mind, intelligence, memory _____
    B. Senses _____
    C. Bowel and bladder functions _____
    D. Nerve cells for voluntary movement _____

48. When traumatic brain injury occurs
    A. Brain tissue is _____
    B. Bleeding can be in the _____ or _____
    C. Spinal cord injuries are _____

49. _____ are the major cause of head injuries in newborns.

50. When caring for a person with paralysis, you must check the person often if he or she is unable to use _____.

51. Range-of-motion exercises are important when caring for a person with paralysis because they will maintain _____ and prevent _____.

52. If the nurse delegates you to raise the head of the bed 45 degrees or more for a person with a spinal cord injury, the person may have signs or symptoms of _____

53. If you are caring for a person with arthritis, what are the benefits of these treatments?
    A. Drugs _____
    B. Heat _____
    C. Exercise _____
    D. Rest and joint care _____

54. How do these assistive devices help a person with arthritis?
    A. Canes and walkers _____
    B. Splints _____
    C. Adaptive and self-help devices _____

55. When caring for a person who has had a hip replacement, what instructions are given to the person to protect the hip?
    A. Positioning legs _____
    B. To sit _____
    C. To bend _____
    D. To reach _____
    E. Toileting _____
    F. Sleeping _____

56. List how these risk factors affect developing osteoporosis.
    A. Women risk increases _____
    B. Family _____
    C. Weight _____

57. Calcium is lost from bone if it does not _____. What happens to the bone when calcium is lost? _____

58. What joints are exercised to help prevent osteoporosis? _____

    What types of exercise are used on these joints?

59. When a person has cast on a fracture, what do these symptoms mean?

    A. Pain _____

    B. Odor _____

    C. Numbness _____

    D. Cool skin _____

    E. Hot skin _____

60. When caring for a person in traction, what would you do in these situations?

    A. Rope is frayed. _____

    B. ROM exercises are performed on _____.

    C. Positioning _____

    D. Redness, drainage, and odor are noted at the pin site. _____

    E. Person complains of numbness.

    _____

61. How should the fractured hip be supported in these situations?

    A. Prevent external rotation _____

    B. Keep leg abducted _____

62. When turning and positioning a person after hip surgery, usually the person is not positioned on

    _____

63. If the person has an internal fixation device, the operative leg is not elevated when sitting in a chair because _____

64. What disease is a common cause of vascular changes that can lead to an amputation? _____

65. Phantom pain after an amputation may occur for a _____ or for _____.

Use the FOCUS ON PRIDE section to complete this statement.

66. To promote independence when a person had disorders discussed in this chapter, it is important to

    A. _____

    B. _____

    C. _____

    D. _____

Optional Learning Exercises

You are caring for Mrs. Huber, who has had a stroke. The next 5 questions relate to Mrs. Huber and her care. Explain the reason(s) the care plan gives each of the following instructions.

67. Position Mrs. Huber in a side-lying position.

    _____

68. Approach Mrs. Huber from the unaffected side.

    _____

69. Mrs. Huber is given a dysphagia diet.

    _____

70. Elastic stockings are applied as part of her care.

    _____

71. Range-of-motion exercises are given.

    _____

You are caring for 2 persons who have arthritis. Read the information about each of them and answer the 2 questions about these persons.

- *Mr. Miller is 78 years old. He worked in construction for many years, where he did heavy physical work. He complains about pain in his hips and right knee. His fingers are deformed by arthritis and interfere with good range of motion.*

- *Mrs. Haxton is 40 years old. She has swelling, warmth, and tenderness in her wrists, several finger joints on both hands, and both knees. She tells you that she has had arthritis for about 10 years and it "comes and goes." At present, Mrs. Haxton has a temperature of 100.2°F and she states she is tired and does not feel well.*

72. Which type of arthritis does Mr. Miller have? _____ His job may have caused

    _____

73. Mrs. Haxton probably has _____ arthritis. She complains of not feeling well because the arthritis affects _____ as well as the joints.

45 Cardiovascular, Respiratory, and Lymphatic Disorders

Fill in the Blank: Key Terms

Apnea
Arrhythmia
Congenital

Dysrhythmia
Hemorrhage
High blood pressure

Hypertension
Lymphedema
Pneumonia

Pre-hypertension
Sleep apnea

1. An inflammation and infection of lung tissue is

   _____.

2. An abnormal heart rhythm is

   _____.

3. Pauses in breathing that occur during sleep is

   _____.

4. When the systolic pressure is 140 mm Hg or higher, or the diastolic pressure is 90 mm Hg or higher, it is

   _____.

5. _____ means to be born with a condition.

6. An excessive loss of blood in a short time is

   _____.

7. A buildup of lymph in the tissues causing edema is

   _____.

8. _____ is when the systolic pressure is between 120 and 139 mm Hg or the diastolic pressure is between 80 and 89 mm Hg.

9. Another name for hypertension is

   _____.

10. _____ is another name for dysrhythmia.

11. The lack or absence of breathing is _____.

Circle the Best Answer

12. The leading cause of death in the United States is
    A. Cardiovascular and respiratory system disorders
    B. Cancer
    C. Strokes
    D. Accidents

13. Hypertension (high blood pressure) would be a reading of
    A. 120/70
    B. 100/60
    C. 140/90
    D. 130/60

14. A risk factor for hypertension that cannot change is
    A. Stress
    B. Being over-weight
    C. Age
    D. Lack of exercise

15. The most common cause of coronary artery disease is
    A. Lack of exercise
    B. Atherosclerosis
    C. Family history
    D. Stress

16. Cardiac rehabilitation includes all of these *except*
    A. Exercise training
    B. Learning about the heart condition
    C. Strict bedrest
    D. Learning how to deal with fears about the future

17. If a person has angina pain, it will usually be relieved by
    A. Resting for 3 to 15 minutes
    B. Taking narcotic drugs
    C. Using oxygen therapy
    D. Getting up and walking for exercise

18. If a person takes a nitroglycerin tablet for angina, you should
    A. Give them a large glass of water to swallow the pill
    B. Take the pills back to the nurses' station
    C. Make sure the nurse is told a pill was taken
    D. Encourage the person to walk around the room

19. When a myocardial infarction occurs, it means that
    A. Part of the heart muscle dies
    B. The heart muscle is not receiving enough oxygen
    C. Pain can be relieved by rest
    D. Blood backs up into the lungs

20. If a person complains of pain or numbness in the back, neck, jaw, or stomach, you should tell the nurse at once because the person
    A. Is having an angina attack
    B. May be having a stroke
    C. May be having a myocardial infarction
    D. Has symptoms of COPD

21. When heart failure occurs, the person may have
    A. Fluid in the lungs (pulmonary edema)
    B. Death of the heart muscle
    C. A lack of oxygen to the heart muscle
    D. Blood clots in the arteries

22. An older person with heart failure is at risk for
    A. Contractures
    B. Skin breakdown
    C. Fractures
    D. Urinary tract infections

23. When a person has a pacemaker
    A. He or she can never take a tub bath or go swimming
    B. He or she may feel dizzy or lightheaded and have fluttering in the chest
    C. The function and battery life of the pacemaker must be checked regularly
    D. It is removed after the heart becomes stronger

24. The most important risk factor for chronic obstructive pulmonary disease (COPD) is
    A. Family history
    B. Respiratory infections
    C. Cigarette smoking
    D. Exercise

25. When a person has COPD, it interferes with
    A. Oxygen (O_2) and carbon dioxide (CO_2) exchange in the lungs
    B. Blood flow to the heart
    C. The function of the kidneys and bladder
    D. Heart rhythm and the strength of the contractions

26. If a person has chronic bronchitis, a common symptom is
    A. Wheezing and tightening in the chest
    B. Shortness of breath on exertion
    C. A smoker's cough in the morning
    D. A high temperature for several days

27. Asthma is often triggered by
    A. Allergies
    B. Warm air
    C. Pauses in breathing during sleep
    D. An excess secretion of mucus

28. If a person has sleep apnea, it is treated by
    A. Administering drugs to promote sleep
    B. Having the person sleep in a high-Fowler's position
    C. Using continuous positive airway pressure (CPAP) while sleeping
    D. Taking several naps during the day

29. If an older person has influenza, he or she may
    A. Have a body temperature below normal
    B. Have an increased appetite
    C. Feel more energy than usual
    D. Have no symptoms of illness

30. Which of these symptoms is more likely to be from a cold rather than the flu?
    A. Stuffy nose
    B. High fever (100°F to 102°F)
    C. Fatigue for 2 to 3 weeks
    D. Bronchitis or pneumonia

31. The flu vaccine would be recommended for all of these persons *except*
    A. A man with diabetes and chronic heart disease
    B. A woman who had a severe reaction to the flu vaccine
    C. A healthy 30 year old
    D. A 75-year-old man in good health

32. When a person has pneumonia, fluid intake is increased to
    A. Decrease the amount of bacteria in the lungs
    B. Dilute medication given to treat the disease
    C. Thin secretions and help reduce fever
    D. Decrease inflammation of the breathing passages

33. Breathing is easier for a person with pneumonia when the person is positioned in
    A. Semi-Fowler's position
    B. Side-lying position
    C. Supine position
    D. A soft chair

34. When a person has lymphedema, it is important that you
    A. Never use an affected arm to take a blood pressure
    B. Keep the affected arm or leg elevated at all times
    C. Keep the person on strict bedrest
    D. Restrict fluid intake

Fill in the Blank

35. Write out the abbreviations.
    A. CAD _____
    B. CDC _____
    C. CHF _____
    D. CO_2 _____
    E. COPD _____
    F. EV-D68 _____
    G. IV _____
    H. MI _____
    I. mm Hg _____
    J. O_2 _____
    K. RBC _____
    L. TB _____
    M. VHF _____
    N. WBC _____

36. What risk factors that increase blood pressure cannot be changed?
    A. _____
    B. _____
    C. _____
    D. _____

37. The most common cause of coronary artery disease (CAD) is _____. When this occurs, _____ collects on the _____.

38. When a person has CAD, what life-style changes are needed?
    A. _____
    B. _____
    C. _____
    D. _____

39. What activities or other factors can cause angina?
    A. _____
    B. _____
    C. _____
    D. _____
    E. _____
    F. _____

40. Where are nitroglycerin tablets kept?
    _____

41. Signs and symptoms of a myocardial infarction may be chest pain that is
    A. _____
    B. _____
    C. _____
    D. _____

42. The goals of cardiac rehabilitation after a myocardial infarction are
    A. _____
    B. _____
    C. _____

43. Older persons with heart failure are at risk for skin breakdown because of
    A. _____
    B. _____
    C. _____

44. How can you help to prevent skin breakdown in older persons with heart failure?
    _____

45. Dysrythmias are caused by changes in the heart's
    _____

46. What changes occur in the lungs when a person has chronic obstructive pulmonary disease (COPD)?
    A. _____
    B. _____
    C. _____
    D. _____

47. If a person has bronchitis or emphysema, the person must stop _____

48. Signs and symptoms of sleep apnea are
    A. _____
    B. _____
    C. _____
    D. _____
    E. _____
    F. _____
    G. _____

49. A common complication of influenza is
    _____

50. What signs and symptoms may be present if a person has active tuberculosis (TB)?
    A. _____
    B. _____
    C. _____
    D. _____
    E. _____
    F. _____
    G. _____
    H. _____
    I. _____

51. Why does TB sometimes become active as a person ages? _____

52. The goals of treating lymphedema are
    A. _____
    B. _____
    C. _____
    D. _____

53. Lymphoma is cancer involving cells in the
    _____

Use the FOCUS ON PRIDE section to complete these statements.

54. When a person makes unhealthy choices, such as smoking, the health team
    A. Teaches the person the
    _____ and
    encourages _____
    B. Cannot force _____
    C. Must be sure the person understands
    _____

55. Color-coded wristbands communicate
    _____ or
    _____

56. If a color-coded bracelet says "limb alert" or "forbidden extremity," it means that an arm must not be used for
    A. _____
    B. _____
    C. _____

Matching

Match the symptom listed with disorders of coronary artery disease.
A. Angina
B. Myocardial infarction
C. Heart failure

57. _____ Chest pain occurs with exertion.

58. _____ Blood flow to the heart is suddenly blocked.

59. _____ Blood backs up into the venous system.

60. _____ Fluid in the lungs.

61. _____ Rest and nitroglycerin often relieves the symptoms.

62. _____ Pain is described as crushing, stabbing, or squeezing.

Match the form of chronic obstructive pulmonary disorder (COPD) with the related symptom.

A. Chronic bronchitis
B. Emphysema
C. Asthma

63. _____ Person develops a barrel chest.

64. _____ Mucus and inflamed breathing passages obstruct airflow.

65. _____ Alveoli become less elastic.

66. _____ Air passages narrow.

67. _____ First symptom is often a smoker's cough in the morning.

68. _____ Normal O_2 and CO_2 exchange cannot occur in affected alveoli.

69. _____ Allergies and air pollutants are common causes.

Optional Learning Exercises

70. A parent with a congenital heart defect is at risk of having a child with one. What are other risk factors that may cause a congenital heart defect?

A. _____

B. _____

C. _____

D. _____

E. _____

71. Why is hypertension called "the silent killer?"

_____

72. Older persons may not have typical symptoms of flu. Older persons may have these symptoms that signal flu.

A. _____

B. _____

C. _____

D. _____

E. _____

46 Digestive and Endocrine Disorders

Fill in the Blank: Key Terms

Emesis   Hyperglycemia   Jaundice
Heartburn   Hypoglycemia   Vomitus

1. High sugar in the blood is

   _____.

2. _____ is when food and
   fluids are expelled from the stomach through the mouth.

3. Low sugar in the blood is

   _____.

4. Another word for vomitus is

   _____.

5. _____ is yellowish color of
   the skin or whites of the eyes.

6. A burning sensation in the chest and sometimes the

   throat is _____.

Circle the Best Answer

7. A risk factor for gastro-esophageal reflux disease
   (GERD) is
   A. Eating small, frequent meals
   B. Alcohol use
   C. Maintaining normal weight
   D. Respiratory illnesses

8. If you are caring for a person with GERD, the person
   may be
   A. Given large, infrequent meals
   B. Instructed not to lie down for 3 hours after eating
   C. Taught to wear tight-fitting clothing
   D. Continuing to eat a normal diet with plenty of
      fatty, fried foods

9. Aspirated vomitus
   A. Can lead to shock
   B. Can obstruct an airway
   C. Contains undigested food
   D. Has a bitter taste

10. If vomitus looks like coffee grounds, you should
    report at once to the nurse because
    A. It signals bleeding
    B. The person may need a diet change
    C. This indicates an infection
    D. The person may need pain medication

11. Diverticular disease may occur because of
    A. A high fiber diet
    B. Regular bowel movements
    C. Aging
    D. Infections

12. Gallstones are
    A. Needed for digestion of fats
    B. Formed in the small intestine
    C. Sometimes cause bile flow to be blocked
    D. Easily passed through the kidneys

13. A symptom of gallstones is
    A. Pain radiating down one or both arms
    B. Diarrhea
    C. Constipation
    D. Pain in the back, abdomen, or right underarm area

14. When hepatitis is contracted by eating or drinking
    food or water contaminated by feces, it is
    A. Hepatitis A   C. Hepatitis C
    B. Hepatitis B   D. Hepatitis D

15. A person with cirrhosis will need good skin care
    because of
    A. Muscle aches
    B. Itching
    C. Nausea and vomiting
    D. Diarrhea or constipation

16. An obese 50 year-old woman with hypertension is
    diagnosed with diabetes. She most likely has
    A. Type 1   C. Gestational
    B. Type 2   D. Hypoglycemia

17. A diabetic complains of thirst and frequent urination.
    You notice the person has a flushed face and rapid,
    deep, and labored respirations. You know these are
    signs and symptoms of
    A. Hyperglycemia   C. Diabetic coma
    B. Hypoglycemia   D. An infection

Fill in the Blank

18. Write out the meaning of the abbreviations.
    A. BMs _____
    B. GERD _____
    C. GI _____
    D. HBV _____
    E. IBD _____
    F. I&O _____
    G. IV _____

19. What life-style changes may be needed for a person
    with GERD?
    A. _____
    B. _____
    C. _____
    D. _____
    E. _____

20. What measures will help the person who is vomiting?
    A. Turn _____.
    B. Place _____.
    C. Move _____.
    D. Provide _____.
    E. Eliminate _____.

21. Risk factors related to diverticular disease are
    A. Age _____
    B. Diet _____
    C. Weight _____

22. A gallbladder attack often occurs suddenly after
    _____.

23. List the characteristics of the types of hepatitis.
    A. Hepatitis A is spread by the
    _____ route.
    B. Hepatitis B is present in the
    _____ of infected persons.
    C. Hepatitis C can be transmitted even when the
    person has _____.
    D. Hepatitis D occurs only in people with
    _____
    E. Hepatitis E is not common in
    _____

24. Signs and symptoms of cirrhosis that may occur are
    A. _____
    B. _____
    C. _____
    D. _____
    E. _____
    F. _____
    G. _____
    H. _____

25. A person with _____ diabetes will be treated with healthy eating, exercise, and sometimes oral drugs.

26. A person with _____ diabetes will be treated with daily insulin therapy as well as healthy diet and exercise.

Use the FOCUS ON PRIDE section to complete these statements.

27. Understanding health problems allows you to safely
    _____

28. When a person has health problems related to lifestyle choices, it is important that this does not affect how you _____.
    Always show _____.

Matching

Match the type of hepatitis with the correct statement.
A. Hepatitis A
B. Hepatitis B
C. Hepatitis C
D. Hepatitis D

29. _____ This hepatitis occurs in person infected with Hepatitis B.

30. _____ Caused by poor sanitation, crowded living conditions.

31. _____ Caused by HBV.

32. _____ Ingested when eating contaminated food or water.

33. _____ Person may have virus but no symptoms.

34. _____ Serious liver damage shows up years later.

Match the symptom with either hypoglycemia or hyperglycemia.
A. Hypoglycemia
B. Hyperglycemia

35. _____ Trembling, shakiness

36. _____ Sweet breath odor

37. _____ Tingling around the mouth

38. _____ Cold, clammy skin

39. _____ Rapid, deep, and labored respirations

40. _____ Leg cramps

41. _____ Flushed face

42. _____ Frequent urination

Optional Learning Exercises

You are caring for several persons with diabetes. Answer these questions about these persons.

Mr. Jones, a 75-year-old African-American man
Ms. Miller, a 45-year-old white, over-weight woman
Mrs. Thorpe, a 32-year-old pregnant woman
Ms. Hernandez, a 60-year-old Hispanic woman with hypertension
Emily F., a 12-year-old girl who has lost 15 pounds recently without dieting

43. Three of these persons are most likely to have type 2 diabetes. They are
    A. _____
    B. _____
    C. _____

44. The 32 year old probably has _____ diabetes. She is at risk for developing

_____ later in life.

45. The 12 year old probably has

_____ diabetes.

46. Which type of diabetes develops rapidly?

_____

47. Mrs. Hernandez has an open wound on her ankle. Why is this wound a concern?

_____

48. Why is Ms. Miller instructed to decrease her food intake? _____

49. Mr. Jones tells you he feels shaky, dizzy, and has a headache when he misses a meal. He probably is experiencing

_____.

50. Why does Emily F. take a snack with her when she goes to school? _____

_____

47 Urinary and Reproductive Disorders

Fill in the Blank: Key Terms

Dialysis   Dysuria   Oliguria   Urinary diversion
Diuresis   Hematuria   Pyuria   Urostomy

1. Scant urine is _____.

2. Difficult or painful urination is _____.

3. A _____ is a surgically created opening between the ureter and the abdomen.

4. _____ is the process of passing urine; large amounts of urine are produced—1000 to 5000 mL a day.

5. A new pathway for urine to exit the body is a

   _____.

6. Blood in the urine is _____.

7. _____ is pus in the urine.

8. The process of removing waste products from the blood is _____.

Circle the Best Answer

9. Women have a higher risk of urinary tract infections because of
   A. Hormone levels in the body
   B. The short female urethra
   C. Bacteria
   D. Prostrate gland secretions

10. If a person has a UTI, the care plan will include
    A. Restricting fluid intake
    B. Assisting the person to ambulate frequently
    C. Straining the urine
    D. Encouraging the person to drink 2000 mL of fluid a day

11. If a man has prostate enlargement, he will probably
    A. Be incontinent of urine
    B. Have frequent voiding at night
    C. Have increased urine output
    D. Have renal failure

12. After surgery to correct benign prostatic hyperplasia (BPH), the care plan may include
    A. A balanced diet to prevent constipation
    B. Increased activity with an exercise plan
    C. Restricted fluid intake
    D. Care of the surgical incision

13. When caring for a person with a urinary diversion, the pouch is changed
    A. Every shift
    B. Every 3 to 4 hours
    C. When the person showers or takes a tub bath
    D. Every 5 to 7 days or if it leaks

14. If you are caring for a person with kidney stones, your care will include
    A. Restricting fluids
    B. Keeping the person on strict bedrest
    C. Straining all urine
    D. Maintaining a strict diet

15. When you care for a person with acute renal failure, the care plan will include
    A. Increasing fluid intake to 2000 to 3000 mL per day
    B. Measuring and recording urine output every hour
    C. Making sure the person does not drink any fluids
    D. Measuring weight weekly

16. Chronic renal failure
    A. Occurs suddenly
    B. Generally improves and kidney function returns to normal within 1 year
    C. Occurs when nephrons of the kidney are destroyed over many years
    D. Has very little effect on the person's over-all health

17. If a person has chronic renal failure, which of these would be included in the care plan?
    A. A diet high in protein, potassium, and sodium
    B. Plenty of exercise
    C. Measures to prevent itching
    D. Frequent bathing with soap

18. A woman who complains about frothy, thick, foul-smelling vaginal discharge most likely has
    A. Gonorrhea   C. Syphilis
    B. Genital warts   D. Trichomoniasis

Fill in the Blank

19. Write out the meaning of the abbreviations.
    A. BPH _____
    B. CKD _____
    C. mL _____
    D. STD _____
    E. TURP _____
    F. UTI _____

20. After a transurethral resection of the prostate (TURP), the person's care plan may include
    A. _____
    B. _____
    C. _____
    D. _____
    E. _____

21. A person with kidney stones needs to drink 2000 to 3000 mL of fluid a day to help

    _____

22. When acute renal failure occurs, there are 2 phases. Name and explain each phase.

    A. At first, _____ occurs. Urine output

    is _____. This

    phase lasts _____.

    B. Then, _____ occurs. Urine

    output is _____.

    This phase lasts _____.

23. When caring for a person with acute renal failure, report to the nurse at once if the person has

    _____

24. You may need to assist a person in chronic renal failure with nutritional needs. List what the care plan is likely to include for the following:

    A. Diet _____

    B. Fluids _____

25. Sexually transmitted diseases are transmitted by

    _____

26. Using _____ prevents the spread of STDs.

27. When caring for a person with an STD, you should

    follow _____ and

    _____

Use the FOCUS ON PRIDE section to complete these statements.

28. You can help to prevent UTIs when giving care to females by always cleaning the perineal area from

    _____

29. When a person has a urinary or reproductive disorder, you protect the person's rights and give respect when you give information only to

    _____

Matching

Match the sexually transmitted disease with the correct statement. Use Table 47-1 to complete the matching.

  A. Herpes
  B. Genital warts
  C. Gonorrhea
  D. Chlamydia
  E. Syphilis
  F. Trichomoniasis

30. _____ Surgical removal if ointment is not effective

31. _____ Sores may have a watery discharge

32. _____ No symptoms in men, only in women

33. _____ May have vaginal bleeding

34. _____ Urinary urgency and frequency is present

35. _____ Treated with anti-viral drugs

36. _____ Painless sores appear on genitals 10 to 90 days after exposure

37. _____ May not show symptoms

Optional Learning Exercises

You give home care to Mrs. Eunice Weber twice a week. She is 92 years old and lives alone. She has severe osteoporosis and uses a walker to move about in her home. She receives Meals on Wheels and spends most of the day sitting on the sofa. She has periods of incontinence or dribbling because of poor bladder control. When you arrive to care for her today, she tells you she is not feeling well. She tells you it burns when she urinates. When she needs to urinate, the urge comes on suddenly and she often does not get to the toilet in time. Answer these questions about Mrs. Weber.

38. You should tell the _____ because these symptoms may mean Mrs. Weber has

    _____

39. When the feeling to urinate comes on suddenly, it is

    called _____.

40. How does Mrs. Weber's immobility affect the following?

    A. Fluid intake _____

    _____

    B. Perineal care _____

    _____

41. Why is Mrs. Weber at high risk for urinary tract infections because she is a woman?

    _____

42. The doctor will probably order _____ to treat the condition.

43. The care plan will probably include "Encourage

    fluids to _____ per day."

Two weeks later you notice that Mrs. Weber has chills. When you take her temperature, it is 102°F. She tells you she has been vomiting since yesterday. You observe her urine and see that it is very cloudy.

44. You report these symptoms to the nurse, because it

    can indicate Mrs. Weber now has _____.
    This means the infection has moved from the

    _____ to the _____.

48 Mental Health Problems

Fill in the Blank: Key Terms

Alcohol abuse
Alcoholism
Anxiety
Compulsion
Defense mechanism
Delusion

Delusion of grandeur
Delusion of
  persecution
Drug abuse
Drug addiction
Flashback

Hallucination
Mental
Mental health
Mental health
  disorder
Mental illness

Obsession
Panic
Personality
Phobia
Psychiatric disorder
Psychosis

Stress
Stressor
Suicide
Suicide contagion
Withdrawal
  syndrome

1. Using a drug for non-medical or non-therapy effects is _____.

2. Alcohol dependence that involves craving, loss of control, physical dependence, and tolerance is _____

3. When a person has an exaggerated belief about one's own importance, wealth, power, or talents, it is called _____

4. A _____ is a disturbance in the ability to cope with or adjust to stress; behavior and function are impaired; also called mental illness or psychiatric disorder.

5. A _____ is any event or factor that causes stress.

6. _____ is relating to the mind. It is something that exists in the mind or is performed by the mind.

7. A recurrent, unwanted thought or idea is an _____

8. The response or change in the body caused by any emotional, physical, social, or economic factor is _____

9. A _____ is an intense fear.

10. A false belief is a _____.

11. Mental _____ is another name for a mental health disorder.

12. A state of severe mental impairment is _____

13. A _____ is seeing, hearing, or feeling something that is not real.

14. The repeating of an act over and over is _____

15. _____ is when the person copes with and adjusts to every-day stresses in ways accepted by society.

16. The set of attitudes, values, behaviors, and traits of a person is _____

17. _____ is a false belief that one is being mistreated, abused, or harassed.

18. An intense and sudden feeling of fear, anxiety, terror, or dread is _____.

19. _____ is another name for emotional illness, mental health disorder, or mental illness.

20. A _____ is an unconscious reaction that blocks unpleasant or threatening feelings.

21. _____ occurs with exposure to suicide or suicidal behaviors within one's family, peer group, or media reports of suicide.

22. Reliving the trauma in thoughts during the day and in nightmares at night is _____.

23. The person's physical and mental response after stopping or severely reducing the use of a substance that was used regularly is _____.

24. When drinking leads to problems but the person is not dependent on alcohol, it is _____.

25. To kill oneself is called _____.

26. _____ is a strong urge or craving to use the substance and cannot stop using. Tolerance develops.

27. A vague, uneasy feeling in response to stress is _____.

Circle the Best Answer

28. The causes of mental health disorders include
    A. Physical illness
    B. Growth and development tasks
    C. Not being able to cope or adjust to stress
    D. Personality development

29. Which of these statements about anxiety is *not* true?
    A. Anxiety often occurs when needs are not met.
    B. All anxiety is normal.
    C. Increases in pulse, respirations, and blood pressure may be due to anxiety.
    D. The anxiety level depends on the stressor.

30. An unhealthy coping mechanism would be
    A. Talking about the problem
    B. Playing music
    C. Smoking
    D. Exercising

31. A student fails a test and blames a friend for not helping with studying. This is an example of a defense mechanism called
    A. Conversion
    B. Projection
    C. Repression
    D. Displacement

32. When a person has a panic disorder
    A. The person cannot function
    B. It occurs gradually
    C. Delusions occur
    D. It continues for many months or years

33. When a person washes his or her hands over and over, it may be a sign of
    A. Schizophrenia
    B. Hallucinations
    C. A phobia
    D. Obsessive-compulsive disorder

34. A person who was abused as a child may have difficulty feeling close to people or trusting people. The person may have
    A. Paranoia
    B. Panic disorder
    C. Post-traumatic stress disorder
    D. Conversion

35. A person you are caring for tells you he is the president of the United States. He has a delusion of grandeur, which is a part of
    A. Obsessive-compulsive disorder
    B. Phobias
    C. Bipolar disorders
    D. Schizophrenia

36. A person with bipolar disorder may
    A. Be more depressed than manic
    B. Be more manic than depressed
    C. Alternate between depression and mania
    D. Have any of the above

37. A safety risk of depression is that the person
    A. May be very sad
    B. Has thoughts of suicide and death
    C. Has depressed body functions
    D. Cannot concentrate

38. Depression may be overlooked in older persons because
    A. It does not occur often in older persons
    B. Depression is very mild in the elderly
    C. The person may be diagnosed with a cognitive disorder
    D. Physical problems are more important

39. A person with an antisocial personality may
    A. Be suspicious and distrust others
    B. Have emotional highs and lows
    C. See, hear, or feel something that is not real
    D. Have no regard for the safety of others

40. All abused drugs
    A. Depress the nervous system
    B. Stimulate the nervous system
    C. Affect the mind and thinking
    D. Are illegal substances

41. When alcohol is ingested, it will
    A. Make the person more alert
    B. Slow down brain activity
    C. Have little effect on the organs of the body
    D. Do permanent damage to organs even in small amounts

42. Older persons have more risks when drinking alcohol because they
    A. Have slower reaction times
    B. Often binge drink
    C. Have a higher tolerance for alcohol
    D. Have increased dementia

43. When a person uses drugs over a period of time, a sign of addiction is
    A. The person uses the substance once or twice a month
    B. Larger amounts of the substance are needed to get the same effect
    C. Using the substance occasionally in a social setting
    D. Being on time for the person's job and meeting family obligations

44. When a young woman eats large amounts of food and then purges the body, she has
    A. Anorexia nervosa
    B. Depression
    C. Anxiety
    D. Bulimia nervosa

45. If a person mentions suicide
    A. It means the person will not act on carrying it out
    B. The person has anxiety
    C. Take the person seriously
    D. It means the person has psychosis

Fill in the Blank

46. Write out the meaning of the abbreviations.
    A. AUD _____
    B. BPD _____
    C. CDC _____
    D. GAD _____
    E. OCD _____
    F. OTC _____
    G. PTSD _____

47. What are causes of mental health disorders?
    A. _____
    B. _____
    C. _____
    D. _____
    E. _____
    F. _____
    G. _____

48. Name the defense mechanism being used in these situations.
    A. A girl fails a test. She blames the other girl for not helping her study.

    _____

    B. A man does not like his boss. He buys the boss an expensive Christmas present.

    _____

    C. A girl complains of a stomach-ache so she will not have to read aloud.

    _____

    D. A child is angry with his teacher. He hits his brother.

    _____

    E. A woman misses work frequently and is often late. She gets a bad evaluation. She says that the boss does not like her.

    _____

    _____

49. What is the phobia in each example?
    A. _____ Being afraid of strangers
    B. _____ Fear of pain or seeing others in pain
    C. _____ Being trapped in an enclosed area
    D. _____ Fear of darkness

50. During a _____, the person may lose touch with reality and believe the trauma is happening all over again. This occurs when the person has

    _____.

51. Below are examples of problems that occur with schizophrenia. Name each one.
    A. A woman says that voices told her to set fire to her apartment. _____
    B. A man believes that others can hear his thoughts on the radio. _____
    C. A woman tells you she owns 3 BMW cars and is the president of McDonald's. _____

Use the FOCUS ON PRIDE section to complete these statements.

52. When caring for a person with mental illness, the team must react quickly to _____.

53. When caring for a person with a mental illness, you can take pride in working as a team when you _____ when the person calls for help.

Optional Learning Exercises

54. Mr. Johnson is very worried about his surgery tomorrow. You notice that he is talking very fast and sweating. You give him directions to collect a urine specimen. Five minutes later, he turns on his call light to ask you to repeat the directions. He tells you he is using the toilet "all the time" because he has diarrhea and frequent urination. The nurse tells you all of these things are signs and symptoms of

    _____

55. You are assigned to care for Mrs. Grand, a new resident. She is getting ready to go to the dining room. You assist her to get dressed and she tells you she wants to wash her hands before going to the dining room. She goes to the bathroom and washes her hands for several minutes. As she leaves the room, she stops to turn off the light. Then she tells you she must wash her hands again. She repeats washing her hands and turning the lights on and off 4 or 5 times. You report this to the nurse, who tells you Mrs. Grand has

    _____

49 Confusion and Dementia

Fill in the Blank: Key Terms

Cognitive function   Delirium   Dementia   Hallucination   Pseudodementia
Confusion   Delusion   Elopement   Paranoia   Sundowning

1. _____ occurs when a person leaves the agency without staff knowledge.

2. A false belief is a _____.

3. Seeing, hearing, smelling, or feeling something that is not real is _____.

4. Increased signs, symptoms, and behavior of AD during hours of darkness is

   _____

5. _____ is a state of temporary but acute mental confusion that comes on suddenly.

6. The loss of cognitive function and social function that interferes with routine personal, social, and occupational activities is _____.

7. _____ is false dementia.

8. _____ involves memory, thinking, reasoning, ability to understand, judgment, and behavior.

9. _____ is a disorder of the mind; the person has false beliefs and suspicion about a person or situation.

10. _____ is a mental state of being disoriented to person, place, situation, or identity.

Circle the Best Answer

11. Nervous system changes from aging
    A. Occur suddenly
    B. Are due to reduced blood flow to the brain
    C. Can be cured
    D. Are usually temporary

12. Delirium
    A. Occurs slowly
    B. Is the result of aging
    C. Cannot be cured
    D. Signals physical changes

13. When a person is confused, it is helpful if you
    A. Repeat the date and time as often as necessary
    B. Change the routine each day to stimulate the person
    C. Keep the drapes pulled during the day
    D. Give complex answers to questions

14. Vision and hearing decrease with confusion, so you should
    A. Speak in a loud voice
    B. Write out directions to the person
    C. Face the person and speak clearly
    D. Keep the lighting dim in the room

15. Dementia can be treated if it is caused by
    A. AIDS
    B. Head injuries or bleeding in the brain
    C. Stroke
    D. Alzheimer's disease

16. Dementia
    A. Is a specific disease
    B. Causes the person to have problems with common activities
    C. Is always temporary and can be cured
    D. Affects most older people

17. The most common type of permanent dementia in older persons is
    A. Alzheimer's disease   C. Depression
    B. Dementia   D. Delirium

18. Depression is often overlooked in older persons because
    A. Signs and symptoms are similar to aging and some drug side effects
    B. Depression is rare in older persons
    C. It is a temporary condition that passes without treatment
    D. It is always the result of a physical problem

19. The most common early symptom of Alzheimer's disease (AD) is
    A. Mood and personality changes
    B. Difficulty remembering newly learned information
    C. Acute confusion and delirium
    D. Wandering and sundowning

20. In mild AD, the person may
    A. Walk slowly with a shuffling gait
    B. Be totally incontinent
    C. Take longer to complete daily tasks
    D. Become agitated and may be violent

21. As AD progresses to moderate AD, the person
    A. Depends on others for care
    B. Has problems with tasks that have multiple steps
    C. Is disoriented to time and place
    D. Has seizures

22. In severe AD, the person may
    A. Forget recent events
    B. Lose impulse control and use foul language or have poor table manners
    C. Be less interested in things or be less outgoing
    D. Not be able to communicate

23. When a person with AD wanders, the major risk is
    A. The person's comfort
    B. Life-threatening accidents can occur
    C. Inconvenience of the family or facility
    D. Making sure the person gets enough rest and sleep

24. When a person with AD has symptoms of sundowning, it may be due to
    A. Being tired or hungry
    B. Having poor judgment
    C. Impaired vision or hearing
    D. The person looking for something or someone

25. When you assist a person with AD to wear prescribed glasses or hearing aids, it helps to prevent
    A. Wandering
    B. Sundowning
    C. Hallucinations or delusions
    D. Paranoia

26. If a person with AD seems afraid or is worried about money, you should
    A. Ignore the worry
    B. Tell them everything is okay
    C. Report the concern to the nurse
    D. Assume the person has paranoia

27. Too much stimuli from being asked too many questions all at once can overwhelm a person and cause
    A. Delusions
    B. Catastrophic reactions
    C. Hallucinations
    D. Sundowning

28. A caregiver may cause agitation and aggression by
    A. Calling the person by name
    B. Selecting tasks and activities specific to the person's cognitive abilities and interests
    C. Encouraging activity early in the day
    D. Rushing the person to complete care quickly

29. When you wish to communicate with the person who has AD or other dementias, you should
    A. Make eye contact to get the person's attention
    B. Give the person an order such as "Sit down and eat"
    C. Ask an open-ended question
    D. Make sure the TV or radio is playing in the background

30. If a person with AD displays sexual behaviors, the nurse may tell you to
    A. Tell the person this behavior is not acceptable
    B. Make sure the person has good hygiene to prevent itching
    C. Avoid caring for the person
    D. Ignore the behavior because the disease causes it

31. What should you do when a person repeats the same motions or repeats the same words over and over?
    A. Remind the person to stop the repeating.
    B. Report this to the nurse immediately.
    C. Take the person for a walk or distract the person with music or picture books.
    D. Isolate the person in his or her room until the repeating behavior stops.

32. A person with AD is encouraged to take part in therapies and activities that
    A. Increase the level of confusion
    B. Help the person to feel useful, worthwhile, and active
    C. Will prevent aggressive behaviors
    D. Improve physical problems such as incontinence and contractures

33. How do AD special care units differ from other areas of a care facility?
    A. Complete care is provided.
    B. Entrances and exits may be locked.
    C. Meals are served in the person's room.
    D. No activities are provided.

34. A person with AD no longer stays in a secured unit when
    A. The condition improves
    B. The family requests a move to another unit
    C. The person cannot sit or walk
    D. Aggressive behaviors disrupt the unit

35. A family who cares for a person with dementia at home
    A. Is encouraged to be with the person at all times
    B. May feel guilty, angry, and upset
    C. Generally does not need any help from others
    D. Should not place the person in a long-term care facility

Fill in the Blank

36. Write out the meaning of the abbreviations.
    A. AD _____
    B. ADL _____
    C. NIA _____

37. Cognitive functioning involves
    A. _____
    B. _____
    C. _____
    D. _____
    E. _____
    F. _____

38. What senses decrease with changes in the nervous system from aging?
    A. _____
    B. _____
    C. _____
    D. _____
    E. _____

39. Some early warning signs of dementia affect these areas. Explain or give an example for each one.
    A. Memory _____
    B. Common tasks _____
    C. Language _____
    D. Judgment _____

40. What substances can cause treatable dementia?
    A. _____
    B. _____

41. Pseudodementia can occur with _____
    and _____.

42. With delirium, the onset is _____.
    It often lasts for about _____.
    It may take _____ for normal mental function to return.

43. In Alzheimer's disease (AD) there is a slow, steady decline in mental functions, including
    A. _____
    B. _____
    C. _____
    D. _____
    E. _____
    F. _____
    G. _____
    H. _____

44. Certain behaviors are common with AD. Name the behavior for each of these examples.
    A. The person becomes more anxious, confused, or restless during the night.

    _____

    B. The person sits in a chair and folds the same napkin over and over.

    _____

    C. The person begins to scream and cry when a visitor asks many questions.

    _____

    D. The person walks away from home and cannot find the way back home.

    _____

    E. The person begins to get upset when a set routine for ADL is changed.

    _____

    F. The person tells you he sees his dog sitting in the room but you do not see anything.

    _____

    G. You frequently find the person looking for lost items in a wastebasket.

    _____

    H. The person tries to hug and kiss other residents of the facility.

    _____

Use the FOCUS ON PRIDE section to complete these statements.

45. You demonstrate personal and professional responsibility when you treat each person as unique, with his or her own

    _____.

46. You show that you respect the rights of a person when you keep personal items _____.
    It is important to protect the person's belongings from

    _____ or

    _____.

47. You help to maintain independence for a person with AD by maintaining the person's _____ when giving ADLs.

Optional Learning Exercises

You are caring for Mr. Harris, a 78 year old who is confused. You know there are ways to help a person to be more oriented. Answer these questions about ways to help a confused person.

48. How can you help to orient Mr. Harris every time you are in contact with him?

    _____

49. What are ways you can help to orient Mr. Harris to time?
    A. _____
    B. _____

50. What are ways you can maintain the day-night cycle?
    A. _____
    B. _____
    C. _____

You are caring for Mrs. Matthews, an 82-year-old resident. The nurse tells you she lived with her daughter for the last 2 years but the family is now concerned for her safety. She left the home when the temperature was 35 °F and was found 2 miles away, wearing a light sweater. On another occasion, she turned on the gas stove and could not remember how to turn it off. Sometimes, she did not recognize her daughter and resisted getting a bath or changing clothes. Since admission to the care facility, she repeatedly tells everyone she must leave to go to her birthday party. She brushes her arms and legs and tells you "bugs" are crawling on her. Answer these questions about Mrs. Matthews and her care.

51. What is the most important reason that Mrs. Matthews is living in a special care unit in the nursing facility?

    _____

    _____

52. Mrs. Matthews is diagnosed with

    _____ stage AD. What activities would indicate she is in this stage?
    A. _____
    B. _____
    C. _____
    D. _____
    E. _____

53. The nurse may encourage Mrs. Matthews's daughter to join a _____ group. How can this be helpful to the daughter?
    A. _____
    B. _____
    C. _____

50 Intellectual and Developmental Disabilities

Fill in the Blank: Key Terms

Birth defect
Developmental disabilities

Disability
Inherited

Intellectual disability
Spastic

1. _____ involves severe limits in intellectual function and adaptive behavior occurring before age 18.

2. An abnormality present at birth that can involve body structure or function is a _____.

3. The uncontrolled contractions of skeletal muscles is _____.

4. That which is passed down from parents to children is _____.

5. A disability that occurs before 22 years of age is _____.

6. Any lost, absent, or impaired physical or mental function is a _____.

Circle the Best Answer

7. Intellectual and developmental disabilities (IDD)
   A. Occur before, during, or after birth
   B. Are usually temporary
   C. Limit function in 3 or more life skills
   D. Are present before the age of 12

8. Developmentally disabled adults
   A. Need life-long assistance, support, and special services
   B. Usually can live independently after they become adults
   C. Always need to be in long-term care in special centers
   D. Generally outgrow the problems as they mature

9. A person is considered to have intellectual disabilities if
   A. The IQ score is below 90
   B. The condition occurs after the age of 18
   C. The person has hallucinations and delusions
   D. The person needs adaptive behaviors to live, work, and play

10. The Arc of the United States is a national organization
    A. Related to Alzheimer's disease
    B. That focuses on people with intellectual and related developmental disabilities
    C. That provides care for people with physical disability
    D. For persons with cerebral palsy

11. Down syndrome (DS) is caused by
    A. An extra chromosome
    B. Head injury during birth
    C. Diseases of the mother during pregnancy
    D. Lack of oxygen to the brain

12. A person with Down syndrome is at risk for
    A. Cerebral palsy
    B. Being underweight
    C. Ear and respiratory infections
    D. Poor nutrition

13. Fragile X syndrome occurs because
    A. Of a birth injury
    B. Of an extra chromosome
    C. Of a change in a gene that makes a protein needed for brain development
    D. The mother had rubella (German measles) during pregnancy

14. A person with autism may
    A. Withdraw from physical contact that is over-stimulating
    B. Have bladder and bowel control problems
    C. Have generalized seizures
    D. Have diplegia or hemiplegia

15. The person with autism
    A. Needs to develop social and work skills
    B. Will outgrow the condition
    C. Will always live in group homes or residential care centers
    D. Will have severe physical problems

16. Cerebral palsy is a group of disorders involving
    A. Intellectual disabilities
    B. Paralysis and injuries or abnormalities in the brain
    C. Abnormal genes from 1 or both parents
    D. An increased risk of developing leukemia

17. When a person has spastic cerebral palsy, the symptoms include
    A. Constant slow weaving or writhing motions
    B. Uncontrolled contractions of skeletal muscles
    C. Using little or no eye contact
    D. A strong attachment to a single item, idea, activity, or person

18. Spina bifida occurs
    A. At birth, due to injury during delivery
    B. Because of traumatic injury in childhood
    C. During the first month of pregnancy
    D. As a result of child abuse

19. Which of these types of spina bifida cause the person to have leg paralysis and lack of bowel and bladder control?
    A. Spina bifida cystica
    B. Myelomeningocele
    C. Spina bifida occulta
    D. Meningocele

20. A shunt placed in the brain of a child with hydrocephalus will
    A. Increase pressure on the brain
    B. Drain fluid from the brain to a body cavity
    C. Cause intellectual disabilities or neurological damage
    D. Cure the hydrocephalus

Fill in the Blank

21. Write out the abbreviations.
    A. ADA _____
    B. CP _____
    C. DS _____
    D. Fragile X _____
    E. IDD _____
    F. IQ _____
    G. SB _____

22. Intellectual and developmental disabilities (IDDs) affect 3 areas of development. They are
    A. _____
    B. _____
    C. _____

23. What genetic conditions can cause intellectual disabilities?
    A. _____
    B. _____

24. Intellectual disabilities may be caused after birth by childhood infections such as
    A. _____
    B. _____
    C. _____
    D. _____
    E. _____
    F. _____

25. According to the Arc of the United States, intellectual disabilities involve the condition being present before _____

26. The Arc beliefs about sexuality include the rights to
    A. _____
    B. _____
    C. _____
    D. _____
    E. _____
    F. _____
    G. _____
    H. _____
    I. _____
    J. _____
    K. _____

27. If a child has Down syndrome (DS), what features are present in these areas?
    A. Head, ears, mouth _____
    B. Eyes _____
    C. Tongue _____
    D. Nose _____
    E. Hands and fingers _____

28. Persons with Down syndrome and other developmental disabilities need therapy in these areas.
    A. _____
    B. _____
    C. _____
    D. _____
    E. _____

29. The most common type of cerebral palsy is _____

30. The goal for a person with developmental disabilities is to be _____

31. What sign of autism is described in each of the following?
    A. May find normal noises painful
    B. May not respond to smiles or eye contact
    C. Shows little pretend or imaginary play
    D. Cannot start or maintain a social conversation

32. Spina bifida is a defect of the _____

33. Which type of spina bifida would cause the problems in each of the examples given?
    A. The person has leg paralysis and a lack of bowel and bladder control. _____
    B. The person may have no symptoms. _____
    C. Nerve damage usually does not occur and surgery corrects the defect.

34. If a hydrochephalus is not treated, pressure increases in the head and causes _____ and _____

Use the FOCUS ON PRIDE section to complete these statements.

35. Persons with developmental disabilities have a right to enjoy and maintain a good quality of life. Such a life involves
    A. _____
    B. _____
    C. _____

36. The goal for children with developmental disabilities is independence _____.

37. Signs of abuse of a developmentally disabled person may be

    A. _____

    B. _____

    C. _____

    D. _____

    E. _____

Optional Learning Exercises

Mr. Murphy is one of the residents you care for. He has Down syndrome. Answer the 2 questions that relate to this person.

38. Mr. Murphy is 40 years old. What disease is a risk for an adult with Down syndrome?

    _____

39. Mr. Murphy is encouraged to eat a well-balanced diet and to attend regular exercise classes. Including these in the care plan will help to prevent the problems of

    _____ and _____.

You care for Mary Reynolds, who has cerebral palsy. Answer the 2 questions about Ms. Reynolds.

40. It is difficult to feed Ms. Reynolds because she drools, grimaces, and moves her head constantly. You notice that the movements become worse during

    _____

41. Because Ms. Reynolds remains in bed or a special chair all the time, she is at special risk for

    _____

    because of immobility and incontinence. She needs to be re-positioned at least every _____.

51 Sexuality

Fill in the Blank: Key Terms

Bisexual   Heterosexual   Sex   Transgender
Erectile dysfunction   Homosexual   Sexual orientation   Transsexual
Gender identity   Impotence   Sexuality   Transvestite

1. A person's sense of feelings of being male, female, or transgender is _____.

2. _____ is a broad term to describe people who express their sexuality or gender in other than the expected way.

3. Another name for impotence is

   _____.

4. _____ is the physical, psychological, social, cultural, and spiritual factors that affect a person's feelings and attitudes about his or her sex.

5. A _____ is a person who dresses and behaves like the other sex for emotional and sexual relief.

6. A person attracted to both sexes is _____.

7. A _____ is a person who believes that he or she is really a member of the other sex.

8. A _____ is a person who is attracted to members of the same sex.

9. The physical activities involving the reproductive organs is _____.

10. A person who is attracted to members of the other sex is _____.

11. The inability of the male to have an erection is erectile dysfunction or

    _____.

12. _____ is the gender (male or female) to which a person is emotionally, romantically, and physically attracted.

Circle the Best Answer

13. Sexuality
    A. Involves the whole person
    B. Is the physical activities involving reproductive organs
    C. Is unimportant in old age
    D. Is done for pleasure or to have children

14. A women who is attracted to men is
    A. Homosexual   C. Lesbian
    B. Heterosexual   D. Bisexual

15. Diabetes, spinal cord injuries, and multiple sclerosis may cause
    A. Impotence
    B. Menopause
    C. Sexual aggression
    D. Heterosexuality

16. Which of these are *not* true about sexuality and older persons?
    A. An orgasm is less forceful than in younger persons.
    B. Arousal takes longer.
    C. Older persons lose sexual needs and desires.
    D. Love, affection, and intimacy are needed throughout life.

17. When older adult couples live in a nursing center, OBRA requires that they
    A. Are allowed to share the same room
    B. Are placed in separate rooms
    C. Are not encouraged to be intimate
    D. Cannot share a bed

18. If a person touches you in the wrong way, you should
    A. Ignore it and realize the person is not responsible
    B. Tell the person you do not like him or her
    C. Politely tell the person that those behaviors make you uncomfortable
    D. Refuse to give care to the person

Fill in the Blank

19. Sexuality develops when the baby's _____.

20. Children know their own sex at age _____.

21. Homosexual males are called _____.

22. Homosexual women are called _____.

23. Sexual function may be affected by chronic illnesses such as
    A. _____
    B. _____
    C. _____
    D. _____

24. What reproductive surgeries may affect sexuality?
    A. Men _____
    B. Women _____

25. Some older people do not have intercourse. They may express their sexual needs or desires by

    _____.

26. What can you do to allow privacy for a person and a partner?

    A. Close _____.

    B. Let the person and partner know _____.

    C. Tell other _____.

    D. Knock _____.

27. Masturbation is a normal _____.

28. If a person becomes sexually aroused, you should allow for _____.

29. What health-related problems may cause a person to touch his or her genitals?

    A. _____ or _____ system disorders

    B. Poor _____

    C. Being _____ or _____ from urine and feces

Use the FOCUS ON PRIDE section to complete these statements.

30. When you are caring for a person, it is important to get consent before touching _____, _____, or _____.

31. If you touch without consent, you may be accused of _____.

32. Sexuality includes _____, _____, _____, _____, and _____ factors.

33. When giving care, you can promote sexuality when you

    A. _____

    B. _____

    C. _____

    D. _____

Optional Learning Exercises

Mr. and Mrs. Davis are 78-year-old residents in a nursing center, where they share a room. They need assistance with ADL but are mentally alert. They are an affectionate couple that cares deeply for each other. Answer this question about meeting their sexuality needs.

34. Mr. Davis has diabetes and high blood pressure. What effect can these disorders have on sexuality?

    _____

52 Caring for Mothers and Babies

Fill in the Blank: Key Terms

Breast-feeding   Episiotomy   Meconium   Postpartum   Umbilical cord
Circumcision   Lochia   Nursing   Prenatal care

1. An _____ is an incision into the perineum.

2. Breast-feeding is also called _____.

3. After childbirth is called _____.

4. _____ is the surgical removal of foreskin from the penis.

5. The vaginal discharge that occurs after childbirth is
_____

6. The structure that carries blood, oxygen, and nutrients from the mother to the fetus is the
_____

7. A dark green to black, tarry bowel movement is
_____

8. Feeding a baby milk from the mother's breast is
_____

9. _____ is the care a woman receives while pregnant.

Circle the Best Answer

10. You lift a newborn by
    A. The arms
    B. Using only 1 hand
    C. Supporting the head and upper back
    D. Using 2 hands—one to support the head and back, the other to support the legs

11. If a baby is lying on a scale, bed, table, or other surface, you should
    A. Place pillows around the baby
    B. Tuck a blanket firmly around the baby
    C. Always keep 1 hand on the baby
    D. Watch the baby carefully if you must walk away

12. Babies should be placed on a firm surface to sleep because
    A. Soft surfaces will not provide enough support to the back
    B. Soft items such as pillows, quilts, or soft toys can cause suffocation
    C. They need a firm support when sleeping on the stomach
    D. The beds are too firm for comfort

13. When a crib is checked for safety, which of these is *not* correct?
    A. There should be no gap or space between the mattress and the crib.
    B. Drop-side latches cannot be easily released by the baby.
    C. Crib slats are spaced no more than 2⅜ inches apart.
    D. There are no cut-outs in the head-board or foot-board to allow the baby's head to get caught.

14. Which of these should be reported to the nurse at once?
    A. The baby has a rectal temperature of 99.6°F.
    B. The baby has a soft, unformed stool after being breast-fed.
    C. The baby turns his or her head to 1 side or puts a hand to 1 ear.
    D. The baby cries when the diaper is wet or when he or she is hungry

15. A breast-fed newborn baby generally nurses
    A. Every 2 to 3 hours
    B. Every 8 to 12 hours
    C. About once an hour for very short periods of time
    D. On a very strict schedule

16. When a mother is breast-feeding, she should avoid
    A. Drinking whole milk
    B. Certain foods that cause the baby to have cramping or diarrhea
    C. Foods that are high in calories or calcium
    D. Any foods with caffeine

17. When the mother is breast-feeding, she should
    A. Position the baby by using a pillow to prop up the baby
    B. Begin by stroking the baby's cheek with her nipple
    C. Nurse only from 1 breast at each feeding
    D. Lay the baby on his or her stomach after feeding

18. When preparing bottles for feeding babies, you should
    A. Prepare and then refrigerate bottles that can be used within 24 hours
    B. Sterilize the bottles by boiling them for 20 minutes
    C. Rinse bottles and nipples that have been used only in cool water
    D. Not use any soap when cleaning the equipment as it can cause serious stomach and intestinal irritation

19. When preparing to give a bottle to a baby
    A. It may be used from the refrigerator without heating
    B. Warm the bottle in warm running tap water
    C. Take the bottle out of the refrigerator and allow it to warm
    D. Heat the bottle in a microwave oven

20. When diapering a baby, report to the nurse if
    A. The stool is soft and unformed
    B. The stool is hard and formed or watery
    C. The diaper is wet 6 to 8 times a day
    D. The baby has 3 stools in 1 day

21. The diaper is changed
    A. Only when stool is present
    B. When the diaper is wet, usually 6 to 8 times a day
    C. Before and after feeding
    D. 3 to 4 times a day

22. The umbilical cord stump falls off
    A. At birth
    B. Within 2 to 3 days after birth
    C. About 2 weeks after birth
    D. About 1 month after birth

23. Circumcision care includes
    A. Washing the area with mild soap and water or commercial wipes
    B. Cleaning the area with a sterile solution
    C. Applying a snug dressing to the area
    D. Cleaning the area once a day

24. Sponge baths are given
    A. To protect the dry skin of an infant
    B. Until the cord site and circumcision heal
    C. Because it is unsafe to give a baby a tub bath
    D. Until the baby is able to support the head without assistance

25. When giving a bath to a baby, the water should be
    A. Room temperature
    B. 75°F to 80°F
    C. 100°F to 105°F
    D. 110°F to 115°F

26. An important safety measure when giving a bath to a baby is
    A. Apply lotion when the bath is finished
    B. Clean the ears and nostrils with cotton swabs
    C. Use a mild soap when bathing the baby
    D. Always keep 1 hand on the baby if you must look away

27. When a baby is breast-fed, the baby is weighed
    A. Once a day
    B. Before and after each feeding
    C. After every diaper change
    D. Once a week

28. When a mother breast-feeds, she
    A. Can expect a menstrual period within 2 to 4 weeks
    B. Cannot get pregnant as long as she continues to breast-feed
    C. Needs to use birth control measures to prevent pregnancy
    D. Will have difficulty losing weight gained during the pregnancy

29. You are caring for a mother who had a baby 4 weeks ago. She tells you she is concerned because she has whitish vaginal drainage. You know that this
    A. Is abnormal and should be reported to the nurse at once
    B. Is unusual because her discharge should be pinkish brown in color
    C. Is normal at this time after having a baby
    D. Can mean she has an infection

30. Report to the nurse if during the postpartum period the mother
    A. Has occasional emotional reactions
    B. Has a whitish vaginal discharge 12 days after delivery
    C. Complains of leg, abdominal, or perineal pain
    D. Has a menstrual period about 4 weeks after the baby is born

Fill in the Blank

31. Write out the meaning of the abbreviations.
    A. BM _____
    B. C _____
    C. C-section _____
    D. F _____
    E. SIDS _____
    F. SUID _____

32. When you hold and cuddle infants or respond to their cries, it helps them learn to feel _____ and _____.

33. You should not place pillows, quilts, or soft toys in the crib because they may cause _____.

34. Babies are not placed on their stomachs for sleep because this position can _____.

35. What signs or symptoms related to each of these may indicate the baby is ill?
    A. Skin color _____
    B. Respirations _____
    C. Eyes _____
    D. Stools _____

36. When a mother is breast-feeding, if the baby finished the last feeding at the right breast, the baby starts the next feeding at the _____ breast.

37. The baby is burped at least twice when breast-feeding. Burping is done
    A. _____
    B. _____

38. Cribs should not have drop-side rails because
    _____

39. Sudden unexpected infant death may occur because of accidental _____ or strangulation
    _____

40. When taking a pulse on a baby, it is taken
    _____

41. When planning meals or grocery shopping for a mother who is breast-feeding, what should you know about her diet?

    A. Calories _____

    B. Dairy group _____

    _____

    C. Calcium _____

    D. What foods should be avoided? _____

    _____ Why? _____

    _____

    E. What foods are used in moderation? _____

    _____ Why? _____

    _____

    F. She should not drink _____.

42. Why is it important to thoroughly rinse baby bottles, caps, and nipples to remove all soap?

    _____

43. You can prevent having air in the neck of the bottle or in the nipple by _____

    _____

44. When you are burping a baby, you should support the _____ for the first _____ months.

45. If you are using cloth diapers, rinse the soiled diaper in _____.

46. When changing a baby's diaper, what observations should be reported and recorded?

    A. _____

    B. _____

    C. _____

    D. _____

47. When diapering a newborn, what should you do if the baby has an unhealed circumcision or a cord stump still attached?

    A. Circumcision _____

    B. Cord stump _____

48. The base of the cord stump is washed with _____ if it is dirty or sticky. The stump heals faster if allowed to _____.

49. When caring for the umbilical cord, you should report the following to the nurse.

    A. _____

    B. _____

    C. _____

    D. _____

50. Petrolatum gauze dressing or jelly is applied to an unhealed circumcision to

    A. _____

    B. _____

51. To protect an infant during a bath, what safety measures are followed?

    A. Room temperature _____

    B. Bath water temperature _____

    C. Never _____.

    D. Always _____.

    E. Hold _____.

52. What steps are used to wash a baby's head?

    A. _____

    B. _____

    C. _____

    D. _____

    E. _____

53. In order to protect a baby from falling when you weigh him or her, always keep _____.

54. Describe the vaginal discharge that occurs after childbirth.

    A. Lochia rubra _____ It is seen during the _____.

    B. Lochia serosa _____ It lasts about _____.

    C. Lochia alba _____ It continues for _____.

55. What signs and symptoms of postpartum complications should be reported to the nurse at once?

    A. _____

    B. _____

    C. _____

    D. _____

    E. _____

    F. _____

    G. _____

    H. _____

    I. _____

    J. _____

    K. _____

Use the FOCUS ON PRIDE section to complete these statements.

56. When you return a newborn to the mother, it is your professional responsibility to follow the agency policy for _____.

57. Parents will learn to be independent and gain confidence by performing _____

    _____.

58. Newborns wear a security bracelet that will signal the agency when he or she is carried _____.

Optional Learning Exercises

You are caring for Marilyn Hansen and her newborn son, Samuel, at home. Answer the questions about their care.

59. Ms. Hansen asks you if the crib she was given is safe. What safety guidelines are important for a crib?

    A. _____

    B. _____

    C. _____

    D. _____

    E. _____

    F. _____

    G. _____

    H. _____

60. Ms. Hansen is breast-feeding. When she strokes the baby's cheek with her nipple, what does the baby do?

    _____

    This is called the _____.

61. Ms. Hansen is having difficulty in removing Samuel from her breast. You tell her that to break the suction she can _____

    _____

62. You notice that Ms. Hansen's nipples are dry and cracking. What can she do to prevent this from happening?

    A. _____

    B. _____

    C. _____

    D. _____

63. When you are changing Samuel's diaper, clean the genital area from _____.

64. The cord stump is still in place. Ms. Hansen asks you when it will fall off. You tell her it dries up and falls off in _____

65. Samuel has been circumcised and Ms. Hansen is concerned because the penis looks red, swollen, and sore. You know that this is _____. However, you should observe the circumcision for signs of

    A. _____ and _____

    B. There should be no _____.

66. Ms. Hansen asks whether she should bathe Samuel in the morning or in the evening. You tell her an evening bath might work well because it

    A. _____

    _____

    B. _____

    _____

53 Assisted Living

Fill in the Blank: Key Terms

Assisted living   Medication reminder   Service plan

1. A _____ is reminding the person to take drugs, observing them being taken as prescribed, and charting that they were taken.

2. A written plan that lists the services needed by the person and who provides them is a

   _____.

3. _____ is a housing option for older persons who need help with activities of daily living but do not need constant care.

Circle the Best Answer

4. Which of these persons would *not* be living in an ALR?
   A. A person who needs medication management or help taking drugs
   B. A person who needs help with shopping, banking, and money management
   C. A person who needs complete help with ADL
   D. A person who needs supervision for dementia

5. When a person lives in an ALR, 1 requirement is
   A. At least 2 rooms and a bath
   B. Both a bathtub and a shower
   C. A door that locks and the person keeps the key
   D. A double or queen-sized bed

6. Environmental requirements in an ALR include
   A. Bathrooms have toilet paper, soap, and cloth towels or a dryer
   B. Pets or animals must be kept in kennels
   C. Hot water temperatures are between 110°F and 130°F
   D. Garbage is stored in covered containers lined with plastic bags that are removed at least once a day

7. Which of these is *not* included in the Assisted Living Residents' Rights?
   A. May take part in religious, social, community, and other activities
   B. Receive privacy in personal care, correspondence, and financial matters
   C. Has a doctor or pharmacist assigned by the facility
   D. Has help in understanding, protecting, and exercising residents' rights

8. A staff member in an ALR would be expected to have training in all of these areas *except*
   A. Assisting with drugs
   B. Needs and goals of ALR residents
   C. Food preparation, service, and storage
   D. Measuring and giving medications

9. Which of these is often a requirement of a resident in an ALR?
   A. The person must be able to leave the building in an emergency.
   B. The person requires skilled nursing services.
   C. The person has complex nursing problems.
   D. The person must not be paralyzed or be chronically ill.

10. Which of these is a service offered in an ALR?
    A. Daily housekeeping
    B. A garage for cars owned by residents
    C. A 24-hour emergency communication system
    D. A bank in the facility

11. Meals in an ALR
    A. Are always served in the person's room
    B. Include the noon meal only
    C. May provide a nutritious snack in the evening
    D. Cannot meet special dietary needs

12. When you assist with housekeeping, you will be expected to
    A. Clean the tub or shower after each use
    B. Put out clean towels and washcloths every week
    C. Use a disinfectant or water and detergent to clean bathroom surfaces once a week
    D. Dust furniture every day

13. A measure you should follow when handling, preparing, or storing foods is
    A. Empty garbage at least once a week
    B. Wash all pots and pans in a dishwasher
    C. Save or discard left-overs
    D. Clean kitchen appliances, counters, tables, and other surfaces once a day

14. When assisting with laundry, a guideline to follow is
    A. Sort and wash items according to the amount of soil on the items
    B. Wear gloves when handling soiled laundry
    C. Use hot water to wash all items
    D. Use the highest setting on the dryer to sanitize the items

15. When you assist a person with medication, it may involve
    A. Opening containers for the person who cannot do so
    B. Measuring the medications for the person
    C. Explaining to the person the action of the medication
    D. Preparing a pill organizer for the person each week

16. If a drug error occurs, you should
    A. Tell the person not to do it again
    B. Make sure the person takes the correct medication at the next scheduled time
    C. Report the error to the nurse
    D. Take all medications away from the person immediately

17. An attendant is needed in an ALR 24 hours a day to
    A. Give care to those who need it
    B. Make sure medications are dispensed when ordered
    C. Assist those who need assistance if an emergency occurs
    D. Provide activities for the residents

18. A resident can be transferred, discharged, or evicted from the ALR for all of these *except*
    A. The ALR closes
    B. The person is a threat to the health and safety of self or others
    C. The person fails to pay for services as agreed upon
    D. The person is not well liked by others in the ALR

19. Which of these is *not* a right of a resident in assisted living?
    A. The right to expect personal care to be confidential
    B. The right to have overnight guests whenever the resident wishes
    C. The right to not to be discriminated against
    D. The right to be take part in developing a service plan

Fill in the Blank

20. Write out the meaning of the abbreviations.
    A. ADL _____
    B. ALR _____

21. When working in an assisted living setting, you should follow _____ when contact with blood, body fluids, secretions, excretions, or potentially contaminated items is likely.

22. Most persons living in ALRs need help with one or more ADL, such as
    A. _____
    B. _____
    C. _____
    D. _____
    E. _____
    F. _____

23. A bathroom in an ALR must provide privacy and
    A. _____
    B. _____
    C. _____
    D. _____
    E. _____

24. The ALR cannot employ a person with a _____.

25. The service plan is a written plan listing
    A. _____
    B. _____
    C. _____

26. The service plan also relates to
    A. _____
    B. _____
    C. _____
    D. _____
    E. _____
    F. _____

27. What 24-hour services are usually provided by the ALR?
    A. _____
    B. _____

28. When you wash eating and cooking items by hand, what is the order in which they are washed?
    _____

29. If you are assisting the person with taking medications, you should know the 6 rights of drug administration. They are
    A. _____
    B. _____
    C. _____
    D. _____
    E. _____
    F. _____

30. If a person is taking his or her drugs and tells you that a pill looks different, what should you do?
    _____

31. If a person needs a medication reminder, it means reminding _____, observing _____, and charting _____.

32. If you are assisting in drug administration, you should report any drug error to the RN. Errors would include:
    A. _____
    B. _____
    C. _____
    D. _____
    E. _____
    F. _____
    G. _____
    H. _____
    I. _____

Use the FOCUS ON PRIDE section to complete these statements.

33. When you are caring for residents in assisted living, your interactions should assure the person and family that you will provide

_____.

34. In order to make the room in an ALR feel home-like, residents are allowed to _____.

35. It is important to know your state's laws when you assist with drugs because if you act beyond those limits, you can lose _____ and your ability to work _____.

Optional Learning Exercises

You are working in an assisting living facility. What would you do in these situations?

36. A resident in the facility has lived there for 2 years and has needed little assistance. He recently had a stroke and now needs care for all of his ADL. Why is he being moved to a nursing facility? _____

_____

37. Mrs. Jenkins tells you she is expecting an important phone call and wants to eat her lunch in her room. What should you do? _____

_____

38. Mr. Shante asks you to get his medicines ready for him to take. What assistance are you allowed to give when the nurse has trained you?

A. _____
B. _____
C. _____
D. _____
E. _____
F. _____
G. _____
H. _____

39. When you are assisting Mrs. Clyde with her medicines, you notice 2 of the labels have an expired date. What should you do? _____

_____

40. Mrs. Johnson asks you when the next meeting of the quilting group will be held. She also asks what days the community crafts fair is planned. Where would you direct her to find this information? _____

_____

Fill in the Blank: Key Terms

Anaphylaxis	Convulsion	First aid	Respiratory arrest	Shock
Cardiac arrest	Fainting	Hemorrhage	Seizure	Sudden cardiac arrest

1. Another term for sudden cardiac arrest (SCA) is
   _____.

2. In _____, breathing stops but the heart action continues for several minutes.

3. The sudden loss of consciousness from an inadequate blood supply to the brain is _____.

4. When the heart and breathing stop suddenly and without warning, it is _____ or cardiac arrest.

5. _____ results when there is not enough blood supply to organs and tissues.

6. Emergency care given to an ill or injured person before medical help arrives is _____.

7. Violent and sudden contractions or tremors of muscle groups is a convulsion or _____.

8. _____ is the excessive loss of blood in a short period of time.

9. A life-threatening sensitivity to an antigen is
   _____.

10. Another term for a seizure is _____.

Circle the Best Answer

11. When an emergency occurs in nursing centers, the nurse determines when to
    A. Call the doctor for orders
    B. Activate the EMS system
    C. Call the supervisor
    D. Assist the person to bed

12. If you find a person lying on the floor, you should
    A. Keep the person lying down
    B. Help the person back to bed
    C. Elevate the head
    D. Help the person to a chair

13. If the nurse instructs you to activate the EMS system, you should do all of these *except*
    A. Tell the operator your location
    B. Explain to the operator what has happened
    C. Describe aid that is being given
    D. Hang up as soon as you have finished giving the information

14. It is important to restore breathing and circulation quickly because
    A. The lungs will be damaged
    B. The person will lose consciousness
    C. Brain and other organ damage occurs within minutes
    D. Hemorrhage will occur

15. Which of these is *not* a major sign of sudden cardiac arrest (SCA)?
    A. Complaints of chest pain
    B. No pulse
    C. No breathing
    D. No response

16. The purpose of chest compressions is to
    A. Deflate the lungs
    B. Increase oxygen in the blood
    C. Force blood through the circulatory system
    D. Help the heart work more effectively

17. In order for chest compressions to be effective, the person must be
    A. In prone position
    B. On a soft surface
    C. Supine on a hard, flat surface
    D. In semi-Fowler's position

18. When preparing to give chest compressions, locate the hands
    A. On the sternum between the nipples
    B. On the upper half of the sternum
    C. Side by side over the sternum
    D. Slightly below the end of the sternum

19. When giving chest compressions to an adult, depress the sternum
    A. About 1 to 1½ inches
    B. No more than 1 inch
    C. At least 2 inches
    D. About 3 inches

20. The purpose of the head tilt–chin lift maneuver is to
    A. Make the person more comfortable
    B. Open the airway
    C. Practice Standard Precautions
    D. Stimulate the heart to beat

21. When a person is given breaths, you should
    A. Allow the person's chin to relax against the neck
    B. Place your mouth loosely over the person's mouth
    C. Give a breath for about 1 second each; you should see the chest rise with each breath
    D. Apply pressure on the chin to close the mouth

22. Barrier device breathing is used
    A. Whenever possible to avoid contact with body fluids
    B. In order to make a better seal for breathing
    C. When you cannot ventilate through the person's mouth
    D. Only when other methods will not work

23. Mouth-to-nose breathing is used when
    A. You cannot breathe through the person's mouth
    B. You want to avoid contact with body fluids
    C. When giving rescue breaths to a child
    D. When chest compressions are not needed

24. If an automated external defibrillator (AED) is available
    A. Use it only after other methods have been unsuccessful
    B. It can be used only by an RN or doctor
    C. Use it as soon as possible
    D. Use it once the person is responsive

25. When an automated external defibrillator (AED) is used, it
    A. Stops the heart
    B. Slows down the heartbeat
    C. Stops ventricular fibrillation and restores a regular heartbeat
    D. Starts the heartbeat

26. CPR is done when the person
    A. Does not respond when you shout, "Are you okay?"
    B. Is not breathing
    C. Is unconscious
    D. Does not respond, is not breathing, and has no pulse

27. Before starting chest compressions
    A. Make sure the person is breathing
    B. Check for a carotid pulse for 5 to 10 seconds
    C. Wait 30 seconds to see if the person regains consciousness
    D. Turn the person to the side

28. When 1-rescuer CPR is started, you first give
    A. 30 chest compressions
    B. 2 breaths
    C. 5 breaths
    D. 15 chest compressions

29. If the person is not breathing or not breathing adequately, give 2 breaths that
    A. Last about 1 second each
    B. Last about 5 seconds each
    C. Last 5 to 10 seconds each
    D. Last 15 seconds each

30. When performing 1-rescuer CPR, chest compressions are at a rate of
    A. 15–30 compressions per minute
    B. 100–120 compressions per minute
    C. 60–80 compressions per minute
    D. 12–20 compressions per minute

31. When performing 1-rescuer CPR, continue cycles of compressions and breathing
    A. For 5 minutes
    B. For 30 minutes
    C. Until an AED arrives
    D. For 4 cycles of 15 compressions and 2 breaths

32. The recovery position is used when
    A. Giving chest compressions
    B. Performing mouth-to-nose breathing
    C. The person is breathing and has a pulse but is not responding
    D. You are preparing to use an AED

33. When giving CPR to children, chest compressions
    A. Move the sternum about ⅓ of an inch
    B. Are done with enough pressure to press down ⅓ the depth of the chest
    C. Are not done
    D. The sternum is compressed ½ to 1 inch

34. When giving breaths to an infant, you should
    A. Tip the head back as far as possible to open the airway
    B. Pinch the nose closed and breathe through the mouth
    C. Cover the infant's mouth and nose with your mouth
    D. Always use a mouth barrier

35. If a person has swallowed poison, you should
    A. Try to have the person vomit
    B. Give the person something to drink or eat
    C. Contact the Poison Control Center as soon as possible
    D. Keep the person warm and in a supine position

36. Which of these is a sign of internal hemorrhage?
    A. Steady flow of blood from a wound
    B. Pain, shock, vomiting blood, or coughing up blood
    C. Bleeding that occurs in spurts
    D. Dried blood at the site of an injury

37. To control external bleeding, you should do all of these *except*
    A. Remove any objects that have pierced or stabbed the person
    B. Place a sterile dressing directly over the wound
    C. Apply pressure with your hand directly over the bleeding site
    D. Bind the wound when bleeding stops

38. If a person tells you she feels faint
    A. Have her lie down in a supine position
    B. Let her walk around to increase circulation
    C. Have her sit or lie down before fainting occurs
    D. If she is lying down, raise her head with pillows

39. If a person is in shock, it is helpful if you
    A. Have the person sit in a chair
    B. Keep the person cool by removing some of the clothing
    C. Stay calm; this helps the person feel more secure
    D. Give the person something to drink or eat

40. Anaphylactic shock occurs because of
    A. Hemorrhage
    B. An allergy to foods, insects, chemicals, or drugs
    C. Sudden cardiac arrest
    D. Seizures

41. If you suspect a person has had a stroke, you should
    A. Position the person in a chair
    B. Begin CPR immediately
    C. Activate the EMS system at once
    D. Take vital signs and report to the nurse

42. If a person has a seizure, you should
    A. Place an object between the teeth
    B. Distract the person to stop the seizure
    C. Position the person in bed
    D. Move furniture, equipment, and sharp objects away from the person

43. If you are assisting a person with burns
    A. Remove burned clothing
    B. Cover the burn wounds with a sterile or clean, cool, moist covering
    C. Give the person plenty of fluids
    D. Apply oils or ointments to the burns

Fill in the Blank

44. Write out the abbreviations.
    A. AED _____
    B. AHA _____
    C. BLS _____
    D. CPR _____
    E. EMS _____
    F. MET _____
    G. RRT _____
    H. SCA _____
    I. VF; V-fib _____

45. If you activate the EMS system, what information should you give to the operator?
    A. _____
    B. _____
    C. _____
    D. _____
    E. _____
    F. _____

46. Chain of Survival actions in the hospital are
    A. _____
    B. _____
    C. _____
    D. _____
    E. _____

47. The 3 major signs of sudden cardiac arrest (SCA) are
    A. _____
    B. _____
    C. _____

48. Rescue breaths are given when there is a _____ but no _____. To give rescue breaths
    A. _____
    B. _____
    C. _____
    D. _____
    E. _____

49. To find the carotid pulse, place _____. Slide your fingers down _____

50. When doing chest compressions, the AHA recommends that you
    A. _____
    B. _____

51. When performing the head tilt–chin lift maneuver, explain how you tilt the head and lift the chin.
    A. Place the palm _____
    B. Tilt _____
    C. Place the fingers _____
    D. Lift _____
    E. Do not close _____

52. When you perform mouth-to-mouth breathing, it is likely you will have contact with _____

53. A bag valve mask is a _____ device. It is squeezed to give _____. It can be connected to an _____

54. Mouth-to-nose breathing is used when
    A. _____
    B. _____
    C. _____
    D. _____
    E. _____

55. When performing CPR, a cycle of _____ compressions is followed by _____ rescue breaths.

56. When defibrillation is used, the AHA recommends that rescuers
    A. Use _____
    B. Minimize _____
    C. Give _____
    D. Check _____

57. When giving CPR to an infant when you are alone, you should
    A. Check _____ and _____ at the same time.
    B. Start CPR if the infant's pulse rate is _____
    C. Give compressions at a rate of _____
    D. Release pressure and allow _____.

58. For children, CPR rules for the following are
    A. Start CPR if the child's heart rate is _____
    B. Give chest compressions with enough pressure to _____
    C. When you give breath, you should see _____

59. After calling the Poison Control Center, what emergency measures should be done when poison is
    A. In the eyes _____
    B. On the skin _____
    C. Inhaled _____
    D. Swallowed _____

60. If firm pressure over the bleeding site does not stop hemorrhage, wrap an _____.

61. Common causes of fainting are
    A. _____
    B. _____
    C. _____
    D. _____

62. Signs and symptoms of shock include
    A. _____
    B. _____
    C. _____
    D. _____
    E. _____
    F. _____
    G. _____
    H. _____

63. Anaphylaxis is an emergency because the reaction occurs within _____

64. Penicillin causes _____ shock in many people.

65. Signs of a stroke include sudden
    A. _____
    B. _____
    C. _____
    D. _____
    E. _____

66. Describe the 2 phases of a generalized tonic-clonic seizure.
    A. Tonic phase _____
    _____
    B. Clonic phase _____

67. The following relate to the emergency care of a person having a seizure.
    A. How do you protect the person's head? _____
    B. How is the person positioned? _____
    C. Why is furniture moved? _____
    D. What 2 times are noted? _____

68. If a person has a concussion, what symptoms may occur related to
    A. Thinking _____
    B. Physical function _____
    C. Mood _____
    D. Sleep _____

69. Repeated concussions can cause chronic problems, such as problems with
    A. _____
    B. _____
    C. _____
    D. _____

70. Partial thickness burns involve the _____. These burns are very painful because _____.

71. Full thickness burns involve _____.

72. When giving emergency care for a burn, apply _____ until pain is relieved. Do not put _____ on burns.

Use the FOCUS ON PRIDE section to complete these statements.

73. You demonstrate professional responsibility when you take a _____ course that you can use to save a life.

74. If a person has an emergency in a public place, you protect the person's right to privacy when you do what you can to _____.

75. When an emergency happens, it is good ethics when you keep the person's _____.

Optional Learning Exercises

You are visiting a neighbor and she is washing dishes. As she washes a glass, it shatters and she has a deep cut on her wrist. Answer the following questions about how you would respond.

76. Your neighbor is crying and walking around the room. What is the best thing you can do to help her?

    _____

    _____

77. Clean rubber gloves are lying on the counter. How can they be useful to you? _____

    _____

    _____

78. What materials in the home could be used to place over the wound? _____

    _____

79. Your neighbor is restless and has a rapid and weak pulse. You notice her skin is cold, moist, and pale. These signs indicate she may be in _____.

80. Her wound is still bleeding and she loses consciousness. What should you do before you continue to give first aid? _____

55 End-of-Life Care

Fill in the Blank: Key Terms

Advance directive   End-of-life care   Post-mortem care   Rigor mortis
Autopsy   Palliative care   Reincarnation   Terminal illness

1. The support and care given during the time surrounding death is _____.

2. The stiffness or rigidity of skeletal muscles that occurs after death is _____.

3. An _____ is a document stating a person's wishes about health care when that person cannot make his or her own decisions.

4. Care of the body after death is _____.

5. An illness or injury for which there is no reasonable expectation of recovery is a _____.

6. _____ is the belief that the spirit or soul is reborn in another human body or in another form of life.

7. The examination of the body after death is an

_____.

8. _____ is care that involves relieving or reducing the intensity of uncomfortable symptoms without producing a cure.

Circle the Best Answer

9. When a person has a terminal illness
   A. The doctor is able to accurately predict when the person will die
   B. Modern medicine can cure the disease
   C. He or she may live longer than expected because of a strong will to live
   D. He or she will die when expected

10. When palliative care is done
    A. The person has an acute illness that can be cured
    B. The focus is on relieving symptoms
    C. Life-saving measures will be taken to prolong life
    D. The person always remains at home

11. Hospice care
    A. Is available only when the person remains at home
    B. Is used when the person is receiving rehabilitation therapy after an illness
    C. Stresses pain relief and comfort
    D. Is given until the person recovers from the illness

12. Practices and attitudes among people from India include
    A. Placing small pillows under the body's neck, feet, and wrists
    B. Wearing white clothing for mourning
    C. Needing a time and place for prayer for the family and the person
    D. Having an aversion to death

13. Children between ages 2 and 6 years may see death as
    A. Final
    B. Punishment for being bad
    C. Suffering and pain
    D. A reunion with those who have died

14. Older persons see death as
    A. A temporary state
    B. Freedom from pain, suffering, and disability
    C. Something that happens to other people
    D. Something that affects plans, hopes, dreams, and ambitions

15. In which stage of dying does the person make promises and make "just one more" request?
    A. Acceptance   C. Depression
    B. Anger   D. Bargaining

16. If a dying person begins to talk about worries and concerns, you should
    A. Call a spiritual leader
    B. Tell the nurse
    C. Listen quietly and use touch
    D. Change the subject to more pleasant topics

17. Care given when a person is dying should be done
    A. Only if the person requests it
    B. To promote physical and psychological comfort
    C. Often, to keep the person active
    D. Only while the person is conscious

18. Because vision fails as death approaches, you should
    A. Explain what you are doing to the person when you are in the room
    B. Have the room lit very brightly
    C. Turn off all lights
    D. Keep the eyes covered at all times

19. Hearing is one of the last functions lost, so it is important to
    A. Ask the person questions while giving care
    B. Talk in a loud voice so the person can hear you
    C. Provide re-assurance and explanations about care
    D. Ask the family to be quiet so they do not disturb the person

20. As death nears, oral hygiene is
    A. Given routinely
    B. More frequent when taking oral fluids is difficult
    C. Very infrequent to avoid disturbing the person
    D. Never given because the person cannot swallow

21. Which of these does *not* occur as death nears?
    A. Body temperature rises.
    B. The skin is cool, pale, and mottled.
    C. Sweating decreases.
    D. Circulation fails.

22. Because of breathing difficulties, the dying person is generally more comfortable in
    A. The supine position
    B. Trendelenburg's position
    C. A prone position
    D. A semi-Fowler's position

23. When a person is dying, you can help the family by
    A. Allowing family members to stay as long as they wish
    B. Staying away from the room and delaying giving care
    C. Telling family members that they need to leave so you can give care
    D. Telling family members that the person dying is not in pain

24. If a person has a living will, it may instruct doctors
    A. Not to start measures that will save the person's life
    B. To start CPR whenever necessary
    C. Not to start measures that prolong dying
    D. Never to activate the EMS system for a person

25. If the doctor writes a "Do Not Resuscitate" (DNR) order, it means that
    A. The person will not be resuscitated
    B. The person will be resuscitated if it is an emergency
    C. The doctor will decide whether or not to resuscitate
    D. The RN may decide that in a particular situation resuscitation is needed

26. A sign that death is near would be
    A. Deep, rapid respirations
    B. Body temperature increases
    C. Muscles tense and contract in spasms
    D. Peristalsis increases

27. When the family wishes to see the body after death, it should
    A. Remain exactly as the person was at death
    B. Be positioned to appear comfortable and natural
    C. Be completely uncovered
    D. Be placed in a semi-Fowler's position

28. When you are assisting with post-mortem care, you should
    A. Place the body in good alignment in side-lying position without pillows
    B. Tape all jewelry in place
    C. Gently pull eyelids over the eyes
    D. Dress the person in his or her regular clothing

29. An ID tag is attached to the big toe or
    A. Wrist   C. Upper arm
    B. Ankle   D. Upper leg

30. A Dying Person's Bill of Last Rights includes all of these *except*
    A. The right to be in denial
    B. The right to touch and be touched
    C. The right to participate in resident and family groups
    D. The right to be angry and sad

Fill in the Blank

31. Write out the abbreviations.
    A. DNR _____
    B. ID _____
    C. OBRA _____

32. It is important to examine your own feelings about death because they will affect _____.

33. When you understand the dying process, you can approach the dying person with _____ _____.

34. Hospice care focuses on these needs of the dying person and families.
    A. _____
    B. _____
    C. _____
    D. _____

35. Religious beliefs strengthen when dying and often provide _____ _____

36. Adults fear death because they fear
    A. _____ and _____
    B. Dying _____
    C. Invasion _____
    D. _____ and _____ from loved ones
    E. _____ and _____ of those left behind

37. Name the 5 stages of dying.
    A. _____
    B. _____
    C. _____
    D. _____
    E. _____

38. The goals of comfort needs are
    A. _____
    B. _____

39. When caring for a dying person, do not ask questions that need long answers because _____.

40. Because crusting and irritation of the nostrils can occur, you should _____ _____

41. What kinds of elimination problems can occur in the dying person?
    A. _____ and _____ incontinence
    B. _____
    C. _____ retention

42. The Patient Self-Determination Act and OBRA give 2 rights that affect the rights of a dying person. They are

    A. _____

    B. _____

43. A living will instructs doctors

    A. _____

    B. _____

44. When a person cannot make health care decisions, the authority to do so is given to the person with

    _____.

45. What are the signs that death is near?

    A. _____

    B. _____

    C. _____

    D. _____

    E. _____

    F. _____

46. The signs of death include no _____ _____. The pupils are _____ and _____.

47. When assisting with post-mortem care, you need this information from the nurse.

    A. _____

    B. _____

    C. _____

    D. _____

    E. _____

48. A Dying Patient's Bill of Last Rights give the person the right to

    A. _____

    B. _____

    C. _____

    D. _____

    E. _____

    F. _____

    G. _____

    H. _____

    I. _____

Use the FOCUS ON PRIDE section to complete these statements.

49. You are giving quality care to a dying person when you

    A. _____

    B. _____

    C. _____

    D. _____

50. According to OBRA, the right to confidentiality before and after death means that

    _____.

51. When a dying person refuses treatment, the health team must respect these choices because of the person's right to _____.

Optional Learning Exercises

You are assigned to care for Mrs. Adams, who is dying. Answer the questions regarding this situation.

52. You find Mrs. Adams crying in her room. When you ask her what is wrong, she tells you no one gave her fresh water this morning and she has not had her bath yet. She tells you just to go away. What stage of dying is she displaying? _____

53. Later in the day, Mrs. Adams tells you she can't wait until she is better to go home and plant her garden. She states that she knows the tests done last week were wrong and she will recover quickly from her illness. Now what stage is she displaying? _____. Why is she displaying 2 different stages so rapidly? _____

54. A minister comes to visit Mrs. Adams while you are giving care. What should you do?

    _____

55. You are working one night and find Mrs. Adams awake during the night. She asks you to sit with her. She begins to talk about her fears, worries, and anxieties. What are 2 things you can do to convey caring to her? _____

56. As Mrs. Adams becomes weaker, a family member is always at her bedside. When the family member asks to assist with her care, you know that this is acceptable because _____

57. Mrs. Adams dies while you are working and the nurse asks you to assist with post-mortem care. As you clean soiled areas, you assist the nurse to turn the body and air is expelled. This occurs because

    _____

58. You wear gloves during post-mortem care to protect you from _____.

Fill in the Blank: Key Terms

Job application
Job interview

1. When an employer asks a job applicant questions about his or her education and career, it is a

   _____.

2. An agency's official form listing questions that require factual answers is a

   _____.

Circle the Best Answer

3. Displaying good work ethics at your clinical experience site may help you find a job because
   A. You will pass the course
   B. It will show you care
   C. You will get better grades
   D. The staff always looks at students as future employees

4. You should be well-groomed when looking for a job because it
   A. Shows you are cooperative
   B. Makes a good first impression
   C. Shows you are respectful
   D. Shows you have values and attitudes that fit with the center

5. How does an employer know you can perform required job skills?
   A. They request proof of successful NATCEP completion and check the state nursing assistant registry.
   B. They will have you give a demonstration of your skills.
   C. You will be asked many questions about performing certain skills.
   D. You will be required to take a written test.

6. Which of these is not an OBRA requirement to work in long-term care?
   A. You must complete a state-approved training and competency evaluation program.
   B. You must have 3 references from former employers.
   C. The employer checks your record in the state nursing assistant registry.
   D. The nursing center cannot hire persons who were convicted of abusing, neglecting, or mistreating a person.

7. You get a job application from
   A. The personnel office or the human resources office
   B. A friend who works at the center
   C. The director of nursing
   D. The receptionist in the lobby of the center

8. You should take a dry run to a job interview to
   A. Show you follow directions well
   B. Show you listen well
   C. Know how long it takes to get from your home to the personnel office
   D. Look over the center to see if you want to work there

9. When you are interviewing, it is correct to
   A. Have a glass of wine before going
   B. Look directly at the interviewer
   C. Wear a sweatsuit and athletic shoes
   D. Shake hands very gently

10. What is a good way to share your list of skills with the interviewer?
    A. Tell the person verbally what you can do.
    B. Ask for a list of skills and check the ones you know.
    C. Prepare a list of your skills and give it to the interviewer.
    D. Tell the interviewer you will send a list as soon as possible.

11. It is important for you to ask questions at the end of the interview because it
    A. Will show the interviewer you are interested in the job
    B. Will help you to decide if the job is right for you
    C. Shows you have good communication skills
    D. Shows you are dependable

12. After an interview, it is advised that you
    A. Send a thank you note within 24 hours of the interview
    B. Call the interviewer every day to see if you are being hired
    C. Wait for the employer to contact you
    D. Call one week after the interview to thank the person for the interview

Fill in the Blank

13. Write out the abbreviations.
    A. EEOC _____
    B. NATCEP _____
    C. OBRA _____

14. List 9 places you can find out about jobs.
    A. _____
    B. _____
    C. _____
    D. _____
    E. _____
    F. _____
    G. _____
    H. _____
    I. _____

15. When an employer requests proof of successful NATCEP completion, give the person these items.

    A. _____

    B. _____

    C. _____

16. If a job application asks you to print in black ink, why is it a poor idea to use blue ink? _____

    _____

    _____

17. Your writing on a job application should be readable so the agency can _____

    _____

18. When a section on a job application does not apply to you, you should _____

    _____

19. When you provide information about employment gaps, it gives the employer a good impression about your _____

20. If you lie on a job application, it is _____.

    If you do this, what can happen? _____

    _____

21. Be prepared to provide these when completing a job application.

    A. _____

    B. _____

    C. _____

    D. _____

22. When you fill out a job application, it is easier to complete if you have a file that contains

    A. _____

    B. _____

    C. _____

    D. _____

    E. _____

    F. _____

    G. _____

    H. _____

    I. _____

    J. _____

23. You should ask questions at the end of an interview because the agency wants to hire someone who

    _____

Use the FOCUS ON PRIDE section to complete these statements.

24. When you ask questions during the interview, it helps you decide if the agency is _____.

    This shows _____

    and _____ responsibility.

25. EEOC limits the questions employers may ask. Appropriate questions they may ask include

    A. _____

    B. _____

    C. _____

26. Even if you have never worked in health care, other work experience gives employers information about your _____,

    _____, and

    _____

Optional Learning Experiences

Applying for a Job in Home Care

27. When the RN is not at the bedside to help you if problems occur, you are expected to be able to

    _____

28. When you arrive at homes on time, you are using

    _____.

    What temptations should be avoided when you are giving home care? _____

    _____

29. When you shop for a person, you should accurately report to the person or family _____

    _____. When you do these things, you are displaying your

    _____

30. You should read the manufacturer's instructions before using any appliance. This shows _____ for the person's property.

31. What questions should you ask if you are interviewing for a job in home care?

    A. _____

    B. _____

    C. _____

    D. _____

    E. _____

    F. _____

Relieving Choking—Adult or Child (Over 1 Year of Age)

Name: _____ Date: _____

Procedure	S	U	Comments
1. Asked the person if he or she was choking. Helped the person if he or she nodded "yes" and could not talk.	_____	_____	_____
2. Had someone call for help.			
a. *In a public area,* had someone activate the EMS system by calling 911. Sent someone to get an automated external defibrillator (AED).	_____	_____	_____
b. *In an agency,* had someone call the Rapid Response Team (RRT) and sent someone to get the defibrillator (AED).	_____	_____	_____
3. Gave abdominal thrusts.			
a. *If the person was standing or sitting:*			
1) Stood or knelt behind the person.	_____	_____	_____
2) Wrapped your arms around the person's waist.	_____	_____	_____
3) Made fist with 1 hand.	_____	_____	_____
4) Placed the thumb side of the fist against the abdomen. The fist was slightly above the navel in the middle of the abdomen and well below the end of the sternum (breastbone).	_____	_____	_____
5) Grasped the fist with your other hand.	_____	_____	_____
6) Pressed your fist into the person's abdomen with a quick, upward thrust.	_____	_____	_____
b. *If the person was lying down but responsive:*			
1) Straddled the person's thighs.	_____	_____	_____
2) Placed the heel of 1 hand against the abdomen. It was in the middle slightly above the navel and well below the end of the sternum (breastbone).	_____	_____	_____
3) Placed your second hand on top of your first hand.	_____	_____	_____
4) Pressed both hands into the abdomen with a quick, upward thrust.	_____	_____	_____
4. Repeated thrusts until the object was expelled or the person became unresponsive.	_____	_____	_____
5. *If the object was dislodged,* encouraged the person to go to the hospital. Injuries could occur from abdominal thrusts.	_____	_____	_____
6. *If the person became unresponsive,* lowered the person to the floor or ground. Positioned the person supine (lying flat on the back). Made sure the Emergency Medical Services (EMS) or RRT was called. If alone, provided 5 cycles (2 minutes) of cardiopulmonary respiration (CPR) first. Then called the EMS or RRT.	_____	_____	_____
7. Started CPR.			
a. Did not check for a pulse. Began with compressions. Gave 30 compressions. Chest compressions helped dislodge an obstruction.	_____	_____	_____
b. Used the head tilt–chin lift method to open the airway. Opened the person's mouth. The mouth was wide open. Looked for an object. Removed the object if you saw it and removed it easily. Used your fingers.	_____	_____	_____
c. Gave 2 breaths.	_____	_____	_____
d. Continued cycles of 30 compressions and 2 breaths. Looked for an object every time you opened the airway for rescue breaths.	_____	_____	_____

Date of Satisfactory Completion _____ Instructor's Initials _____

Procedure—cont'd	S	U	Comments

8. *If you relieved choking in an unresponsive person:*
   a. Checked for a response, breathing, and a pulse.
      1) *If no response, no normal breathing, and no pulse*—continued CPR. Attached an AED. _____ _____ _____
      2) *If no response and no normal breathing but there was a pulse*—gave rescue breaths. For an adult, gave 1 breath every 5 to 6 seconds (12 to 20 breaths per minute). Checked for a pulse every 2 minutes. If no pulse, began CPR. _____ _____ _____
      3) *If the person had normal breathing and a pulse*—placed the person in the recovery position if there was no response. Continued to check the person until help arrived. Encouraged the person to go to the hospital if the person responded. _____ _____ _____

Date of Satisfactory Completion _____   Instructor's Initials _____

Relieving Choking—In the Infant (Less Than 1 Year of Age)

Name: _____   Date: _____

Procedure	S	U	Comments

Procedure

1. Had someone call for help.
   a. *In a public area,* had someone activate the Emergency Medical Services (EMS) systems by calling 911. Sent someone to get an automated external defibrillator (AED).
   b. *In an agency,* had someone call the agency's Rapid Response Team (RRT) and got a defibrillator (AED).
2. Knelt next to the infant. Or sat with the infant in your lap.
3. Exposed the infant's chest and back. Performed this step only if it was done easily.
4. Held the infant face down over your forearm. (Supported your arm on your thigh or lap.) The infant's head was lower than the chest. Supported the head and jaw with your hand.
5. Gave up to 5 forceful back slaps (back blows). Used the heel of your hand. Gave the back slaps between the shoulder blades. (Stopped the back slaps if the object was expelled.)
6. Turned the infant as a unit.
   a. Continued to support the infant's face, jaw, head, neck, and chest with 1 hand.
   b. Supported the back and the back of the infant's head with your other hand. Your palm supported the back of the head.
   c. Turned the infant as a unit. The infant was in a back-lying position on your forearm. Your forearm rested on your thigh. The infant's head was lower than the chest.
7. Gave up to 5 chest thrusts. The chest thrusts were quick and downward.
   a. Placed two fingers in the center of the chest just below the nipple line.
   b. Gave chest thrusts at a rate of about 1 every second.
   c. Stopped chest thrusts if the object was expelled.
8. Continued giving 5 back slaps followed by 5 chest thrusts until:
   a. The object was expelled.
   b. The infant became unresponsive.
9. *If the infant became unresponsive:*
   a. Sent someone to activate the EMS system or RRT if not already done. If alone, did so after 2 minutes of cardiopulmonary resuscitation (CPR).
   b. Placed the infant on a firm, flat surface.
   c. Started CPR. Began with compressions. Gave 30 compressions.
   d. Opened the airway. Used the head tilt–chin lift method. Opened the infant's mouth. Looked for an object. Removed the object if you saw it and could remove it easily. Used your fingers.
   e. Gave 2 breaths.
   f. Continued cycles of 30 compressions and 2 breaths. Looked for an object. Removed the object if you saw it and could remove it easily. Used your fingers.
   g. Continued CPR until help arrived or until choking was relieved.

Date of Satisfactory Completion _____   Instructor's Initials _____

Using a Fire Extinguisher

Name: _____   Date: _____

Procedure	S	U	Comments
1. Pulled the fire alarm.	___	___	_____
2. Got the nearest fire extinguisher.	___	___	_____
3. Carried it upright.	___	___	_____
4. Took it to the fire.	___	___	_____
5. Followed the word *PASS*.			
a. *P*—for *pull the safety pin*. This unlocked the handle.	___	___	_____
b. *A*—for *aim low*. Directed the hose or nozzle at the base of the fire. Did not try to spray the tops of the flames.	___	___	_____
c. *S*—for *squeeze the lever*. Squeezed or pushed down on the lever, handle, or button to start the stream. Released the lever, handle, or button to stop the stream.	___	___	_____
d. *S*—for *sweep back and forth*. Swept the stream back and forth (side to side) at the base of the fire.	___	___	_____

Date of Satisfactory Completion _____   Instructor's Initials _____

Using a Transfer/Gait Belt

Name: _____   Date: _____

Procedure	S	U	Comments

Quality of Life
- Knocked before entering the person's room.
- Addressed the person by name.
- Explained the procedure before starting and during the procedure.
- Handled the person gently during the procedure.

Pre-Procedure
1. Saw *Promoting Safety and Comfort: Transfer/Gait Belts.*
2. Practiced hand hygiene.
3. Obtained a transfer/gait belt of the correct type and size.
4. Identified the person. Checked the identification (ID) bracelet against the assignment sheet. Used 2 identifiers. Also called the person by name.
5. Provided for privacy.

Procedure
6. Assisted the person to sitting position.
7. Applied the belt. Held the belt by the buckle. Wrapped the belt around the person's waist. Applied the belt over clothing. Did not apply it over bare skin.
   a. *For a belt with a metal buckle:*
      1) Inserted the belt's metal tip into the buckle. Passed the belt through the side with the teeth first.
      2) Brought the belt tip across the front of the buckle. Inserted the tip through the buckle's smooth side.
   b. *For a belt with a quick-release buckle,* pushed the belt ends together to secure the buckle.
8. Tightened the belt so it was snug. It did not cause discomfort or impair breathing. You were able to slide your open, flat hand under the belt. Asked the person about his or her comfort.
9. Made sure that a woman's breasts were not caught under the belt.
10. Placed the buckle off-center in the front or off-center in the back for the person's comfort. A quick-release buckle was turned around to the person's back out of his or her reach. The buckle was not over the spine.
11. Tucked any excess strap into the belt.
12. Completed the transfer or ambulation procedure. Grasped the belt from underneath with 2 hands. Or grasped the belt by the handles.

Post-Procedure
13. Removed the belt after completing the transfer or ambulation. The person was not left alone wearing the belt.
    a. *For a belt with a metal buckle:*
       1) Brought the belt strap back through the buckle's smooth side.
       2) Pulled the belt through the side with the teeth.
    b. *For a belt with a quick-release buckle,* pushed inward on the quick-release buttons.
    c. Removed the belt from the person's waist. Avoided dragging the belt across the waist.
14. Provided for comfort.
15. Placed the call light and other needed items within reach.

Date of Satisfactory Completion _____   Instructor's Initials _____

Post-Procedure—cont'd

	S	U	Comments
16. Unscreened the person.	___	___	_____
17. Completed a safety check of the room.	___	___	_____
18. Returned the transfer/gait belt to its proper place.	___	___	_____
19. Practiced hand hygiene.	___	___	_____
20. Reported and recorded your observations.	___	___	_____

Date of Satisfactory Completion _____   Instructor's Initials _____

Helping the Falling Person

Name: _____   Date: _____

Procedure	S	U	Comments
1. Stood behind the person with your feet apart. Kept your back straight.	___	___	_____
2. Brought the person close to your body as fast as possible. Used the transfer/gait belt. Or wrapped your arms around the person's waist. If necessary, you held the person under the arms.	___	___	_____
3. Moved your leg so the person's buttocks rested on it. Moved the leg near the person.	___	___	_____
4. Lowered the person to the floor. The person slid down your leg to the floor. Bent at your hips and knees as you lowered the person.	___	___	_____
5. Called a nurse to check the person. Stayed with the person.	___	___	_____
6. Helped the nurse return the person to bed. Asked other staff to help, if needed.	___	___	_____

Post-Procedure

	S	U	Comments
7. Provided for comfort.	___	___	_____
8. Placed the call light and other needed items within reach.	___	___	_____
9. Raised or lowered bed rails. Followed the care plan.	___	___	_____
10. Completed a safety check of the room.	___	___	_____
11. Practiced hand hygiene.	___	___	_____
12. Reported and recorded the following:			
• How the fall occurred	___	___	_____
• How far the person walked	___	___	_____
• How activity was tolerated before the fall	___	___	_____
• Complaints before the fall	___	___	_____
• How much help the person needed while walking	___	___	_____
13. Completed an incident report.	___	___	_____

Date of Satisfactory Completion _____   Instructor's Initials _____

Applying Restraints

VIDEO   **VIDEO CLIP**

Name: _____   Date: _____

Procedure	S	U	Comments

Quality of Life
- Knocked before entering the person's room.
- Addressed the person by name.
- Introduced yourself by name and title.
- Explained the procedure before starting and during the procedure.
- Protected the person's rights during the procedure.
- Handled the person gently during the procedure.

Pre-Procedure
1. Followed *Delegation Guidelines: Applying Restraints.* Saw *Promoting Safety and Comfort: Applying Restraints.*
2. Collected the following as instructed by the nurse.
   - Correct type and size of restraint
   - Padding for skin and bony areas
   - Bed rail pads or gap protectors (if needed)
3. Practiced hand hygiene.
4. Identified the person. Checked the ID (identification) bracelet against the assignment sheet. Used 2 identifiers. Also called the person by name.
5. Provided for privacy.

Procedure
6. Positioned the person for comfort and good alignment.
7. Placed the bed rail pads or gap protectors (if needed) on the bed if the person was in bed. Followed the manufacturer's instructions.
8. Padded bony areas. Followed the nurse's instructions and the care plan.
9. Read the manufacturer's instructions. Noted the front and back of the restraint.
10. *For wrist restraints:*
    a. Applied the restraint following the manufacturer's instructions. Placed the soft or foam part toward the skin.
    b. Secured the restraint so it was snug but not tight. Made sure you could slide 1 finger under the restraint. Followed the manufacturer's instructions. Adjusted the straps if the restraint was too loose or too tight. Checked for snugness again.
    c. Secured the straps to the movable part of the bed frame out of the person's reach. Used the buckle or quick-release tie.
    d. Repeated the following for the other wrist.
       1) Applied the restraint following the manufacturer's instructions. Placed the soft or foam part toward the skin.
       2) Secured the restraint so it was snug but not tight. Made sure you could slide 1 finger under the restraint. Followed the manufacturer's instructions. Adjusted the straps if the restraint was too loose or too tight. Checked for snugness again.
       3) Secured the straps to the movable part of the bed frame out of the person's reach. Used the buckle or quick-release tie.
11. *For mitt restraints:*
    a. Cleaned and dried the person's hands.
    b. Inserted the person's hand into the restraint with the palm down. Followed the manufacturer's instructions.

Date of Satisfactory Completion _____   Instructor's Initials _____

Procedure—cont'd   S   U   **Comments**

    c. Wrapped the wrist strap around the smallest part of the wrist. Secured the strap with the hook-and-loop closure.   ____ ____ _____

    d. Secured the restraint to the bed if directed to do so. Secured the straps to the movable part of the bed frame out of the person's reach. Used the buckle or a quick-release tie.   ____ ____ _____

    e. Checked for snugness. Slid 1 finger between the restraint and the wrist. Followed the manufacturer's instructions. Adjusted the straps if the restraint was too loose or too tight. Checked for snugness again. ____ ____ _____

    f. Repeated the following for the other hand.

      1) Inserted the person's hand into the restraint with the palm down. Followed the manufacturer's instructions. ____ ____ _____

      2) Wrapped the wrist strap around the smallest part of the wrist. Secured the strap with the hook-and-loop closure. ____ ____ _____

      3) Secured the restraint to the bed if directed to do so. Secured the straps to the movable part of the bed frame out of the person's reach. Used the buckle or a quick-release tie. ____ ____ _____

      4) Checked for snugness. Slid 1 finger between the restraint and the wrist. Followed the manufacturer's instructions. Adjusted the straps if the restraint was too loose or too tight. ____ ____ _____

12. *For a belt restraint:*

    a. Assisted the person to a sitting position. ____ ____ _____

    b. Applied the restraint. Followed the manufacturer's instructions. ____ ____ _____

    c. Removed wrinkles or creases from the front and back of the restraint. ____ ____ _____

    d. Brought the ties through the slots in the back. ____ ____ _____

    e. Positioned the straps at a 45-degree angle between the wheelchair seat and sides. If in bed, helped the person lie down. ____ ____ _____

    f. Made sure the person was comfortable and in good alignment. ____ ____ _____

    g. Secured the straps to the movable part of the bed frame. Used the buckle or a quick-release tie. The buckle or tie was out of the person's reach. For a wheelchair, criss-crossed and secured the straps. ____ ____ _____

    h. Checked for snugness. Slid an open hand between the restraint and the person. Adjusted the restraint if it was too loose or too tight. Checked for snugness again. ____ ____ _____

13. *For a vest restraint:*

    a. Assisted the person to a sitting position. If in a wheelchair:

      1) Positioned him or her as far back in the wheelchair as possible.

      2) Made sure the buttocks were against the chair back. ____ ____ _____

    b. Applied the restraint. Followed the manufacturer's instructions. The "V" part of the vest crossed in front. ____ ____ _____

    c. Brought the straps through the slots. ____ ____ _____

    d. Removed wrinkles in the front and back. ____ ____ _____

    e. Positioned the straps at a 45-degree angle between the wheelchair seat and sides. If in bed, helped the person lie down. ____ ____ _____

    f. Made sure the person was comfortable and in good alignment. ____ ____ _____

    g. Secured the straps to the movable part of the bed frame at waist level. Used the buckle or a quick-release tie. The buckle or tie was out of the person's reach. For a wheelchair, criss-crossed and secured the straps. ____ ____ _____

    h. Checked for snugness. Slid an open hand between the restraint and the person. Adjusted the restraint if it was too loose or too tight. Checked for snugness again. ____ ____ _____

Date of Satisfactory Completion _____   Instructor's Initials _____

Procedure—cont'd	S	U	Comments

14. *For a jacket restraint:*

a. Assisted the person to a sitting position. If in a wheelchair:

   1) Positioned him or her as far back in the wheelchair as possible. ___ ___ _____

   2) Made sure the buttocks were against the chair back. ___ ___ _____

b. Applied the restraint. Followed the manufacturer's instructions. The jacket opening went in the back. ___ ___ _____

c. Closed the back with the zipper, ties, or hook-and-loop closures. ___ ___ _____

d. Made sure the side seams were under the arms. Removed wrinkles in the front and back. ___ ___ _____

e. Positioned the straps at a 45-degree angle between the wheelchair seat and sides. If in bed, helped the person lie down. ___ ___ _____

f. Made sure the person was comfortable and in good alignment. ___ ___ _____

g. Secured the straps to the movable part of the bed frame at waist level. Used the buckle or quick-release tie. The buckle or tie was out of the person's reach. For a wheelchair, criss-crossed and secured the straps. ___ ___ _____

h. Checked for snugness. Slid an open hand between the restraint and the person. Adjusted the restraint if it was too loose or too tight. Checked for snugness again. ___ ___ _____

15. *For elbow restraints:*

a. Released the adjustment straps (hook-and-loop). ___ ___ _____

b. Wrapped a splint over 1 arm. The splint was centered over the elbow. ___ ___ _____

c. Secured the hook fastener to the quilted material. If necessary to hold the splint in place, pinned the splint to the person's clothing at the top and bottom of the splint. ___ ___ _____

d. Checked for snugness. Slid 2 fingers between the splint and the person's arm. Adjusted the splint if it was too loose or too tight. Checked for snugness again. ___ ___ _____

e. Repeated for the other arm:

   1) Released the adjustment straps (hook-and-loop). ___ ___ _____

   2) Wrapped a splint over 1 arm. The splint was centered over the elbow. ___ ___ _____

   3) Secured the hook fastener to the quilted material. If necessary to hold the splint in place, pinned the splint to the person's clothing at the top and bottom of the splint. ___ ___ _____

   4) Checked for snugness. Slid 2 fingers between the splint and the person's arm. Adjusted the splint if it was too loose or too tight. Checked for snugness again. ___ ___ _____

Post-Procedure

16. Positioned the person as the nurse directed. ___ ___ _____

17. Provided for comfort. ___ ___ _____

18. Placed the call light and other need items within the person's reach. ___ ___ _____

19. Raised or lowered bed rails. Followed the care plan and the manufacturer's instructions for restraints. ___ ___ _____

20. Unscreened the person. ___ ___ _____

21. Completed a safety check of the room. ___ ___ _____

22. Practiced hand hygiene. ___ ___ _____

Date of Satisfactory Completion _____   Instructor's Initials _____

Post-Procedure—cont'd   S   U   **Comments**

23. Checked the person and the restraint at least every 15 minutes or
    as often as directed by the nurse and the care plan. Reported and
    recorded your observations.
    a. *For wrist or mitt restraints or elbow splints:* checked the pulse,
       color, and temperature of restrained parts.   _____   _____   _____
    b. *For vest, jacket, or belt restraint:* checked the person's breathing.
       *Called for the nurse at once if the person was not breathing or was
       having problems breathing.* Made sure the restraint was properly
       positioned in the front and back.   _____   _____   _____
24. Did the following at least every 2 hours for at least 10 minutes.
    a. Removed or released the restraint.   _____   _____   _____
    b. Measured vital signs.   _____   _____   _____
    c. Re-positioned the person.   _____   _____   _____
    d. Met food, fluid, hygiene, and elimination needs.   _____   _____   _____
    e. Gave skin care.   _____   _____   _____
    f. Performed range-of-motion (ROM) exercises or helped the
       person walk. Followed the care plan.   _____   _____   _____
    g. Provided for physical and emotional support.   _____   _____   _____
    h. Re-applied the restraint.   _____   _____   _____
25. Completed a safety check of the room.   _____   _____   _____
26. Practiced hand hygiene.   _____   _____   _____
27. Reported and recorded your observations and the care given.   _____   _____   _____

Date of Satisfactory Completion _____   Instructor's Initials _____

Hand-Washing

Name: _____   Date: _____

Procedure	S	U	Comments
1. Saw *Promoting Safety and Comfort: Hand Hygiene.*	____	____	_____
2. Made sure you had soap, paper towels, an orangewood stick or nail file, and a wastebasket. Collected missing items.	____	____	_____
3. Pushed your watch up your arm 4 to 5 inches. Pushed long uniform sleeves up too.	____	____	_____
4. Stood away from the sink so your clothes did not touch the sink. Stood so the soap and faucet were easy to reach.	____	____	_____
5. Turned on and adjusted the water until it felt warm.	____	____	_____
6. Wet your wrists and hands. Kept your hands lower than your elbows. Was sure to wet the area 3 to 4 inches above your wrists.	____	____	_____
7. Applied about 1 teaspoon of soap to your hands.	____	____	_____
8. Rubbed your palms together and interlaced your fingers to work up a good lather. Lathered your wrists, hands, and fingers. Kept your hands lower than your elbows. This step should have lasted at least 15 to 20 seconds.	____	____	_____
9. Washed each hand and wrist thoroughly. Cleaned the back of your fingers and between your fingers.	____	____	_____
10. Cleaned under the fingernails. Rubbed your fingernails against your palms.	____	____	_____
11. Cleaned under the fingernails with a nail file or orangewood stick. Did this for the first hand-washing of the day and when your hands were highly soiled.	____	____	_____
12. Rinsed your wrists, hands, and fingers well. Water flowed from above the wrists to your fingertips.	____	____	_____
13. Repeated steps 7 through 12, if needed.			
a. Applied about 1 teaspoon of soap to your hands.	____	____	_____
b. Rubbed your palms together and interlaced your fingers to work up a good lather. Lathered your wrists, hands, and fingers. Kept your hands lower than your elbows. This step should have lasted at least 15 to 20 seconds.	____	____	_____
c. Washed each hand and wrist thoroughly. Cleaned the back of your fingers and between your fingers.	____	____	_____
d. Cleaned under the fingernails. Rubbed your fingertips against your palms.	____	____	_____
e. Cleaned under the fingernails with a nail file or orangewood stick. Did this for the first hand-washing of the day and when your hands were highly soiled.	____	____	_____
f. Rinsed your wrists, hands, and fingers well. Water flowed from above the wrists to your fingertips.	____	____	_____
14. Dried your wrists and hands with clean, dry paper towels. Patted dry starting at your fingertips.	____	____	_____
15. Discarded the paper towels into the wastebasket.	____	____	_____
16. Turned off faucets with clean, dry paper towels. This prevented you from contaminating your hands. Used a clean paper towel for each faucet. Or used knee or foot controls to turn off the faucet.	____	____	_____
17. Discarded the paper towels into the wastebasket.	____	____	_____

Date of Satisfactory Completion _____   Instructor's Initials _____

Using an Alcohol-Based Hand Rub

Name: _____   Date: _____

Procedure	S	U	Comments
1. Saw *Promoting Safety and Comfort: Hand Hygiene.*	____	____	_____
2. Applied a palmful of an alcohol-based hand rub into a cupped hand.	____	____	_____
3. Rubbed your palms together.	____	____	_____
4. Rubbed the palm of 1 hand over the back of the other. Did the same for the other hand.	____	____	_____
5. Rubbed your palms together with your fingers interlaced.	____	____	_____
6. Interlocked your fingers. Rubbed your fingers back and forth.	____	____	_____
7. Rubbed the thumb of 1 hand into the palm of the other. Did the same for the other thumb.	____	____	_____
8. Rubbed the fingers of 1 hand into the palm of the other hand. Used a circular motion. Did the same for the fingers of the other hand.	____	____	_____
9. Continued rubbing your hands until they were dry.	____	____	_____

Date of Satisfactory Completion _____   Instructor's Initials _____

Donning and Removing Personal Protective Equipment (PPE)

Name: _____   Date: _____

Procedure	S	U	Comments

Procedure

1. Followed *Delegation Guidelines: Transmission-Based Precautions.*
   Saw *Promoting Safety and Comfort:*
   a. *Transmission-Based Precautions*   ___ ___ _____
   b. *Goggles and Face Shields*   ___ ___ _____
   c. *Gloves*   ___ ___ _____
   d. *Donning and Removing PPE*   ___ ___ _____
2. Removed your watch and all jewelry.   ___ ___ _____
3. Rolled up uniform sleeves.   ___ ___ _____
4. Practiced hand hygiene.   ___ ___ _____
5. Put on a gown.
   a. Held a clean gown out in front of you.   ___ ___ _____
   b. Unfolded the gown. Faced the back of the gown. Did not
      shake it.   ___ ___ _____
   c. Put your hands and arms through the sleeves. ___ ___ _____
   d. Made sure the gown covered you from your neck to your
      knees. It covered your arms to the end of your wrists. ___ ___ _____
   e. Tied the strings at the back of the neck. ___ ___ _____
   f. Overlapped the back of the gown. Made sure it covered your
      uniform. The gown was snug, not loose.   ___ ___ _____
   g. Tied the waist strings. Tied them at the back or the side. Did
      not tie them in front.   ___ ___ _____
6. Put on a mask or respirator.
   a. Picked up a mask by its upper ties. Did not touch the part that
      covered your face.   ___ ___ _____
   b. Placed the mask over your nose and mouth. ___ ___ _____
   c. Placed the upper strings above your ears. Tied them at the
      back in the middle of your head.   ___ ___ _____
   d. Tied the lower strings at the back of your neck. The lower part
      of the mask was under your chin.   ___ ___ _____
   e. Pinched the metal band around your nose. The top of the mask
      was snug over your nose. If you wore eyeglasses, the mask was
      snug under the bottom of the eyeglasses. ___ ___ _____
   f. Made sure the mask was snug over your face and under
      your chin.   ___ ___ _____
7. Put on goggles or a face shield (if needed and was not part of
   the mask).
   a. Placed the device over your face and eyes. Touched only the
      ties or the elastic bands.   ___ ___ _____
   b. Adjusted the device to fit.   ___ ___ _____
8. Put on gloves. Made sure the gloves covered the wrists of
   the gown.   ___ ___ _____
9. Provided care.   ___ ___ _____
10. Removed and discarded the PPE. Practiced hand hygiene
    between each step if your hands became contaminated.
    a. *Method 1: Gloves, goggles, or face shield, gown, mask or respirator.*
       1) Removed and discarded the gloves.
          a) Made sure that glove touched only glove. ___ ___ _____
          b) Grasped a glove at the palm. Grasped it on the outside. ___ ___ _____
          c) Pulled the glove down over your hand so it was
             inside out.   ___ ___ _____
          d) Held the removed glove with your other gloved hand. ___ ___ _____
          e) Reached inside the other glove. Used the first 2 fingers
             of the ungloved hand.   ___ ___ _____

Date of Satisfactory Completion _____   Instructor's Initials _____

Procedure—cont'd	**S**	**U**	**Comments**
f) Pulled the glove down (inside out) over your hand and the other glove.	_____	_____	_____
g) Discarded the gloves.	_____	_____	_____
2) Removed and discarded the goggles or face shield if worn.			
a) Lifted the headband from the back. Did not touch the front of the device.	_____	_____	_____
b) Discarded the device. If re-usable, followed agency policy.	_____	_____	_____
3) Removed and discarded the gown. Did not touch the outside of the gown.			
a) Untied the neck and then the waist strings.	_____	_____	_____
b) Pulled the gown down and away from your neck and shoulders. Only touched the inside of the gown.	_____	_____	_____
c) Turned the gown inside out as it was removed. Held it at the inside shoulder seams and brought your hands together.	_____	_____	_____
d) Folded or rolled up the gown away from you. Kept it inside out. Did not let the gown touch the floor.	_____	_____	_____
e) Discarded the gown.	_____	_____	_____
4) Removed and discarded the mask if worn. (NOTE: Removed a respirator after leaving the room and closing the door.)			
a) Untied the lower strings of the mask.	_____	_____	_____
b) Untied the top strings.	_____	_____	_____
c) Held the top strings. Removed the mask.	_____	_____	_____
d) Discarded the mask.	_____	_____	_____
b. *Method 2: Gown and gloves, goggles or face shield, mask or respirator.*			
1) Removed and discarded the gown and gloves.			
a) Grasped the gown in front with your gloved hands. Pulled away from your body so the ties broke. Only touched the outside of the gown.	_____	_____	_____
b) Folded or rolled the gown inside out into a bundle while removing the gown. Kept it inside out. Did not let the gown touch the floor.	_____	_____	_____
c) Peeled off your gloves as you removed the gown. Only touched the inside of the gloves and the gown with your bare hands.	_____	_____	_____
d) Discarded the gown and gloves.	_____	_____	_____
2) Removed and discarded the goggles or face shield.			
a) Lifted the headband from the back. Did not touch the front of the device.	_____	_____	_____
b) Discarded the device. If re-usable, followed agency policy.	_____	_____	_____
3) Removed and discarded the mask if worn. (NOTE: Removed a respirator after leaving the room and closing the door.)			
a) Untied the lower strings of the mask.	_____	_____	_____
b) Untied the top strings.	_____	_____	_____
c) Held the top strings. Removed the mask.	_____	_____	_____
d) Discarded the mask.	_____	_____	_____
11. Practiced hand hygiene after removing all PPE.	_____	_____	_____

Date of Satisfactory Completion _____   Instructor's Initials _____

Double-Bagging

Name: _____   Date: _____

Procedure	S	U	Comments
1. Asked a co-worker to help you. He or she stood outside the doorway. You were in the room.	____	____	_____
2. Placed soiled linen, re-usable items, disposable supplies, and trash in the right containers. Containers were lined with leak-proof biohazard bags. Those were the *dirty (contaminated)* bags.	____	____	_____
3. Sealed the *dirty* bags securely.	____	____	_____
4. Asked your co-worker to make a wide cuff on a *clean* bag. It was held wide open. The cuff protected the hands from contamination.	____	____	_____
5. Placed the *dirty* bag into the *clean* bag. Did not touch the outside of the *clean* bag.	____	____	_____
6. Asked your co-worker to seal the *clean* bag. Had the bag labeled with the BIOHAZARD symbol.	____	____	_____
7. Repeated the following steps for other *dirty* bags.			
a. Sealed the *dirty* bags securely.	____	____	_____
b. Asked your co-worker to make a wide cuff on a *clean* bag. It was held wide open. The cuff protected the hands from contamination.	____	____	_____
c. Placed the *dirty* bag into the *clean* bag. Did not touch the outside of the *clean* bag.	____	____	_____
d. Asked your co-worker to seal the *clean* bag. Had the bag labeled with the BIOHAZARD symbol.	____	____	_____
8. Asked your co-worker to take or send the bags to the appropriate department for disposal, disinfection, or sterilization.	____	____	_____

Date of Satisfactory Completion _____   Instructor's Initials _____

Sterile Gloving

Name: _____   Date: _____

Procedure	S	U	Comments
1. Followed *Delegation Guidelines: Assisting With Sterile Procedures.* Saw *Promoting Safety and Comfort:*			
a. *Assisting With Sterile Procedures*	___	___	_____
b. *Sterile Gloving*	___	___	_____
2. Practiced hand hygiene.	___	___	_____
3. Inspected the package of sterile gloves for sterility.			
a. Checked the expiration date.	___	___	_____
b. Saw if the package was dry.	___	___	_____
c. Checked for tears, holes, punctures, and watermarks.	___	___	_____
4. Arranged a work surface.			
a. Made sure you had enough room.	___	___	_____
b. Arranged the work surface at waist level and within your vision.	___	___	_____
c. Cleaned and dried the work surface.	___	___	_____
d. Did not reach over or turn your back on the work surface.	___	___	_____
5. Opened the package. Grasped the flaps. Gently peeled them back.	___	___	_____
6. Removed the inner package. Placed it on your work surface.	___	___	_____
7. Read the manufacturer's instructions on the inner package. It may have been labeled *left, right, up,* and *down.*	___	___	_____
8. Arranged the inner package for left, right, up, and down. The left glove was on your left. The right glove was on your right. The cuffs were near you, the fingers pointed away from you.	___	___	_____
9. Grasped the folded edges of the inner package. Used the thumb and index finger of each hand.	___	___	_____
10. Folded back the inner package to expose the gloves. Did not touch or otherwise contaminate the inside package or the gloves. The inside of the inner package was a sterile field.	___	___	_____
11. Noted that each glove had a cuff about 2 to 3 inches wide. The cuffs and insides of the gloves were *not sterile.*	___	___	_____
12. Put on the right glove if you were right-handed. Put on the left glove if you were left-handed.			
a. Picked up the glove with your other hand. Used your thumb and index and middle fingers.	___	___	_____
b. Touched only the glove and the inside of the glove.	___	___	_____
c. Turned the hand to be gloved palm side up.	___	___	_____
d. Lifted the cuff up. Slid your fingers and hand into the glove.	___	___	_____
e. Pulled the glove up over your hand. If some fingers got stuck, left them that way until the other glove was on. *Did not use your ungloved hand to straighten the glove. Did not let the outside of the glove touch any non-sterile surface.*	___	___	_____
f. Left the cuff turned down.	___	___	_____
13. Put on the other glove. Used your gloved hand.			
a. Reached under the cuff of the second glove. Used the 4 fingers of your gloved hand. Kept your gloved thumb close to your gloved palm.	___	___	_____
b. Put on the second glove. Your gloved hand did not touch the cuff or any surface. Held the thumb of your first gloved hand away from the second gloved palm.	___	___	_____
14. Adjusted each glove with the other hand. The gloves were smooth and comfortable.	___	___	_____
15. Slid your fingers under the cuffs to pull them up.	___	___	_____
16. Touched only sterile items.	___	___	_____
17. Removed and discarded the gloves.	___	___	_____
18. Practiced hand hygiene.	___	___	_____

Date of Satisfactory Completion _____   Instructor's Initials _____

Raising the Person's Head and Shoulders

Name: _____   Date: _____

Quality of Life	S	U	Comments
• Knocked before entering the person's room.	___	___	___
• Addressed the person by name.	___	___	___
• Introduced yourself by name and title.	___	___	___
• Explained the procedure before starting and during the procedure.	___	___	___
• Protected the person's rights during the procedure.	___	___	___
• Handled the person gently during the procedure.	___	___	___

Pre-Procedure

1. Followed *Delegation Guidelines:*
   a. *Preventing Work-Related Injuries*   ___ ___ ___
   b. *Moving Persons in Bed*   ___ ___ ___
   Saw *Promoting Safety and Comfort:*
   a. *Safely Moving the Person*   ___ ___ ___
   b. *Preventing Work-Related Injuries*   ___ ___ ___
2. Asked a co-worker to assist if needed.   ___ ___ ___
3. Practiced hand hygiene.   ___ ___ ___
4. Identified the person. Checked the ID (identification) bracelet against the assignment sheet. Used 2 identifiers. Also called the person by name.   ___ ___ ___
5. Provided for privacy.   ___ ___ ___
6. Locked the brakes on bed wheels.   ___ ___ ___
7. Raised the bed for body mechanics. Bed rails were up if used.   ___ ___ ___

Procedure

8. Had your co-worker stand on the other side of the bed. Lowered the bed rails if up.   ___ ___
9. Asked the person to put the near arm under your near arm and behind your shoulder. His or her hand rested on top of your shoulder. If you were standing on the right side, the person's right hand rested on your right shoulder. The person did the same with your co-worker. The person's left hand rested on your co-worker's left shoulder.   ___ ___
10. Placed your arm nearest to the person under his or her arm. Your hand was on the person's shoulder. Your co-worker did the same.   ___ ___ ___
11. Placed your free arm under the person's neck and shoulders. Your co-worker did the same. Supported the neck.   ___ ___ ___
12. Helped the person rise to a sitting or semi-sitting position on the "count of 3."   ___ ___ ___
13. Used the arm and hand that supported the person's neck and shoulders to give care. Your co-worker supported the person.   ___ ___ ___
14. Helped the person lie down. Provided support with your locked arm. Your co-worker did the same.   ___ ___ ___

Post-Procedure

15. Provided for comfort.   ___ ___ ___
16. Placed the call light and other needed items within reach.   ___ ___ ___
17. Lowered the bed to a safe and comfortable level appropriate for the person. Followed the care plan.   ___ ___ ___
18. Raised or lowered bed rails. Followed the care plan.   ___ ___ ___
19. Unscreened the person.   ___ ___ ___
20. Completed a safety check of the room.   ___ ___ ___
21. Practiced hand hygiene.   ___ ___ ___
22. Reported and recorded your observations.   ___ ___ ___

Date of Satisfactory Completion _____   Instructor's Initials _____

Moving the Person Up In Bed

Name: _____   Date: _____

Quality of Life	S	U	Comments
• Knocked before entering the person's room.	____	____	_____
• Addressed the person by name.	____	____	_____
• Introduced yourself by name and title.	____	____	_____
• Explained the procedure before starting and during the procedure.	____	____	_____
• Protected the person's rights during the procedure.	____	____	_____
• Handled the person gently during the procedure.	____	____	_____

Pre-Procedure

1. Followed *Delegation Guidelines:*
   a. *Preventing Work-Related Injuries*
   b. *Moving Persons in Bed*
   Saw *Promoting Safety and Comfort:*
   a. *Safely Moving the Person*
   b. *Preventing Work-Related Injuries*
2. Asked a co-worker to help you.
3. Practiced hand hygiene.
4. Identified the person. Checked the ID (identification) bracelet against the assignment sheet. Used 2 identifiers. Also called the person by name.
5. Provided for privacy.
6. Locked brakes on the bed wheels.
7. Raised the bed for body mechanics. Bed rails were up if used.

Procedure

8. Lowered the head of the bed to a level appropriate for the person. It was as flat as possible.
9. Stood on 1 side of the bed. Your co-worker stood on the other side.
10. Lowered the bed rails if up.
11. Removed pillows as directed by the nurse. Placed a pillow against the head-board if the person could be without it.
12. Stood with a wide base of support. Pointed the foot near the head of the bed toward the head of the bed. Faced the head of the bed.
13. Bent your hips and knees. Kept your back straight.
14. Placed 1 arm under the person's shoulder and 1 arm under the thighs. Your co-worker did the same. Grasped each other's forearms.
15. Asked the person to grasp the trapeze.
16. Had the person flex both knees.
17. Explained that:
    a. You will count "1, 2, 3."
    b. The move will be on "3."
    c. On "3," the person pushes against the bed with the feet if able. And the person pulls up with the trapeze.
18. Moved the person to the head of the bed on the "count of 3." Shifted your weight from your rear leg to your front leg. Your co-worker did the same.
19. Repeated the following steps if necessary.
    a. Stood with a wide base of support. Pointed the foot near the head of the bed toward the head of the bed. Faced the head of the bed.
    b. Bent your hips and knees. Kept your back straight.
    c. Placed 1 arm under the person's shoulder and 1 arm under the thighs. Your co-worker did the same. Grasped each other's forearms.

Date of Satisfactory Completion _____   Instructor's Initials _____

	S	U	Comments
Procedure—cont'd			
d. Asked the person to grasp the trapeze.	___	___	_____
e. Had the person flex both knees.	___	___	_____
f. Explained that:			
1) You will count "1, 2, 3."	___	___	_____
2) The move will be on "3."	___	___	_____
3) On "3," the person pushes against the bed with the feet if able. And the person pulls up with the trapeze.	___	___	_____
g. Moved the person to the head of the bed on the "count of 3." Shifted your weight from your rear leg to your front leg. Your co-worker did the same.	___	___	_____
Post-Procedure			
20. Placed the pillow under the person's head and shoulders. Straightened linens.	___	___	_____
21. Positioned the person in good alignment. Raised the head of the bed to a level appropriate for the person.	___	___	_____
22. Provided for comfort.	___	___	_____
23. Placed the call light and other needed items within reach.	___	___	_____
24. Lowered the bed to a safe and comfortable level appropriate for the person. Followed the care plan.	___	___	_____
25. Raised or lowered bed rails. Followed the care plan.	___	___	_____
26. Unscreened the person.	___	___	_____
27. Completed a safety check of the room.	___	___	_____
28. Practiced hand hygiene.	___	___	_____
29. Reported and recorded your observations.	___	___	_____

Date of Satisfactory Completion _____ Instructor's Initials _____

Moving the Person Up in Bed With an Assist Device

Name: _____   Date: _____

Quality of Life	S	U	Comments

Quality of Life
- Knocked before entering the person's room.
- Addressed the person by name.
- Introduced yourself by name and title.
- Explained the procedure before starting and during the procedure.
- Protected the person's rights during the procedure.
- Handled the person gently during the procedure.

Pre-Procedure
1. Followed *Delegation Guidelines:*
   a. *Preventing Work-Related Injuries*
   b. *Moving Persons in Bed*
   Saw *Promoting Safety and Comfort:*
   a. *Safely Moving the Person*
   b. *Preventing Work-Related Injuries*
   c. *Moving the Person Up in Bed*
   d. *Moving the Person Up in Bed With an Assist Device*
2. Asked a co-worker to help you.
3. Practiced hand hygiene.
4. Identified the person. Checked the ID (identification) bracelet against the assignment sheet. Used 2 identifiers. Also called the person by name.
5. Provided for privacy.
6. Locked brakes on the bed wheels.
7. Raised the bed for body mechanics. Bed rails were up if used.

Procedure
8. Lowered the head of the bed to a level appropriate for the person. It was as flat as possible.
9. Stood on 1 side of the bed. Your co-worker stood on the other side.
10. Lowered the bed rails if up.
11. Removed pillows as directed by the nurse. Placed a pillow against the head-board if the person could be without it.
12. Stood with a wide base of support. Pointed the foot near the head of the bed toward the head of the bed. Faced the head of the bed.
13. Rolled the sides of the assist device up close to the person. (NOTE: Omitted this step if the device had handles.)
14. Grasped the rolled-up assist device firmly near the person's shoulders and hips. Or grasped it by the handles. Supported the head.
15. Bent your hips and knees.
16. Moved the person up in bed on the "count of 3." Shifted your weight from your rear leg to your front leg.
17. Repeated the following steps if necessary.
    a. Stood with a wide base of support. Pointed the foot near the head of the bed toward the head of the bed. Faced the head of the bed.
    b. Rolled the sides of the assist device firmly near the person. (NOTE: Omitted this step if the device had handles.)
    c. Grasped the rolled-up assist device firmly near the person's shoulders and hips. Or grasped it by the handles. Supported the head.

Date of Satisfactory Completion _____   Instructor's Initials _____

Procedure—cont'd	S	U	Comments
d. Bent your hips and knees.	___	___	___
e. Moved the person up in bed on the "count of 3." Shifted your weight from your rear leg to your front leg.	___	___	___
18. Unrolled the assist device. (NOTE: Omitted this step if the device had handles.) Removed the slide sheet if used.	___	___	___

Post-Procedure

	S	U	Comments
19. Placed the pillow under the person's head and shoulders. Straightened linens.	___	___	___
20. Positioned the person in good alignment. Raised the head of the bed to a level appropriate for the person.	___	___	___
21. Provided for comfort.	___	___	___
22. Placed the call light and other needed items within reach.	___	___	___
23. Lowered the bed to a safe and comfortable level appropriate for the person. Followed the care plan.	___	___	___
24. Raised or lowered bed rails. Followed the care plan.	___	___	___
25. Unscreened the person.	___	___	___
26. Completed a safety check of the room.	___	___	___
27. Practiced hand hygiene.	___	___	___
28. Reported and recorded your observations.	___	___	___

Date of Satisfactory Completion _____ Instructor's Initials _____

Moving the Person to the Side of the Bed

Name: _____   Date: _____

	S	U	Comments

Quality of Life
- Knocked before entering the person's room.
- Addressed the person by name.
- Introduced yourself by name and title.
- Explained the procedure before starting and during the procedure.
- Protected the person's rights during the procedure.
- Handled the person gently during the procedure.

Pre-Procedure
1. Followed *Delegation Guidelines:*
   a. *Preventing Work-Related Injuries*
   b. *Moving Persons in Bed*
   Saw *Promoting Safety and Comfort:*
   a. *Safely Moving the Person*
   b. *Preventing Work-Related Injuries*
   c. *Moving the Person to the Side of the Bed*
2. Asked 1 or 2 co-workers to help you if you used an assist device.
3. Practiced hand hygiene.
4. Identified the person. Checked the ID (identification) bracelet against the assignment sheet. Used 2 identifiers. Also called the person by name.
5. Provided for privacy.
6. Locked brakes on the bed wheels.
7. Raised the bed for body mechanics. Bed rails were up if used.

Procedure
8. Lowered the head of the bed to a level appropriate for the person. It was as flat as possible.
9. Stood on the side of the bed to which you will move the person.
10. Lowered the bed rail near you if bed rails were used.
11. Removed pillows as directed by the nurse.
12. Crossed the person's arms over the chest.
13. Stood with your feet about 12 inches apart. One foot was in front of the other. Flexed your knees.
14. *Method 1—Moving the person in segments:*
    a. Placed your arm under the person's neck and shoulders. Grasped the far shoulder.
    b. Placed your other arm under the mid-back.
    c. Moved the upper part of the person's body toward you. Rocked backward and shifted your weight to your rear leg.
    d. Placed 1 arm under the person's waist and 1 under the thighs.
    e. Rocked backward to move the lower part of the person toward you.
    f. Repeated the procedure for the legs and feet.
       1) Placed 1 arm under the person's thighs.
       2) Placed your other arm under the person's calves.
       3) Rocked backward to move the legs and feet of the person toward you.
15. *Method 2—Moving the person with a drawsheet:*
    a. Rolled up the drawsheet close to the person.
    b. Grasped the rolled-up drawsheet near the person's shoulders and hips. Your co-worker did the same. Supported the person's head.

Date of Satisfactory Completion _____   Instructor's Initials _____

Procedure—cont'd	S	U	Comments
c. Rocked backward on the "count of 3," moving the person toward you. Your co-worker rocked backward slightly and then forward toward you while keeping the arms straight.	___	___	_____
d. Unrolled the drawsheet. Removed any wrinkles.	___	___	_____

Post-Procedure

	S	U	Comments
16. Placed the pillow under the person's head and shoulders. Straightened linens.	___	___	_____
17. Positioned the person in good alignment.	___	___	_____
18. Provided for comfort.	___	___	_____
19. Placed the call light and other needed items within reach.	___	___	_____
20. Lowered the bed to a safe and comfortable level appropriate for the person. Followed the care plan.	___	___	_____
21. Raised or lowered bed rails. Followed the care plan.	___	___	_____
22. Unscreened the person.	___	___	_____
23. Completed a safety check of the room.	___	___	_____
24. Practiced hand hygiene.	___	___	_____
25. Reported and recorded your observations.	___	___	_____

Date of Satisfactory Completion _____   Instructor's Initials _____

Turning and Re-Positioning the Person

Name: _____ Date: _____

	S	U	Comments
Quality of Life			
• Knocked before entering the person's room.	___	___	_____
• Addressed the person by name.	___	___	_____
• Introduced yourself by name and title.	___	___	_____
• Explained the procedure before starting and during the procedure.	___	___	_____
• Protected the person's rights during the procedure.	___	___	_____
• Handled the person gently during the procedure.	___	___	_____

Pre-Procedure

1. Followed *Delegation Guidelines:*
   a. *Preventing Work-Related Injuries*
   b. *Moving Persons in Bed*
   c. *Turning Persons*
   Saw *Promoting Safety and Comfort:*
   a. *Safely Moving the Person*
   b. *Preventing Work-Related Injuries*
   c. *Moving the Person to the Side of the Bed*
   d. *Turning Persons*
2. Practiced hand hygiene.
3. Identified the person. Checked the ID (identification) bracelet against the assignment sheet. Used 2 identifiers. Also called the person by name.
4. Provided for privacy.
5. Locked brakes on the bed wheels.
6. Raised the bed for body mechanics. Bed rails were up if used.

Procedure

7. Lowered the head of the bed to a level appropriate for the person. It was as flat as possible.
8. Stood on the side of the bed opposite to where you will turn the person.
9. Lowered the bed rail.
10. Moved the person to the side near you.
11. Crossed the person's arms over the chest. Crossed the leg near you over the far leg.
12. *Turning the person away from you:*
    a. Stood with a wide base of support. Flexed the knees.
    b. Placed 1 hand on the person's shoulder. Placed the other on the hip near you.
    c. Rolled the person gently away from you toward the raised bed rail.
    d. Shifted your weight from your rear leg to your front leg.
13. *Turning the person toward you:*
    a. Raised the bed rail.
    b. Went to the other side of the bed. Lowered the bed rail.
    c. Stood with a wide base of support. Flexed your knees.
    d. Placed 1 hand on the person's shoulder. Placed the other on the far hip.
    e. Pulled the person toward you gently.

Date of Satisfactory Completion _____ Instructor's Initials _____

Procedure—cont'd   S   U   **Comments**

14. Positioned the person. Followed the nurse's directions and the
    care plan. The following are common.
    a. Placed a pillow under the head and neck.   ____   ____   _____
    b. Adjusted the shoulder. The person should not be on an arm. ____   ____   _____
    c. Placed a small pillow under the upper hand and arm.   ____   ____   _____
    d. Positioned a pillow against the back.   ____   ____   _____
    e. Flexed the upper knee. Positioned the upper leg in front of the
       lower leg.   ____   ____   _____
    f. Supported the upper leg and thigh on pillows. Made sure the
       ankle was supported.   ____   ____   _____

Post-Procedure
15. Provided for comfort.   ____   ____   _____
16. Placed the call light and other needed items within reach. ____   ____   _____
17. Lowered the bed to a safe and comfortable level appropriate for
    the person. Followed the care plan.   ____   ____   _____
18. Raised or lowered bed rails. Followed the care plan.   ____   ____   _____
19. Unscreened the person.   ____   ____   _____
20. Completed a safety check of the room.   ____   ____   _____
21. Practiced hand hygiene.   ____   ____   _____
22. Reported and recorded your observations.   ____   ____   _____

Date of Satisfactory Completion _____   Instructor's Initials _____

Logrolling the Person

NATCEP™   VIDEO

Name: _____   Date: _____

	S	U	Comments

Quality of Life
- Knocked before entering the person's room.
- Addressed the person by name.
- Introduced yourself by name and title.
- Explained the procedure before starting and during the procedure.
- Protected the person's rights during the procedure.
- Handled the person gently during the procedure.

Pre-Procedure
1. Followed *Delegation Guidelines:*
   a. *Preventing Work-Related Injuries*
   b. *Moving Persons in Bed*
   c. *Turning Persons*
   Saw *Promoting Safety and Comfort:*
   a. *Safely Moving the Person*
   b. *Preventing Work-Related Injuries*
   c. *Turning Persons*
   d. *Logrolling*
2. Asked a co-worker to help you.
3. Practiced hand hygiene.
4. Identified the person. Checked the identification (ID) bracelet against the assignment sheet. Used 2 identifiers. Also called the person by name.
5. Provided for privacy.
6. Locked brakes on the bed wheels.
7. Raised the bed for body mechanics. Bed rails were up if used.

Procedure
8. Made sure the bed was flat.
9. Stood on the side opposite to which you turned the person. Your co-worker stood on the other side.
10. Lowered the bed rails if used.
11. Moved the person as a unit to the side of the bed near you. Used the assist device. (If the person had a spinal cord injury or had spinal cord surgery, assisted the nurse as directed.)
12. Placed the person's arms across the chest. Placed a pillow between the knees.
13. Raised the bed rail if used.
14. Went to the other side.
15. Stood near the shoulders and chest. Your co-worker stood near the hips and thighs.
16. Stood with a wide base of support. One foot was in front of the other.
17. Asked the person to hold his or her body rigid.
18. Rolled the person toward you. Or used the assist device. Turned the person as a unit.
19. Positioned the person in good alignment. Used pillows as directed by the nurse and care plan. The following is common (unless the spinal cord was involved).
   a. Placed a pillow under the head and neck if allowed.
   b. Adjusted the shoulder. The person was not on an arm.
   c. Placed a small pillow under the upper hand and arm.
   d. Positioned a pillow against the back.

Date of Satisfactory Completion _____   Instructor's Initials _____

	S	U	Comments

Procedure—cont'd

    e. Flexed the upper knee. Positioned the upper leg in front of the lower leg.

    f. Supported the upper leg and thigh on pillows. Made sure the ankle was supported.

Post-Procedure

20. Provided for comfort.
21. Placed the call light and other needed items within reach.
22. Lowered the bed to a safe and comfortable level appropriate for the person. Followed the care plan.
23. Raised or lowered bed rails. Followed the care plan.
24. Unscreened the person.
25. Completed a safety check of the room.
26. Practiced hand hygiene.
27. Reported and recorded your observations.

Date of Satisfactory Completion _____   Instructor's Initials _____

Sitting on the Side of the Bed (Dangling)

Name: _____   Date: _____

	S	U	Comments

Quality of Life
- Knocked before entering the person's room.
- Addressed the person by name.
- Introduced yourself by name and title.
- Explained the procedure before starting and during the procedure.
- Protected the person's rights during the procedure.
- Handled the person gently during the procedure.

Pre-Procedure
1. Followed *Delegation Guidelines:*
   a. *Preventing Work-Related Injuries*
   b. *Dangling*
   Saw *Promoting Safety and Comfort:*
   a. *Safely Moving the Person*
   b. *Preventing Work-Related Injuries*
   c. *Dangling*
2. Asked a co-worker to help you.
3. Practiced hand hygiene.
4. Identified the person. Checked the identification (ID) bracelet against the assignment sheet. Used 2 identifiers. Also called the person by name.
5. Provided for privacy.
6. Decided which side of the bed to use.
7. Moved furniture to provide moving space.
8. Locked brakes on the bed wheels.
9. Raised the bed for body mechanics. Bed rails were up if used.

Procedure
10. Lowered the bed rail if up.
11. Positioned the person in a side-lying position facing you. The person laid on the strong side.
12. Raised the head of the bed to a sitting position.
13. Stood by the person's hips. Faced the foot of the bed.
14. Stood with your feet apart. The foot near the head of the bed was in front of the other foot.
15. Slid 1 arm under the person's neck and shoulders. Grasped the far shoulder. Placed your other hand over the thighs near the knees.
16. Pivoted toward the foot of the bed while moving the person's legs and feet over the side of the bed. As the legs went over the edge of the mattress, the trunk was upright.
17. Asked the person to hold on to the edge of the mattress. This supported the person in the sitting position. If possible, raised a half-length bed rail (on the person's strong side) for the person to grasp. Had your co-worker support the person at all times.
18. Did not leave the person alone. Provided support at all times.
19. Checked the person's condition.
    a. Asked how the person felt. Asked if the person felt dizzy or light-headed.
    b. Checked the pulse and respirations.
    c. Checked for difficulty breathing.
    d. Noted if the skin was pale or bluish in color.
20. Reversed the procedure to return the person to bed. (Or prepared the person to walk or for a transfer to a chair or wheelchair. The person's feet were flat on the floor. Supported the person at all times.)

Date of Satisfactory Completion _____   Instructor's Initials _____

Procedure—cont'd	S	U	Comments
21. Lowered the head of the bed after the person returned to bed. Helped him or her move to the center of the bed.	_____	_____	_____
22. Positioned the person in good alignment.	_____	_____	_____

Post-Procedure

	S	U	Comments
23. Provided for comfort.	_____	_____	_____
24. Placed the call light and other needed items within reach.	_____	_____	_____
25. Lowered the bed to a safe and comfortable level appropriate for the person. Followed the care plan.	_____	_____	_____
26. Raised or lowered bed rails. Followed the care plan.	_____	_____	_____
27. Returned furniture to its proper place.	_____	_____	_____
28. Unscreened the person.	_____	_____	_____
29. Completed a safety check of the room.	_____	_____	_____
30. Practiced hand hygiene.	_____	_____	_____
31. Reported and recorded your observations.	_____	_____	_____

NATCEP VIDEO VIDEO CLIP

Transferring the Person to a Chair or Wheelchair

Name: _____ Date: _____

	S	U	Comments
Quality of Life			
• Knocked before entering the person's room.			
• Addressed the person by name.			
• Introduced yourself by name and title.			
• Explained the procedure before starting and during the procedure.			
• Protected the person's rights during the procedure.			
• Handled the person gently during the procedure.			

Pre-Procedure
1. Followed *Delegation Guidelines:*
   a. *Safely Transferring the Person*
   b. *Stand and Pivot Transfers*
   Saw *Promoting Safety and Comfort:*
   a. *Transfer Belts*
   b. *Safely Transferring the Person*
   c. *Stand and Pivot Transfer*
   d. *Bed to Chair or Wheelchair Transfers*
2. Collected the following:
   • Wheelchair or arm chair
   • Bath blanket
   • Lap blanket (if used)
   • Robe and non-skid footwear
   • Paper or sheet
   • Transfer belt (if needed)
   • Seat cushion (if needed)
3. Practiced hand hygiene.
4. Identified the person. Checked the identification (ID) bracelet against the assignment sheet. Used 2 identifiers. Also called the person by name.
5. Provided for privacy.
6. Decided which side of the bed to use. Moved furniture for a safe transfer.

Procedure
7. Raised the wheelchair footplates. Removed or swung front rigging out of the way if possible. Positioned the chair or wheelchair near the bed on the person's strong side.
   a. If at the head of the bed, it faced the foot of the bed.
   b. If at the foot of the bed, it faced the head of the bed.
   c. The armrest almost touched the bed.
8. Placed a folded bath blanket or cushion on the seat (if needed).
9. Locked (braked) the wheelchair wheels.
10. Fan-folded top linens to the foot of the bed.
11. Placed the paper or sheet under the person's feet. (This protected linens from footwear.) Put footwear on the person.
12. Lowered the bed to a safe and comfortable level for the person. Locked (braked) the bed wheels.
13. Helped the person sit on the side of the bed. His or her feet were flat on the floor.
14. Helped the person put on a robe.
15. Applied the transfer belt if needed. It was applied at the waist over clothing.

Date of Satisfactory Completion _____   Instructor's Initials _____

Procedure—cont'd	S	U	Comments

16. *Method 1: Using a transfer belt:*
   a. Stood in front of the person.
   b. Had the person hold on to the mattress.
   c. Made sure the person's feet were flat on the floor.
   d. Had the person lean forward.
   e. Grasped the transfer belt at each side. Grasped the handles or grasped the belt from underneath.
   f. Prevented the person from sliding or falling. Did one of the following:
      1) Braced your knees against the person's knees. Blocked his or her feet with your feet.
      2) Used the knee and foot of 1 leg to block the person's weak leg or foot. Placed your other foot slightly behind you for balance.
      3) Straddled your legs around the person's weak leg.
   g. Explained the following:
      1) You will count "1, 2, 3."
      2) The move will be on "3."
      3) On "3," the person pushes down on the mattress and stands.
   h. Asked the person to push down on the mattress and to stand on the "count of 3." Assisted the person to a standing position as you straightened your knees.
17. *Method 2: No transfer belt.* (NOTE: Used this method only if directed by the nurse and the care plan.)
   a. Followed steps 16, a–c.
      1) Stood in front of the person.
      2) Had the person hold on to the mattress.
      3) Made sure the person's feet were flat on the floor.
   b. Placed your hands under the person's arms. Your hands were around the person's shoulder blades.
   c. Had the person lean forward.
   d. Prevented the person from sliding or falling. Did one of the following:
      1) Braced your knees against the person's knees. Blocked his or her feet with your feet.
      2) Used the knee and foot of 1 leg to block the person's weak leg or foot. Placed your other foot slightly behind you for balance.
      3) Straddled your legs around the person's weak leg.
   e. Explained the "count of 3."
      1) You will count "1, 2, 3".
      2) The move will be on "3."
      3) On "3," the person pushes down on the mattress and stands.
   f. Asked the person to push down on the mattress and to stand on the "count of 3." Assisted the person up into a standing position as you straightened your knees.
18. Supported the person in the standing position. Held the transfer belt or kept your hands around the person's shoulder blades. Continued to prevent the person from sliding or falling.
19. Helped the person pivot (turn) so he or she could grasp the far arm of the chair or wheelchair. The legs touched the edge of the seat.
20. Continued to help the person pivot (turn) until the other armrest was grasped.
21. Lowered him or her into the chair or wheelchair as you bent your hips and knees. To assist, the person leaned forward and bent his or her elbows and knees.

Date of Satisfactory Completion _____ Instructor's Initials _____

Procedure—cont'd	**S**	**U**	**Comments**
22. Made sure the hips were to the back of the seat. Positioned the person in good alignment.	_____	_____	_____
23. Attached the wheelchair front rigging. Positioned the person's feet on the footplates.	_____	_____	_____
24. Covered the person's lap and legs with a lap blanket (if used). Kept the blanket off the floor and the wheels.	_____	_____	_____
25. Removed the transfer belt if used.	_____	_____	_____
26. Positioned the chair as the person preferred. Locked (braked) the wheelchair wheels according to the care plan.	_____	_____	_____

Post-Procedure			
27. Provided for comfort.	_____	_____	_____
28. Placed the call light and other needed items within reach.	_____	_____	_____
29. Unscreened the person.	_____	_____	_____
30. Completed a safety check of the room.	_____	_____	_____
31. Practiced hand hygiene.	_____	_____	_____
32. Reported and recorded your observations.	_____	_____	_____
33. Saw procedure: *Transferring the Person From a Chair or Wheelchair to Bed* to return the person to bed.	_____	_____	_____

Date of Satisfactory Completion _____   Instructor's Initials _____

NATCEP™ Transferring the Person From a Chair or Wheelchair to Bed

Name: _____   Date: _____

Quality of Life	S	U	Comments
• Knocked before entering the person's room.			
• Addressed the person by name.			
• Introduced yourself by name and title.			
• Explained the procedure before starting and during the procedure.			
• Protected the person's rights during the procedure.			
• Handled the person gently during the procedure.			

Pre-Procedure

1. Followed *Delegation Guidelines:*
   a. *Safely Transferring the Person*
   b. *Stand and Pivot Transfers*
   Saw *Promoting Safety and Comfort:*
   a. *Transfer Belts*
   b. *Safely Transferring the Person*
   c. *Stand and Pivot Transfer*
   d. *Bed to Chair or Wheelchair Transfers*
2. Collected a transfer belt if needed.
3. Practiced hand hygiene.
4. Identified the person. Checked the identification (ID) bracelet against the assignment sheet. Used 2 identifiers. Called the person by name.
5. Provided privacy.

Procedure

6. Moved furniture for moving space.
7. Raised the head of the bed to a sitting position. Lowered the bed to a safe and comfortable level for the person. When the person transferred to the bed, his or her feet were flat on the floor while sitting on the side of the bed.
8. Moved the call light so it would be on the strong side when the person was in bed.
9. Positioned the chair or wheelchair so the person's strong side was next to the bed. Had a co-worker help you if necessary.
10. Locked (braked) the wheelchair and bed wheels.
11. Removed and folded the lap blanket.
12. Removed the person's feet from the footplates. Raised the footplates. Removed or swung front rigging out of the way. Put non-skid footwear on the person if needed.
13. Applied the transfer belt if needed.
14. Made sure the person's feet were flat on the floor.
15. Stood in front of the person.
16. Had the person hold on to the armrests. (If the nurse directed you to do so, placed your arms under the person's arms. Your hands were around the shoulder blades.)
17. Had the person lean forward.
18. Grasped the transfer belt on each side if using it. Grasped underneath the belt.
19. Prevented the person from sliding or falling. Did one of the following:
    a. Braced your knees against the person's knees. Blocked his or her feet with your feet.
    b. Used the knee and foot of 1 leg to block the person's weak leg or foot. Placed your other foot slightly behind you for balance.
    c. Straddled your legs around the person's weak leg.

Date of Satisfactory Completion _____   Instructor's Initials _____

Procedure—cont'd   **S**   **U**   **Comments**

20. Explained the count of "3."
   a. You will count "1, 2, 3."   ____   ____   _____
   b. The move will be on "3."   ____   ____   _____
21. Asked the person to push down on the armrest on the
   "count of 3." Assisted the person into a standing position
   as you straightened your knees.   ____   ____   _____
22. Supported the person in the standing position. Held the
   transfer belt or kept your hands around the person's shoulder
   blades. Continued to prevent the person from sliding or falling.   ____   ____   _____
23. Helped the person pivot (turn) so he or she can reach the
   edge of the mattress. The legs touched the mattress.   ____   ____   _____
24. Continued to help the person pivot (turn) until he or she reached
   the mattress with both hands.   ____   ____   _____
25. Lowered him or her onto the bed as you bent your hips
   and knees. To assist, the person leaned forward and bent the
   elbows and knees.
26. Removed the transfer belt.   ____   ____   _____
27. Removed the robe and footwear.   ____   ____   _____
28. Helped the person lie down.   ____   ____   _____

Post-Procedure
29. Provided for comfort.
30. Placed the call light and other needed items within reach.   ____   ____   _____
31. Raised or lowered bed rails. Followed the care plan.   ____   ____   _____
32. Arranged furniture to meet the person's needs.   ____   ____   _____
33. Unscreened the person.   ____   ____   _____
34. Completed a safety check of the room.   ____   ____   _____
35. Practiced hand hygiene.   ____   ____   _____
36. Reported and recorded your observations.   ____   ____   _____

Date of Satisfactory Completion _____   Instructor's Initials _____

Transferring the Person To and From the Toilet

Name: _____   Date: _____

	S	U	Comments
Quality of Life			
• Knocked before entering the person's room.	___	___	_____
• Addressed the person by name.	___	___	_____
• Introduced yourself by name and title.	___	___	_____
• Explained the procedure before starting and during the procedure.	___	___	_____
• Protected the person's rights during the procedure.	___	___	_____
• Handled the person gently during the procedure.	___	___	_____

Pre-Procedure

1. Followed *Delegation Guidelines:*
   a. *Safely Transferring the Person* ___ ___ _____
   b. *Stand and Pivot Transfers* ___ ___ _____
   Saw *Promoting Safety and Comfort:*
   a. *Transfer Belts* ___ ___ _____
   b. *Safely Transferring the Person* ___ ___ _____
   c. *Stand and Pivot Transfer* ___ ___ _____
   d. *Bed to Chair or Wheelchair Transfers* ___ ___ _____
   e. *Transferring the Person To and From the Toilet* ___ ___ _____
2. Practiced hand hygiene.

Procedure

3. Placed non-skid footwear on the person.
4. Positioned the wheelchair next to the toilet if there is enough room. If not, positioned the chair at a right angle (90-degree angle) to the toilet. It is best if the person's strong side is near the toilet. ___ ___ _____
5. Locked (braked) the wheelchair wheels. ___ ___ _____
6. Raised the footplates. Removed or swung front rigging out of the way. ___ ___ _____
7. Applied the transfer belt. ___ ___ _____
8. Helped the person unfasten clothing. ___ ___ _____
9. Used the transfer belt to help the person stand and to pivot (turn) to the toilet. The person used the grab bars to pivot (turn) to the toilet. ___ ___ _____
10. Supported the person with the transfer belt while he or she lowered clothing. Or had the person hold on to the grab bars for support. Lowered the person's clothing. ___ ___ _____
11. Used the transfer belt to lower the person onto the toilet seat. Checked for proper positioning on the toilet. ___ ___ _____
12. Removed the transfer belt. ___ ___ _____
13. Told the person you would stay nearby. Reminded the person to use the call light or call for you when help was needed. Stayed with the person if required by the care plan. ___ ___ _____
14. Closed the bathroom door for privacy. ___ ___ _____
15. Stayed near the bathroom. Completed other tasks in the person's room. Checked on the person every 5 minutes. ___ ___ _____
16. Knocked on the bathroom door when the person called for you. ___ ___ _____
17. Helped with wiping, perineal care, flushing, and hand-washing as needed. Wore gloves and practiced hand hygiene after removing the gloves. ___ ___ _____
18. Applied the transfer belt. ___ ___ _____
19. Used the transfer belt to help the person stand. ___ ___ _____
20. Helped the person raise and secure clothing. ___ ___ _____
21. Used the transfer belt to transfer the person to the wheelchair. ___ ___ _____
22. Made sure the person's buttocks were to the back of the seat. Positioned the person in good alignment. ___ ___ _____

Date of Satisfactory Completion _____   Instructor's Initials _____

Procedure—cont'd

	S	U	Comments
23. Positioned the person's feet on the footplates.	___	___	_____
24. Removed the transfer belt.	___	___	_____
25. Covered the person's lap and legs with a lap blanket. Kept the blanket off the floor and wheels.	___	___	_____
26. Positioned the chair as the person preferred. Locked (braked) the wheelchair wheels according to the care plan.	___	___	_____

Post-Procedure

	S	U	Comments
27. Provided for comfort.	___	___	_____
28. Placed the call light and other needed items within reach.	___	___	_____
29. Unscreened the person.	___	___	_____
30. Completed a safety check of the room.	___	___	_____
31. Practiced hand hygiene.	___	___	_____
32. Reported and recorded your observations.	___	___	_____

Date of Satisfactory Completion _____   Instructor's Initials _____

Moving the Person to a Stretcher

Name: _____   Date: _____

	S	U	Comments
Quality of Life			
• Knocked before entering the person's room.	___	___	_____
• Addressed the person by name.	___	___	_____
• Introduced yourself by name and title.	___	___	_____
• Explained the procedure before starting and during the procedure.	___	___	_____
• Protected the person's rights during the procedure.	___	___	_____
• Handled the person gently during the procedure.	___	___	_____

Pre-Procedure

1. Followed *Delegation Guidelines:*
   a. *Safely Transferring the Person*   ___ ___ _____
   b. *Moving the Person to a Stretcher*   ___ ___ _____
   Saw *Promoting Safety and Comfort:*
   a. *Safely Transferring the Person*   ___ ___ _____
   b. *Moving the Person to a Stretcher*   ___ ___ _____
2. Asked 1 or 2 staff members to help you.   ___ ___ _____
3. Collected the following:
   • Stretcher covered with a sheet or bath blanket   ___ ___ _____
   • Bath blanket   ___ ___ _____
   • Pillow(s) if needed   ___ ___ _____
   • Slide sheet, lateral transfer device with slide board, drawsheet, or other assist device   ___ ___ _____
4. Practiced hand hygiene.   ___ ___ _____
5. Identified the person. Checked the identification (ID) bracelet against the assignment sheet. Used 2 identifiers. Also called the person by name.   ___ ___ _____
6. Provided for privacy.   ___ ___ _____
7. Raised the bed and stretcher for body mechanics.   ___ ___ _____

Procedure

8. Positioned yourself and co-workers.
   a. 1 or 2 workers stood on the side of the bed where the stretcher was.   ___ ___ _____
   b. 1 worker stood on the other side of the bed.   ___ ___ _____
9. Lowered the head of the bed. It was as flat as possible.   ___ ___ _____
10. Lowered the bed rails if used.   ___ ___ _____
11. Covered the person with a bath blanket. Fan-folded top linens to the foot of the bed.   ___ ___ _____
12. Positioned the assist device. Or loosened the drawsheet on each side.   ___ ___ _____
13. Used the assist device to move the person to the side of the bed. This was the side where the stretcher was.   ___ ___ _____
14. Protected the person from falling. Held the far arm and leg.   ___ ___ _____
15. Had your co-workers position the stretcher next to the bed. They stood behind the stretcher.   ___ ___ _____
16. Locked (braked) the bed and stretcher wheels.   ___ ___ _____
17. Grasped the assist device.   ___ ___ _____
18. Transferred the person to the stretcher on the "count of 3." Centered the person on the stretcher.   ___ ___ _____
19. Placed a pillow or pillows under the person's head and shoulder if allowed. Raised the head of the stretcher if allowed.   ___ ___ _____
20. Covered the person. Provided for comfort.   ___ ___ _____
21. Fastened the safety straps. Raised the side rails.   ___ ___ _____
22. Unlocked (released the brakes) the stretcher wheels. Transported the person.   ___ ___ _____

Date of Satisfactory Completion _____   Instructor's Initials _____

Post-Procedure   S   U   **Comments**

23. Practiced hand hygiene.   ___   ___   _____
24. Reported and recorded:
    • The time of the transport   ___   ___   _____
    • Where the person was transported to   ___   ___   _____
    • Who went with him or her   ___   ___   _____
    • How the transfer was tolerated   ___   ___   _____
25. Reversed the procedure to return the person to bed.   ___   ___   _____

Date of Satisfactory Completion _____   Instructor's Initials _____

Transferring the Person Using a Stand-Assist Mechanical Lift

Name: _____   Date: _____

	S	U	Comments
Quality of Life			
• Knocked before entering the person's room.	___	___	_____
• Addressed the person by name.	___	___	_____
• Introduced yourself by name and title.	___	___	_____
• Explained the procedure before starting and during the procedure.	___	___	_____
• Protected the person's rights during the procedure.	___	___	_____
• Handled the person gently during the procedure.	___	___	_____

Pre-Procedure

1. Followed *Delegation Guidelines:*
   a. *Safely Transferring the Person*
   b. *Using a Mechanical Lift*
   Saw *Promoting Safety and Comfort:*
   a. *Safely Transferring the Person*
   b. *Using a Mechanical Lift*
2. Asked a co-worker to help you (if needed).
3. Collected the following:
   • Stand-assist mechanical lift and sling
   • Arm chair or wheelchair
   • Footwear
   • Bath blanket or cushion
   • Lap blanket (if used)
4. Practiced hand hygiene.
5. Identified the person. Checked the identification (ID) bracelet against the assignment sheet. Used 2 identifiers. Also called the person by name.
6. Provided for privacy.

Procedure

7. Placed the chair (wheelchair) at the head of the bed. It was even with the head-board and about 1 foot away from the bed. Locked (braked) the wheelchair wheels. Placed a folded bath blanket or cushion in the seat if needed.
8. Assisted the person to a seated position on the side of the bed. The person was seated on the side of the bed with the feet flat on the floor. Bed wheels were locked.
9. Put footwear on the person.
10. Applied the sling.
    a. Positioned the sling at the lower back.
    b. Brought the straps around to the front of the chest. The straps were positioned under the arms.
    c. Secured the waist belt around the person's waist. Adjusted the belt so it was snug but not tight.
11. Positioned the lift in front of the person.
12. Widened the lift's base.
13. Locked (braked) the lift's wheels.
14. Directed the person to place his or her feet on the foot plate and the knees against the knee pad. Assisted as needed. If the lift had a knee strap, secured the strap around the legs. Adjusted the strap so it was snug but not tight.
15. Attached the sling to the sling hooks.
16. Directed the person to grasp the lift's hand grips.
17. Unlocked (released the brakes) the lift's wheels.

Date of Satisfactory Completion _____   Instructor's Initials _____

Procedure—cont'd   S   U   **Comments**

18. Raised the person slightly off the bed. Checked that the sling was
secure, the feet were on the foot plate, and the knees were against
the knee pad. If not, lowered the person. Corrected the problem
before proceeding.   _____   _____ _____

19. Raised the lift until the person was clear of the bed. Or raised the
person to a standing position. Followed the care plan.   _____   _____ _____

20. Adjusted the base's width to move from the bed to the chair
(wheelchair) if needed. Kept the base in the wide or open position
as much as possible.   _____   _____ _____

21. Moved the lift to the chair (wheelchair). The person's back was
toward the seat.   _____   _____ _____

22. Lowered the person into the chair (wheelchair). Guided the
person into the seat.   _____   _____ _____

23. Locked (braked) the lift's wheels.   _____   _____ _____

24. Unhooked the sling from the sling hooks.   _____   _____ _____

25. Unbuckled the waist belt. Removed the sling.   _____   _____ _____

26. Unlocked (released the brakes) the lift's wheels.   _____   _____ _____

27. Directed the person to lift the feet off of the footplate. Assisted as
needed. Moved the lift. Positioned the person's feet flat on the
floor or on the wheelchair footplates.   _____   _____ _____

28. Covered the person's lap and legs with a lap blanket (if used).
Kept it off the floor.   _____   _____ _____

Post-Procedure

29. Provided for comfort.   _____   _____ _____

30. Placed the call light and other needed items within reach. _____   _____ _____

31. Unscreened the person.   _____   _____ _____

32. Completed a safety check of the room.   _____   _____ _____

33. Practiced hand hygiene.   _____   _____ _____

34. Reported and recorded your observations.   _____   _____ _____

35. Reversed the procedure to return the person to bed.   _____   _____ _____

Date of Satisfactory Completion _____   Instructor's Initials _____

Transferring the Person Using a Full-Sling Mechanical Lift

VIDEO   VIDEO CLIP

Name: _____   Date: _____

Quality of Life	S	U	Comments

Quality of Life
- Knocked before entering the person's room.
- Addressed the person by name.
- Introduced yourself by name and title.
- Explained the procedure before starting and during the procedure.
- Protected the person's rights during the procedure.
- Handled the person gently during the procedure.

Pre-Procedure
1. Followed *Delegation Guidelines:*
   a. *Safely Transferring the Person*
   b. *Using a Mechanical Lift*
   Saw *Promoting Safety and Comfort:*
   a. *Safely Transferring the Person*
   b. *Using a Mechanical Lift*
2. Asked a co-worker to help you.
3. Collected the following:
   - Full-sling mechanical lift and sling
   - Arm chair or wheelchair
   - Footwear
   - Bath blanket or cushion
   - Lap blanket (if used)
4. Practiced hand hygiene.
5. Identified the person. Checked the identification (ID) bracelet against the assignment sheet. Used 2 identifiers. Also called the person by name.
6. Provided for privacy.
7. Raised the bed for body mechanics. Bed rails were up if used.

Procedure
8. Lowered the head of the bed to a level appropriate for the person. It is as flat as possible.
9. Stood on 1 side of the bed. Your co-worker stood on the other side.
10. Lowered the bed rails if up. Locked (braked) the bed wheels.
11. Centered the sling under the person. To position the sling, turned the person from side to side. Followed the manufacturer's instructions to position the sling.
12. Positioned the person in the semi-Fowler's position.
13. Placed the chair (wheelchair) at the head of the bed. It was even with the head-board and about 1 foot away from the bed. Placed a folded bath blanket or cushion in the seat if needed.
14. Lowered the bed so it was level with the chair.
15. Raised the lift to position it over the person.
16. Positioned the lift over the person.
17. Widened the lift's base. Locked (braked) the lift wheels.
18. Attached the sling to the sling hooks.
19. Raised the head of the bed to a comfortable level for the person.
20. Crossed the person's arms over the chest.
21. Unlocked (released the brakes) the lift wheels.
22. Raised the person slightly from the bed. Checked that the sling was secure. If not, lowered the person. Corrected the problem before proceeding.
23. Raised the lift until the person and sling were free of the bed.
24. Had your co-worker support the person's legs as you moved the lift and the person away from the bed.

Date of Satisfactory Completion _____   Instructor's Initials _____

Procedure—cont'd

	S	U	Comments
25. Adjusted the base's width to move from the bed to the chair (wheelchair) if needed. Kept the base in the wide or open position as much as possible.	___	___	_____
26. Positioned the lift so the person's back was toward the chair (wheelchair).	___	___	_____
27. Positioned the chair (wheelchair) so you could lower the person into it. Locked (braked) the wheelchair wheels.	___	___	_____
28. Lowered the person into the chair (wheelchair). Guided the person into the seat.	___	___	_____
29. Locked (braked) the lift wheels.	___	___	_____
30. Unhooked the sling. Removed the sling from under the person unless otherwise indicated.	___	___	_____
31. Put footwear on the person. Positioned the person's feet flat on the floor or on the wheelchair footplates.	___	___	_____
32. Covered the person's lap and legs with a lap blanket (if used). Kept it off the floor and wheels.	___	___	_____
33. Positioned the chair (wheelchair) as the person preferred. Locked (braked) the wheelchair wheels according to the care plan.	___	___	_____

Post-Procedure

	S	U	Comments
34. Provided for comfort.	___	___	_____
35. Placed the call light and other needed items within reach.	___	___	_____
36. Unscreened the person.	___	___	_____
37. Completed a safety check of the room.	___	___	_____
38. Practiced hand hygiene.	___	___	_____
39. Reported and recorded your observations.	___	___	_____
40. Reversed the procedure to return the person to bed.	___	___	_____

Date of Satisfactory Completion _____ Instructor's Initials _____

Making a Closed Bed

Name: _____   Date: _____

	S	U	Comments
Quality of Life			
• Knocked before entering the person's room.	___	___	_____
• Addressed the person by name.	___	___	_____
• Introduced yourself by name and title.	___	___	_____
• Explained the procedure before starting and during the procedure.	___	___	_____
• Protected the person's rights during the procedure.	___	___	_____
• Handled the person gently during the procedure.	___	___	_____

Pre-Procedure

1. Followed *Delegation Guidelines: Making Beds.* Saw *Promoting Safety and Comfort: Making Beds.* ___ ___ _____
2. Practiced hand hygiene. ___ ___ _____
3. Collected clean linens.
   - Mattress pad (if needed) ___ ___ _____
   - Bottom sheet (flat sheet or fitted sheet) ___ ___ _____
   - Waterproof drawsheet (if needed) ___ ___ _____
   - Cotton drawsheet (if needed) ___ ___ _____
   - Waterproof pad (if needed) ___ ___ _____
   - Top sheet ___ ___ _____
   - Blanket ___ ___ _____
   - A pillowcase for each pillow ___ ___ _____
   - Bath towel ___ ___ _____
   - Hand towel ___ ___ _____
   - Washcloth ___ ___ _____
   - Gown or pajamas ___ ___ _____
   - Gloves ___ ___ _____
   - Laundry bag ___ ___ _____
   - Paper towels (as a barrier for clean linens) ___ ___ _____
4. Placed linens on a clean surface. Used the paper towels as a barrier between the clean surface and the clean linens if required by agency policy. ___ ___ _____
5. Raised the bed for body mechanics. Bed rails are down. ___ ___ _____

Procedure

6. Put on gloves. ___ ___ _____
7. Removed linens. Rolled each piece away from you. Placed each piece in a laundry bag. (NOTE: Discarded the incontinence product, disposable bed protector, and disposable drawsheet in the trash. Did not put them in the laundry bag.) ___ ___ _____
8. Cleaned the bed frame and mattress (if this was your job). ___ ___ _____
9. Removed and discarded the gloves. Practiced hand hygiene. ___ ___ _____
10. Moved the mattress to the head of the bed. ___ ___ _____
11. Put the mattress pad on the mattress. It was even with the top of the mattress. ___ ___ _____
12. Placed the bottom set on the mattress pad. Unfolded it length-wise. Placed the center crease in the middle of the bed. If using a flat sheet:
    a. Positioned the lower edge even with the bottom of the mattress. ___ ___ _____
    b. Placed the large hem at the top and the small hem at the bottom. ___ ___ _____
    c. Faced hem-stitching downward, away from the person. ___ ___ _____
13. Opened the sheet. Fan-folded it to the other side of the bed. ___ ___ _____
14. Tucked the corners of a fitted sheet over the mattress at the top and then foot of the bed. For a flat sheet, tucked the top of the sheet under the mattress. The sheet was tight and smooth. ___ ___ _____
15. Made a mitered corner at the top if using a flat sheet. ___ ___ _____

Date of Satisfactory Completion _____   Instructor's Initials _____

Procedure—cont'd	**S**	**U**	**Comments**

16. *If using a cotton drawsheet:*
    a. Placed the drawsheet on the bed. It was in the middle of the mattress.
    b. Opened the drawsheet. Fan-folded it to the other side of the bed.
    c. Tucked the drawsheet under the mattress.
17. *If using waterproof and cotton drawsheets:*
    a. Placed the waterproof drawsheet on the bed. It was in the middle of the mattress.
    b. Opened the waterproof drawsheet. Fan-folded it to the other side of the bed.
    c. Placed a cotton drawsheet over the waterproof drawsheet. It covered the entire waterproof drawsheet.
    d. Opened the cotton drawsheet. Fan-folded it to the other side of the bed.
    e. Tucked both drawsheets under the mattress. Or tucked each in separately.
18. Went to the other side of the bed.
19. Mitered the top corner of the flat bottom sheet.
20. Pulled the bottom sheet tight so there were no wrinkles. Tucked in the sheet.
21. Pulled the drawsheets tight so there were no wrinkles. Tucked both in together or separately.
22. *If using a waterproof pad*, placed the waterproof pad on the bed. It was in the middle of the mattress.
23. Went to the other side of the bed.
24. Put the top sheet on the bed.
    a. Unfolded it length-wise. Placed the center crease in the middle.
    b. Placed the large hem even with the top of the mattress.
    c. Opened the sheet. Fan-folded it to the other side.
    d. Faced hem-stitching outward, away from the person.
    e. Did not tuck the bottom in yet.
    f. Never tucked top linens in on the sides.
25. Placed the blanket on the bed.
    a. Unfolded it so the center crease was in the middle.
    b. Put the upper hem about 6 to 8 inches from the top of the mattress.
    c. Opened the blanket. Fan-folded it to the other side.
    d. If steps 31 and 32 were not done, turned the top sheet down over the blanket. Hem-stitching was down, away from the person.
26. Placed the bedspread on the bed.
    a. Unfolded it so the center crease was in the middle.
    b. Placed the upper hem even with the top of the mattress.
    c. Opened and fan-folded the bedspread to the other side.
    d. Made sure the bedspread facing the door was even. It covered all top linens.
27. Tucked in top linens together at the foot of the bed so they were smooth and tight. Made a mitered corner. Left the side of the top linens untucked.
28. Went to the other side.
29. Straightened all top linens. Worked from the head of the bed to the foot.
30. Tucked in top linens together at the foot of the bed. Made a mitered corner. Left the side of top linens untucked.

Date of Satisfactory Completion _____   Instructor's Initials _____

Procedure—cont'd   S   U   Comments

31. Turned the top hem of the bedspread under the blanket to
    form a cuff.   _____ _____ _____
32. Turned the top sheet down over the bedspread. Hem-stitching
    was down. (Steps 31 and 32 are not done in some agencies.
    The bedspread covers the pillow. If so, tucked the bedspread
    under the pillow.)   _____ _____ _____
33. Put the pillowcase on the pillow. Folded extra material under the
    pillow at the seam end of the pillowcase.   _____ _____ _____
34. Placed the pillow on the bed. The open end of the pillowcase was
    away from the door. The seam was toward the head of the bed. _____ _____ _____

Post-Procedure

35. Provided for comfort. NOTE: Omitted this step if the bed was
    prepared for a new patient or resident.   _____ _____ _____
36. Attached the call light to the bed. Or placed it within the person's
    reach.   _____ _____ _____
37. Lowered the bed to a safe and comfortable level for the person.
    Locked (braked) the bed wheels.   _____ _____ _____
38. Put the towels, washcloth, gown or pajamas, and bath blanket in
    the bedside stand.   _____ _____ _____
39. Completed a safety check of the room.   _____ _____ _____
40. Followed agency policy for used linens.   _____ _____ _____
41. Practiced hand hygiene.   _____ _____ _____

Date of Satisfactory Completion _____   Instructor's Initials _____

Making an Open Bed

Name: _____   Date: _____

Quality of Life	S	U	Comments
• Knocked before entering the person's room.	___	___	_____
• Addressed the person by name.	___	___	_____
• Introduced yourself by name and title.	___	___	_____
• Explained the procedure before starting and during the procedure.	___	___	_____
• Protected the person's rights during the procedure.	___	___	_____
• Handled the person gently during the procedure.	___	___	_____

Pre-Procedure

1. Followed *Delegation Guidelines: Making Beds.*
   Saw *Promoting Safety and Comfort: Making Beds.*
2. Practiced hand hygiene.
3. Collected clean linens.
   - Mattress pad (if needed)
   - Bottom sheet (flat sheet or fitted sheet)
   - Waterproof drawsheet (if needed)
   - Cotton drawsheet (if needed)
   - Waterproof pad (if needed)
   - Top sheet
   - Blanket
   - A pillowcase for each pillow
   - Bath towel
   - Hand towel
   - Washcloth
   - Gown or pajamas
   - Gloves
   - Laundry bag
   - Paper towels (as a barrier for clean linens)

Procedure

4. Made a closed bed.
   a. Placed linens on a clean surface. Used the paper towels as a barrier between the clean surface and the clean linens if required by agency policy.
   b. Raised the bed for body mechanics. Bed rails were down.
   c. Put on gloves.
   d. Removed linens. Rolled each piece away from you. Placed each piece in a laundry bag. (NOTE: Discarded the incontinence product, disposable bed protector, and disposable drawsheet in the trash. Did not put them in the laundry bag.)
   e. Cleaned the bed frame and mattress (if this was your job).
   f. Removed and discarded the gloves. Practiced hand hygiene.
   g. Moved the mattress to the head of the bed.
   h. Put the mattress pad on the mattress. It was even with the top of the mattress.
   i. Placed the bottom set on the mattress pad. Unfolded it length-wise. Placed the center crease in the middle of the bed. If using a flat sheet:
      1) Positioned the lower edge even with the bottom of the mattress.
      2) Placed the large hem at the top and small hem at the bottom.
      3) Faced hem-stitching downward, away from the person.

Date of Satisfactory Completion _____   Instructor's Initials _____

Procedure—cont'd   S   U   Comments

   j. Opened the sheet. Fan-folded it to the other side of the bed.

   k. Tucked the corners of a fitted sheet over the mattress at the top and then foot of the bed. For a flat sheet, tucked the top of the sheet under the mattress. The sheet was tight and smooth.

   l. Made a mitered corner at the top if using a flat sheet.

  m. *If using a cotton drawsheet:*
      1) Placed the drawsheet on the bed. It was in the middle of the mattress.
      2) Opened the drawsheet. Fan-folded it to the other side of the bed.
      3) Tucked the drawsheet under the mattress.

   n. *If using waterproof and cotton drawsheets:*
      1) Placed the waterproof drawsheet on the bed. It was in the middle of the mattress.
      2) Opened the waterproof drawsheet. Fan-folded it to the other side of the bed.
      3) Placed a cotton drawsheet over the waterproof drawsheet. It covered the entire waterproof drawsheet.
      4) Opened the cotton drawsheet. Fan-folded it to the other side of the bed.
      5) Tucked both drawsheets under the mattress. Or tucked each in separately.

   o. Went to the other side of the bed.

   p. Mitered the top corner of the flat bottom sheet.

   q. Pulled the bottom sheet tight so there were no wrinkles. Tucked in the sheet.

   r. Pulled the drawsheets tight so there were no wrinkles. Tucked both in together or separately.

   s. *If using a waterproof pad*, placed the waterproof pad on the bed. It was in the middle of the mattress.

   t. Went to the other side of the bed.

   u. Put the top sheet on the bed.
      1) Unfolded it length-wise. Placed the center crease in the middle.
      2) Placed the large hem even with the top of the mattress.
      3) Opened the sheet. Fan-folded it to the other side.
      4) Faced hem-stitching outward, away from the person.
      5) Did not tuck the bottom in yet.
      6) Never tucked top linens in on the sides.

   v. Placed the blanket on the bed.
      1) Unfolded it so the center crease was in the middle.
      2) Put the upper hem about 6 to 8 inches from the top of the mattress.
      3) Opened the blanket. Fan-folded it to the other side.
      4) If step 4, aa and bb was not done, turned the top sheet down over the blanket. Hem-stitching was down, away from the person.

   w. Placed the bedspread on the bed.
      1) Unfolded it so the center crease was in the middle.
      2) Placed the upper hem even with the top of the mattress.
      3) Opened and fan-folded the bedspread to the other side.
      4) Made sure the bedspread facing the door was even. It covered all top linens.

   x. Tucked in top linens together at the foot of the bed so they were smooth and tight. Made a mitered corner. Left the side of the top linens untucked.

   y. Went to the other side.

Date of Satisfactory Completion _____   Instructor's Initials _____

Procedure—cont'd	**S**	**U**	**Comments**
z. Straightened all top linens. Worked from the head of the bed to the foot.	_____	_____	_____
aa. Tucked in top linens together at the foot of the bed. Made a mitered corner. Left the side of top linens untucked.	_____	_____	_____
bb. Turned the top hem of the bedspread under the blanket to form a cuff.	_____	_____	_____
5. Fan-folded top linens to the foot of the bed.	_____	_____	_____

Post-Procedure

	S	**U**	**Comments**
6. Attached the call light to the bed. Or placed it within the person's reach.	_____	_____	_____
7. Lowered the bed to a safe and comfortable level for the person.	_____	_____	_____
8. Put the towels, washcloth, gown or pajamas, and bath blanket in the bedside stand.	_____	_____	_____
9. Provided for comfort.	_____	_____	_____
10. Completed a safety check of the room.	_____	_____	_____
11. Followed agency policy for dirty linens.	_____	_____	_____
12. Practiced hand hygiene.	_____	_____	_____

Date of Satisfactory Completion _____   Instructor's Initials _____

Making an Occupied Bed

Name: _____   Date: _____

Quality of Life	S	U	Comments

- Knocked before entering the person's room.
- Addressed the person by name.
- Introduced yourself by name and title.
- Explained the procedure before starting and during the procedure.
- Protected the person's rights during the procedure.
- Handled the person gently during the procedure.

Pre-Procedure

1. Followed *Delegation Guidelines: Making Beds*.
   Saw *Promoting Safety and Comfort*:
   a. *Making Beds*
   b. *The Occupied Bed*
2. Practiced hand hygiene.
3. Collected the following:
   - Gloves
   - Laundry bag
   - Clean linens
   - Paper towels (as a barrier for clean linens)
4. Placed linens on a clean surface. Used the paper towels as a barrier between the clean surface and clean linens if required by agency policy.
5. Identified the person. Checked the identification (ID) bracelet against the assignment sheet. Used 2 identifiers. Also called the person by name.
6. Provided for privacy.
7. Removed the call light.
8. Raised the bed for body mechanics. Bed rails were up if used. Bed wheels were locked (braked).
9. Lowered the head of the bed. It was as flat as possible.

Procedure

10. Practiced hand hygiene. Put on gloves.
11. Loosened top linens at the foot of the bed.
12. Lowered the bed rail near you if up.
13. Folded and removed the bedspread. Folded and removed the blanket the same way. Placed each piece over the chair.
14. Covered the person with a bath blanket. Used the one in the bedside stand.
    a. Unfolded the bath blanket over the top sheet.
    b. Asked the person to hold the bath blanket. If he or she could not, tucked the top part under the person's shoulders.
    c. Grasped the top sheet under the bath blanket at the shoulders. Brought the sheet down toward the foot of the bed. Removed the sheet from under the blanket.
15. Positioned the person on his or her side facing away from you. Adjusted the pillow for comfort.
16. Loosened bottom linens from the head to the foot of the bed.
17. Fan-folded bottom linens 1 at a time toward the person. Started with the cotton drawsheet. If the mattress pad was re-used, did not fan-fold it.
18. Removed and discarded the gloves. Practiced hand hygiene. Put on clean gloves.

Date of Satisfactory Completion _____   Instructor's Initials _____

Procedure—cont'd

	S	U	Comments

19. Placed a clean mattress pad on the bed. Unfolded it length-wise. The center crease was in the middle. Fan-folded the top part toward the person. If the mattress pad was re-used, straightened and smoothed any wrinkles.

20. Placed the bottom sheet on the mattress pad. Hem-stitching was away from the person. Unfolded the sheet so the crease was in the middle. If a flat sheet was used, the small hem was even with the bottom of the mattress. Fan-folded the top part toward the person.

21. Tucked the corners of a fitted sheet over the mattress. If a flat sheet was used, made a mitered corner at the head of the bed. Tucked the sheet under the mattress from the head to the foot.

22. *If using a cotton drawsheet:*
    a. Placed the drawsheet on the bed. It was in the middle of the mattress.
    b. Opened the drawsheet. If used with a waterproof drawsheet, it covered the entire waterproof drawsheet.
    c. Fan-folded it toward the person.
    d. Tucked in excess fabric.

23. *If using a waterproof pad:*
    a. Placed the waterproof pad on the bed. It was in the middle of the mattress.
    b. Fan-folded it toward the person.

24. *If re-using the waterproof drawsheet:*
    a. Pulled the drawsheet toward you over the bottom sheet.
    b. Tucked excess material under the mattress.
    c. Placed the cotton drawsheet over the waterproof drawsheet. It covered the entire waterproof drawsheet. Fan-folded the top part toward the person. Tucked in excess fabric.

25. *If using a clean waterproof drawsheet:*
    a. Placed the waterproof drawsheet on the bed. It was in the middle of the mattress.
    b. Fan-folded the top part toward the person.
    c. Tucked in excess material.
    d. Placed the cotton drawsheet over the waterproof drawsheet. It covered the entire waterproof drawsheet. Fan-folded the top part toward the person. Tucked in excess fabric.

26. Explained to the person that he or she would roll over a "bump." Assured the person that he or she would not fall.

27. Helped the person turn to the other side. Adjusted the pillow for comfort.

28. Raised the bed rail. Went to the other side and lowered the bed rail.

29. Loosened bottom linens. Removed 1 piece at a time. Placed each piece in the laundry bag. (NOTE: Discarded the disposable bed protector, incontinence product, and disposable drawsheet in the trash. Did not put them in the laundry bag.)

30. Removed and discarded the gloves. Practiced hand hygiene.

31. Straightened and smoothed the mattress pad.

32. Pulled the clean bottom sheet toward you. Tucked the corners of a fitted sheet over the mattress. If using a flat sheet, made a mitered corner at the top. Tucked the sheet under the mattress from the head to the foot of the bed.

33. Pulled the drawsheets tightly toward you. Tucked in the drawsheets.

34. Positioned the person supine in the center of the bed. Adjusted the pillow for comfort.

Date of Satisfactory Completion _____   Instructor's Initials _____

Procedure—cont'd	S	U	Comments
35. Put the top sheet on the bed. Unfolded it length-wise. The crease was in the middle. The large hem was even with the top of the mattress. Hem-stitching was on the outside.	___	___	_____
36. Asked the person to hold the top sheet so you could remove the bath blanket. Or tucked the top sheet under the person's shoulders. Removed the bath blanket. Placed it in the laundry bag.	___	___	_____
37. Placed the blanket on the bed. Unfolded it so the crease was in the middle and it covered the person. The upper hem was 6 to 8 inches from the top of the mattress.	___	___	_____
38. Placed the bedspread on the bed. Unfolded it so the center crease was in the middle and it covered the person. The top hem was even with the mattress top.	___	___	_____
39. Turned the top hem of the bedspread under the blanket to make a cuff.	___	___	_____
40. Brought the top sheet down over the bedspread to form a cuff.	___	___	_____
41. Went to the foot of the bed.	___	___	_____
42. Made a toe pleat. Made a 2-inch pleat across the foot of the bed. The pleat was about 6 to 8 inches from the foot of the bed.	___	___	_____
43. Lifted the mattress corner with 1 arm. Tucked all top linens under the bottom of the mattress. Made a mitered corner. Left the side of the top linens untucked.	___	___	_____
44. Raised the bed rail. Went to the other side and lowered the bed rail.	___	___	_____
45. Straightened and smoothed top linens.	___	___	_____
46. Tucked all top linens under the bottom of the mattress. Made a mitered corner. Left the side of the top linens untucked.	___	___	_____
47. Changed the pillowcase(s).	___	___	_____
Post-Procedure			
48. Provided for comfort.	___	___	_____
49. Placed the call light and other needed items within reach.	___	___	_____
50. Lowered the bed to a safe and comfortable level for the person. The bed wheels were locked (braked).	___	___	_____
51. Raised or lowered bed rails. Followed the care plan.	___	___	_____
52. Put the clean towels, washcloth, gown or pajamas, and bath blanket in the bedside stand.	___	___	_____
53. Unscreened the person.	___	___	_____
54. Completed a safety check of the room.	___	___	_____
55. Followed agency policy for used linens.	___	___	_____
56. Practiced hand hygiene.	___	___	_____

Date of Satisfactory Completion _____   Instructor's Initials _____

Making a Surgical Bed

VIDEO   VIDEO CLIP

Name: _____   Date: _____

Pre-Procedure	S	U	Comments

1. Followed *Delegation Guidelines: Making Beds*.
   Saw *Promoting Safety and Comfort:*
   a. *Making Beds*
   b. *The Surgical Bed*
2. Practiced hand hygiene.
3. Collected the following:
   - Clean linens
   - Gloves
   - Laundry bag
   - Equipment requested by the nurse
   - Paper towels (as a barrier for clean linens)
4. Placed linens on a clean surface. Used the paper towels as a barrier between the clean surface and clean linens if required by agency policy.
5. Removed the call light.
6. Raised the bed for body mechanics.

Procedure

7. Removed all linens from the bed. Placed them in the laundry bag. Wore gloves. Practiced hand hygiene after removing and discarding them.
8. Made a closed bed. Did not tuck top linens under the mattress.
9. Folded all top linens at the foot of the bed back onto the bed. The fold was even with the edge of the mattress.
10. Knew on which side of the bed the stretcher would be placed. Fan-folded linens length-wise to the other side of the bed.
11. Put a pillowcase on each pillow.
12. Placed the pillow(s) on a clean surface.

Post-Procedure

13. Left the bed in its highest position.
14. Left both bed rails down.
15. Placed the clean towels, washcloth, gown or pajamas, and bath blanket in the bedside stand.
16. Moved furniture away from the bed. Allowed room for the stretcher and the staff.
17. Did not attach the call light to the bed.
18. Completed a safety check of the room.
19. Followed agency policy for used linens.
20. Practiced hand hygiene.

Date of Satisfactory Completion _____   Instructor's Initials _____

Assisting the Person to Brush and Floss the Teeth

Name: _____   Date: _____

	S	U	Comments
Quality of Life			
• Knocked before entering the person's room.	___	___	_____
• Addressed the person by name.	___	___	_____
• Introduced yourself by name and title.	___	___	_____
• Explained the procedure before starting and during the procedure.	___	___	_____
• Protected the person's rights during the procedure.	___	___	_____
• Handled the person gently during the procedure.	___	___	_____

Pre-Procedure

1. Followed *Delegation Guidelines: Oral Hygiene.* Saw *Promoting Safety and Comfort: Oral Hygiene.*   ___ ___ _____
2. Practiced hand hygiene.   ___ ___ _____
3. Collected the following:
   - Toothbrush with soft bristles   ___ ___ _____
   - Toothpaste   ___ ___ _____
   - Mouthwash (or solution noted on care plan)   ___ ___ _____
   - Dental floss (if used)   ___ ___ _____
   - Water cup with cool water   ___ ___ _____
   - Straw   ___ ___ _____
   - Kidney basin   ___ ___ _____
   - Hand towel   ___ ___ _____
   - Paper towels   ___ ___ _____
   - Gloves   ___ ___ _____
4. Placed the paper towels on the over-bed table. Arranged items on top of them.   ___ ___ _____
5. Identified the person. Checked the ID (identification) bracelet against the assignment sheet. Used 2 identifiers. Also called the person by name.   ___ ___ _____
6. Provided for privacy.   ___ ___ _____
7. Lowered the bed rail near you if up.   ___ ___ _____

Procedure

8. Positioned the person to allow brushing with ease.   ___ ___ _____
9. Placed the towel over the person's chest. This protected garments and linens from spills.   ___ ___ _____
10. Adjusted the over-bed table in front of the person.   ___ ___ _____
11. Allowed the person to perform oral hygiene. This included brushing the teeth and tongue, rinsing the mouth, flossing, and using mouthwash or other solution.   ___ ___ _____
12. Removed the towel when the person was done.   ___ ___ _____
13. Moved the over-bed table to the side of the bed.   ___ ___ _____

Post-Procedure

14. Provided for comfort.   ___ ___ _____
15. Placed the call light and other needed items within reach.   ___ ___ _____
16. Raised or lowered bed rails. Followed the care plan.   ___ ___ _____
17. Rinsed the toothbrush. Cleaned, rinsed, and dried equipment. Returned the toothbrush and equipment to their proper place. Wore gloves.   ___ ___ _____
18. Wiped the over-bed table with the paper towels. Discarded the paper towels.   ___ ___ _____
19. Unscreened the person.   ___ ___ _____
20. Completed a safety check of the room.   ___ ___ _____
21. Followed agency policy for dirty linens.   ___ ___ _____
22. Removed and discarded the gloves. Practiced hand hygiene.   ___ ___ _____
23. Reported and recorded your observations.   ___ ___ _____

Date of Satisfactory Completion _____   Instructor's Initials _____

Brushing and Flossing the Person's Teeth

Name: _____ Date: _____

	S	U	Comments

Quality of Life
- Knocked before entering the person's room.
- Addressed the person by name.
- Introduced yourself by name and title.
- Explained the procedure before starting and during the procedure.
- Protected the person's rights during the procedure.
- Handled the person gently during the procedure.

Pre-Procedure
1. Followed *Delegation Guidelines: Oral Hygiene.*
   Saw *Promoting Safety and Comfort: Oral Hygiene.*
2. Practiced hand hygiene.
3. Collected the following:
   - Toothbrush with soft bristles
   - Toothpaste
   - Mouthwash (or solution noted on care plan)
   - Dental floss (if used)
   - Water cup with cool water
   - Straw
   - Kidney basin
   - Hand towel
   - Paper towels
   - Gloves
4. Placed the paper towels on the over-bed table. Arranged items on top of them.
5. Identified the person. Checked the ID (identification) bracelet against the assignment sheet. Used 2 identifiers. Also called the person by name.
6. Provided for privacy.
7. Raised the bed for body mechanics. Bed rails were up if used.

Procedure
8. Lowered the bed rail near you if up.
9. Assisted the person to a sitting position or side-lying position near you. (NOTE: Some state competency tests require that the person be at a 75- to 90-degree angle.)
10. Placed the towel across the person's chest.
11. Adjusted the over-bed table so you could reach it with ease.
12. Practiced hand hygiene. Put on the gloves.
13. Held the toothbrush over the kidney basin. Poured some water over the brush.
14. Applied toothpaste to the toothbrush.
15. Brushed the teeth gently. Brushed the inner, outer, and chewing surfaces of upper and lower teeth.
16. Brushed the tongue gently.
17. Allowed the person to rinse the mouth with water. Held the kidney basin under the person's chin. Repeated this step as needed.
18. Flossed the person's teeth (optional).
    a. Broke off an 18-inch piece of dental floss from the dispenser.
    b. Held the floss between the middle fingers of each hand.
    c. Stretched the floss with your thumbs. Held the floss between your thumbs and index fingers.
    d. Started at the upper back tooth on the right side. Worked around to the left side.

Date of Satisfactory Completion _____ Instructor's Initials _____

Procedure—cont'd	S	U	Comments
e. Rubbed gently against the side of the tooth. Used up-and-down motions. Did not jerk or snap the floss against the tooth. Worked from the top of the crown to the gum line.	____	____	____
f. Moved to a new section of floss after every second tooth.	____	____	____
g. Flossed the lower teeth. Used gentle up-and-down motions as for the upper teeth. Started on the right side. Worked around to the left side.	____	____	____
19. Allowed the person to use mouthwash or other solution. Held the kidney basin under the chin.	____	____	____
20. Wiped the person's mouth. Removed the towel.	____	____	____
21. Removed and discarded the gloves. Practiced hand hygiene.	____	____	____

Post-Procedure

	S	U	Comments
22. Provided for comfort.	____	____	____
23. Placed the call light and other needed items within reach.	____	____	____
24. Lowered the bed to a safe and comfortable level appropriate for the person. Followed the care plan.	____	____	____
25. Raised or lowered bed rails. Followed the care plan.	____	____	____
26. Rinsed the toothbrush. Cleaned, rinsed, and dried equipment. Returned the toothbrush and equipment to their proper place. Wore gloves.	____	____	____
27. Wiped off the over-bed table with the paper towels. Discarded the paper towels.	____	____	____
28. Unscreened the person.	____	____	____
29. Completed a safety check of the room.	____	____	____
30. Followed agency policy for used linens.	____	____	____
31. Removed and discarded the gloves. Practiced hand hygiene.	____	____	____
32. Reported and recorded your observations.	____	____	____

Date of Satisfactory Completion _____ Instructor's Initials _____

Providing Mouth Care for the Unconscious Person

Name: _____   Date: _____

Quality of Life	S	U	Comments
• Knocked before entering the person's room.			
• Addressed the person by name.			
• Introduced yourself by name and title.			
• Explained the procedure before starting and during the procedure.			
• Protected the person's rights during the procedure.			
• Handled the person gently during the procedure.			

Pre-Procedure

1. Followed *Delegation Guidelines: Oral Hygiene.*
   Saw *Promoting Safety and Comfort:*
   a. *Oral Hygiene*
   b. *Mouth Care for the Unconscious Person*
2. Practiced hand hygiene.
3. Collected the following:
   • Cleaning agent (checked care plan)
   • Sponge swabs
   • Padded tongue blade
   • Water cup with cool water
   • Hand towel
   • Kidney basin
   • Lip lubricant
   • Paper towels
   • Gloves
4. Placed the paper towels on the over-bed table. Arranged items on top of them.
5. Identified the person. Checked the ID (identification) bracelet against the assignment sheet. Used 2 identifiers. Also called the person by name.
6. Provided for privacy.
7. Raised the bed for body mechanics. Bed rails were up if used.

Procedure

8. Lowered the bed rail near you.
9. Positioned the person in a side-lying position near you. Turned the person's head well to the side.
10. Put on the gloves.
11. Placed the towel under the person's face.
12. Placed the kidney basin under the person's chin.
13. Separated the upper and lower teeth. Used the padded tongue blade. Was gentle. Never used force. If you had problems, asked the nurse for help.
14. Cleaned the mouth using sponge swabs moistened with the cleaning agent.
    a. Cleaned the chewing and inner surfaces of the teeth.
    b. Cleaned the gums and outer surfaces of the teeth.
    c. Swabbed the roof of the mouth, inside of the cheek, and the lips.
    d. Swabbed the tongue.
    e. Moistened a clean swab. Swabbed the mouth to rinse.
    f. Placed used swabs in the kidney basin.
15. Removed the kidney basin and supplies.
16. Wiped the person's mouth. Removed the towel.
17. Applied lubricant to the lips.
18. Removed and discarded the gloves. Practiced hand hygiene.

Date of Satisfactory Completion _____   Instructor's Initials _____

Post-Procedure	S	U	Comments
19. Provided for comfort.	___	___	_____
20. Placed the call light and other needed items within reach.	___	___	_____
21. Lowered the bed to a safe and comfortable level for the person. Followed the care plan.	___	___	_____
22. Raised or lowered bed rails. Followed the care plan.	___	___	_____
23. Cleaned, rinsed, dried, and returned equipment to its proper place. Discarded disposable items. (Wore gloves.)	___	___	_____
24. Wiped off the over-bed table with paper towels. Discarded the paper towels.	___	___	_____
25. Unscreened the person.	___	___	_____
26. Completed a safety check of the room.	___	___	_____
27. Told the person that you were leaving the room. Told the person when you would return.	___	___	_____
28. Followed agency policy for dirty linens.	___	___	_____
29. Removed and discarded the gloves. Practiced hand hygiene.	___	___	_____
30. Reported and recorded your observations.	___	___	_____

Date of Satisfactory Completion _____   Instructor's Initials _____

Providing Denture Care

Name: _____   Date: _____

Quality of Life	S	U	Comments
• Knocked before entering the person's room.	___	___	_____
• Addressed the person by name.	___	___	_____
• Introduced yourself by name and title.	___	___	_____
• Explained the procedure before starting and during the procedure.	___	___	_____
• Protected the person's rights during the procedure.	___	___	_____
• Handled the person gently during the procedure.	___	___	_____

Pre-Procedure

1. Followed *Delegation Guidelines: Oral Hygiene.*
   Saw *Promoting Safety and Comfort:*
   a. *Oral Hygiene*
   b. *Denture Care*
2. Practiced hand hygiene.
3. Collected the following:
   - Denture brush or toothbrush (for cleaning dentures)
   - Denture cup labeled with the person's name and room and bed number
   - Denture cleaning agent
   - Soft-bristled toothbrush or sponge swabs (for oral hygiene)
   - Toothpaste
   - Water cup with cool water
   - Straw
   - Mouthwash (or other noted solution)
   - Kidney basin
   - 2 hand towels
   - Gauze squares
   - Paper towels
   - Gloves
4. Placed the paper towels on the over-bed table. Arranged items on top of them.
5. Identified the person. Checked the ID (identification) bracelet against the assignment sheet. Used 2 identifiers. Also called the person by name.
6. Provided for privacy.

Procedure

7. Lined the bottom of the sink with a towel. Did not use paper towels. Filled the sink half-way with water.
8. Raised the bed for body mechanics.
9. Lowered the bed rail near you if up.
10. Practiced hand hygiene. Put on gloves.
11. Placed the towel over the person's chest.
12. Asked the person to remove the dentures. Carefully placed them in the kidney basin.
13. Removed the dentures if the person could not do so. Used gauze squares to get a good grip on the slippery dentures.
    a. Grasped the upper denture with your thumb and index finger. Moved it up and down slightly to break the seal. Gently removed the denture. Placed it in the kidney basin.
    b. Grasped and removed the lower denture with your thumb and index finger. Turned it slightly and lifted it out of the person's mouth. Placed it in the kidney basin.
14. Followed the care plan for raising side rails.
15. Took the kidney basin, denture cup, denture brush, and denture cleaning agent to the sink.

Date of Satisfactory Completion _____   Instructor's Initials _____

Procedure—cont'd

	S	U	Comments
16. Rinsed the denture cup and lid.			
17. Rinsed each denture under cool or warm running water. Followed center policy for water temperature.			
18. Returned dentures to the kidney basin.			
19. Applied the denture cleaning agent to the brush.			
20. Brushed the dentures. Brushed the inner, outer, and chewing surfaces and all surfaces that touched the gums.			
21. Rinsed the dentures under running water. Used warm or cool water as directed by the cleaning agent manufacturer.			
22. Placed dentures in the denture cup. Covered the dentures with cool or warm water. Followed center policy for water temperature.			
23. Cleaned the kidney basin.			
24. Took the denture cup and kidney basin to the over-bed table.			
25. Lowered the bed rail if up.			
26. Positioned the person for oral hygiene.			
27. Cleaned the person's gums and tongue. Brushed any natural teeth. Used toothpaste and the toothbrush (or sponge swab).			
28. Had the person use mouthwash (or noted solution). Held the kidney basin under the chin.			
29. Asked the person to insert the dentures. Inserted them if the person could not.			
a. Held the upper denture firmly with your thumb and index finger. Raised the upper lip with the other hand. Inserted the denture. Gently pressed on the denture with your index fingers to make sure it was in place.			
b. Held the lower denture with your thumb and index finger. Pulled the lower lip down slightly. Inserted the denture. Gently pressed down on it to make sure it was in place.			
30. Placed the denture cup in the top drawer of the bedside stand if the dentures were not worn. The dentures were in water or in a denture soaking solution.			
31. Wiped the person's mouth. Removed the towel.			
32. Removed and discarded the gloves. Practiced hand hygiene.			

Post-Procedure

	S	U	Comments
33. Assisted with hand-washing.			
34. Provided for comfort.			
35. Placed the call light and other needed items within reach.			
36. Lowered the bed to a safe and comfortable level appropriate for the person. Followed the care plan.			
37. Raised or lowered bed rails. Followed the care plan.			
38. Removed the towel from the sink. Drained the sink.			
39. Rinsed the brushes. Cleaned, rinsed, and dried equipment. Returned brushes and equipment to their proper place. Discarded disposable items. Wore gloves for this step.			
40. Wiped off the over-bed table with the paper towels. Discarded the paper towels.			
41. Unscreened the person.			
42. Completed a safety check of the room.			
43. Followed center policy for dirty linens.			
44. Removed and discarded the gloves. Practiced hand hygiene.			
45. Reported and recorded your observations.			

Date of Satisfactory Completion _____   Instructor's Initials _____

Giving a Complete Bed Bath

NATCEP™ · VIDEO · VIDEO CLIP

Name: _____   Date: _____

	S	U	Comments

Quality of Life
- Knocked before entering the person's room.
- Addressed the person by name.
- Introduced yourself by name and title.
- Explained the procedure before starting and during the procedure.
- Protected the person's rights during the procedure.
- Handled the person gently during the procedure.

Pre-Procedure
1. Followed *Delegation Guidelines: Bathing*.
   Saw *Promoting Safety and Comfort:*
   a. *Personal Hygiene*
   b. *Bathing*
2. Practiced hand hygiene.
3. Identified the person. Checked the identification (ID) bracelet against the assignment sheet. Used 2 identifiers. Also called the person by name.
4. Collected clean linens. Placed linens on a clean surface.
5. Collected the following:
   - Wash basin
   - Soap
   - Bath thermometer
   - Orangewood stick or nail file
   - Washcloth (and at least 4 washcloths for perineal care)
   - 2 bath towels and 2 hand towels
   - Bath blanket
   - Clothing or sleepwear
   - Lotion
   - Powder
   - Deodorant or antiperspirant
   - Brush and comb
   - Other grooming items as requested
   - Paper towels
   - Gloves
6. Covered the over-bed table with paper towels. Arranged items on the over-bed table. Adjusted the height as needed.
7. Provided for privacy.
8. Raised the bed for body mechanics. Bed rails were up if used. Lowered the bed rail near you if up.

Procedure
9. Practiced hand hygiene. Put on gloves.
10. Removed the sleepwear. Did not expose the person. Followed agency policy for used sleepwear.
11. Covered the person with a bath blanket. Removed top linens.
12. Lowered the head of the bed. It was as flat as possible. The person had at least 1 pillow.
13. Filled the wash basin ⅔ (two-thirds) full with water. Raised the bed rail before leaving the bedside. Followed the care plan for water temperature. Water temperature was 110°F to 115°F (43.3°C to 46.1°C) for adults. Measured water temperature. Used the bath thermometer. Or dipped your elbow or inner wrist into the basin to test the water.
14. Lowered the bed rail near you if up.

Date of Satisfactory Completion _____   Instructor's Initials _____

Procedure—cont'd	S	U	Comments
15. Asked the person to check the water temperature. Adjusted the water temperature if too hot or too cold. Raised the bed rail before leaving the bedside. Lowered the bed rail when you returned.	___	___	_____
16. Placed the basin on the over-bed table.	___	___	_____
17. Placed a hand towel over the person's chest.	___	___	_____
18. Made a mitt with the washcloth. Used a mitt for the entire bath.	___	___	_____
19. Washed around the person's eyes with water. Did not use soap.			
a. Cleaned the far eye. Gently wiped from the inner to the outer aspect of the eye with a corner of the mitt.	___	___	_____
b. Cleaned around the eye near you. Used a clean part of the washcloth for each stroke.	___	___	_____
20. Asked the person if you should use soap to wash the face.	___	___	_____
21. Washed the face, ears, and neck. Rinsed and patted dry with the towel on the chest.	___	___	_____
22. Helped the person move to the side of the bed near you.	___	___	_____
23. Exposed the far arm. Placed a bath towel length-wise under the arm. Applied soap to the washcloth.	___	___	_____
24. Supported the arm with your palm under the person's elbow. His or her forearm rested on your forearm.			
25. Washed the arm, shoulder, and underarm. Used long, firm strokes. Rinsed and patted dry.	___	___	_____
26. Placed the basin on the towel. Put the person's hand into the water. Washed the hand well. Cleaned under the fingernails with an orangewood stick or nail file.	___	___	_____
27. Had the person exercise the hand and fingers.	___	___	_____
28. Removed the basin. Dried the hand well. Covered the arm with the bath blanket.	___	___	_____
29. Repeated for the near arm.			
a. Placed a bath towel length-wise under the near arm.	___	___	_____
b. Supported the arm with your palm under the person's elbow. His or her forearm rested on your forearm.	___	___	_____
c. Washed the arm, shoulder, and underarm. Used long, firm strokes. Rinsed and patted dry.	___	___	_____
d. Placed the basin on the towel. Put the person's hand into the water. Washed the hand well. Cleaned under the fingernails with an orangewood stick or nail file.	___	___	_____
e. Had the person exercise the hand and fingers.			
f. Removed the basin. Dried the hand well. Covered the arm with the bath blanket.	___	___	_____
30. Placed a bath towel over the chest cross-wise. Held the towel in place. Pulled the bath blanket from under the towel to the waist. Applied soap to the washcloth.	___	___	_____
31. Lifted the towel slightly and washed the chest. Did not expose the person. Rinsed and patted dry, especially under the breasts.	___	___	_____
32. Moved the towel length-wise over the chest and abdomen. Did not expose the person. Pulled the bath blanket down to the pubic area. Applied soap to the washcloth.	___	___	_____
33. Lifted the towel slightly and washed the abdomen. Rinsed and patted dry.	___	___	_____
34. Pulled the bath blanket up to the shoulders. Covered both arms. Removed the towel.	___	___	_____
35. Changed soapy or cool water. Measured bath water temperature. Water temperature was 110°F to 115°F (43.3°C to 46.1°C) for adults. Used the bath thermometer. Or dipped your elbow or inner wrist into the basin to test the water. If bed rails were used, raised the bed rail near you before leaving the bedside. Lowered it when you returned.	___	___	_____

Date of Satisfactory Completion _____   Instructor's Initials _____

Procedure—cont'd   S   U   **Comments**

36. Uncovered the far leg. Did not expose the genital area. Placed a towel length-wise under the foot and leg. Applied soap to the washcloth.   _____   _____   _____

37. Bent the knee and supported the leg with your arm. Washed it with long, firm strokes. Rinsed and patted dry.   _____   _____   _____

38. Placed the basin on the towel near the foot.   _____   _____   _____

39. Lifted the leg slightly. Slid the basin under the foot.   _____   _____   _____

40. Placed the foot in the basin. Used an orangewood stick or nail file to clean under toenails if necessary. If the person could not bend the knees:

   a. Washed the foot. Carefully separated the toes. Rinsed and patted dry.   _____   _____   _____

   b. Cleaned under the toenails with the orangewood stick or nail file if necessary.   _____   _____   _____

41. Removed the basin. Dried the leg and foot. Applied lotion to the foot if directed by the nurse and care plan. Covered the leg with the bath blanket. Removed the towel.   _____   _____   _____

42. Repeated for the near leg.

   a. Uncovered the near leg. Did not expose the genital area. Placed a towel length-wise under the foot and leg.   _____   _____   _____

   b. Bent the knee and supported the leg with your arm. Washed it with long, firm strokes. Rinsed and patted dry.   _____   _____   _____

   c. Placed the basin on the towel near the foot.   _____   _____   _____

   d. Lifted the leg slightly. Slid the basin under the foot.   _____   _____   _____

   e. Placed the foot in the basin. Used an orangewood stick or nail file to clean under toenails if necessary. If the person could not bend the knee:

      1) Washed the foot. Carefully separated the toes. Rinsed and patted dry.   _____   _____   _____

      2) Cleaned under the toenails with an orangewood stick or nail file if necessary.   _____   _____   _____

   f. Removed the basin. Dried the leg and foot. Applied lotion to the foot if directed by the nurse and care plan. Covered the leg with the bath blanket. Removed the towel.   _____   _____   _____

43. Changed the water. Measured water temperature. Water temperature was 110°F to 115°F (43.3°C to 46.1°C) for adults. Used the bath thermometer. Or dipped your elbow or inner wrist into the basin to test the water. Raised the bed rail near you before leaving the bedside. Lowered it when you returned.   _____   _____   _____

44. Turned the person onto the side away from you. The person was covered with the bath blanket.   _____   _____   _____

45. Uncovered the back and buttocks. Did not expose the person. Placed a towel length-wise on the bed along the back. Applied soap to the washcloth.   _____   _____   _____

46. Washed the back. Worked from the back of the neck to the lower end of the buttocks. Used long, firm, continuous strokes. Rinsed and dried well.   _____   _____   _____

47. Turned the person onto his or her back.   _____   _____   _____

48. Changed the water for perineal care. Water temperature was 105°F to 109°F (40.5°C to 42.7°C). Followed the care plan for water temperature. Measured water temperature according to agency policy. (Some state competency tests also require changing gloves and hand hygiene completed at this time.) Raised the bed rail near you before leaving the bedside. Lowered it when you returned.   _____   _____   _____

49. Allowed the person to perform perineal care if able. Provided perineal care if the person could not do so. At least 4 washcloths were used. (Practiced hand hygiene and wore gloves for perineal care.)   _____   _____   _____

Date of Satisfactory Completion _____   Instructor's Initials _____

	S	U	Comments

Procedure—cont'd

50. Removed and discarded the gloves. Practiced hand hygiene.
51. Gave a back massage.
52. Applied deodorant or antiperspirant. Applied lotion and powder as requested. Saw *Promoting Safety and Comfort: Bathing.*
53. Put clean garments on the person.
54. Combed and brushed the hair.
55. Made the bed.

Post-Procedure

56. Provided for comfort.
57. Placed the call light and other needed items within reach.
58. Lowered the bed to a safe and comfortable level for the person. Followed the care plan.
59. Raised or lowered bed rails. Followed the care plan.
60. Put on clean gloves.
61. Emptied, cleaned, rinsed, and dried the wash basin. Returned it and other supplies to their proper place.
62. Wiped off the over-bed table with paper towels. Discarded the paper towels.
63. Unscreened the person.
64. Completed a safety check of the room.
65. Followed center policy for used linens.
66. Removed and discarded the gloves. Practiced hand hygiene.
67. Reported and recorded your observations.

Date of Satisfactory Completion _____   Instructor's Initials _____

Assisting With the Partial Bath

NATCEP™ VIDEO

Name: _____   Date: _____

Quality of Life	S	U	Comments

Quality of Life
- Knocked before entering the person's room.
- Addressed the person by name.
- Introduced yourself by name and title.
- Explained the procedure before starting and during the procedure.
- Protected the person's rights during the procedure.
- Handled the person gently during the procedure.

Pre-Procedure
1. Followed *Delegation Guidelines: Bathing.*
   Saw *Promoting Safety and Comfort:*
   a. *Bathing*
   b. *Personal Hygiene*
2. Did the following:
   a. Practiced hand hygiene.
   b. Identified the person. Checked the identification (ID) bracelet against the assignment sheet. Used 2 identifiers. Also called the person by name.
   c. Collected clean linens. Placed linens on a clean surface.
   d. Collected the following:
      - Wash basin
      - Soap
      - Bath thermometer
      - Orangewood stick or nail file
      - Washcloth (and at least 4 washcloths for perineal care).
      - 2 bath towels and 2 hand towels
      - Bath blanket
      - Clothing or sleepwear
      - Lotion
      - Powder
      - Deodorant or antiperspirant
      - Brush and comb
      - Other grooming items as requested
      - Paper towels
      - Gloves
   e. Covered the over-bed table with paper towels. Arranged items on the over-bed table. Adjusted the height as needed.
   f. Provided for privacy.

Procedure
3. Made sure the bed was in the lowest position.
4. Practiced hand hygiene. Put on gloves.
5. Covered the person with a bath blanket. Removed top linens.
6. Filled the wash basin ⅔ (two-thirds) full with water. Water temperature was 110°F to 115°F (43.3°C to 46.1°C) or as directed by the nurse. Measured water temperature with the bath thermometer. Or tested bath water by dipping your elbow or inner wrist into the basin.
7. Asked the person to check the water temperature. Adjusted if it was too hot or too cold.
8. Placed the basin on the over-bed table.
9. Positioned the person in Fowler's position. Or assisted him or her to sit at the bedside.
10. Adjusted the over-bed table so the person could reach the basin and supplies.

Date of Satisfactory Completion _____   Instructor's Initials _____

Procedure—cont'd	S	U	Comments
11. Helped the person undress. Used the bath blanket for privacy and warmth.	___	___	_____
12. Asked the person to wash easy-to-reach body parts. Explained that you would wash the back and areas the person could not reach.	___	___	_____
13. Placed the call light within reach. Asked him or her to signal when help was needed or bathing was completed.	___	___	_____
14. Removed and discarded the gloves. Practiced hand hygiene. Then left the room.	___	___	_____
15. Returned when the call light was on. Knocked before entering. Practiced hand hygiene.	___	___	_____
16. Changed the bath water. Measured bath water temperature (110°F to 115°F or 43.3°C to 46.1°C or as directed by the nurse). Used the bath thermometer. Or tested the water by dipping your elbow or inner wrist into the basin.	___	___	_____
17. Raised the bed for body mechanics. The far bed rail was up if used.	___	___	_____
18. Asked what was washed. Put on gloves. Washed and dried areas the person could not reach. The face, hands, underarms, back, buttocks, and perineal area were washed for the partial bath.	___	___	_____
19. Removed and discarded the gloves. Practiced hand hygiene.	___	___	_____
20. Gave a back massage.	___	___	_____
21. Applied lotion, powder, and deodorant or antiperspirant as requested.	___	___	_____
22. Helped the person put on clean garments.	___	___	_____
23. Assisted with hair care and other grooming needs.	___	___	_____
24. Made the bed.	___	___	_____

Post-Procedure

	S	U	Comments
25. Provided for comfort.	___	___	_____
26. Placed the call light and other needed items within reach.	___	___	_____
27. Lowered the bed to a safe and comfortable level appropriate for the person. Followed the care plan.	___	___	_____
28. Raised or lowered bed rails. Followed the care plan.	___	___	_____
29. Put on clean gloves.	___	___	_____
30. Emptied, cleaned, rinsed, and dried the bath basin. Returned it and supplies to their proper place.	___	___	_____
31. Wiped off the over-bed table with the paper towels. Discarded the paper towels.	___	___	_____
32. Unscreened the person.	___	___	_____
33. Completed a safety check of the room.	___	___	_____
34. Followed center policy for used linens.	___	___	_____
35. Removed and discarded the gloves. Practiced hand hygiene.	___	___	_____
36. Reported and recorded your observations.	___	___	_____

Date of Satisfactory Completion _____   Instructor's Initials _____

Assisting With a Tub Bath or Shower

Name: _____ Date: _____

Quality of Life	S	U	Comments
• Knocked before entering the person's room.	___	___	_____
• Addressed the person by name.	___	___	_____
• Introduced yourself by name and title.	___	___	_____
• Explained the procedure before starting and during the procedure.	___	___	_____
• Protected the person's rights during the procedure.	___	___	_____
• Handled the person gently during the procedure.	___	___	_____

Pre-Procedure

	S	U	Comments
1. Followed *Delegation Guidelines:*			
a. *Bathing*	___	___	_____
b. *Tub Baths and Showers*	___	___	_____
Saw *Promoting Safety and Comfort:*			
a. *Personal Hygiene*	___	___	_____
b. *Bathing*	___	___	_____
c. *Tub Baths and Showers*	___	___	_____
2. Reserved the tub or shower room.	___	___	_____
3. Practiced hand hygiene.	___	___	_____
4. Identified the person. Checked the identification (ID) bracelet against the assignment sheet. Used 2 identifiers. Also called the person by name.	___	___	_____
5. Collected the following:			
• Washcloth and 2 bath towels	___	___	_____
• Bath blanket	___	___	_____
• Soap	___	___	_____
• Bath thermometer (for tub bath)	___	___	_____
• Clothing or sleepwear	___	___	_____
• Grooming items as requested	___	___	_____
• Robe and non-skid footwear	___	___	_____
• Rubber bath mat if needed	___	___	_____
• Disposable bath mat	___	___	_____
• Gloves	___	___	_____
• Wheelchair, shower chair, transfer bench, and so on as needed	___	___	_____

Procedure

	S	U	Comments
6. Placed items in the tub or shower room. Used the space provided or a chair.	___	___	_____
7. Cleaned, disinfected, and dried the tub or shower (wore gloves for this step).	___	___	_____
8. Placed a rubber bath mat in the tub or on the shower floor. Did not block the drain.	___	___	_____
9. Placed the disposable bath mat on the floor in front of the tub or shower.	___	___	_____
10. Placed the OCCUPIED sign on the door.	___	___	_____
11. Returned to the person's room. Provided for privacy. Practiced hand hygiene.	___	___	_____
12. Helped the person sit on the side of the bed.	___	___	_____
13. Helped the person put on a robe and non-skid footwear. Or the person left on clothing.	___	___	_____
14. Assisted or transported the person to the tub or shower room.	___	___	_____
15. Had the person sit on a chair if he or she walked to the tub or shower room.	___	___	_____
16. Provided for privacy.	___	___	_____

Date of Satisfactory Completion _____ Instructor's Initials _____

Procedure—cont'd   S   U   **Comments**

17. *For a tub bath:*
    a. Filled the tub halfway with warm water (usually 105°F; 40.5°C). Followed the care plan for water temperature.   _____ _____ _____
    b. Measured water temperature. Used the bath thermometer or checked the digital display.   _____ _____ _____
    c. Asked the person to check the water temperature. Adjusted the water temperature if it was too hot or too cold.   _____ _____ _____
18. *For a shower:*
    a. Turned on the shower.   _____ _____ _____
    b. Adjusted water temperature and pressure. Checked the digital display.   _____ _____ _____
    c. Asked the person to check the water temperature. Adjusted the water if too hot or too cold.   _____ _____ _____
19. Helped the person undress and removed footwear.   _____ _____ _____
20. Helped the person into the tub or shower. Positioned the shower chair and locked (braked) the wheels.   _____ _____ _____
21. Assisted with washing as necessary. Wore gloves.   _____ _____ _____
22. Asked the person to use the call light when done or when help is needed. Reminded the person that a tub bath lasts no longer than 20 minutes.   _____ _____ _____
23. Placed a towel across the chair.   _____ _____ _____
24. Left the room if the person could bathe alone. If not, stayed in the room or nearby. Removed and discarded the gloves and practiced hand hygiene if you left the room.   _____ _____ _____
25. Checked the person at least every 5 minutes.   _____ _____ _____
26. Returned when he or she signaled for you. Knocked before entering. Practiced hand hygiene.   _____ _____ _____
27. Turned off the shower or drained the tub. Covered the person with the bath blanket while the tub drained.   _____ _____ _____
28. Helped the person out of the shower or tub and onto a chair.   _____ _____ _____
29. Helped the person dry off. Patted gently. Dried under the breasts, between skin folds, in the perineal area, and between the toes.   _____ _____ _____
30. Assisted with lotion and other grooming items as needed.   _____ _____ _____
31. Helped the person dress and put on footwear.   _____ _____ _____
32. Helped the person return to the room. Provided for privacy.   _____ _____ _____
33. Assisted the person to a chair or into bed.   _____ _____ _____
34. Provided a back massage if the person returned to bed.   _____ _____ _____
35. Assisted with hair care and other grooming needs.   _____ _____ _____

Post-Procedure
36. Provided for comfort.   _____ _____ _____
37. Placed the call light and other needed items within reach.   _____ _____ _____
38. Raised or lowered bed rails. Followed the care plan.   _____ _____ _____
39. Unscreened the person.   _____ _____ _____
40. Completed a safety check of the room.   _____ _____ _____
41. Cleaned, disinfected, and dried the tub or shower. Removed soiled linens. Wore gloves.   _____ _____ _____
42. Discarded disposable items. Put the UNOCCUPIED sign on the door. Returned supplies to their proper place.   _____ _____ _____
43. Followed center policy for dirty linens.   _____ _____ _____
44. Removed and discarded the gloves. Practiced hand hygiene.   _____ _____ _____
45. Reported and recorded your observations.   _____ _____ _____

Date of Satisfactory Completion _____   Instructor's Initials _____

NATCEP™ VIDEO VIDEO CLIP   Giving Female Perineal Care

Name: _____   Date: _____

Quality of Life	S	U	Comments
• Knocked before entering the person's room.	____	____	_____
• Addressed the person by name.	____	____	_____
• Introduced yourself by name and title.	____	____	_____
• Explained the procedure before starting and during the procedure.	____	____	_____
• Protected the person's rights during the procedure.	____	____	_____
• Handled the person gently during the procedure.	____	____	_____

Pre-Procedure

1. Followed *Delegation Guidelines: Perineal Care.*
   Saw *Promoting Safety and Comfort:*
   a. *Personal Hygiene*   ____ ____ _____
   b. *Perineal Care*   ____ ____ _____
2. Practiced hand hygiene.   ____ ____ _____
3. Collected the following:
   - Soap or other cleaning agent as directed   ____ ____ _____
   - At least 4 washcloths   ____ ____ _____
   - Bath towel   ____ ____ _____
   - Bath blanket   ____ ____ _____
   - Bath thermometer   ____ ____ _____
   - Wash basin   ____ ____ _____
   - Waterproof pad   ____ ____ _____
   - Gloves   ____ ____ _____
   - Laundry bag   ____ ____ _____
   - Paper towels   ____ ____ _____
4. Covered the over-bed table with paper towels. Arranged items on top of them.   ____ ____ _____
5. Identified the person. Checked the identification (ID) bracelet against the assignment sheet. Used 2 identifiers. Also called the person by name.   ____ ____ _____
6. Provided for privacy.   ____ ____ _____
7. Raised the bed for body mechanics.
   Bed rails were up if used.   ____ ____ _____

Procedure

8. Lowered the bed rail near you if up.   ____ ____ _____
9. Practiced hand hygiene. Put on gloves.   ____ ____ _____
10. Covered the person with a bath blanket. Moved top linens to the foot of the bed.   ____ ____ _____
11. Positioned the person on her back.   ____ ____ _____
12. Draped the person.   ____ ____ _____
13. Raised the bed rail if used.   ____ ____ _____
14. Filled the wash basin. Water temperature was 105°F to 109°F (40.5°C to 42.7°C). Followed the care plan for water temperature. Measured water temperature according to agency policy.   ____ ____ _____
15. Asked the person to check the water temperature. Adjusted if it was too hot or too cold. Raised the bed rail before leaving the bedside. Lowered it when you returned.   ____ ____ _____
16. Placed the basin on the over-bed table.   ____ ____ _____
17. Lowered the bed rail if up.   ____ ____ _____
18. Helped the person flex her knees and spread her legs. Or helped her spread her legs as much as possible with the knees straight.   ____ ____ _____
19. Folded the corner of the bath blanket between her legs onto her abdomen.   ____ ____ _____
20. Placed a waterproof pad under her buttocks. Removed any wet or soiled incontinence products.   ____ ____ _____

Date of Satisfactory Completion _____   Instructor's Initials _____

Procedure—cont'd | S | U | Comments

17. *For a tub bath:*
    a. Filled the tub halfway with warm water (usually 105°F; 40.5°C). Followed the care plan for water temperature.
    b. Measured water temperature. Used the bath thermometer or checked the digital display.
    c. Asked the person to check the water temperature. Adjusted the water temperature if it was too hot or too cold.
18. *For a shower:*
    a. Turned on the shower.
    b. Adjusted water temperature and pressure. Checked the digital display.
    c. Asked the person to check the water temperature. Adjusted the water if too hot or too cold.
19. Helped the person undress and removed footwear.
20. Helped the person into the tub or shower. Positioned the shower chair and locked (braked) the wheels.
21. Assisted with washing as necessary. Wore gloves.
22. Asked the person to use the call light when done or when help is needed. Reminded the person that a tub bath lasts no longer than 20 minutes.
23. Placed a towel across the chair.
24. Left the room if the person could bathe alone. If not, stayed in the room or nearby. Removed and discarded the gloves and practiced hand hygiene if you left the room.
25. Checked the person at least every 5 minutes.
26. Returned when he or she signaled for you. Knocked before entering. Practiced hand hygiene.
27. Turned off the shower or drained the tub. Covered the person with the bath blanket while the tub drained.
28. Helped the person out of the shower or tub and onto a chair.
29. Helped the person dry off. Patted gently. Dried under the breasts, between skin folds, in the perineal area, and between the toes.
30. Assisted with lotion and other grooming items as needed.
31. Helped the person dress and put on footwear.
32. Helped the person return to the room. Provided for privacy.
33. Assisted the person to a chair or into bed.
34. Provided a back massage if the person returned to bed.
35. Assisted with hair care and other grooming needs.

Post-Procedure
36. Provided for comfort.
37. Placed the call light and other needed items within reach.
38. Raised or lowered bed rails. Followed the care plan.
39. Unscreened the person.
40. Completed a safety check of the room.
41. Cleaned, disinfected, and dried the tub or shower. Removed soiled linens. Wore gloves.
42. Discarded disposable items. Put the UNOCCUPIED sign on the door. Returned supplies to their proper place.
43. Followed center policy for dirty linens.
44. Removed and discarded the gloves. Practiced hand hygiene.
45. Reported and recorded your observations.

Date of Satisfactory Completion _____   Instructor's Initials _____

NATCEP   VIDEO   VIDEO CLIP   **Giving Female Perineal Care**

Name: _____   Date: _____

	S	U	Comments

Quality of Life
- Knocked before entering the person's room.
- Addressed the person by name.
- Introduced yourself by name and title.
- Explained the procedure before starting and during the procedure.
- Protected the person's rights during the procedure.
- Handled the person gently during the procedure.

Pre-Procedure
1. Followed *Delegation Guidelines: Perineal Care.*
   Saw *Promoting Safety and Comfort:*
   a. *Personal Hygiene*
   b. *Perineal Care*
2. Practiced hand hygiene.
3. Collected the following:
   - Soap or other cleaning agent as directed
   - At least 4 washcloths
   - Bath towel
   - Bath blanket
   - Bath thermometer
   - Wash basin
   - Waterproof pad
   - Gloves
   - Laundry bag
   - Paper towels
4. Covered the over-bed table with paper towels. Arranged items on top of them.
5. Identified the person. Checked the identification (ID) bracelet against the assignment sheet. Used 2 identifiers. Also called the person by name.
6. Provided for privacy.
7. Raised the bed for body mechanics.
   Bed rails were up if used.

Procedure
8. Lowered the bed rail near you if up.
9. Practiced hand hygiene. Put on gloves.
10. Covered the person with a bath blanket. Moved top linens to the foot of the bed.
11. Positioned the person on her back.
12. Draped the person.
13. Raised the bed rail if used.
14. Filled the wash basin. Water temperature was 105°F to 109°F (40.5°C to 42.7°C). Followed the care plan for water temperature. Measured water temperature according to agency policy.
15. Asked the person to check the water temperature. Adjusted if it was too hot or too cold. Raised the bed rail before leaving the bedside. Lowered it when you returned.
16. Placed the basin on the over-bed table.
17. Lowered the bed rail if up.
18. Helped the person flex her knees and spread her legs. Or helped her spread her legs as much as possible with the knees straight.
19. Folded the corner of the bath blanket between her legs onto her abdomen.
20. Placed a waterproof pad under her buttocks. Removed any wet or soiled incontinence products.

Date of Satisfactory Completion _____   Instructor's Initials _____

Procedure—cont'd	**S**	**U**	**Comments**
21. Removed and discarded the gloves. Practiced hand hygiene. Put on clean gloves.	_____	_____	_____
22. Wet the washcloths.	_____	_____	_____
23. Squeezed out water from a washcloth. Made a mitted washcloth. Applied soap. (Squeezed out excess water every time you changed washcloths. Did not place used washcloths back in the basin. Put used washcloths in the laundry bag.)	_____	_____	_____
24. Cleaned the perineum. Changed washcloths as needed.			
a. Spread the labia.	_____	_____	_____
b. Cleaned 1 side of the labia. Cleaned downward from front to back (top to bottom) with 1 stroke. Used 1 part of a washcloth.	_____	_____	_____
c. Cleaned the other side of the labia. Cleaned downward from front to back (top to bottom) with 1 stroke. Used a clean part of a washcloth.	_____	_____	_____
d. Cleaned the vaginal area. Cleaned downward from front to back (top to bottom) with 1 stroke. Used a clean part of a washcloth.	_____	_____	_____
25. Rinsed the perineum using a clean washcloth. Changed washcloths as needed.			
a. Separated the labia.	_____	_____	_____
b. Rinsed 1 side of the labia. Rinsed downward from front to back (top to bottom) with 1 stroke. Used 1 part of a washcloth.	_____	_____	_____
c. Rinsed the other side of the labia. Rinsed downward from front to back (top to bottom) with 1 stroke. Used a clean part of a washcloth.	_____	_____	_____
d. Rinsed the vaginal area. Rinsed downward front to back (top to bottom) with 1 stroke. Used a clean part of a washcloth.	_____	_____	_____
26. Patted the perineal area dry with the towel. Dried from front to back.	_____	_____	_____
27. Folded the blanket back between her legs.	_____	_____	_____
28. Helped the person lower her legs and turn onto her side away from you.	_____	_____	_____
29. Applied soap to a mitted washcloth. Used a clean washcloth.	_____	_____	_____
30. Cleaned and rinsed the rectal area.	_____	_____	_____
a. Cleaned from the vagina to the anus with 1 stroke. Used part of the washcloth.	_____	_____	_____
b. Repeated until the area is clean. Used a clean part of the washcloth for each stroke. Used more than 1 washcloth if needed.			
1) Applied soap to a mitted washcloth.	_____	_____	_____
2) Cleaned the rectal area. Cleaned from the vagina to the anus with 1 stroke.	_____	_____	_____
31. Patted the rectal area dry with the towel. Dried from the vagina to the anus.	_____	_____	_____
32. Removed the waterproof pad.	_____	_____	_____
33. Removed and discarded the gloves. Practiced hand hygiene. Put on clean gloves.	_____	_____	_____
34. Provided clean and dry linens and incontinence products as needed.	_____	_____	_____

Post-Procedure

	S	**U**	**Comments**
35. Covered the person. Removed the bath blanket.	_____	_____	_____
36. Provided for comfort.	_____	_____	_____
37. Placed the call light and other needed items within reach.	_____	_____	_____
38. Lowered the bed to a safe and comfortable level appropriate for the person. Followed the care plan.	_____	_____	_____
39. Raised or lowered bed rails. Followed the care plan.	_____	_____	_____
40. Emptied, cleaned, rinsed, and dried the wash basin.	_____	_____	_____

Date of Satisfactory Completion _____   Instructor's Initials _____

Post-Procedure—cont'd   S   U   **Comments**

41. Returned the basin and supplies to their proper place.   ____   ____   _____
42. Wiped off the over-bed table with the paper towels.
    Discarded the paper towels.   ____   ____   _____
43. Unscreened the person.   ____   ____   _____
44. Completed a safety check of the room.   ____   ____   _____
45. Followed agency policy for used linens.   ____   ____   _____
46. Removed and discarded the gloves. Practiced hand hygiene. ____   ____   _____
47. Reported and recorded your observations.   ____   ____   _____

Date of Satisfactory Completion _____   Instructor's Initials _____

Giving Male Perineal Care

NATCEP™ VIDEO VIDEO CLIP

Name: _____   Date: _____

Quality of Life	S	U	Comments
• Knocked before entering the person's room.	___	___	_____
• Addressed the person by name.	___	___	_____
• Introduced yourself by name and title.	___	___	_____
• Explained the procedure before starting and during the procedure.	___	___	_____
• Protected the person's rights during the procedure.	___	___	_____
• Handled the person gently during the procedure.	___	___	_____

Procedure

1. Followed these steps and draped the person.
   a. Followed *Delegation Guidelines: Perineal Care.* Saw *Promoting Safety and Comfort: Personal Hygiene and Perineal Care.*
   b. Practiced hand hygiene.
   c. Collected the following:
      • Soap or other cleansing agent as directed
      • At least 4 washcloths
      • Bath towel
      • Bath blanket
      • Bath thermometer
      • Wash basin
      • Waterproof pad
      • Gloves
      • Laundry bag
      • Paper towels
   d. Covered the over-bed table with paper towels. Arranged items on top of them.
   e. Identified the person. Checked the identification (ID) bracelet against the assignment sheet. Used 2 identifiers. Also called the person by name.
   f. Provided for privacy.
   g. Raised the bed for body mechanics. Bed rails were up if used.
   h. Lowered the bed rail near you if up.
   i. Practiced hand hygiene. Put on gloves.
   j. Covered the person with a bath blanket. Moved top linens to the foot of the bed.
   k. Positioned the person on his back.
   l. Draped the person.
   m. Raised the bed rail if used.
   n. Filled the wash basin. Water temperature was 105°F to 109°F (40.5°C to 42.7°C). Followed the care plan for water temperature. Measured water temperature according to agency policy.
   o. Asked the person to check the water temperature. Adjusted the water temperature if it was too hot or too cold. Raised the bed rail before leaving the bedside. Lowered it when you returned.
   p. Placed the basin on the over-bed table.
   q. Lowered the bed rail if up.
2. Folded the corner of the bath blanket between the legs onto his abdomen.
3. Placed a waterproof pad under the buttocks. Removed any wet or soiled incontinence products.
4. Removed and discarded the gloves. Practiced hand hygiene. Put on clean gloves.
5. Retracted the foreskin if the person was uncircumcised.
6. Grasped the penis.

Date of Satisfactory Completion _____   Instructor's Initials _____

Procedure—cont'd   S   U   **Comments**

7. Cleaned the tip. Used a circular motion. Started at the meatus of
   the urethra and worked outward. Repeated as needed. Used a
   clean part of the washcloth each time.   _____   _____   _____

8. Rinsed the area with another washcloth. Used the same
   circular motion.   _____   _____   _____

9. Returned the foreskin to its natural position immediately
   after rinsing.   _____   _____   _____

10. Cleaned the shaft of the penis. Used firm downward strokes.
    Rinsed the area.   _____   _____   _____

11. Helped the person flex his knees and spread his legs. Or helped
    him spread his legs as much as possible with his knees straight. _____   _____   _____

12. Cleaned the scrotum. Rinsed well. Observed for redness and
    irritation of the skin folds.   _____   _____   _____

13. Patted dry the penis and the scrotum. Used the towel.   _____   _____   _____

14. Folded the bath blanket back between his legs.   _____   _____   _____

15. Helped him lower his legs and turn onto his side away from you. _____   _____   _____

16. Cleaned the rectal area. Cleaned from scrotum (front or top) to the
    anus (back or bottom). Rinsed and dried well.   _____   _____   _____

17. Removed the waterproof pad.   _____   _____   _____

18. Removed and discarded the gloves. Practiced hand hygiene.
    Put on clean gloves.   _____   _____   _____

19. Provided clean and dry linens and incontinence products.   _____   _____   _____

20. Did the following:
    a. Covered the person. Removed the bath blanket.   _____   _____   _____
    b. Provided for comfort.   _____   _____   _____
    c. Placed the call light and other needed items within reach.   _____   _____   _____
    d. Lowered the bed to a safe and comfortable level appropriate
       for the person. Followed the care plan.   _____   _____   _____
    e. Raised or lowered bed rails. Followed the care plan.   _____   _____   _____
    f. Emptied, cleaned, rinsed, and dried the wash basin.   _____   _____   _____
    g. Returned the basin and supplies to their proper place.   _____   _____   _____
    h. Wiped off the over-bed table with the paper towels. Discarded
       the paper towels.   _____   _____   _____
    i. Unscreened the person.   _____   _____   _____
    j. Completed a safety check of the room.   _____   _____   _____
    k. Followed agency policy for used linens.   _____   _____   _____
    l. Removed and discarded the gloves. Practiced hand hygiene.   _____   _____   _____
    m. Reported and recorded your observations.   _____   _____   _____

Date of Satisfactory Completion _____   Instructor's Initials _____

NATCEP ▶ VIDEO ▶ VIDEO CLIP ## Brushing and Combing Hair

Name: _____   Date: _____

	S	U	Comments
Quality of Life			
• Knocked before entering the person's room.	___	___	_____
• Addressed the person by name.	___	___	_____
• Introduced yourself by name and title.	___	___	_____
• Explained the procedure before starting and during the procedure.	___	___	_____
• Protected the person's rights during the procedure.	___	___	_____
• Handled the person gently during the procedure.	___	___	_____

Pre-Procedure

1. Followed *Delegation Guidelines: Brushing and Combing Hair*. Saw *Promoting Safety and Comfort: Brushing and Combing Hair*.
2. Practiced hand hygiene.
3. Identified the person. Checked the ID (identification) bracelet against the assignment sheet. Used 2 identifiers. Also called the person by name.
4. Asked the person how to style hair.
5. Collected the following:
   • Comb and brush
   • Bath towel
   • Other hair care items as requested
6. Arranged items on the bedside stand.
7. Provided for privacy.

Procedure

8. Lowered the bed rail if up.
9. Positioned the person.
   a. *In a chair*—Helped the person to the chair. The person put on a robe and non-skid footwear while up.
   b. *In bed*—Raised the bed for body mechanics. Bed rails were up if used. Lowered the bed rail near you. Assisted the person to a semi-Fowler's position if allowed.
10. Placed a towel across the person's back and shoulders or across the pillow.
11. Asked the person to remove eyeglasses. Put them in the eyeglass case. Put the case inside the bedside stand.
12. *Brushed and combed hair that was not matted or tangled.*
   a. Used the comb to part the hair.
      1) Parted hair down the middle into 2 sides.
      2) Divided 1 side into 2 smaller sections.
   b. Brushed 1 of the small sections of hair. Started at the scalp and brushed toward the hair ends. Did the same for the other small section of hair.
   c. Repeated for the other side.
      1) Divided side into 2 smaller sections.
      2) Brushed 1 of the small sections of hair. Started at the scalp and brushed toward the hair ends. Did the same for the other small section of hair.
13. *Brushed or combed matted or tangled hair.*
   a. Took a small section of hair near the ends.
   b. Combed or brushed through to the hair ends.
   c. Added small sections of hair as you worked up to the scalp.
   d. Combed or brushed through each longer section to the hair ends.
14. Styled the hair as the person preferred.
15. Removed the towel.
16. Allowed the person to put on the eyeglasses.

Date of Satisfactory Completion _____   Instructor's Initials _____

Post-Procedure

	S	U	Comments
17. Provided for comfort.	___	___	_____
18. Placed the call light and other needed items within reach.	___	___	_____
19. Lowered the bed to a safe and comfortable level for the person. Followed the care plan.	___	___	_____
20. Raised or lowered bed rails. Followed the care plan.	___	___	_____
21. Removed hair from the brush or comb. Cleaned and returned hair care items to their proper place. Wore gloves for this step. Removed and discarded the gloves. Practiced hand hygiene.	___	___	_____
22. Unscreened the person.	___	___	_____
23. Completed a safety check of the room.	___	___	_____
24. Followed agency policy for used linens.	___	___	_____
25. Practiced hand hygiene.	___	___	_____

Date of Satisfactory Completion _____   Instructor's Initials _____

Shampooing the Person's Hair

VIDEO   VIDEO CLIP

Name: _____   Date: _____

Quality of Life	S	U	Comments
• Knocked before entering the person's room.	___	___	_____
• Addressed the person by name.	___	___	_____
• Introduced yourself by name and title.	___	___	_____
• Explained the procedure before starting and during the procedure.	___	___	_____
• Protected the person's rights during the procedure.	___	___	_____
• Handled the person gently during the procedure.	___	___	_____

Pre-Procedure

1. Followed *Delegation Guidelines: Shampooing.* Saw *Promoting Safety and Comfort: Shampooing.*   ___ ___ _____
2. Practiced hand hygiene.   ___ ___ _____
3. Collected the following:
   - 2 bath towels   ___ ___ _____
   - Washcloth   ___ ___ _____
   - Shampoo   ___ ___ _____
   - Hair conditioner (if requested)   ___ ___ _____
   - Bath thermometer   ___ ___ _____
   - Pitcher or hand-held nozzle (if needed)   ___ ___ _____
   - Shampoo tray (if needed)   ___ ___ _____
   - Basin or pan (if needed)   ___ ___ _____
   - Waterproof pad (if needed)   ___ ___ _____
   - Gloves (if needed)   ___ ___ _____
   - Comb and brush   ___ ___ _____
   - Hair dryer   ___ ___ _____
4. Arranged items nearby.   ___ ___ _____
5. Identified the person. Checked the ID (identification) bracelet against the assignment sheet. Used 2 identifiers. Also called the person by name.   ___ ___ _____
6. Provided for privacy.   ___ ___ _____
7. Raised the bed for body mechanics for a shampoo in bed. Bed rails were up if used.   ___ ___ _____
8. Practiced hand hygiene.   ___ ___ _____

Procedure

9. Lowered the bed rail near you if up.   ___ ___ _____
10. Covered the person's chest with a bath towel.   ___ ___ _____
11. Brushed and combed the hair to remove snarls and tangles.   ___ ___ _____
12. Positioned the person for the method used.   ___ ___ _____
    For a shampoo in bed:
    a. Lowered the head of the bed and removed the pillow.   ___ ___ _____
    b. Placed the waterproof pad and shampoo tray under the head and shoulders.   ___ ___ _____
    c. Supported the head and neck with a folded towel if necessary.   ___ ___ _____
13. Raised the bed rail if used.   ___ ___ _____
14. Obtained water. Water temperature was 105°F (40.5°C), usually. Tested water temperature according to agency policy. Also asked the nurse to check the water. Adjusted the water temperature as needed. Raised the bed rail before leaving the bedside.   ___ ___ _____
15. Lowered the bed rail near you if up.   ___ ___ _____
16. Put on gloves (if needed).   ___ ___ _____
17. Asked the person to hold a washcloth over the eyes. It did not cover the nose and mouth. (NOTE: A damp washcloth is easier to hold. It does not slip. However, your agency may have required a dry washcloth.)   ___ ___ _____

Date of Satisfactory Completion _____   Instructor's Initials _____

Procedure—cont'd

	S	U	Comments
18. Used the water pitcher or nozzle to wet the hair.	___	___	_____
19. Applied a small amount of shampoo.	___	___	_____
20. Worked up a lather with both hands. Started at the hairline. Worked toward the back of the head.	___	___	_____
21. Massaged the scalp with your fingertips. Did not scratch the scalp with your fingernails.	___	___	_____
22. Rinsed the hair until the water ran clear.	___	___	_____
23. Repeated the following steps:			
a. Applied a small amount of shampoo.	___	___	_____
b. Worked up a lather with both hands. Started at the hairline. Worked toward the back of the head.	___	___	_____
c. Massaged the scalp with your fingertips. Did not scratch the scalp with your fingernails.	___	___	_____
d. Rinsed the hair until the water ran clear.	___	___	_____
24. Applied conditioner. Followed directions on the container.	___	___	_____
25. Squeezed water from the person's hair.	___	___	_____
26. Covered the hair with a bath towel.	___	___	_____
27. Removed the shampoo tray, basin, and waterproof pad.	___	___	_____
28. Dried the person's face with a towel. Used the towel on the person's chest.	___	___	_____
29. Helped the person raise the head if appropriate. For the person in bed, raised the head of the bed.	___	___	_____
30. Rubbed the hair and scalp with the towel. Rubbed gently. Used the second towel if the first one was wet.	___	___	_____
31. Combed the hair to remove snarls and tangles.	___	___	_____
32. Dried and styled hair.	___	___	_____
33. Removed and discarded the gloves (if used). Practiced hand hygiene.	___	___	_____

Post-Procedure

	S	U	Comments
34. Provided for comfort.	___	___	_____
35. Placed the call light and other needed items within reach.	___	___	_____
36. Lowered the bed to a safe and comfortable level for the person. Followed the care plan.	___	___	_____
37. Raised or lowered bed rails. Followed the care plan.	___	___	_____
38. Unscreened the person.	___	___	_____
39. Completed a safety check of the room.	___	___	_____
40. Cleaned, rinsed, dried, and returned equipment to its proper place. Remembered to clean the comb and brush. Wore gloves for this step. Discarded disposable items. Removed and discarded the gloves.	___	___	_____
41. Followed agency policy for used linens.	___	___	_____
42. Practiced hand hygiene.	___	___	_____
43. Reported and recorded your observations.	___	___	_____

Date of Satisfactory Completion _____   Instructor's Initials _____

Shaving the Person's Face With a Safety Razor

Name: _____ Date: _____

	S	U	Comments

Quality of Life
- Knocked before entering the person's room.
- Addressed the person by name.
- Introduced yourself by name and title.
- Explained the procedure before starting and during the procedure.
- Protected the person's rights during the procedure.
- Handled the person gently during the procedure.

Pre-Procedure
1. Followed *Delegation Guidelines: Shaving*. Saw *Promoting Safety and Comfort: Shaving*.
2. Practiced hand hygiene.
3. Collected the following:
   - Wash basin
   - Bath towel
   - Hand towel
   - Washcloth
   - Safety razor
   - Mirror
   - Shaving cream, soap, or lotion
   - Shaving brush
   - After-shave or lotion
   - Tissues or paper towels
   - Gloves
4. Arranged paper towels and supplies on the over-bed table.
5. Identified the person. Checked the ID (identification) bracelet against the assignment sheet. Used 2 identifiers. Also called the person by name.
6. Provided for privacy.
7. Raised the bed for body mechanics. Bed rails are up if used.

Procedure
8. Filled the wash basin with warm water.
9. Placed the basin on the over-bed table.
10. Lowered the bed rail near you if up.
11. Practiced hand hygiene. Put on gloves.
12. Assisted the person to semi-Fowler's position if allowed or the supine position.
13. Adjusted lighting to clearly see the person's face.
14. Placed the towel over the person's chest and shoulders.
15. Adjusted the over-bed table for easy reach.
16. Tightened the razor blade to the shaver if necessary.
17. Washed the person's face. Did not dry.
18. Wet the washcloth or towel. Wrung it out.
19. Applied the washcloth or towel to the face for a few minutes.
20. Applied shaving cream with your hands. Or used a shaving brush to apply lather.
21. Held the skin taut with 1 hand.
22. Shaved in the direction of hair growth. Used shorter strokes around the chin and lips.
23. Rinsed the razor often. Wiped it with tissues or paper towels.
24. Applied direct pressure to any bleeding areas.
25. Washed off any remaining shaving cream or soap. Patted dry with a towel.

Date of Satisfactory Completion _____ Instructor's Initials _____

Procedure—cont'd	**S**	**U**	**Comments**
26. Applied after-shave or lotion if requested. (If there were nicks or cuts, did not apply after-shave or lotion.)	_____	_____	_____
27. Removed and discarded the towels and gloves. Practiced hand hygiene.	_____	_____	_____

Post-Procedure

28. Provided for comfort.	_____	_____	_____
29. Placed the call light and other needed items within reach.	_____	_____	_____
30. Lowered the bed to a safe and comfortable level for the person. Followed the care plan.	_____	_____	_____
31. Raised or lowered bed rails. Followed the care plan.	_____	_____	_____
32. Cleaned, rinsed, dried, and returned equipment and supplies to their proper place. Discarded the razor blade or disposable razor into the sharps container. Discarded other disposable items. Wore gloves.	_____	_____	_____
33. Wiped off the over-bed table with paper towels. Discarded the paper towels.	_____	_____	_____
34. Unscreened the person.	_____	_____	_____
35. Completed a safety check of the room.	_____	_____	_____
36. Followed agency policy for used linens.	_____	_____	_____
37. Removed and discarded the gloves. Practiced hand hygiene.	_____	_____	_____
38. Reported nicks, cuts, irritation, or bleeding to the nurse at once. Also reported and recorded other observations.	_____	_____	_____

Date of Satisfactory Completion _____   Instructor's Initials _____

Giving Nail and Foot Care

Name: _____   Date: _____

	S	U	Comments
Quality of Life			
• Knocked before entering the person's room.	___	___	_____
• Addressed the person by name.	___	___	_____
• Introduced yourself by name and title.	___	___	_____
• Explained the procedure before starting and during the procedure.	___	___	_____
• Protected the person's rights during the procedure.	___	___	_____
• Handled the person gently during the procedure.	___	___	_____

Pre-Procedure

1. Followed *Delegation Guidelines: Nail and Foot Care.* Saw *Promoting Safety and Comfort: Nail and Foot Care.* ___ ___ _____
2. Practiced hand hygiene. ___ ___ _____
3. Collected the following:
   - Wash basin or whirlpool foot bath ___ ___ _____
   - Soap ___ ___ _____
   - Bath thermometer ___ ___ _____
   - Bath towel ___ ___ _____
   - Hand towel ___ ___ _____
   - Washcloth ___ ___ _____
   - Kidney basin ___ ___ _____
   - Nail clippers ___ ___ _____
   - Orangewood stick ___ ___ _____
   - Emery board or nail file ___ ___ _____
   - Lotion for the hands ___ ___ _____
   - Lotion or petroleum jelly for the feet ___ ___ _____
   - Paper towels ___ ___ _____
   - Bath mat ___ ___ _____
   - Gloves ___ ___ _____
4. Arranged paper towels and other items on the over-bed table. ___ ___ _____
5. Identified the person. Checked the ID (identification) bracelet against the assignment sheet. Used 2 identifiers. Also called the person by name. ___ ___ _____
6. Provided for privacy. ___ ___ _____
7. Assisted the person to the bedside chair. Removed footwear and socks or stockings. Placed the call light and other needed items within reach. ___ ___ _____

Procedure

8. Placed the bath mat under the feet. ___ ___ _____
9. Filled the wash basin or whirlpool foot bath ⅔ (two-thirds) full with water. The nurse told you what water temperature to use. (Measured water temperature with a bath thermometer. Or tested it by dipping your elbow or inner wrist into the basin. Followed agency policy.) Also asked the person to check the water temperature. Adjusted the water temperature as needed. ___ ___ _____
10. Placed the basin or foot bath on the bath mat. ___ ___ _____
11. Put on gloves. ___ ___ _____
12. Helped the person put his or her bare feet into the basin or foot bath. Both feet were completely covered by water. ___ ___ _____
13. Adjusted the over-bed table in front of the person. ___ ___ _____
14. Filled the kidney basin ⅔ (two-thirds) full with water. The nurse told you what water temperature to use. (Measured water temperature with a bath thermometer. Or tested it by dipping your elbow or inner wrist into the basin. Followed agency policy.) Also asked the person to check the water temperature. Adjusted the water temperature as needed. ___ ___ _____

Date of Satisfactory Completion _____   Instructor's Initials _____

Procedure—cont'd	S	U	Comments
15. Placed the kidney basin on the over-bed table.	___	___	_____
16. Placed the person's fingers into the basin. Positioned the arms for comfort.	___	___	_____
17. Allowed the fingers to soak for 5 to 10 minutes. Allowed the feet to soak for 15 to 20 minutes. Re-warmed water as needed.	___	___	_____
18. Removed the kidney basin.	___	___	_____
19. Dried the hands between the fingers thoroughly.	___	___	_____
20. Cleaned under the fingernails with the orangewood stick. Used a towel to wipe the orangewood stick after each nail.	___	___	_____
21. Pushed cuticles back with the orangewood stick or a washcloth.	___	___	_____
22. Clipped fingernails straight across with nail clippers.	___	___	_____
23. Filed and shaped nails with an emery board or nail file. Nails were smooth with no rough edges. Checked each nail for smoothness. Filed as needed.	___	___	_____
24. Applied lotion to the hands. Warmed lotion before applying it.	___	___	_____
25. Moved the over-bed table to the side.	___	___	_____
26. Removed and discarded the gloves. Practiced hand hygiene. Put on clean gloves. (NOTE: Some state competency tests require clean gloves for foot care.)	___	___	_____
27. Lifted a foot out of the water. Supported the foot and ankle with 1 hand. With your other hand, washed the foot and between the toes with soap and a washcloth. Returned the foot to the water for rinsing. Made sure you rinsed between the toes.	___	___	_____
28. Repeated for the other foot. Lifted foot out of the water. Supported the foot and ankle with 1 hand. With your other hand, washed the foot and between the toes with soap and a washcloth. Returned the foot to the water for rinsing. Made sure you rinsed between the toes.	___	___	_____
29. Removed the feet from the basin or foot bath. Dried thoroughly, especially between the toes. Supported the foot and ankle as needed.	___	___	_____
30. Applied lotion or petroleum jelly to the tops, soles, and heels of the feet. Did not apply between the toes. Warmed lotion or petroleum jelly before applying it. Removed excess lotion or petroleum jelly with a towel. Supported the foot and ankle as needed.	___	___	_____
31. Removed and discarded the gloves. Practiced hand hygiene.	___	___	_____
32. Helped the person put on non-skid footwear.	___	___	_____

Post-Procedure

	S	U	Comments
33. Provided for comfort.	___	___	_____
34. Placed the call light and other needed items within reach.	___	___	_____
35. Raised or lowered bed rails. Followed the care plan.	___	___	_____
36. Cleaned, rinsed, dried, and returned equipment and supplies to their proper place. Discarded disposable items. Wore gloves.	___	___	_____
37. Unscreened the person.	___	___	_____
38. Completed a safety check of the room.	___	___	_____
39. Followed agency policy for used linens.	___	___	_____
40. Removed and discarded the gloves. Practiced hand hygiene.	___	___	_____
41. Reported and recorded your observations.	___	___	_____

Date of Satisfactory Completion _____   Instructor's Initials _____

Undressing the Person

Name: _____   Date: _____

	S	U	Comments

Quality of Life
- Knocked before entering the person's room.
- Addressed the person by name.
- Introduced yourself by name and title.
- Explained the procedure before starting and during the procedure.
- Protected the person's rights during the procedure.
- Handled the person gently during the procedure.

Pre-Procedure
1. Followed *Delegation Guidelines: Dressing and Undressing.* Saw *Promoting Safety and Comfort: Dressing and Undressing.*
2. Asked a co-worker to help turn and position the person if needed.
3. Practiced hand hygiene.
4. Collected a bath blanket and clothing as requested by the person.
5. Identified the person. Checked the ID (identification) bracelet against the assignment sheet. Used 2 identifiers. Also called the person by name.
6. Provided for privacy.
7. Raised the bed for body mechanics. Bed rails were up if used.
8. Lowered the bed rail on the person's weak side.
9. Positioned the person supine.
10. Covered the person with a bath blanket. Fan-folded linens to the foot of the bed.

Procedure
11. Removed garments that open in the back.
    a. Raised the head and shoulders. Or turned the person onto the side away from you.
    b. Undid buttons, zippers, ties, or snaps.
    c. Brought the sides of the garment to the sides of the person. For a side-lying position, tucked the far side under the person. Folded the near side onto the chest.
    d. Positioned the person supine.
    e. Slid the garment off the shoulder on the strong side. Removed it from the arm.
    f. Removed the garment from the weak side.
12. Removed garments that open in the front.
    a. Undid buttons, zippers, ties, or snaps.
    b. Slid the garment off the shoulder and arm on the strong side.
    c. Assisted the person to sit up or raised the head and shoulders. Brought the garment over to the weak side.
    d. Lowered the head and shoulders. Removed the garment from the weak side.
    e. If you could not raise the head and shoulders:
        1) Turned the person toward you. Tucked the removed part under the person.
        2) Turned the person onto the side away from you.
        3) Pulled the side of the garment out from under the person. Made sure the person did not lie on it when supine.
        4) Returned the person to the supine position.
        5) Removed the garment from the weak side.

Date of Satisfactory Completion _____   Instructor's Initials _____

Procedure—cont'd   S   U   **Comments**

13. Removed pullover garments.
    a. Undid any buttons, zippers, ties, or snaps.   _____   _____   _____
    b. Removed the garment from the strong side.   _____   _____   _____
    c. Raised the head and shoulders. Or turned the person onto the
       side away from you. Brought the garment up to the
       person's neck.   _____   _____   _____
    d. Brought the garment over the person's head.   _____   _____   _____
    e. Removed the garment from the weak side.   _____   _____   _____
    f. Positioned the person in the supine position.   _____   _____   _____
14. Removed pants or slacks.
    a. Removed footwear and socks.   _____   _____   _____
    b. Positioned the person supine.   _____   _____   _____
    c. Undid buttons, zippers, ties, snaps, or buckles.   _____   _____   _____
    d. Removed the belt.   _____   _____   _____
    e. Asked the person to lift the buttocks off the bed. Slid the pants
       down over the hips and buttocks. Had the person lower the
       hips and buttocks.   _____   _____   _____
    f. If the person could not raise the hips off the bed:
       1) Turned the person toward you.   _____   _____   _____
       2) Slid the pants off the hip and buttocks on the strong side.   _____   _____   _____
       3) Turned the person away from you.   _____   _____   _____
       4) Slid the pants off the hip and buttocks on the weak side.   _____   _____   _____
    g. Slid the pants down the legs and over the feet.   _____   _____   _____
15. Dressed the person.   _____   _____   _____

Post-Procedure
16. Provided for comfort.   _____   _____   _____
17. Placed the call light and other needed items within reach.   _____   _____   _____
18. Lowered the bed to a safe and comfortable level for the person.
    Followed the care plan.   _____   _____   _____
19. Raised or lowered bed rails. Followed the care plan.   _____   _____   _____
20. Unscreened the person.   _____   _____   _____
21. Completed a safety check of the room.   _____   _____   _____
22. Followed agency policy for soiled clothing.   _____   _____   _____
23. Practiced hand hygiene.   _____   _____   _____
24. Reported and recorded your observations.   _____   _____   _____

Date of Satisfactory Completion _____   Instructor's Initials _____

NATCEP™ VIDEO   **Dressing the Person**
Name: _____   Date: _____

Quality of Life	S	U	Comments
• Knocked before entering the person's room.	___	___	_____
• Addressed the person by name.	___	___	_____
• Introduced yourself by name and title.	___	___	_____
• Explained the procedure before starting and during the procedure.	___	___	_____
• Protected the person's rights during the procedure.	___	___	_____
• Handled the person gently during the procedure.	___	___	_____

Pre-Procedure

1. Followed *Delegation Guidelines: Dressing and Undressing*. Saw *Promoting Safety and Comfort: Dressing and Undressing*.   ___ ___ _____
2. Asked a co-worker to help turn and position the person if needed.   ___ ___ _____
3. Practiced hand hygiene.   ___ ___ _____
4. Asked the person what he or she would like to wear.   ___ ___ _____
5. Got a bath blanket and clothing requested by the person.   ___ ___ _____
6. Identified the person. Checked the ID (identification) bracelet against the assignment sheet. Used 2 identifiers. Also called the person by name.   ___ ___ _____
7. Provided for privacy.   ___ ___ _____
8. Raised the bed for body mechanics. Bed rails were up if used.   ___ ___ _____
9. Lowered the bed rail (if up) on the person's weak side.   ___ ___ _____
10. Positioned the person supine.   ___ ___ _____
11. Covered the person with a bath blanket. Fan-folded linens to the foot of the bed.   ___ ___ _____
12. Undressed the person.   ___ ___ _____
13. Raised the bed rail and went to the other side of the bed. This was the person's strong side. Lowered the bed rail near you if up.   ___ ___ _____

Procedure

14. Put on garments that open in the back.
    a. Slid the garment onto the arm and shoulder of the weak side.   ___ ___ _____
    b. Slid the garment onto the arm and shoulder of the strong side.   ___ ___ _____
    c. Raised the person's head and shoulders.   ___ ___ _____
    d. Brought the sides to the back.   ___ ___ _____
    e. If you could not raise the person's head and shoulders:
       1) Turned the person toward you.   ___ ___ _____
       2) Brought 1 side of the garment to the person's back.   ___ ___ _____
       3) Turned the person away from you.   ___ ___ _____
       4) Brought the other side to the person's back.   ___ ___ _____
    f. Fastened buttons, zippers, ties, snaps, or other closures.   ___ ___ _____
    g. Positioned the person supine.   ___ ___ _____
15. Put on garments that open in the front.
    a. Slid the garment onto the arm and shoulder on the weak side.   ___ ___ _____
    b. Raised the head and shoulders. Brought the side of the garment around to the back. Lowered the person down. Slid the garment onto the arm and shoulder of the strong arm.   ___ ___ _____
    c. If the person could not raise the head and shoulders:
       1) Turned the person toward you.   ___ ___ _____
       2) Tucked the garment under him or her.   ___ ___ _____
       3) Turned the person away from you.   ___ ___ _____
       4) Pulled the garment out from under him or her.   ___ ___ _____
       5) Turned the person back to the supine position.   ___ ___ _____
       6) Slid the garment over the arm and shoulder of the strong arm.   ___ ___ _____
    d. Fastened buttons, zippers, ties, snaps, or other closures.   ___ ___ _____

Date of Satisfactory Completion _____   Instructor's Initials _____

Procedure—cont'd	**S**	**U**	**Comments**
16. Put on pullover garments.			
a. Positioned the person supine.	_____	_____	_____
b. Slid the arm and shoulder of the garment onto the weak side.	_____	_____	_____
c. Raised the person's head and shoulders.	_____	_____	_____
d. Brought the neck of the garment over the head.	_____	_____	_____
e. Slid the arm and shoulder of the garment onto the strong side.	_____	_____	_____
f. Brought the garment down.	_____	_____	_____
g. If the person could not assume a semi-sitting position:			
1) Brought the neck of the garment over the head.	_____	_____	_____
2) Slid the arm and shoulder of the garment onto the strong side.	_____	_____	_____
3) Turned the person onto the strong side.	_____	_____	_____
4) Pulled the garment down on the person's weak side.	_____	_____	_____
5) Turned the person onto the weak side.	_____	_____	_____
6) Pulled the garment down on the person's strong side.	_____	_____	_____
7) Positioned the person supine.	_____	_____	_____
17. Put on pants or slacks.			
a. Slid the pants over the feet and up the legs.	_____	_____	_____
b. Asked the person to raise the hips and buttocks off the bed.	_____	_____	_____
c. Brought the pants up over the buttock and hip on the weak side.	_____	_____	_____
d. Pulled the pants over the buttock and hip on the strong side.	_____	_____	_____
e. If the person could not raise the hips and buttocks:			
1) Turned the person onto the strong side.	_____	_____	_____
2) Pulled the pants over the buttock and hip on the weak side.	_____	_____	_____
3) Turned the person onto the weak side.	_____	_____	_____
4) Pulled the pants over the buttock and hip on the strong side.	_____	_____	_____
5) Positioned the person supine.	_____	_____	_____
f. Fastened buttons, zippers, ties, snaps, a belt buckle, or other closures.	_____	_____	_____
18. Put socks and non-skid footwear on the person.	_____	_____	_____
19. Helped the person get out of bed. If the person stayed in bed, covered the person. Removed the bath blanket.	_____	_____	_____

Post-Procedure

	S	**U**	**Comments**
20. Provided for comfort.	_____	_____	_____
21. Placed the call light and other needed items within reach.	_____	_____	_____
22. Lowered the bed to a safe and comfortable level for the person. Followed the care plan.	_____	_____	_____
23. Raised or lowered bed rails. Followed the care plan.	_____	_____	_____
24. Unscreened the person.	_____	_____	_____
25. Completed a safety check of the room.	_____	_____	_____
26. Followed agency policy for soiled clothing.	_____	_____	_____
27. Practiced hand hygiene.	_____	_____	_____
28. Reported and recorded your observations.	_____	_____	_____

Date of Satisfactory Completion _____   Instructor's Initials _____

Changing a Patient Gown on a Person With an Intravenous (IV)

Name: _____   Date: _____

	S	U	Comments
Quality of Life			
• Knocked before entering the person's room.	___	___	_____
• Addressed the person by name.	___	___	_____
• Introduced yourself by name and title.	___	___	_____
• Explained the procedure before starting and during the procedure.	___	___	_____
• Protected the person's rights during the procedure.	___	___	_____
• Handled the person gently during the procedure.	___	___	_____

Pre-Procedure

1. Followed *Delegation Guidelines: Changing Patient Gowns*. Saw *Promoting Safety and Comfort: Changing Patient Gowns*. ___ ___ _____
2. Practiced hand hygiene. ___ ___ _____
3. Got a clean gown and bath blanket. ___ ___ _____
4. Identified the person. Checked the ID (identification) bracelet against the assignment sheet. Used 2 identifiers. Also called the person by name. ___ ___ _____
5. Provided for privacy. ___ ___ _____
6. Raised the bed for body mechanics. Bed rails were up if used. ___ ___ _____

Procedure

7. Lowered the bed rail near you (if up). ___ ___ _____
8. Covered the person with a bath blanket. Fan-folded linens to the foot of the bed. ___ ___ _____
9. Untied the gown. Freed parts that the person was lying on. ___ ___ _____
10. Removed the gown from the arm with *no IV*. ___ ___ _____
11. Gathered up the sleeve of the arm *with the IV*. Slid it over the IV site and tubing. Removed the arm and hand from the sleeve. ___ ___ _____
12. Kept the sleeve gathered. Slid your arm along the tubing to the bag. ___ ___ _____
13. Removed the bag from the pole. Slid the bag and tubing through the sleeve. Did not pull on the tubing. Kept the bag above the person. ___ ___ _____
14. Hung the IV bag on the pole. ___ ___ _____
15. Gathered the sleeve of the clean gown that went on the arm with the IV infusion. ___ ___ _____
16. Removed the bag from the pole. Slipped the sleeve over the bag at the shoulder part of the gown. Hung the bag. ___ ___ _____
17. Slid the gathered sleeve over the tubing, hand, arm, and IV site. Then slid it onto the shoulder. ___ ___ _____
18. Put the other side of the gown on the person. Fastened the gown. ___ ___ _____
19. Covered the person. Removed the bath blanket. ___ ___ _____

Post-Procedure

20. Provided for comfort. ___ ___ _____
21. Placed the call light and other needed items within reach. ___ ___ _____
22. Lowered the bed to a safe and comfortable level for the person. Followed the care plan. ___ ___ _____
23. Raised or lowered bed rails. Followed the care plan. ___ ___ _____
24. Unscreened the person. ___ ___ _____
25. Completed a safety check of the room. ___ ___ _____
26. Followed agency policy for used linens. ___ ___ _____
27. Practiced hand hygiene. ___ ___ _____
28. Asked the nurse to check the flow rate. ___ ___ _____
29. Reported and recorded your observations. ___ ___ _____

Date of Satisfactory Completion _____   Instructor's Initials _____

Giving the Bedpan

Name: _____   Date: _____

	S	U	Comments

Quality of Life
- Knocked before entering the person's room.
- Addressed the person by name.
- Introduced yourself by name and title.
- Explained the procedure before starting and during the procedure.
- Protected the person's rights during the procedure.
- Handled the person gently during the procedure.

Pre-Procedure
1. Followed *Delegation Guidelines: Bedpans.*
   Saw *Promoting Safety and Comfort:*
   a. *Urinary Elimination*
   b. *Bedpans*
2. Provided for privacy.
3. Practiced hand hygiene.
4. Put on gloves.
5. Collected the following:
   - Bedpan
   - Bedpan cover
   - Toilet tissue
   - Waterproof pad (if required by agency policy)
6. Arranged equipment on the chair or bed.

Procedure
7. Lowered the bed rail near you (if up).
8. Lowered the head of the bed. Positioned the person supine. Or raised the head of the bed slightly for the person's comfort.
9. Folded the top linens and gown out of the way. Kept the lower body covered.
10. Asked the person to flex the knees and raised the buttocks. He or she did so by pushing against the mattress with the feet.
11. Slid your hand under the lower back. Helped raise the buttocks. If used a waterproof pad, placed it under the buttocks.
12. Slid the bedpan under the person.
13. If the person could not assist in getting on the bedpan:
    a. Placed the waterproof pad under the buttocks if using one.
    b. Turned the person onto the side away from you.
    c. Placed the bedpan firmly against the buttocks.
    d. Held the bedpan securely. Turned the person onto his or her back.
    e. Made sure the bedpan was centered under the person.
14. Covered the person.
15. Raised the head of the bed so the person was in a sitting position (Fowler's position) for a standard bedpan. (NOTE: Some state competency tests require removing gloves and hand-washing before you raise the head of the bed.)
16. Made sure the person was correctly positioned on the bedpan.
17. Raised the bed rail if used.
18. Placed the toilet tissue and call light within reach. (NOTE: For some state competency tests you ask the person to use hand wipes to clean the hands after wiping with toilet paper.)
19. Asked the person to signal when done or when help was needed.
20. Removed and discarded the gloves. Practiced hand hygiene.
21. Left the room and closed the door.
22. Returned when the person signaled. Or checked on the person every 5 minutes. Knocked before entering.

Date of Satisfactory Completion _____   Instructor's Initials _____

Procedure—cont'd	S	U	Comments
23. Practiced hand hygiene. Put on gloves.			
24. Raised the bed for body mechanics. Lowered the bed rail (if used) and lowered the head of the bed.			
25. Asked the person to raise the buttocks. Removed the bedpan. Or held the bedpan and turned the person onto the side away from you.			
26. Cleaned the genital area if the person did not do so.			
a. Cleaned from the meatus (front or top) to the anus (back or bottom) with toilet tissue. Used fresh tissue for each wipe.			
b. Provided perineal care if needed.			
c. Removed and discarded the waterproof pad if using one.			
27. Covered the bedpan. Took it to the bathroom. Raised the bed rail (if used) before leaving the bedside.			
28. Noted the color, amount (output), and character of urine or feces.			
29. Emptied the bedpan contents into the toilet and flushed.			
30. Rinsed the bedpan. Poured the rinse into the toilet and flushed.			
31. Cleaned the bedpan with a disinfectant. Poured disinfectant into the toilet and flushed.			
32. Removed and discarded the gloves. Practiced hand hygiene and put on clean gloves.			
33. Returned the bedpan and clean cover to the bedside stand.			
34. Helped the person with hand-washing. Wore gloves for this step.			
35. Removed and discarded the gloves. Practiced hand hygiene.			

Post-Procedure

	S	U	Comments
36. Provided for comfort.			
37. Placed the call light and other needed items within reach.			
38. Lowered the bed to a safe and comfortable level for the person. Followed the care plan.			
39. Raised or lowered bed rails. Followed the care plan.			
40. Unscreened the person.			
41. Completed a safety check of the room.			
42. Followed agency policy for used linens.			
43. Practiced hand hygiene.			
44. Reported and recorded your observations.			

Date of Satisfactory Completion _____   Instructor's Initials _____

Giving the Urinal

Name: _____   Date: _____

	S	U	Comments

Quality of Life
- Knocked before entering the person's room.
- Addressed the person by name.
- Introduced yourself by name and title.
- Explained the procedure before starting and during the procedure.
- Protected the person's rights during the procedure.
- Handled the person gently during the procedure.

Pre-Procedure
1. Followed *Delegation Guidelines: Urinals.*
   Saw *Promoting Safety and Comfort:*
   a. *Urinary Elimination*
   b. *Urinals*
2. Provided for privacy.
3. Determined if the man would stand, sit, or lie in bed.
4. Practiced hand hygiene.
5. Put on gloves.
6. Collected the following:
   - Urinal
   - Non-skid footwear if the man would stand to void

Procedure
7. *Using the urinal in bed:*
   a. Gave him the urinal if he was in bed.
   b. Reminded him to tilt the bottom down to prevent spills.
8. *Standing to use the urinal:*
   a. Helped him sit on the side of the bed.
   b. Put non-skid footwear on him.
   c. Helped him stand. Provided support if he was unsteady.
   d. Gave him the urinal.
9. *Positioning the urinal (in bed or standing):*
   a. Helped the person stand if he would stand.
      1) Helped him sit on the side of the bed.
      2) Put non-skid footwear on him.
      3) Helped him stand. Provided support if he was unsteady.
   b. Positioned the urinal.
   c. Placed the penis in the urinal if he could not do so.
   d. Covered him for privacy.
10. Placed the call light within reach. Asked him to signal when done or when help was needed.
11. Provided for privacy.
12. Removed and discarded the gloves. Practiced hand hygiene.
13. Left the room and closed the door.
14. Returned when he signaled for you. Or checked on him every 5 minutes. Knocked before entering.
15. Practiced hand hygiene. Put on gloves.
16. Closed the cap on the urinal. Took it to the bathroom.
17. Noted the color, amount (output), and clarity of urine.
18. Emptied the urinal into the toilet and flushed.
19. Rinsed the urinal with cold water. Poured rinse into the toilet and flushed.
20. Cleaned the urinal with a disinfectant. Poured disinfectant into the toilet and flushed.
21. Returned the urinal to its proper place.

Date of Satisfactory Completion _____   Instructor's Initials _____

Procedure—cont'd	S	U	Comments
22. Removed and discarded the soiled gloves. Practiced hand hygiene and put on clean gloves.	___	___	_____
23. Assisted with hand-washing.	___	___	_____
24. Removed and discarded the gloves. Practiced hand hygiene.	___	___	_____

Post-Procedure			
25. Provided for comfort.	___	___	_____
26. Placed the call light and other needed items within reach.	___	___	_____
27. Raised or lowered bed rails. Followed the care plan.	___	___	_____
28. Unscreened him.	___	___	_____
29. Completed a safety check of the room.	___	___	_____
30. Followed agency policy for used linens.	___	___	_____
31. Practiced hand hygiene.	___	___	_____
32. Reported and recorded your observations.	___	___	_____

Date of Satisfactory Completion _____   Instructor's Initials _____

VIDEO VIDEO CLIP

Helping the Person to the Commode

Name: _____   Date: _____

	S	U	Comments

Quality of Life
- Knocked before entering the person's room.
- Addressed the person by name.
- Introduced yourself by name and title.
- Explained the procedure before starting and during the procedure.
- Protected the person's rights during the procedure.
- Handled the person gently during the procedure.

Pre-Procedure
1. Followed *Delegation Guidelines: Commodes.* Saw *Promoting Safety and Comfort:*
   a. *Urinary Elimination*
   b. *Commodes*
2. Provided for privacy.
3. Practiced hand hygiene.
4. Put on gloves.
5. Collected the following:
   - Commode
   - Toilet tissue
   - Bath blanket
   - Transfer belt
   - Robe and non-skid footwear

Procedure
6. Brought the commode next to the bed.
7. Helped the person sit on the side of the bed. Lowered the bed rail if used.
8. Helped the person put on a robe and non-skid footwear.
9. Applied the transfer belt.
10. Assisted the person to the commode. Used the transfer belt.
11. Removed the transfer belt. Covered the person with a bath blanket for warmth.
12. Placed the toilet tissue and call light within reach.
13. Asked the person to signal when done or when help was needed. (Stayed with the person if necessary. Was respectful. Provided as much privacy as possible.)
14. Removed and discarded the gloves. Practiced hand hygiene.
15. Left the room. Closed the door.
16. Returned when the person signaled. Or checked on the person every 5 minutes. Knocked before entering.
17. Practiced hand hygiene. Put on gloves.
18. Helped the person clean the genital area as needed. Removed and discarded the gloves. Practiced hand hygiene.
19. Applied the transfer belt. Helped the person back to bed; used the transfer belt. Removed the transfer belt, robe, and footwear. Raised the bed rail if used.
20. Put on clean gloves. Removed and covered the commode container. Cleaned the commode.
21. Took the container to the bathroom.
22. Observed urine and feces for color, amount (output), and character.
23. Emptied the container contents into the toilet and flushed.
24. Rinsed the container. Poured the rinse into the toilet and flushed.
25. Cleaned and disinfected the container. Poured disinfectant into the toilet and flushed.
26. Returned the container to the commode. Closed the lid on the commode. Cleaned other parts of the commode if necessary.

Date of Satisfactory Completion _____   Instructor's Initials _____

Procedure—cont'd

	S	U	Comments
27. Returned other supplies to their proper place.	___	___	___
28. Removed and discarded the gloves. Practiced hand hygiene and put on clean gloves.	___	___	___
29. Assisted with hand-washing.	___	___	___
30. Removed and discarded the gloves. Practiced hand hygiene.	___	___	___

Post-Procedure

	S	U	Comments
31. Provided for comfort.	___	___	___
32. Placed the call light and other needed items within reach.	___	___	___
33. Raised or lowered bed rails. Followed the care plan.	___	___	___
34. Unscreened the person.	___	___	___
35. Completed a safety check of the room.	___	___	___
36. Followed center policy for used linens.	___	___	___
37. Practiced hand hygiene.	___	___	___
38. Reported and recorded your observations.	___	___	___

Date of Satisfactory Completion _____   Instructor's Initials _____

NATCEP™   VIDEO   VIDEO CLIP   **Applying Incontinence Products**
Name: _____   Date: _____

	S	U	Comments

Quality of Life
- Knocked before entering the person's room.
- Addressed the person by name.
- Introduced yourself by name and title.
- Explained the procedure before starting and during the procedure.
- Protected the person's rights during the procedure.
- Handled the person gently during the procedure.

Pre-Procedure
1. Followed *Delegation Guidelines: Applying Incontinence Products.*
   Saw *Promoting Safety and Comfort:*
   a. *Urinary Elimination*
   b. *Applying Incontinence Products*
2. Practiced hand hygiene.
3. Collected the following:
   - Incontinence product as directed by the nurse
   - Barrier cream or moisturizer as directed by the nurse
   - Cleanser
   - Items for perineal care
   - Paper towels
   - Trash bags
   - Gloves
   - Non-skid footwear if the person stands
4. Covered the over-bed table with paper towels. Arranged items on top of them.
5. Identified the person. Checked the ID (identification) bracelet against the assignment sheet. Used 2 identifiers. Also called the person by name.
6. Marked the date, time, and your initials on the new product. Followed agency policy.
7. Provided for privacy.
8. Filled the wash basin. Water temperature was 105°F to 109°F (40.5°C to 42.7°C). Measured water temperature according to agency policy. Asked the person to check the water temperature. Adjusted water temperature as needed.
9. Raised the bed for body mechanics. Bed rails were up if used. (Omitted this step if the person stood.)

Procedure
10. Lowered the head of the bed. The bed was as flat as possible.
11. Lowered the bed rail near you if up.
12. Practiced hand hygiene. Put on the gloves.
13. Covered the person with a bath blanket. Lowered top linens to the foot of the bed. Lowered the pants or slacks (omitted this step if the person was standing).
14. *To apply an incontinence brief with the person in bed:*
    a. Placed a waterproof pad under the buttocks. Asked the person to raise the buttocks off the bed. Or turned the person from side to side.
    b. Loosened the tabs on each side of the used brief.
    c. Turned the person onto the side away from you.
    d. Removed the brief from front to back (top to bottom). Observed the urine as you rolled the product up.
    e. Placed the used brief in the trash bag. Set the bag aside.
    f. Performed perineal care wearing clean gloves. Applied the barrier cream or moisturizer.

Date of Satisfactory Completion _____   Instructor's Initials _____

Procedure—cont'd	**S**	**U**	**Comments**

g. Opened the new brief. Folded it in half length-wise along the center.

h. Inserted the brief between the legs from front to back (top to bottom).

i. Unfolded and spread the back panel.

j. Centered the brief in the perineal area.

k. Turned the person onto his or her back.

l. Unfolded and spread the front panel. Provided a "cup" shape in the perineal area. For a man, positioned the penis downward.

m. Made sure the brief was positioned high in the groin folds. This allowed the brief to fit the shape of the body.

n. Secured the brief.
   1) Pulled the lower tape tab forward on the side near you. Attached it at a slightly upward angle. Did the same for the other side.
   2) Pulled the upper tape tab forward on the side near you. Attached it in a horizontal manner. Did the same for the other side.

o. Smoothed out all wrinkles and folds.

15. *To apply a pad and undergarment with the person in bed:*
   a. Placed a waterproof pad under the buttocks. Asked the person to raise the buttocks off the bed. Or turned the person from side to side.

   b. Turned the person onto the side away from you.

   c. Pulled the undergarment down. The waistband was over the knee.

   d. Removed the used pad from the front to back (top to bottom). Observed the urine as you rolled the product up.

   e. Placed the used pad in the trash bag. Set the bag aside.

   f. Performed perineal care wearing clean gloves. Applied the barrier cream or moisturizer.

   g. Folded the new pad in half length-wise along the center.

   h. Inserted the pad between the legs from front to back (top to bottom).

   i. Unfolded and spread the back panel.

   j. Centered the pad in the perineal area.

   k. Pulled the garment up at the back.

   l. Turned the person onto his or her back.

   m. Unfolded and spread the front panel. For a man, positioned the penis downward.

   n. Pulled the garment up in front.

   o. Checked and adjusted the pad and undergarment for a good fit.

16. *To apply pull-on underwear with the person standing:*
   a. Helped the person put on non-skid footwear.

   b. Helped the person stand. Removed the pants or slacks.

   c. Tore the side seams to remove the used underwear.

   d. Removed the underwear from front to back (top to bottom). Observed the urine as you rolled the underwear up.

   e. Placed the used underwear in the trash bag. Set the bag aside.

   f. Performed perineal care wearing clean gloves. Applied barrier cream or moisturizer.

   g. Had the person sit on the side of the bed.

   h. Slid the new underwear over the feet to past the knees.

   i. Helped the person stand.

   j. Pulled the underwear up.

   k. Checked for a good fit.

Date of Satisfactory Completion _____   Instructor's Initials _____

Procedure—cont'd

	S	U	Comments
17. Asked about comfort. Asked if the product felt too loose or too tight. Checked for wrinkles or creases. Made sure the product did not rub or irritate the groin. Adjusted the product as needed.	____	____	_____
18. Removed and discarded the gloves. Practiced hand hygiene.	____	____	_____
19. Raised or put on pants or slacks.	____	____	_____

Post-Procedure

20. Provided for comfort.	____	____	_____
21. Placed the call light and other needed items within reach.	____	____	_____
22. Lowered the bed to a safe and comfortable level for the person. Followed the care plan.	____	____	_____
23. Raised or lowered bed rails. Followed the care plan.	____	____	_____
24. Unscreened the person.	____	____	_____
25. Practiced hand hygiene. Put on clean gloves.	____	____	_____
26. Estimated the amount of urine in the used product: small, moderate, large. Opened the product to observe for urine color and blood.	____	____	_____
27. Cleaned, rinsed, dried, and returned the wash basin and other equipment. Returned items to their proper place.	____	____	_____
28. Removed and discarded the gloves. Practiced hand hygiene.	____	____	_____
29. Completed a safety check of the room.	____	____	_____
30. Reported and recorded your observations.	____	____	_____

Date of Satisfactory Completion _____   Instructor's Initials _____

Giving Catheter Care

Name: _____   Date: _____

Quality of Life	S	U	Comments
• Knocked before entering the person's room.	_____	_____	_____
• Addressed the person by name.	_____	_____	_____
• Introduced yourself by name and title.	_____	_____	_____
• Explained the procedure before starting and during the procedure.	_____	_____	_____
• Protected the person's rights during the procedure.	_____	_____	_____
• Handled the person gently during the procedure.	_____	_____	_____

Pre-Procedure

1. Followed *Delegation Guidelines:*
   a. *Perineal Care*   _____ _____ _____
   b. *Catheters*   _____ _____ _____
   Saw *Promoting Safety and Comfort:*
   a. *Perineal Care*   _____ _____ _____
   b. *Urinary Catheters*   _____ _____ _____
   c. *Catheter Care*   _____ _____ _____
2. Practiced hand hygiene.   _____ _____ _____
3. Collected the following:
   • Items for perineal care   _____ _____ _____
   • Gloves   _____ _____ _____
   • Bath blanket   _____ _____ _____
4. Covered the over-bed table with paper towels. Arranged items on top of them.   _____ _____ _____
5. Identified the person. Checked the ID (identification) bracelet against the assignment sheet. Used 2 identifiers. Also called the person by name.   _____ _____ _____
6. Provided for privacy.   _____ _____ _____
7. Filled the wash basin. Water temperature was 105°F to 109°F (40.5°C to 42.7°C). Measured water temperature according to agency policy. Asked the person to check the water temperature. Adjusted water temperature as needed.   _____ _____ _____
8. Raised the bed for body mechanics. Bed rails were up if used.   _____ _____ _____
9. Lowered the bed rail near you if up.   _____ _____ _____

Procedure

10. Practiced hand hygiene. Put on the gloves.   _____ _____ _____
11. Covered the person with a bath blanket. Fan-folded top linens to the foot of the bed.   _____ _____ _____
12. Positioned and draped the person for perineal care.   _____ _____ _____
13. Folded back the bath blanket to expose the perineal area.   _____ _____ _____
14. Asked the person to flex the knees and raise the buttocks off the bed. Placed the waterproof pad under the buttocks.   _____ _____ _____
15. Checked the drainage tubing. Made sure it was not kinked and that urine could flow freely.   _____ _____ _____
16. Separated the labia (female). In an uncircumcised male, retracted the foreskin. Checked for crusts, abnormal drainage, or secretions.   _____ _____ _____
17. Gave perineal care. Kept the foreskin of the uncircumcised male retracted through step 24.   _____ _____ _____
18. Applied soap to clean, wet washcloth.   _____ _____ _____
19. Held the catheter at the meatus. Did so for steps 20 through 24.   _____ _____ _____
20. Washed around the catheter at the meatus. Used a circular motion.   _____ _____ _____
21. Cleaned the catheter from the meatus down the catheter at least 4 inches. Cleaned downward, away from the meatus with 1 stroke. Did not tug or pull on the catheter. Repeated as needed with a clean area of the washcloth. Used a clean washcloth if needed.   _____ _____ _____

Date of Satisfactory Completion _____   Instructor's Initials _____

Procedure—cont'd	S	U	Comments

Procedure—cont'd

22. Rinsed around the catheter at the meatus with a clean washcloth.
23. Rinsed the catheter from the meatus down the catheter at least 4 inches. Rinsed downward, away from the meatus with 1 stroke. Did not tug or pull on the catheter. Repeated as needed with a clean area of the washcloth. Used a clean washcloth if needed.
24. Patted dry the areas washed. Dried from the meatus down the catheter at least 4 inches. Did not tug or pull on the catheter.
25. Returned the foreskin (uncircumcised male) to its natural position.
26. Patted dry perineal area. Dried from front to back (top to bottom).
27. Secured the catheter. Positioned the tubing in a straight line or coiled on the bed. Followed the nurse's directions.
28. Removed the waterproof pad.
29. Covered the person. Removed the bath blanket.
30. Removed and discarded the gloves. Practiced hand hygiene.

Post-Procedure

31. Provided for comfort.
32. Placed the call light and other needed items within reach.
33. Lowered the bed to a safe and comfortable level for the person. Followed the care plan.
34. Raised or lowered bed rails. Followed the care plan.
35. Cleaned, rinsed, dried, and returned equipment to its proper place. Discarded disposable items. Wore gloves for this step.
36. Unscreened the person.
37. Completed a safety check of the room.
38. Followed center policy for used linens.
39. Removed and discarded the gloves. Practiced hand hygiene.
40. Reported and recorded your observations.

Date of Satisfactory Completion _____ Instructor's Initials _____

Changing a Leg Bag to a Standard Drainage Bag

Name: _____   Date: _____

	S	U	Comments
Quality of Life			
• Knocked before entering the person's room.			
• Addressed the person by name.			
• Introduced yourself by name and title.			
• Explained the procedure before starting and during the procedure.			
• Protected the person's rights during the procedure.			
• Handled the person gently during the procedure.			

Pre-Procedure

1. Followed *Delegation Guidelines: Urine Drainage Systems.*
   Saw *Promoting Safety and Comfort:*
   a. *Urinary Catheters*
   b. *Urine Drainage Systems*
2. Practiced hand hygiene.
3. Collected the following:
   • Gloves
   • Standard drainage bag and tubing
   • Antiseptic wipes
   • Waterproof pad
   • Sterile cap and plug
   • Catheter clamp
   • Paper towels
   • Bedpan
   • Bath blanket
4. Arranged paper towels and equipment on the over-bed table.
5. Identified the person. Checked the ID (identification) bracelet against the assignment sheet. Used 2 identifiers. Also called the person by name.
6. Provided for privacy.

Procedure

7. Had the person sit on the side of the bed.
8. Practiced hand hygiene. Put on gloves.
9. Exposed the catheter and leg bag.
10. Clamped the catheter. This prevented urine from draining from the catheter into the drainage tubing.
11. Allowed urine to drain from below the clamp into the drainage tubing. This emptied the lower end of the catheter.
12. Helped the person to lie down.
13. Raised the bed rails if used. Raised the bed for body mechanics.
14. Lowered the bed rail near you if up.
15. Covered the person with a bath blanket. Fan-folded top linens to the foot of the bed. Exposed the catheter and leg bag.
16. Placed the waterproof pad under the person's leg.
17. Opened the antiseptic wipes. Placed them on paper towels.
18. Opened the package with the sterile cap and plug. Placed the package on the paper towels. Did not let anything touch the sterile cap or plug.
19. Opened the package with the standard drainage bag and tubing.
20. Attached the standard drainage bag to the bed frame.
21. Disconnected the catheter from the drainage tubing. Did not allow anything to touch the ends.

Date of Satisfactory Completion _____   Instructor's Initials _____

Procedure—cont'd	S	U	Comments
22. Inserted the sterile plug into the catheter end. Touched only the end of the plug. Did not touch the part that went inside the catheter. (If you contaminated the end of the catheter, wiped the end with an antiseptic wipe. Did so before you inserted the sterile plug.)	___	___	_____
23. Placed the sterile cap on the end of the leg bag drainage tube. (If you contaminated the tubing end, wiped the end with an antiseptic wipe. Did so before you applied the sterile cap.)	___	___	_____
24. Removed the cap from the new standard drainage tubing.	___	___	_____
25. Removed the sterile plug from the catheter.	___	___	_____
26. Inserted the end of the drainage tubing into the catheter.	___	___	_____
27. Removed the clamp from the catheter.	___	___	_____
28. Positioned drainage tubing in a straight line or coiled on the bed. Followed the nurse's directions. Secured the tubing to the bottom linens.	___	___	_____
29. Removed the leg bag. Placed it in the bedpan.	___	___	_____
30. Removed and discarded the waterproof pad.	___	___	_____
31. Covered the person. Removed the bath blanket.	___	___	_____
32. Took the bedpan to the bathroom.	___	___	_____
33. Removed and discarded the gloves. Practiced hand hygiene.	___	___	_____

Post-Procedure

	S	U	Comments
34. Provided for comfort.	___	___	_____
35. Placed the call light and other needed items within reach.	___	___	_____
36. Lowered the bed to a safe and comfortable level for the person. Followed the care plan.	___	___	_____
37. Raised or lowered bed rails. Followed the care plan.	___	___	_____
38. Unscreened the person.	___	___	_____
39. Put on clean gloves. Discarded disposable items.	___	___	_____
40. Emptied the drainage bag.	___	___	_____
41. Discarded the drainage tubing and leg bag following center policy. Or cleaned the bag following center policy.	___	___	_____
42. Cleaned and disinfected the bedpan. Placed it in a clean cover.	___	___	_____
43. Returned the bedpan and other supplies to their proper place.	___	___	_____
44. Removed and discarded the gloves. Practiced hand hygiene.	___	___	_____
45. Completed a safety check of the room.	___	___	_____
46. Followed center policy for used linens.	___	___	_____
47. Practiced hand hygiene.	___	___	_____
48. Reported and recorded your observations.	___	___	_____

Date of Satisfactory Completion _____   Instructor's Initials _____

Emptying a Urine Drainage Bag

Name: _____   Date: _____

	S	U	Comments

Quality of Life
- Knocked before entering the person's room.
- Addressed the person by name.
- Introduced yourself by name and title.
- Explained the procedure before starting and during the procedure.
- Protected the person's rights during the procedure.
- Handled the person gently during the procedure.

Pre-Procedure
1. Followed *Delegation Guidelines: Urine Drainage Systems*. Saw *Promoting Safety and Comfort*:
   a. *Urinary Catheters*
   b. *Urine Drainage Systems*
2. Collected the following:
   - Graduate (measuring container)
   - Gloves
   - Paper towels
   - Antiseptic wipes
3. Practiced hand hygiene.
4. Identified the person. Checked the ID (identification) bracelet against the assignment sheet. Used 2 identifiers. Also called the person by name.
5. Provided for privacy.

Procedure
6. Put on the gloves.
7. Placed paper towel on the floor. Placed graduate on top of it.
8. Positioned the graduate under the drainage bag.
9. Opened the clamp on the drain.
10. Allowed all urine to drain into the graduate. Did not let the drain touch the graduate.
11. Cleaned the end of the drain with an antiseptic wipe.
12. Closed and positioned the clamp.
13. Measured the urine.
14. Removed and discarded the paper towel.
15. Emptied the contents of the graduate into the toilet and flushed.
16. Rinsed the graduate. Emptied the rinse into the toilet and flushed.
17. Cleaned and disinfected the graduate.
18. Returned the graduate to its proper place.
19. Removed and discarded the gloves. Practiced hand hygiene.
20. Recorded the time and amount of the urine on the intake and output (I&O) record.

Post-Procedure
21. Provided for comfort.
22. Placed the call light and other needed items within reach.
23. Unscreened the person.
24. Completed a safety check of the room.
25. Reported and recorded the amount of urine and other observations.

Date of Satisfactory Completion _____   Instructor's Initials _____

Removing an Indwelling Catheter

Name: _____ Date: _____

	S	U	Comments
Quality of Life			
• Knocked before entering the person's room.	___	___	_____
• Addressed the person by name.	___	___	_____
• Introduced yourself by name and title.	___	___	_____
• Explained the procedure before starting and during the procedure.	___	___	_____
• Protected the person's rights during the procedure.	___	___	_____
• Handled the person gently during the procedure.	___	___	_____

Pre-Procedure

1. Followed *Delegation Guidelines: Removing Indwelling Catheters.* Saw *Promoting Safety and Comfort:*
   a. *Urinary Catheters*
   b. *Removing Indwelling Catheters*
2. Practiced hand hygiene.
3. Collected the following:
   • Disposable towel
   • Syringe in the size directed by the nurse
   • Disposable bag
   • Gloves
   • Bath blanket
4. Identified the person. Checked the ID (identification) bracelet against the assignment sheet. Used 2 identifiers. Also called the person by name.
5. Provided for privacy.
6. Raised the bed for body mechanics. Bed rails were up if used.

Procedure

7. Lowered the bed rail near you if up.
8. Practiced hand hygiene. Put on gloves.
9. Positioned and draped the person as for perineal care.
10. Covered the person with a bath blanket.
11. Checked the size of balloon. Knew the amount of water in the balloon. Made sure the syringe was large enough to withdraw all the water from the balloon.
12. Removed the tape or tube holder securing the catheter to the person.
13. Positioned the towel.
    a. Female—between her legs
    b. Male—over his thighs
14. Removed all the water from the balloon.
    a. Slid the syringe plunger up and down several times. This loosened the plunger.
    b. Pulled the plunger back to the 0.5 (one-half) mL mark.
    c. Attached the syringe to the catheter's balloon port gently. Used only enough force to get the syringe to stay in the port.
    d. Allowed the water to drain into the syringe. Waited at least 30 seconds to allow the full amount to drain. Did not pull back on the plunger. If the water was draining slow or not at all, called the nurse. Did not remove the catheter if there was water in the balloon. The nurse may have had you:
       1. Gently reposition the syringe in the port.
       2. Re-position the person.
       3. Pull back on the syringe gently and slowly. Forceful pulling would collapse the catheter.

Date of Satisfactory Completion _____ Instructor's Initials _____

Procedure—cont'd	S	U	Comments
15. Pulled the catheter straight out once all the water was removed. Removed the catheter gently.	___ ___	___	_____
16. Discarded the catheter into the bag.	___	___	_____
17. Dried the perineal area with the towel. Discarded the disposable towel in the bag.	___	___	_____
18. Removed and discarded the gloves. Practiced hand hygiene.	___	___	_____
19. Covered the person. Removed the bath blanket.	___	___	_____

Post-Procedure			
20. Provided for privacy.	___	___	_____
21. Placed the call light and other needed items within reach.	___	___	_____
22. Lowered the bed to a safe and comfortable level for the person. Followed the care plan.	___	___	_____
23. Raised or lowered bed rails. Followed the care plan.	___	___	_____
24. Unscreened the person.	___	___	_____
25. Put on clean gloves. Discarded disposable items. Discarded the syringe according to agency policy.	___	___	_____
26. Emptied the drainage bag. Noted the amount of urine.	___	___	_____
27. Discarded the drainage tubing and bag following agency policy.	___	___	_____
28. Removed and discarded the gloves. Practiced hand hygiene.	___	___	_____
29. Completed a safety check of the room.	___	___	_____
30. Practiced hand hygiene.	___	___	_____
31. Reported and recorded your observations.	___	___	_____

Date of Satisfactory Completion _____   Instructor's Initials _____

Applying a Condom Catheter

VIDEO　　VIDEO CLIP

Name: _____　　　Date: _____

	S	U	Comments

Quality of Life
- Knocked before entering the person's room.
- Addressed the person by name.
- Introduced yourself by name and title.
- Explained the procedure before starting and during the procedure.
- Protected the person's rights during the procedure.
- Handled the person gently during the procedure.

Pre-Procedure
1. Followed *Delegation Guidelines:*
   a. *Perineal Care*
   b. *Condom Catheters*
   Saw *Promoting Safety and Comfort:*
   a. *Perineal Care*
   b. *Urinary Catheters*
   c. *Condom Catheters*
2. Practiced hand hygiene.
3. Collected the following:
   - Condom catheter
   - Elastic tape
   - Standard drainage bag or leg bag
   - Cap for the drainage bag
   - Basin of warm water
   - Soap
   - Towel and washcloths
   - Bath blanket
   - Gloves
   - Waterproof pad
   - Paper towels
4. Covered the over-bed table with paper towels. Arranged items on top of them.
5. Identified the person. Checked the ID (identification) bracelet against the assignment sheet. Used 2 identifiers. Also called the person by name.
6. Provided for privacy.
7. Raised the bed for body mechanics. Bed rails were up if used.

Procedure
8. Lowered the bed rail near you if up.
9. Practiced hand hygiene. Put on the gloves.
10. Covered the person with a bath blanket. Lowered top linens to the knees.
11. Asked the person to raise his buttocks off the bed. Or turned him onto his side away from you.
12. Slid the waterproof pad under his buttocks.
13. Had the person lower his buttocks. Or turned him onto his back.
14. Secured the standard drainage bag to the bed frame. Or had a leg bag ready. Closed the drain.
15. Exposed the genital area.
16. Removed the condom catheter.
    a. Removed the tape. Rolled the sheath off the penis.
    b. Disconnected the drainage tubing from the condom. Capped the drainage tube.
    c. Discarded the tape and condom.

Date of Satisfactory Completion _____　　Instructor's Initials _____

Procedure—cont'd	S	U	Comments
17. Provided perineal care. Observed the penis for reddened areas, skin breakdown, and irritations.	___	___	_____
18. Removed and discarded the gloves. Practiced hand hygiene. Put on clean gloves.	___	___	_____
19. Removed the protective backing from the condom. This exposed the adhesive strip.	___	___	_____
20. Held the penis firmly. Rolled the condom onto the penis. Left a 1-inch space between the penis and the end of the catheter.	___	___	_____
21. Secured the condom.			
a. *For a self-adhering condom:* pressed the condom to the penis.	___	___	_____
b. *For a condom secured with elastic tape:* applied elastic tape in a spiral. Did not apply tape completely around the penis.	___	___	_____
22. Made sure the penis tip did not touch the condom. Made sure the condom was not twisted.	___	___	_____
23. Connected the condom to the drainage tubing. Coiled and secured excess tubing on the bed. Or attached a leg bag.	___	___	_____
24. Removed the waterproof pad and gloves. Discarded them. Practiced hand hygiene.	___	___	_____
25. Covered the person. Removed the bath blanket.	___	___	_____

Post-Procedure

	S	U	Comments
26. Provided for comfort.	___	___	_____
27. Placed the call light and other needed items within reach.	___	___	_____
28. Lowered the bed to a safe and comfortable level for the person. Followed the care plan.	___	___	_____
29. Raised or lowered bed rails. Followed the care plan.	___	___	_____
30. Unscreened the person.	___	___	_____
31. Practiced hand hygiene. Put on clean gloves.	___	___	_____
32. Measured and recorded the amount of urine in the bag. Cleaned and discarded the drainage bag.	___	___	_____
33. Cleaned, rinsed, dried, and returned the wash basin and other equipment. Returned items to their proper place.	___	___	_____
34. Removed and discarded the gloves. Practiced hand hygiene.	___	___	_____
35. Completed a safety check of the room.	___	___	_____
36. Reported and recorded your observations.	___	___	_____

Date of Satisfactory Completion _____   Instructor's Initials _____

Checking for and Removing a Fecal Impaction

Name: _____   Date: _____

	S	U	Comments

Quality of Life
- Knocked before entering the person's room.
- Addressed the person by name.
- Introduced yourself by name and title.
- Explained the procedure before starting and during the procedure.
- Protected the person's rights during the procedure.
- Handled the person gently during the procedure.

Pre-Procedure
1. Followed *Delegation Guidelines:*
   a. *Bowel Elimination*
   b. *Fecal Impaction*
   Saw *Promoting Safety and Comfort:*
   a. *Bowel Elimination*
   b. *Fecal Impaction*
2. Practiced hand hygiene.
3. Collected the following:
   - Bedpan and cover
   - Bath blanket
   - Toilet tissue
   - Gloves
   - Lubricant
   - Waterproof pad
   - Basin of warm water
   - Soap
   - Washcloth
   - Bath towel
4. Practiced hand hygiene.
5. Identified the person. Checked the ID (identification) bracelet against the assignment sheet. Used 2 identifiers. Also called the person by name.
6. Provided for privacy.
7. Raised the bed for body mechanics. Bed rails were up if used.

Procedure
8. Lowered the bed rail near you if up.
9. Covered the person with a bath blanket. Fan-folded top linens to the foot of the bed.
10. Positioned the person in Sims' position or in a left side-lying position.
11. Checked the person's pulse. Noted the rate and rhythm.
12. Practiced hand hygiene. Put on the gloves.
13. Placed the waterproof pad under the buttocks.
14. Exposed the anal area.
15. Lubricated your gloved index finger.
16. Asked the person to take a deep breath through his or her mouth.
17. Inserted the gloved finger while the person was taking a deep breath.
18. Checked for a fecal mass. Removed your finger and wiped the area with toilet tissue if:
    a. You did not feel a fecal mass.
    b. You felt a fecal mass but did not remove the impaction.
19. Removed the impaction.
    a. Hooked your index finger around a small piece of feces.
    b. Removed your finger and the feces.
    c. Dropped the stool into the bedpan.

Date of Satisfactory Completion _____   Instructor's Initials _____

Procedure—cont'd	S	U	Comments

Procedure—cont'd

    d. Cleaned your finger with toilet tissue. Placed the toilet
       tissue in the bedpan.

    e. Repeated until you no longer felt feces.

      1) Hooked your index finger around a small piece of feces.

      2) Removed your finger and the feces.

      3) Dropped the stool into the bedpan.

      4) Cleaned your finger with toilet tissue. Placed the toilet
         tissue in the bedpan.

    f. *Checked the person's pulse at intervals. Used your clean*
      gloved hand. Noted rate and rhythm. Stopped the procedure
      if the pulse rate slowed or if the rhythm was irregular.

20. Wiped the anal area with toilet tissue.

21. Removed and discarded the gloves. Practiced hand hygiene.
    Put on clean gloves.

22. Helped the person onto the bedpan. Raised the head of the
    bed and raised the bed rail if used. Or assisted the person to
    the bathroom or commode. The person wore a robe and
    non-skid footwear when up. The bed was in a low position
    safe and comfortable for the person.

23. Placed the call light and toilet tissue within reach. Reminded
    the person not to flush the toilet.

24. Discarded disposable items.

25. Removed and discarded the gloves. Practiced hand hygiene.

26. Left the room if the person could be left alone.

27. Returned when the person signaled. Or checked on the person
    every 5 minutes. Knocked before entering.

28. Practiced hand hygiene and put on gloves. Lowered the
    bed rail if up.

29. Observed stools for amount, color, consistency, shape, and odor.

30. Provided perineal care as needed.

31. Removed the waterproof pad.

32. Emptied, rinsed, cleaned, and disinfected equipment. If the
    person had a bowel movement (BM), flushed the toilet after
    the nurse observed it.

33. Returned equipment to its proper place.

34. Removed and discarded the gloves. Practiced hand hygiene
    after removing and discarding the gloves.

35. Assisted with hand-washing. Wore gloves for this step.
    Practiced hand hygiene after removing and discarding the gloves.

36. Covered the person. Removed the bath blanket.

Post-Procedure

37. Provided for comfort.

38. Placed the call light and other needed items within reach.

39. Lowered the bed to a safe and comfortable level for the person.
    Followed the care plan.

40. Raised or lowered bed rails. Followed the care plan.

41. Unscreened the person.

42. Completed a safety check of the room.

43. Followed agency policy for used linens and used supplies.

44. Practiced hand hygiene.

45. Reported and recorded your observations.

Date of Satisfactory Completion _____   Instructor's Initials _____

Giving a Cleansing Enema

Name: _____   Date: _____

	S	U	Comments

Quality of Life
- Knocked before entering the person's room.
- Addressed the person by name.
- Introduced yourself by name and title.
- Explained the procedure before starting and during the procedure.
- Protected the person's rights during the procedure.
- Handled the person gently during the procedure.

Pre-Procedure
1. Followed *Delegation Guidelines:*
   a. *Bowel Elimination*
   b. *Enemas*
   Saw *Promoting Safety and Comfort:*
   a. *Bowel Elimination*
   b. *Enemas*
2. Practiced hand hygiene.
3. Collected the following before going to the person's room.
   - Disposable enema kit as directed by the nurse (enema bag, tube, clamp, and waterproof pad)
   - Bath thermometer
   - Waterproof pad (if not part of the enema kit)
   - Water-soluble lubricant
   - 3 to 5 milliliters (1 teaspoon) castile soap or 1 to 2 teaspoons of salt
   - IV (intravenous) pole
   - Gloves
4. Arranged items in the person's room and bathroom.
5. Practiced hand hygiene.
6. Identified the person. Checked the ID (identification) bracelet against the assignment sheet. Used 2 identifiers. Also called the person by name.
7. Put on gloves.
8. Collected the following:
   - Commode or bedpan and cover
   - Toilet tissue
   - Bath blanket
   - Robe and non-skid footwear
   - Paper towels
9. Removed and discarded the gloves. Practiced hand hygiene. Put on clean gloves.
10. Provided for privacy.
11. Raised the bed for body mechanics. Bed rails were up if used.

Procedure
12. Lowered the bed rail near you if up.
13. Covered the person with a bath blanket. Fan-folded top linens to the foot of the bed.
14. Positioned the IV pole so the enema bag was 12 inches above the anus. Or it was at the height directed by the nurse.
15. Raised the bed rail if used.
16. Prepared the enema.
    a. Closed the clamp on the tube.
    b. Adjusted water flow until it was lukewarm.
    c. Filled the enema bag for the amount ordered.
    d. Measured water temperature with the bath thermometer. The nurse told you what water temperature to use.

Date of Satisfactory Completion _____   Instructor's Initials _____

Procedure—cont'd	S	U	Comments
e. Prepared the solution as directed by the nurse.			
1) *Tap water:* added nothing.	___	___	_____
2) *Saline enema:* added salt as directed.	___	___	_____
3) *Soapsuds enema (SSE):* added castile soap as directed.	___	___	_____
f. Stirred the solution with the bath thermometer. Scooped off any suds (SSE).	___	___	_____
g. Sealed the bag.	___	___	_____
h. Hung the bag on the IV pole.	___	___	_____
17. Lowered the bed rail near you if up.	___	___	_____
18. Positioned the person in Sims' position or in left side-lying position.	___	___	_____
19. Placed a waterproof pad under the buttocks.	___	___	_____
20. Exposed the anal area.	___	___	_____
21. Placed the bedpan behind the person.	___	___	_____
22. Positioned the enema tube in the bedpan. Removed the cap from the tubing.	___	___	_____
23. Opened the clamp. Allowed solution to flow through the tube to remove air. Clamped the tube.	___	___	_____
24. Lubricated the tube 2 to 4 inches from the tip.	___	___	_____
25. Separated the buttocks to see the anus.	___	___	_____
26. Asked the person to take a deep breath through the mouth.	___	___	_____
27. Inserted the tube gently 2 to 4 inches into the adult's rectum. Did this when the person was exhaling. Stopped if the person complained of pain, you felt resistance, or bleeding occurred.	___	___	_____
28. Checked the amount of solution in the bag.	___	___	_____
29. Unclamped the tube. Gave the solution slowly.	___	___	_____
30. Asked the person to take slow, deep breaths. This helped the person relax.	___	___	_____
31. Clamped the tube if the person needed to have a bowel movement (BM), had cramping, or started to expel solution. Also clamped the tube if the person was sweating or complained of nausea or weakness. Unclamped when symptoms subsided.	___	___	_____
32. Gave the amount of solution ordered. Stopped if the person did not tolerate the procedure.	___	___	_____
33. Clamped the tube before it emptied. This prevented air from entering the bowel.	___	___	_____
34. Held toilet tissue around the tube and against the anus. Removed the tube.	___	___	_____
35. Discarded toilet tissue into the bedpan.	___	___	_____
36. Wrapped the tubing tip with paper towels. Placed it inside the enema bag.	___	___	_____
37. Encouraged retention of the enema for the time ordered.	___	___	_____
38. Assisted the person to the bathroom or commode. The person wore a robe and non-skid footwear when up. The bed was at a low level that was safe and comfortable for the person. Or helped the person onto the bedpan. Raised the head of the bed. Raised or lowered bed rails according to the care plan.	___	___	_____
39. Placed the call light and toilet tissue within reach. Reminded the person not to flush the toilet.	___	___	_____
40. Discarded disposable items.	___	___	_____
41. Removed and discarded the gloves. Practiced hand hygiene.	___	___	_____
42. Left the room if the person could be left alone.	___	___	_____
43. Returned when the person signaled. Or checked on the person every 5 minutes. Knocked before entering the room or bathroom.	___	___	_____
44. Practiced hand hygiene and put on gloves. Lowered the bed rail if up.	___	___	_____
45. Observed enema results for amount, color, consistency, shape, and odor. Called the nurse to observe results.	___	___	_____

Date of Satisfactory Completion _____   Instructor's Initials _____

Procedure—cont'd	S	U	Comments
46. Provided perineal care as needed.			
47. Removed the waterproof pad.	___	___	_____
48. Emptied, rinsed, cleaned, and disinfected equipment. Flushed the toilet after the nurse observed the results.	___	___	_____
49. Returned equipment to its proper place.	___	___	_____
50. Removed and discarded the gloves. Practiced hand hygiene.	___	___	_____
51. Assisted with hand-washing. Wore gloves for this step. Practiced hand hygiene after removing and discarding the gloves.	___	___	_____
52. Covered the person. Removed the bath blanket.	___	___	_____

Post-Procedure

	S	U	Comments
53. Provided for comfort.	___	___	_____
54. Placed the call light and other needed items within reach.	___	___	_____
55. Lowered the bed to a safe and comfortable level for the person. Followed the care plan.	___	___	_____
56. Raised or lowered bed rails. Followed the care plan.	___	___	_____
57. Unscreened the person.	___	___	_____
58. Completed a safety check of the room.	___	___	_____
59. Followed center policy for used linens and used supplies.	___	___	_____
60. Practiced hand hygiene.	___	___	_____
61. Reported and recorded your observations.	___	___	_____

Date of Satisfactory Completion _____   Instructor's Initials _____

Giving a Small-Volume Enema

Name: _____   Date: _____

Quality of Life	S	U	Comments
• Knocked before entering the person's room.	___	___	_____
• Addressed the person by name.	___	___	_____
• Introduced yourself by name and title.	___	___	_____
• Explained the procedure before starting and during the procedure.	___	___	_____
• Protected the person's rights during the procedure.	___	___	_____
• Handled the person gently during the procedure.	___	___	_____

Pre-Procedure

1. Followed *Delegation Guidelines:*
   a. *Bowel Elimination*   ___ ___ _____
   b. *Enemas*   ___ ___ _____
   Saw *Promoting Safety and Comfort:*
   a. *Bowel Elimination*   ___ ___ _____
   b. *Enemas*   ___ ___ _____
2. Practiced hand hygiene.   ___ ___ _____
3. Collected the following before going to the person's room.
   • Small-volume enema   ___ ___ _____
   • Waterproof pad   ___ ___ _____
   • Gloves   ___ ___ _____
4. Arranged items in the person's room.   ___ ___ _____
5. Practiced hand hygiene.   ___ ___ _____
6. Identified the person. Checked the ID (identification) bracelet against the assignment sheet. Used 2 identifiers. Also called the person by name.   ___ ___ _____
7. Put on gloves.   ___ ___ _____
8. Collected the following:
   • Commode or bedpan   ___ ___ _____
   • Toilet tissue   ___ ___ _____
   • Bath blanket   ___ ___ _____
9. Removed and discarded the gloves. Practiced hand hygiene. Put on clean gloves.   ___ ___ _____
10. Provided for privacy.   ___ ___ _____
11. Raised the bed for body mechanics. Bed rails were up if used.   ___ ___ _____

Procedure

12. Lowered the bed rail near you if up.   ___ ___ _____
13. Covered the person with a bath blanket. Fan-folded top linens to the foot of the bed.   ___ ___ _____
14. Positioned the person in Sims' position or in left side-lying position.   ___ ___ _____
15. Placed a waterproof pad under the buttocks.   ___ ___ _____
16. Exposed the anal area.   ___ ___ _____
17. Placed the bedpan near the person.   ___ ___ _____
18. Removed the cap from the enema tip.   ___ ___ _____
19. Separated the buttocks to see the anus. ___ ___ _____
20. Asked the person to take a deep breath through the mouth.   ___ ___ _____
21. Inserted the enema tip 2 inches into the adult's rectum. Did this when the person was exhaling. Inserted the tip gently. Stopped if the person complained of pain, you felt resistance, or bleeding occurred.   ___ ___ _____
22. Squeezed and rolled up the container gently. Released pressure on the bottle after you removed the tip from the rectum.   ___ ___ _____
23. Put the container into the box, tip first. Discarded the container and box.   ___ ___ _____

Date of Satisfactory Completion _____   Instructor's Initials _____

Procedure—cont'd   S   U   **Comments**

24. Assisted the person to the bathroom or commode when he or she had the urge to have a bowel movement (BM). The person wore a robe and non-skid footwear when up. The bed was at a low level that was safe and comfortable for the person. Or helped the person onto the bedpan and raised the head of the bed. Raised or lowered bed rails according to the care plan.
25. Placed the call light and toilet tissue within reach. Reminded the person not to flush the toilet.
26. Discarded disposable items.
27. Removed and discarded the gloves. Practiced hand hygiene.
28. Left the room if the person could be left alone.
29. Returned when the person signaled. Or checked on the person every 5 minutes. Knocked before entering the room or bathroom.
30. Practiced hand hygiene. Put on gloves.
31. Lowered the bed rail if up.
32. Observed enema results for amount, color, consistency, shape, and odor. Called the nurse to observe results.
33. Provided perineal care as needed.
34. Removed the waterproof pad.
35. Emptied, rinsed, cleaned, and disinfected equipment. Flushed the toilet after the nurse observed the results.
36. Returned equipment to its proper place.
37. Removed and discarded the gloves. Practiced hand hygiene.
38. Assisted with hand-washing. Wore gloves for this step. Practiced hand hygiene after removing and discarding the gloves.
39. Covered the person. Removed the bath blanket.

Post-Procedure
40. Provided for comfort.
41. Placed the call light and other needed items within reach.
42. Lowered the bed to a safe and comfortable level for the person. Followed the care plan.
43. Raised or lowered bed rails. Followed the care plan.
44. Unscreened the person.
45. Completed a safety check of the room.
46. Followed center policy for used linens and used supplies.
47. Practiced hand hygiene.
48. Reported and recorded your observations.

Date of Satisfactory Completion _____   Instructor's Initials _____

Giving an Oil-Retention Enema

Name: _____   Date: _____

Quality of Life	S	U	Comments
• Knocked before entering the person's room.	____	____	_____
• Addressed the person by name.	____	____	_____
• Introduced yourself by name and title.	____	____	_____
• Explained the procedure before starting and during the procedure.	____	____	_____
• Protected the person's rights during the procedure.	____	____	_____
• Handled the person gently during the procedure.	____	____	_____

Pre-Procedure

1. Followed *Delegation Guidelines:*
   a. *Bowel Elimination*
   b. *Enemas*
   Saw *Promoting Safety and Comfort:*
   a. *Bowel Elimination*
   b. *Enemas*
2. Practiced hand hygiene.
3. Collected the following before going to the person's room.
   • Oil-retention enema
   • Waterproof pad
   • Gloves
   • Bath blanket
4. Arranged items in the person's room.
5. Practiced hand hygiene.
6. Identified the person. Checked the ID (identification) bracelet against the assignment sheet. Used 2 identifiers. Also called the person by name.
7. Provided for privacy.
8. Raised the bed for body mechanics. Bed rails were up if used.

Procedure

9. Put on gloves.
10. Completed the following steps.
    a. Lowered the bed rail near you if up.
    b. Covered the person with a bath blanket. Fan-folded top linens to the foot of the bed.
    c. Positioned the person in Sims' or in left side-lying position.
    d. Placed the waterproof pad under the buttocks.
    e. Exposed the anal area.
    f. Positioned the bedpan near the person.
    g. Removed the cap from the enema tip.
    h. Separated the buttocks to see the anus.
    i. Asked the person to take a deep breath through the mouth.
    j. Inserted the enema tip 2 inches into the adult's rectum. Did this when the person was exhaling. Inserted the tip gently. Stopped if the person complained of pain, you felt resistance, or bleeding occurred.
    k. Squeezed and rolled up the container gently. Released pressure on the bottle after you removed the tip from the rectum.
    l. Put the container into the box, tip first.
11. Covered the person. Left him or her in the Sims' or left side-lying position.
12. Encouraged retention of the enema for the time ordered.
13. Placed more waterproof pads on the bed if needed.
14. Removed and discarded the gloves. Practiced hand hygiene.

Date of Satisfactory Completion _____   Instructor's Initials _____

Post-Procedure

	S	U	Comments
15. Provided for comfort.	_____	_____	_____
16. Placed the call light and other needed items within reach.	_____	_____	_____
17. Lowered the bed to a safe and comfortable level for the person.	_____	_____	_____
18. Raised or lowered bed rails. Followed the care plan.	_____	_____	_____
19. Unscreened the person.	_____	_____	_____
20. Completed a safety check of the room.	_____	_____	_____
21. Followed center policy for used linens and used supplies.	_____	_____	_____
22. Practiced hand hygiene.	_____	_____	_____
23. Reported and recorded your observations.	_____	_____	_____
24. Checked the person often.	_____	_____	_____

Date of Satisfactory Completion _____   Instructor's Initials _____

Giving an Oil-Retention Enema

VIDEO

Name: _____   Date: _____

Quality of Life	S	U	Comments

Quality of Life
- Knocked before entering the person's room.
- Addressed the person by name.
- Introduced yourself by name and title.
- Explained the procedure before starting and during the procedure.
- Protected the person's rights during the procedure.
- Handled the person gently during the procedure.

Pre-Procedure
1. Followed *Delegation Guidelines:*
   a. *Bowel Elimination*
   b. *Enemas*
   Saw *Promoting Safety and Comfort:*
   a. *Bowel Elimination*
   b. *Enemas*
2. Practiced hand hygiene.
3. Collected the following before going to the person's room.
   - Oil-retention enema
   - Waterproof pad
   - Gloves
   - Bath blanket
4. Arranged items in the person's room.
5. Practiced hand hygiene.
6. Identified the person. Checked the ID (identification) bracelet against the assignment sheet. Used 2 identifiers. Also called the person by name.
7. Provided for privacy.
8. Raised the bed for body mechanics. Bed rails were up if used.

Procedure
9. Put on gloves.
10. Completed the following steps.
    a. Lowered the bed rail near you if up.
    b. Covered the person with a bath blanket. Fan-folded top linens to the foot of the bed.
    c. Positioned the person in Sims' or in left side-lying position.
    d. Placed the waterproof pad under the buttocks.
    e. Exposed the anal area.
    f. Positioned the bedpan near the person.
    g. Removed the cap from the enema tip.
    h. Separated the buttocks to see the anus.
    i. Asked the person to take a deep breath through the mouth.
    j. Inserted the enema tip 2 inches into the adult's rectum. Did this when the person was exhaling. Inserted the tip gently. Stopped if the person complained of pain, you felt resistance, or bleeding occurred.
    k. Squeezed and rolled up the container gently. Released pressure on the bottle after you removed the tip from the rectum.
    l. Put the container into the box, tip first.
11. Covered the person. Left him or her in the Sims' or left side-lying position.
12. Encouraged retention of the enema for the time ordered.
13. Placed more waterproof pads on the bed if needed.
14. Removed and discarded the gloves. Practiced hand hygiene.

Date of Satisfactory Completion _____   Instructor's Initials _____

Post-Procedure

	S	U	Comments
15. Provided for comfort.	_____	_____	_____
16. Placed the call light and other needed items within reach.	_____	_____	_____
17. Lowered the bed to a safe and comfortable level for the person.	_____	_____	_____
18. Raised or lowered bed rails. Followed the care plan.	_____	_____	_____
19. Unscreened the person.	_____	_____	_____
20. Completed a safety check of the room.	_____	_____	_____
21. Followed center policy for used linens and used supplies.	_____	_____	_____
22. Practiced hand hygiene.	_____	_____	_____
23. Reported and recorded your observations.	_____	_____	_____
24. Checked the person often.	_____	_____	_____

Date of Satisfactory Completion _____   Instructor's Initials _____

Changing an Ostomy Pouch

Name: _____   Date: _____

	S	U	Comments

Quality of Life
- Knocked before entering the person's room.
- Addressed the person by name.
- Introduced yourself by name and title.
- Explained the procedure before starting and during the procedure.
- Protected the person's rights during the procedure.
- Handled the person gently during the procedure.

Pre-Procedure
1. Followed *Delegation Guidelines:*
   a. *Bowel Elimination*
   b. *Ostomy Pouches*
   Saw *Promoting Safety and Comfort:*
   a. *Bowel Elimination*
   b. *Ostomy Pouches*
2. Practiced hand hygiene.
3. Collected the following before going to the person's room.
   - Clean pouch with skin barrier
   - Pouch clamp, clip, or wire closure
   - Clean ostomy belt (if used)
   - Gauze pads or washcloths
   - Adhesive remover wipes
   - Skin paste (optional)
   - Pouch deodorant
   - Disposable bag
   - Gloves
   - Paper towels
4. Placed the paper towels on the over-bed table. Arranged supplies on top of the paper towels.
5. Practiced hand hygiene.
6. Identified the person. Checked the ID (identification) bracelet against the assignment sheet. Used 2 identifiers. Also called the person by name.
7. Put on gloves.
8. Collected the following:
   - Bedpan with cover
   - Waterproof pad
   - Bath blanket
   - Wash basin with warm water
9. Removed and discarded the gloves. Practiced hand hygiene. Put on clean gloves.
10. Provided for privacy.
11. Raised the bed for body mechanics. Bed rails were up if used.

Procedure
12. Lowered the bed rail near you if up.
13. Covered the person with a bath blanket. Fan-folded top linens to the foot of the bed.
14. Placed a waterproof pad under the buttocks.
15. Disconnected the pouch from the belt if one was worn. Removed the belt.
16. Removed and placed the pouch and skin barrier in the bedpan. Gently pushed the skin down and lifted up on the barrier. Used adhesive remover wipes if necessary.

Date of Satisfactory Completion _____   Instructor's Initials _____

Procedure—cont'd	S	U	Comments
17. Wiped the stoma and around it with a gauze pad. This removed excess stool and mucus. Discarded the gauze pad into the disposable bag.	___	___	_____
18. Wet the gauze or the washcloth.	___	___	_____
19. Washed the stoma and around it with a gauze pad or washcloth. Washed gently. Did not scrub or rub the skin.	___	___	_____
20. Patted dry with a gauze pad or towel.	___	___	_____
21. Observed the stoma and the skin around the stoma. Reported bleeding, skin irritation, or skin breakdown.	___	___	_____
22. Removed the backing from the new pouch.	___	___	_____
23. Applied a thin layer of paste around the pouch opening. Allowed it to dry following the manufacturer's instructions.	___	___	_____
24. Pulled the skin around the stoma taut. The skin was wrinkle-free.	___	___	_____
25. Centered the pouch over the stoma. The drain was downward.	___	___	_____
26. Pressed around the pouch and skin barrier so it sealed to the skin. Applied gentle pressure with your fingers. Started at the bottom and worked up around the sides to the top.	___	___	_____
27. Maintained the pressure for 1 to 2 minutes. This allowed the adhesive on the skin barrier to activate. Followed the manufacturer's instructions.	___	___	_____
28. Tugged downward on the pouch gently. Made sure pouch was secure.	___	___	_____
29. Added deodorant to the pouch (if used).	___	___	_____
30. Closed the pouch at the bottom. Used a clamp, clip, or wire closure.	___	___	_____
31. Attached the ostomy belt if used. The belt was not too tight. You were able to slide 2 fingers under the belt.	___	___	_____
32. Removed the waterproof pad.	___	___	_____
33. Discarded disposable supplies into the disposable bag.	___	___	_____
34. Removed and discarded the gloves. Practiced hand hygiene.	___	___	_____
35. Covered the person. Removed the bath blanket.	___	___	_____

Post-Procedure

	S	U	Comments
36. Provided for comfort.	___	___	_____
37. Placed the call light and other needed items within reach.	___	___	_____
38. Lowered the bed to a safe and comfortable level for the person. Followed the care plan.	___	___	_____
39. Raised or lowered bed rails. Followed the care plan.	___	___	_____
40. Unscreened the person.	___	___	_____
41. Practiced hand hygiene. Put on gloves.	___	___	_____
42. Took the bedpan and disposable bag into the bathroom.	___	___	_____
43. Emptied the pouch and bedpan into the toilet. Observed the color, amount, consistency, and odor of stools. Flushed the toilet.	___	___	_____
44. Discarded the pouch into the disposable bag. Discarded the disposable bag.	___	___	_____
45. Emptied, rinsed, cleaned, and disinfected equipment. Returned equipment to its proper place.	___	___	_____
46. Removed and discarded gloves. Practiced hand hygiene.	___	___	_____
47. Completed a safety check of the room.	___	___	_____
48. Followed center policy for used linens.	___	___	_____
49. Practiced hand hygiene.	___	___	_____
50. Reported and recorded your observations.	___	___	_____

Date of Satisfactory Completion _____   Instructor's Initials _____

Measuring Intake and Output

NATCEP™ VIDEO VIDEO CLIP

Name: _____   Date: _____

	S	U	Comments
Quality of Life			
• Knocked before entering the person's room.	___	___	_____
• Addressed the person by name.	___	___	_____
• Introduced yourself by name and title.	___	___	_____
• Explained the procedure before starting and during the procedure.	___	___	_____
• Protected the person's rights during the procedure.	___	___	_____
• Handled the person gently during the procedure.	___	___	_____

Pre-Procedure

1. Followed *Delegation Guidelines: Intake and Output*.
   Saw *Promoting Safety and Comfort: Intake and Output*.   ___ ___ _____
2. Practiced hand hygiene.   ___ ___ _____
3. Collected the following:
   - Intake and output (I&O) record   ___ ___ _____
   - Graduates   ___ ___ _____
   - Gloves   ___ ___ _____

Procedure

4. Put on gloves.   ___ ___ _____
5. Measured intake.
   a. Poured liquid remaining in the container into the graduate.
      Avoided spills and splashes on the outside of the graduate.   ___ ___ _____
   b. Measured the amount at eye level. Kept the container
      level.   ___ ___ _____
   c. Checked the serving amount on the I&O record. Or checked
      the serving size of each container.   ___ ___ _____
   d. Subtracted the remaining amount from the full serving
      amount. Noted the amount.   ___ ___ _____
   e. Poured fluid in the graduate back into the container.   ___ ___ _____
   f. Repeated steps for each liquid.
      1) Poured liquid remaining in the container into the graduate.
         Avoided spills and splashes on the outside of the graduate.   ___ ___ _____
      2) Measured the amount at eye level on a flat surface. Kept
         the graduate level.   ___ ___ _____
      3) Checked the serving amount on the I&O record. Or
         checked the serving size of each container.   ___ ___ _____
      4) Subtracted the remaining amount from the full serving
         amount. Noted the amount.   ___ ___ _____
      5) Poured fluid in the graduate back into the container.   ___ ___ _____
   g. Added the amounts from each liquid together.   ___ ___ _____
   h. Recorded the time and amount on the I&O record.   ___ ___ _____
6. Measured output as follows:
   a. Poured fluid into the graduate used to measure output.
      Avoided spills and splashes on the outside of the graduate.   ___ ___ _____
   b. Measured the amount at eye level. Kept the container
      level.   ___ ___ _____
   c. Disposed of fluid in the toilet. Avoided splashes.   ___ ___ _____
7. Cleaned and rinsed the graduates. Disposed of rinse into the
   toilet. Returned the graduates to their proper place.   ___ ___ _____
8. Cleaned, rinsed, and disinfected voiding receptacle or drainage
   container. Disposed of the rinse into the toilet. Returned item
   to its proper place.   ___ ___ _____
9. Removed and discarded the gloves. Practiced hand hygiene.   ___ ___ _____
10. Recorded the output amount on the person's I&O record.   ___ ___ _____

Date of Satisfactory Completion _____   Instructor's Initials _____

Post-Procedure   S   U   **Comments**
11. Provided for comfort.
12. Placed the call light and other items within reach.
13. Completed a safety check of the room.
14. Reported and recorded your observations.

Date of Satisfactory Completion _____   Instructor's Initials _____

Preparing the Person for a Meal

VIDEO   Name: _____   Date: _____

Quality of Life	S	U	Comments

- Knocked before entering the person's room.
- Addressed the person by name.
- Introduced yourself by name and title.
- Explained the procedure before starting and during the procedure.
- Protected the person's rights during the procedure.
- Handled the person gently during the procedure.

Pre-Procedure

1. Followed *Delegation Guidelines: Preparing for Meals.*
   Saw *Promoting Safety and Comfort: Preparing for Meals.*
2. Practiced hand hygiene.
3. Collected the following:
   - Equipment for oral hygiene
   - Bedpan and cover, urinal, commode, or specimen pan
   - Toilet tissue
   - Wash basin
   - Soap
   - Washcloth
   - Towel
   - Gloves
4. Provided for privacy.

Procedure

5. Made sure eyeglasses and hearing aids were in place.
6. Assisted with oral hygiene. Made sure dentures were in place. Wore gloves and practiced hand hygiene after removing and discarding gloves.
7. Assisted with elimination. Made sure the incontinent person was clean and dry. Wore gloves and practiced hand hygiene after removing and discarding the gloves.
8. Assisted with hand-washing. Wore gloves and practiced hand hygiene after removing and discarding them.
9. *Did the following if the person ate in bed.*
   a. Raised the head of the bed to a comfortable position—Fowler's (45 to 60 degrees) or high-Fowler's (60 to 90 degrees). (NOTE: Some state competency tests require that the person sit upright at least 45 degrees to eat, others require 75 to 90 degrees.)
   b. Removed items from the over-bed table. Cleaned the over-bed table.
   c. Adjusted the over-bed table in front of the person.
10. *Did the following if the person sat in a chair.*
    a. Positioned the person in a chair or wheelchair.
    b. Removed items from the over-bed table. Cleaned the table.
    c. Adjusted the over-bed table in front of the person.
11. Assisted the person to the dining area. (This was for the person who ate in dining area.)

Post-Procedure

12. Provided for comfort.
13. Placed the call light and other needed items within reach.
14. Emptied, cleaned, rinsed, and disinfected equipment. Returned equipment to its proper place. Wore gloves and practiced hand hygiene after removing and discarding them.

Date of Satisfactory Completion _____   Instructor's Initials _____

Post-Procedure—cont'd   S   U   **Comments**

15. Straightened the room. Eliminated unpleasant noise,
    odors, or equipment.   _____ _____ _____
16. Unscreened the person.   _____ _____ _____
17. Completed a safety check of the room.   _____ _____ _____
18. Practiced hand hygiene.   _____ _____ _____

Date of Satisfactory Completion _____   Instructor's Initials _____

Serving Meal Trays

Name: _____   Date: _____

	S	U	Comments

Quality of Life
- Knocked before entering the person's room.
- Addressed the person by name.
- Introduced yourself by name and title.
- Explained the procedure before starting and during the procedure.
- Protected the person's rights during the procedure.
- Handled the person gently during the procedure.

Pre-Procedure
1. Followed *Delegation Guidelines: Serving Meal Trays.* Saw *Promoting Safety and Comfort: Serving Meal Trays.*
2. Practiced hand hygiene.

Procedure
3. Made sure the tray was complete. Checked items on the tray with the dietary card. Made sure adaptive equipment (assistive devices) were included.
4. Identified the person. Checked the ID (identification) bracelet against the dietary card. Used 2 identifiers. Also called the person by name.
5. Placed the tray within the person's reach. Adjusted the over-bed table as needed.
6. Removed food covers. Opened cartons, cut meat into bite-sized pieces, buttered bread, and so on as needed. Seasoned food as the person preferred and as allowed on the care plan.
7. Placed the napkin, clothes protector, adaptive equipment (assistive devices), and eating utensils within reach.
8. Placed the call light within reach.
9. Did the following when the person was done eating.
   a. Measured and recorded fluid intake if ordered.
   b. Noted the amount and type of foods eaten.
   c. Checked for and removed any food in the mouth (pocketing). Wore gloves. Practiced hand hygiene after removing and discarding them.
   d. Removed the tray.
   e. Cleaned spills. Changed used linens and clothing.
   f. Helped the person return to bed if needed.
   g. Assisted with oral hygiene and hand-washing. Wore gloves. Decontaminated your hands after removing the gloves.

Post-Procedure
10. Provided for comfort.
11. Placed the call light and other needed items within reach.
12. Raised or lowered bed rails. Followed the care plan.
13. Completed a safety check of the room.
14. Followed center policy for used linens.
15. Practiced hand hygiene.
16. Reported and recorded your observations.

Date of Satisfactory Completion _____   Instructor's Initials _____

Feeding the Person

Name: _____   Date: _____

Quality of Life	S	U	Comments
• Knocked before entering the person's room.	___	___	_____
• Addressed the person by name.	___	___	_____
• Introduced yourself by name and title.	___	___	_____
• Explained the procedure before starting and during the procedure.	___	___	_____
• Protected the person's rights during the procedure.	___	___	_____
• Handled the person gently during the procedure.	___	___	_____

Pre-Procedure

1. Followed *Delegation Guidelines: Feeding the Person.* Saw *Promoting Safety and Comfort: Feeding the Person.*   ___ ___ _____
2. Practiced hand hygiene.   ___ ___ _____
3. Positioned the person in a comfortable position for eating—sitting in a chair or in Fowler's (45 to 60 degrees) or high-Fowler's (60 to 90 degrees). (NOTE: Some state competency tests require that the person sit upright at least 45 degrees, others require 75 to 90 degrees.)   ___ ___ _____
4. Got the tray. Placed the tray on the over-bed table or dining table where the person could reach it.   ___ ___ _____

Procedure

5. Made sure the tray was complete. Checked items on the tray with the dietary card.   ___ ___ _____
6. Identified the person. Checked the ID (identification) bracelet with the dietary card. Used 2 identifiers. Also called the person by name.   ___ ___ _____
7. Draped a napkin across the person's chest and underneath the chin. Cleaned the person's hands with a hand wipe.   ___ ___ _____
8. Told the person what foods and fluids were on the tray.   ___ ___ _____
9. Prepared food for eating. Cut food into bite-sized pieces. Seasoned foods as the person preferred and was allowed on the care plan.   ___ ___ _____
10. Placed a chair where you could sit comfortably. Sat facing the person at eye level.   ___ ___ _____
11. Served foods in the order the person preferred. Identified foods as you served them. Alternated between solid and liquid foods. Used a spoon for safety. Allowed enough time for chewing and swallowing. Did not rush the person. Also offered water, coffee, tea, or other fluids on the tray.   ___ ___ _____
12. Checked the person's mouth before offering more food or fluids. Made sure the person's mouth was empty between bites and swallows. Asked if the person was ready for the next bite or drink.   ___ ___ _____
13. Used straws (if allowed) for liquids if the person could not drink out of a glass or cup. Had 1 straw for each liquid. Provided short straws for weak persons. Followed the care plan for using straws.   ___ ___ _____
14. Wiped the person's hands, face, and mouth as needed during the meal. Used a napkin or hand wipe.   ___ ___ _____
15. Followed the care plan if the person had dysphagia. (Some persons with dysphagia cannot use a straw.) Gave thickened liquids with a spoon.   ___ ___ _____
16. Talked with the person in a pleasant manner.   ___ ___ _____
17. Encouraged the person to eat as much as possible.   ___ ___ _____
18. Wiped the person's mouth with a napkin or a hand wipe. Discarded the napkin or hand wipe.   ___ ___ _____
19. Noted how much and which foods were eaten.   ___ ___ _____

Date of Satisfactory Completion _____   Instructor's Initials _____

Procedure—cont'd	**S**	**U**	**Comments**
20. Measured and recorded fluid intake if ordered.	____	____	_____
21. Removed the tray.	____	____	_____
22. Took the person back to his or her room (if in a dining area).	____	____	_____
23. Assisted with oral hygiene and hand-washing. Wore gloves. Provided for privacy. Practiced hand hygiene after removing and discarding the gloves.	____	____	_____

Post-Procedure			
24. Provided for comfort.	____	____	_____
25. Placed the call light and other needed items within reach.	____	____	_____
26. Raised or lowered bed rails. Followed the care plan.	____	____	_____
27. Completed a safety check of the room.	____	____	_____
28. Returned the food tray to the food cart.	____	____	_____
29. Practiced hand hygiene.	____	____	_____
30. Reported and recorded your observations.	____	____	_____

Date of Satisfactory Completion _____ Instructor's Initials _____

NATCEP™ Providing Drinking Water

Name: _____ Date: _____

	S	U	Comments

Quality of Life
- Knocked before entering the person's room.
- Addressed the person by name.
- Introduced yourself by name and title.
- Explained the procedure before starting and during the procedure.
- Protected the person's rights during the procedure.
- Handled the person gently during the procedure.

Pre-Procedure
1. Followed *Delegation Guidelines: Providing Drinking Water*. Saw *Promoting Safety and Comfort: Providing Drinking Water*.
2. Obtained a list of persons who have special fluid orders from the nurse. Or used your assignment sheet.
3. Practiced hand hygiene.
4. Collected the following:
   - Cart
   - Ice chest filled with ice
   - Cover for ice chest
   - Scoop
   - Paper towels
   - Water mugs for patient or resident use
   - Large water pitcher filled with cold water (optional depending on agency procedure)
   - Towel for the scoop
5. Covered the cart with paper towels. Arranged equipment on top of the paper towels.

Procedure
6. Took the cart to the person's room door. Did not take the cart into the room.
7. Checked the person's fluid orders. Used the list from the nurse.
8. Identified the person. Checked the ID (identification) bracelet against the fluid order sheet or your assignment sheet. Used 2 identifiers. Also called the person by name.
9. Took the mug from the person's over-bed table. Emptied it into the bathroom sink.
10. Determined if a new mug was needed.
11. Used the scoop to fill the mug with ice. Did not let the scoop touch the mug, lid, or straw.
12. Placed the scoop on the towel.
13. Filled the mug with water. Got water from the bathroom or used the larger water pitcher on the cart.
14. Placed the mug on the over-bed table.
15. Made sure the mug was within the person's reach.

Post-Procedure
16. Provided for comfort.
17. Placed the call light and other needed items within reach.
18. Completed a safety check of the room.
19. Practiced hand hygiene.
20. Repeated for each resident.
    a. Took the cart to the person's room door. Did not take the cart into the room.
    b. Checked the person's fluid orders. Used the list from the nurse.

Date of Satisfactory Completion _____   Instructor's Initials _____

	S	U	Comments
Post-Procedure—cont'd			
c. Identified the person. Checked the ID bracelet against the fluid order sheet or your assignment sheet. Used 2 identifiers. Also called the person by name.	____	____	_____
d. Took the mug from the person's over-bed table. Emptied it into the bathroom sink.	____	____	_____
e. Determined if a new mug was needed.	____	____	_____
f. Used the scoop to fill the mug with ice. Did not let the scoop touch the mug, lid, or straw.	____	____	_____
g. Placed the scoop on the towel.	____	____	_____
h. Filled the mug with water. Got water from the bathroom or the large water pitcher on the cart.	____	____	_____
i. Placed the mug on the over-bed table.	____	____	_____
j. Made sure the mug was within the person's reach.	____	____	_____
k. Provided for comfort.	____	____	_____
l. Placed the call light and other needed items within reach.	____	____	_____
m. Completed a safety check of the room.	____	____	_____
n. Practiced hand hygiene.	____	____	_____

Date of Satisfactory Completion _____   Instructor's Initials _____

Taking a Temperature With an Electronic Thermometer

NATCEP™   VIDEO   VIDEO CLIP

Name: _____   Date: _____

	S	U	Comments

Quality of Life
- Knocked before entering the person's room.
- Addressed the person by name.
- Introduced yourself by name and title.
- Explained the procedure before starting and during the procedure.
- Protected the person's rights during the procedure.
- Handled the person gently during the procedure.

Pre-Procedure
1. Followed *Delegation Guidelines: Taking Temperatures.* Saw *Promoting Safety and Comfort: Taking Temperatures.*
2. For an oral temperature, asked the person not to eat, drink, smoke, or chew gum for at least 15 to 20 minutes before the measurement or as required by agency policy.
3. Practiced hand hygiene.
4. Collected the following:
   - Thermometer—electronic or tympanic membrane
   - Probe (blue for an oral or axillary temperature, red for a rectal temperature)
   - Probe covers
   - Toilet tissue (rectal temperature)
   - Water-soluble lubricant (rectal temperature)
   - Gloves
   - Towel (axillary temperature)
5. Plugged the probe into the thermometer if using an electronic thermometer.
6. Practiced hand hygiene.
7. Identified the person. Checked the ID (identification) bracelet against the assignment sheet. Used 2 identifiers. Also called the person by name.

Procedure
8. Provided for privacy. Positioned the person for an oral, rectal, axillary, or tympanic membrane temperature. The Sims' position was used for a rectal temperature.
9. Put on the gloves if contact with blood, body fluids, secretions, or excretions was likely.
10. Inserted the probe into the probe cover.
11. *For an oral temperature:*
    a. Asked the person to open the mouth and raise the tongue.
    b. Placed the covered probe at the base of the tongue and to 1 side.
    c. Asked the person to lower the tongue and close the mouth.
12. *For a rectal temperature:*
    a. Placed some lubricant on a tissue.
    b. Lubricated the end of the covered probe.
    c. Exposed the anal area.
    d. Raised the upper buttock.
    e. Inserted the probe ½ inch into the rectum.
    f. Held the probe in place.
13. *For an axillary temperature:*
    a. Helped the person remove an arm from the gown. Did not expose the person.
    b. Dried the axilla with a towel.
    c. Placed the covered probe in the axilla.
    d. Placed the person's arm over the chest.
    e. Held the probe in place.

Date of Satisfactory Completion _____   Instructor's Initials _____

Procedure—cont'd	S	U	Comments

Procedure—cont'd

14. *For a tympanic membrane temperature:*
    a. Asked the person to turn his or her head so the ear was in front of you. ___ ___ _____
    b. Pulled up and back on the adult's ear to straighten the ear canal. ___ ___ _____
    c. Inserted the covered probe gently. ___ ___ _____
15. Started the thermometer. ___ ___ _____
16. Held the probe in place until you heard a tone or saw a flashing or steady light. ___ ___ _____
17. Read the temperature on the display. ___ ___ _____
18. Removed the probe. Pressed the eject button to discard the cover. ___ ___ _____
19. Noted the person's name, temperature, and temperature site on your note pad or assignment sheet. ___ ___ _____
20. Returned the probe to the holder. ___ ___ _____
21. Helped the person put the gown back on (axillary temperature). For a rectal temperature:
    a. Wiped the anal area with toilet tissue to remove lubricant. ___ ___ _____
    b. Covered the person. ___ ___ _____
    c. Disposed of used toilet tissue. ___ ___ _____
    d. Removed and discarded the gloves. Practiced hand hygiene. ___ ___ _____

Post-Procedure

22. Provided for comfort. ___ ___ _____
23. Placed the call light and other needed items within reach. ___ ___ _____
24. Unscreened the person. ___ ___ _____
25. Completed a safety check of the room. ___ ___ _____
26. Returned the thermometer to the charging unit. ___ ___ _____
27. Practiced hand hygiene. ___ ___ _____
28. Reported and recorded the temperature. Noted the temperature site when reporting and recording. Reported an abnormal temperature at once. ___ ___ _____

Date of Satisfactory Completion _____ Instructor's Initials _____

Taking a Temperature With a Glass Thermometer

Name: _____   Date: _____

Quality of Life	S	U	Comments
• Knocked before entering the person's room.			
• Addressed the person by name.			
• Introduced yourself by name and title.			
• Explained the procedure before starting and during the procedure.			
• Protected the person's rights during the procedure.			
• Handled the person gently during the procedure.			

Pre-Procedure

1. Followed *Delegation Guidelines: Taking Temperatures*.
   Saw *Promoting Safety and Comfort:*
   a. *Taking Temperatures*
   b. *Glass Thermometers*
2. For an oral temperature, asked the person not to eat, drink, smoke, or chew gum for at least 15 to 20 minutes before the measurement or as required by agency policy.
3. Practiced hand hygiene.
4. Collected the following:
   • Oral or rectal thermometer and holder
   • Tissues
   • Plastic covers if used
   • Gloves
   • Toilet tissue (rectal temperature)
   • Water-soluble lubricant (rectal temperature)
   • Towel (axillary temperature)
5. Practiced hand hygiene.
6. Identified the person. Checked the ID (identification) bracelet against the assignment sheet. Used 2 identifiers. Also called the person by name.
7. Provided for privacy.

Procedure

8. Put on the gloves.
9. Rinsed the thermometer under cold running water if it was soaking in disinfectant. Dried it with tissues.
10. Checked for breaks, cracks, or chips.
11. Shook down the thermometer below the lowest number. Held the device by the stem.
12. Inserted it into a plastic cover if used.
13. *For an oral temperature:*
    a. Asked the person to moisten his or her lips.
    b. Placed the bulb end of the thermometer under the tongue and to 1 side.
    c. Asked the person to close the lips around the thermometer to hold it in place.
    d. Asked the person not to talk. Reminded the person not to bite down on the thermometer.
    e. Left it in place for 2 to 3 minutes or as required by agency policy.
14. *For a rectal temperature:*
    a. Positioned the person in the Sims' position.
    b. Put a small amount of lubricant on a tissue.
    c. Lubricated the bulb end of the thermometer.
    d. Folded back top linens to expose the anal area.
    e. Raised the upper buttock to expose the anus.

Date of Satisfactory Completion _____   Instructor's Initials _____

Procedure—cont'd	S	U	Comments

f. Inserted the thermometer 1 inch into the rectum.
Did not force the thermometer. _____ _____ _____

g. Held the thermometer in place for 2 minutes or as required by
agency policy. Did not let go of it while it was in the rectum. _____ _____ _____

15. *For an axillary temperature:*

  a. Helped the person remove an arm from the gown. Did not
  expose the person. _____ _____ _____

  b. Dried the axilla with the towel. _____ _____ _____

  c. Placed the bulb end of the thermometer in the center of the axilla. _____ _____ _____

  d. Asked the person to place the arm over the chest to hold the
  thermometer in place if he or she could not help. _____ _____ _____

  e. Left the thermometer in place for 5 to 10 minutes or as
  required by agency policy. _____ _____ _____

16. Removed the thermometer. _____ _____ _____

17. *For an oral or axillary temperature:*

  a. Used a tissue to remove the plastic cover. _____ _____ _____

  b. Wiped the thermometer with a tissue if no cover was used.
  Wiped from the stem to the bulb end. _____ _____ _____

  c. Discarded the tissue and cover (if used). _____ _____ _____

  d. Read the thermometer. _____ _____ _____

  e. Helped the person put the gown back on (axillary temperature). _____ _____ _____

18. *For a rectal temperature:*

  a. Used toilet tissue to remove the plastic cover. _____ _____ _____

  b. Wiped the thermometer with toilet tissue if no cover was used.
  Wiped from the stem to the bulb end. _____ _____ _____

  c. Placed used toilet tissue on several thicknesses of clean toilet
  tissue. Discarded the cover (if used). _____ _____ _____

  d. Read the thermometer. _____ _____ _____

  e. Placed the thermometer on clean toilet tissue. _____ _____ _____

  f. Wiped the anal area with toilet tissue to remove lubricant and
  any feces. Set the used toilet tissue on several thicknesses of
  clean toilet tissue. _____ _____ _____

  g. Covered the person. _____ _____ _____

  h. Discarded tissue and disposed of toilet tissue in the toilet. _____ _____ _____

  i. Removed and discarded the glove. Practiced hand hygiene. _____ _____ _____

19. Noted the person's name and temperature on your note pad or
assignment sheet. _____ _____ _____

20. Shook down the thermometer. _____ _____ _____

21. Cleaned the thermometer following agency policy. (Wore gloves.)
Returned it to the holder. _____ _____ _____

22. Removed and discarded the gloves. Practiced hand hygiene. _____ _____ _____

Post-Procedure

23. Provided for comfort. _____ _____ _____

24. Placed the call light and other needed items within reach. _____ _____ _____

25. Unscreened the person. _____ _____ _____

26. Completed a safety check of the room. _____ _____ _____

27. Practiced hand hygiene. _____ _____ _____

28. Reported and recorded the temperature. Noted the temperature
site when reporting and recording. Reported an abnormal
temperature at once. _____ _____ _____

Date of Satisfactory Completion _____   Instructor's Initials _____

Taking a Radial Pulse

Name: _____   Date: _____

	S	U	Comments

Quality of Life
- Knocked before entering the person's room.
- Addressed the person by name.
- Introduced yourself by name and title.
- Explained the procedure before starting and during the procedure.
- Protected the person's rights during the procedure.
- Handled the person gently during the procedure.

Pre-Procedure
1. Followed *Delegation Guidelines: Taking Pulses.* Saw *Promoting Safety and Comfort: Taking Pulses.*
2. Practiced hand hygiene.
3. Identified the person. Checked the ID (identification) bracelet against the assignment sheet. Used 2 identifiers. Also called the person by name.
4. Provided for privacy.

Procedure
5. Had the person sit or lie down.
6. Located the radial pulse on the thumb side of the person's wrist. Used your first 2 or 3 middle fingertips.
7. Noted if the pulse was strong or weak, regular or irregular.
8. Counted the pulse for 30 seconds. Multiplied the number of beats by 2 for the number of pulses in 60 seconds (1 minute).
9. Counted the pulse for 1 minute if:
   a. Directed by the nurse and care plan.
   b. Required by agency policy.
   c. The pulse was irregular.
   d. Required for your state competency test.
10. Noted the following on your note pad or assignment sheet.
    a. The person's name
    b. Pulse rate
    c. Pulse strength
    d. If the pulse was regular or irregular

Post-Procedure
11. Provided for comfort.
12. Placed the call light and other needed items within reach.
13. Unscreened the person.
14. Completed a safety check of the room.
15. Practiced hand hygiene.
16. Reported and recorded the pulse rate and your observations. Reported an abnormal pulse at once.

Date of Satisfactory Completion _____   Instructor's Initials _____

Taking an Apical Pulse

Name: _____   Date: _____

	S	U	Comments

Quality of Life
- Knocked before entering the person's room.
- Addressed the person by name.
- Introduced yourself by name and title.
- Explained the procedure before starting and during the procedure.
- Protected the person's rights during the procedure.
- Handled the person gently during the procedure.

Pre-Procedure
1. Followed *Delegation Guidelines: Taking Pulses.*
   Saw *Promoting Safety and Comfort: Using a Stethoscope.*
2. Practiced hand hygiene.
3. Collected a stethoscope and antiseptic wipes.
4. Practiced hand hygiene.
5. Identified the person. Checked the ID (identification) bracelet against the assignment sheet. Used 2 identifiers. Also called the person by name.
6. Provided for privacy.

Procedure
7. Cleaned the stethoscope ear-pieces and chest-piece with the wipes.
8. Had the person sit or lie down.
9. Exposed the nipple area of the left chest. Exposed a woman's breasts only to the extent necessary.
10. Warmed the diaphragm in your palm.
11. Placed the ear-pieces in your ears.
12. Found the apical pulse. Placed the diaphragm 2 to 3 inches to the left of the breastbone and below the left nipple.
13. Counted the pulse for 1 minute. Noted if it was regular or irregular.
14. Covered the person. Removed the ear-pieces.
15. Noted the person's name and pulse on your note pad or assignment sheet. Noted if the pulse was regular or irregular.

Post-Procedure
16. Provided for comfort.
17. Placed the call light and other needed items within reach.
18. Unscreened the person.
19. Completed a safety check of the room.
20. Cleaned the ear-pieces and chest-piece with the wipes.
21. Returned the stethoscope to its proper place.
22. Practiced hand hygiene.
23. Reported and recorded your observations. Recorded the pulse rate with *Ap* for apical. Reported an abnormal pulse rate at once.

Date of Satisfactory Completion _____   Instructor's Initials _____

Taking an Apical-Radial Pulse

Name: _____   Date: _____

	S	U	Comments

Quality of Life
- Knocked before entering the person's room.
- Addressed the person by name.
- Introduced yourself by name and title.
- Explained the procedure before starting and during the procedure.
- Protected the person's rights during the procedure.
- Handled the person gently during the procedure.

Pre-Procedure
1. Followed *Delegation Guidelines: Taking Pulses*.
   Saw *Promoting Safety and Comfort:*
   a. *Using a Stethoscope*
   b. *Taking Pulses*
2. Asked a co-worker to help you.
3. Practiced hand hygiene.
4. Collected a stethoscope and antiseptic wipes.
5. Practiced hand hygiene.
6. Identified the person. Checked the ID (identification) bracelet against the assignment sheet. Used 2 identifiers. Also called the person by name.
7. Provided for privacy.

Procedure
8. Cleaned the stethoscope ear-pieces and chest-piece with the wipes.
9. Had the person sit or lie down.
10. Exposed the nipple area of the left chest. Exposed a woman's breasts to the extent necessary.
11. Warmed the diaphragm in your palm.
12. Placed the ear-pieces in your ears.
13. Found the apical pulse. Your helper found the radial pulse.
14. Gave the signal to begin counting.
15. Counted the apical pulse for 1 minute. Your co-worker counted the radial pulse for 1 minute.
16. Gave the signal to stop counting. Asked your co-worker for the radial pulse.
17. Covered the person. Removed the stethoscope ear-pieces.
18. Noted the person's name and apical and radial pulses on your note pad or assignment sheet. Subtracted the radial pulse from the apical pulse for the pulse deficit. Noted if the pulses were regular or irregular.

Post-Procedure
19. Provided for comfort.
20. Placed the call light and other needed items within reach.
21. Unscreened the person.
22. Completed a safety check of the room.
23. Cleaned the ear-pieces and chest-piece with the wipes.
24. Returned the stethoscope to its proper place.
25. Practiced hand hygiene.
26. Reported and recorded your observations. (Reported an abnormal pulse at once.) Included:
    a. The apical and radial pulse rates.
    b. The pulse deficit.

Date of Satisfactory Completion _____   Instructor's Initials _____

Counting Respirations

Name: _____   Date: _____

Procedure	S	U	Comments
1. Followed *Delegation Guidelines: Counting Respirations.*	___	___	_____
2. Kept your fingers or stethoscope over the pulse site.	___	___	_____
3. Did not tell the person you were counting respirations.	___	___	_____
4. Began counting when the chest rose. Counted each rise and fall of the chest as 1 respiration.	___	___	_____
5. Noted the following:			
a. If respirations were regular	___	___	_____
b. If both sides of the chest rose equally	___	___	_____
c. The depth of the respirations	___	___	_____
d. If the person had any pain or difficulty breathing	___	___	_____
e. An abnormal respiratory pattern	___	___	_____
6. Counted respirations for 30 seconds. Multiplied the number by 2 for the number of respirations in 60 seconds (1 minute).	___	___	_____
7. Counted respirations for 1 minute if:			
a. Directed by the nurse and care plan.	___	___	_____
b. Required by agency policy.	___	___	_____
c. They were abnormal or irregular.	___	___	_____
d. Required for your state competency test.	___	___	_____
8. Noted the person's name, respiratory rate, and other observations on your note pad or assignment sheet.	___	___	_____

Post-Procedure

	S	U	Comments
9. Provided for comfort.	___	___	_____
10. Placed the call light and other needed items within reach.	___	___	_____
11. Unscreened the person.	___	___	_____
12. Completed a safety check of the room.	___	___	_____
13. Practiced hand hygiene.	___	___	_____
14. Reported and recorded the respiratory rate and your observations. Reported abnormal respirations at once.	___	___	_____

Date of Satisfactory Completion _____   Instructor's Initials _____

Measuring Blood Pressure

Name: _____   Date: _____

	S	U	Comments

Quality of Life
- Knocked before entering the person's room.
- Addressed the person by name.
- Introduced yourself by name and title.
- Explained the procedure before starting and during the procedure.
- Protected the person's rights during the procedure.
- Handled the person gently during the procedure.

Pre-Procedure
1. Followed *Delegation Guidelines: Measuring Blood Pressure.*
   Saw *Promoting Safety and Comfort:*
   a. *Using a Stethoscope*
   b. *Blood Pressure Equipment*
2. Practiced hand hygiene.
3. Collected the following:
   - Sphygmomanometer
   - Stethoscope
   - Antiseptic wipes
4. Practiced hand hygiene.
5. Identified the person. Checked the ID (identification) bracelet
   against the assignment sheet. Used 2 identifiers. Also called
   the person by name.
6. Provided for privacy.

Procedure
7. Wiped the stethoscope ear-pieces and chest-piece with the wipes.
   Warmed the diaphragm in your palm.
8. Had the person sit or lie down.
9. Positioned the person's arm level with the heart. The palm was up.
10. Stood no more than 3 feet away from the manometer. The mercury
    type was vertical, on a flat service. The aneroid type was directly in
    front of you.
11. Exposed the upper arm.
12. Squeezed the cuff to expel any air. Closed the valve on the bulb.
13. Found the brachial artery at the inner aspect of the elbow. (The
    brachial artery is on the little finger side of the arm.) Used
    your fingertips.
14. Located the arrow on the cuff. Aligned the arrow on the cuff over
    the brachial artery. Wrapped the cuff around the upper arm at
    least 1 inch above the elbow. It was even and snug.
15. Placed the stethoscope ear-pieces in your ears. Placed the
    diaphragm over the brachial artery. Did not place it under the cuff.
16. Found the radial pulse for Methods 1 and 2.
17. *Method 1:*
    a. Inflated the cuff until you could no longer feel the pulse.
       Noted this point.
    b. Inflated the cuff 30 mm Hg beyond the point where you
       last felt the pulse.
18. *Method 2:*
    a. Inflated the cuff until you no longer felt the pulse.
       Noted this point.
    b. Inflated the cuff 30 mm Hg beyond the point where you
       last felt the pulse.
    c. Deflated the cuff slowly. Noted the point where you felt the pulse.
    d. Waited 30 seconds.
    e. Inflated the cuff 30 mm Hg beyond the point where you
       felt the pulse return.

Date of Satisfactory Completion _____   Instructor's Initials _____

Procedure—cont'd   S   U   **Comments**

19. *Method 3:*
    a. Inflated the cuff 160 mm Hg to 180 mm Hg.   ___   ___   _____
    b. Deflated the cuff if you heard a blood pressure (BP) sound.
        Re-inflated the cuff to 200 mm Hg.   ___   ___   _____
20. Deflated the cuff at an even rate of 2 to 4 millimeters per second.
    Turned the valve counter-clockwise to deflate the cuff.   ___   ___   _____
21. Noted the point where you heard the first sound. This was the
    systolic reading. It was near the point where the radial pulse
    disappeared (Method 1) or returned (Method 2).   ___   ___   _____
22. Continued to deflate the cuff. Noted the point where the sound
    disappeared. This was the diastolic reading.   ___   ___   _____
23. Deflated the cuff completely. Removed it from the person's arm.
    Removed the stethoscope ear-pieces from your ears.   ___   ___   _____
24. Noted the person's name and BP on your note pad or
    assignment sheet.   ___   ___   _____
25. Returned the cuff to the case or the wall holder.   ___   ___   _____

Post-Procedure
26. Provided for comfort.   ___   ___   _____
27. Placed the call light and other needed items within reach.   ___   ___   _____
28. Unscreened the person.   ___   ___   _____
29. Completed a safety check of the room.   ___   ___   _____
30. Cleaned the ear-pieces and chest-piece with the wipes.   ___   ___   _____
31. Returned the equipment to its proper place.   ___   ___   _____
32. Practiced hand hygiene.   ___   ___   _____
33. Reported and recorded the BP. Noted which arm was used.
    Reported an abnormal BP at once.   ___   ___   _____

Date of Satisfactory Completion _____   Instructor's Initials _____

Performing Range-of-Motion Exercises

Name: _____ Date: _____

	S	U	Comments

Quality of Life
- Knocked before entering the person's room.
- Addressed the person by name.
- Introduced yourself by name and title.
- Explained the procedure before starting and during the procedure.
- Protected the person's rights during the procedure.
- Handled the person gently during the procedure.

Pre-Procedure
1. Followed *Delegation Guidelines: Range-of-Motion Exercises*. Saw *Promoting Safety and Comfort: Range-of-Motion Exercises*.
2. Practiced hand hygiene.
3. Identified the person. Checked the ID (identification) bracelet against the assignment sheet. Used 2 identifiers. Also called the person by name.
4. Obtained a bath blanket.
5. Provided for privacy.
6. Raised the bed for body mechanics. Bed rails were up if used.

Procedure
7. Lowered the bed rail near you if up.
8. Positioned the person supine.
9. Covered the person with a bath blanket. Fan-folded top linens to the foot of the bed.
10. Exercised the neck *if allowed by your agency and if the nurse instructed you to do so.*
    a. Placed your hands over the person's ears to support the head. Supported the jaw with your fingers.
    b. Flexion—brought the head forward. The chin touched the chest.
    c. Extension—straightened the head.
    d. Hyperextension—brought the head backward until the chin pointed up.
    e. Rotation—turned the head from side to side.
    f. Lateral flexion—moved the head to the right and to the left.
    g. Repeated flexion, extension, hyperextension, rotation, and lateral flexion 5 times—or the number of times stated on the care plan.
11. Exercised the shoulder.
    a. Grasped the wrist with 1 hand. Grasped the elbow with the other hand.
    b. Flexion—raised the arm straight in front and over the head.
    c. Extension—brought the arm down to the side.
    d. Hyperextension—moved the arm behind the body. (Did this if the person was sitting in a straight-backed chair or was standing.)
    e. Abduction—moved the straight arm away from the side of the body.
    f. Adduction—moved the straight arm to the side of the body.
    g. Internal rotation—bent the elbow. Placed it at the same level as the shoulder. Moved the forearm and hand so the fingers pointed down.
    h. External rotation—moved the forearm and hand so the fingers pointed up.
    i. Repeated flexion, extension, hyperextension, abduction, adduction, and internal and external rotation 5 times—or the number of times stated on the care plan.

Date of Satisfactory Completion _____ Instructor's Initials _____

Procedure—cont'd	S	U	Comments

12. Exercised the elbow.
a. Grasped the person's wrist with 1 hand. Grasped the elbow
   with your other hand. _____ _____ _____
b. Flexion—bent the arm so the same-side shoulder was touched. _____ _____ _____
c. Extension—straightened the arm. _____ _____ _____
d. Repeated flexion and extension 5 times—or the number of
   times stated on the care plan. _____ _____ _____

13. Exercised the forearm.
a. Continued to support the wrist and elbow. _____ _____ _____
b. Pronation—turned the hand so the palm was down. _____ _____ _____
c. Supination—turned the hand so the palm was up. _____ _____ _____
d. Repeated pronation and supination 5 times—or the number
   of times stated on the care plan. _____ _____ _____

14. Exercised the wrist.
a. Held the wrist with both of your hands. _____ _____ _____
b. Flexion—bent the hand down. _____ _____ _____
c. Extension—straightened the hand. _____ _____ _____
d. Hyperextension—bent the hand back. _____ _____ _____
e. Radial flexion—turned the hand toward the thumb. _____ _____ _____
f. Ulnar flexion—turned the hand toward the little finger. _____ _____ _____
g. Repeated flexion, extension, hyperextension, and radial and
   ulnar flexion 5 times—or the number of times stated
   on the care plan. _____ _____ _____

15. Exercised the thumb.
a. Held the person's hand with 1 hand. Held the thumb with
   your other hand. _____ _____ _____
b. Abduction—moved the thumb out from the inner part of
   the index finger. _____ _____ _____
c. Adduction—moved the thumb back next to the index finger. _____ _____ _____
d. Opposition—touched each finger with the thumb. _____ _____ _____
e. Flexion—bent the thumb into the hand. _____ _____ _____
f. Extension—moved the thumb out to the side of the fingers. _____ _____ _____
g. Repeated abduction, adduction, opposition, flexion, and
   extension 5 times—or the number of times stated on
   the care plan. _____ _____ _____

16. Exercised the fingers.
a. Abduction—spread the fingers and the thumb apart. _____ _____ _____
b. Adduction—brought the fingers and thumb together. _____ _____ _____
c. Flexion—made a fist. _____ _____ _____
d. Extension—straightened the fingers so the fingers, hand,
   and arm were straight. _____ _____ _____
e. Repeated abduction, adduction, flexion, and extension
   5 times—or the number of times stated on the care plan. _____ _____ _____

17. Exercised the hip.
a. Supported the leg. Placed 1 hand under the knee. Placed
   your other hand under the ankle. _____ _____ _____
b. Flexion—raised the leg. _____ _____ _____
c. Extension—straightened the leg. _____ _____ _____
d. Hyperextension—moved the leg behind the body. (Did this
   if the person was standing.) _____ _____ _____
e. Abduction—moved the leg away from the body. _____ _____ _____
f. Adduction—moved the leg toward the other leg. _____ _____ _____
g. Internal rotation—turned the leg inward. _____ _____ _____
h. External rotation—turned the leg outward. _____ _____ _____
i. Repeated flexion, extension, hyperextension, abduction,
   adduction, and internal and external rotation 5 times—or the
   number of times stated on the care plan. _____ _____ _____

Date of Satisfactory Completion _____   Instructor's Initials _____

Procedure—cont'd	**S**	**U**	**Comments**

18. Exercised the knee.
    a. Supported the knee. Placed 1 hand under the knee. Placed your other hand under the ankle. _____ _____ _____
    b. Flexion—bent the knee. _____ _____ _____
    c. Extension—straightened the knee. _____ _____ _____
    d. Repeated flexion and extension of the knee 5 times—or the number of times stated on the care plan. _____ _____ _____
19. Exercised the ankle.
    a. Supported the foot and ankle. Placed 1 hand under the foot. Placed your other hand under the ankle. _____ _____ _____
    b. Dorsiflexion—pulled the foot forward. Pushed down on the heel at the same time. _____ _____ _____
    c. Plantar flexion—turned the foot down. Or pointed the toes. _____ _____ _____
    d. Repeated dorsiflexion and plantar flexion 5 times—or the number of times stated on the care plan. _____ _____ _____
20. Exercised the foot.
    a. Continued to support the foot and ankle. _____ _____ _____
    b. Pronation—turned the outside of the foot up and the inside down. _____ _____ _____
    c. Supination—turned the inside of the foot up and the outside down. _____ _____ _____
    d. Repeated pronation and supination 5 times—or the number of times stated on the care plan. _____ _____ _____
21. Exercised the toes.
    a. Flexion—curled the toes. _____ _____ _____
    b. Extension—straightened the toes. _____ _____ _____
    c. Abduction—spread the toes apart. _____ _____ _____
    d. Adduction—pulled the toes together. _____ _____ _____
    e. Repeated flexion, extension, abduction, and adduction 5 times—or the number of times stated on the care plan. _____ _____ _____
22. Covered the leg. Raised the bed rail if used. _____ _____ _____
23. Went to the other side. Lowered the bed rail near you if up. _____ _____ _____
24. Repeated exercises.
    a. Exercised the shoulder.
       1) Grasped the wrist with 1 hand. Grasped the elbow with the other hand. _____ _____ _____
       2) Flexion—raised the arm straight in front and over the head. _____ _____ _____
       3) Extension—brought the arm down to the side. _____ _____ _____
       4) Hyperextension—moved the arm behind the body. (Did this if the person was sitting in a straight-backed chair or was standing.) _____ _____ _____
       5) Abduction—moved the straight arm away from the side of the body. _____ _____ _____
       6) Adduction—Moved the straight arm to the side of the body. _____ _____ _____
       7) Internal rotation—bent the elbow. Placed it at the same level as the shoulder. Moved the forearm down toward the body. _____ _____ _____
       8) External rotation—moved the forearm toward the head. _____ _____ _____
       9) Repeated flexion, extension, hyperextension, abduction, adduction, and internal and external rotation 5 times—or the number of times stated on the care plan. _____ _____ _____
    b. Exercised the elbow.
       1) Grasped the person's wrist with 1 hand. Grasped the elbow with your other hand. _____ _____ _____
       2) Flexion—bent the arm so the same-side shoulder was touched. _____ _____ _____
       3) Extension—straightened the arm. _____ _____ _____
       4) Repeated flexion and extension 5 times—or the number of times stated on the care plan. _____ _____ _____

Date of Satisfactory Completion _____   Instructor's Initials _____

Procedure—cont'd   S   U   **Comments**

   c. Exercised the forearm.
     1) Continued to support the wrist and elbow.   _____ _____ _____
     2) Pronation—turned the hand so the palm was down.   _____ _____ _____
     3) Supination—turned the hand so the palm was up.   _____ _____ _____
     4) Repeated pronation and supination 5 times—or the
        number of times stated on the care plan.   _____ _____ _____
   d. Exercised the wrist.
     1) Held the wrist with both of your hands.   _____ _____ _____
     2) Flexion—bent the hand down.   _____ _____ _____
     3) Extension—straightened the hand.   _____ _____ _____
     4) Hyperextension—bent the hand back.   _____ _____ _____
     5) Radial flexion—turned the hand toward the thumb.   _____ _____ _____
     6) Ulnar flexion—turned the hand toward the little finger.   _____ _____ _____
     7) Repeated flexion, extension, hyperextension, and radial
        and ulnar flexion 5 times—or the number of times
        stated on the care plan.   _____ _____ _____
   e. Exercised the thumb.
     1) Held the person's hand with 1 hand. Held the thumb
        with your other hand.   _____ _____ _____
     2) Abduction—moved the thumb out from the inner part of
        the index finger.   _____ _____ _____
     3) Adduction—moved the thumb back next to the index finger.   _____ _____ _____
     4) Opposition—touched each finger with the thumb.   _____ _____ _____
     5) Flexion—bent the thumb into the hand.   _____ _____ _____
     6) Extension—moved the thumb out to the side of the fingers.   _____ _____ _____
     7) Repeated abduction, adduction, opposition, flexion, and
        extension 5 times—or the number of times stated on
        the care plan.   _____ _____ _____
   f. Exercised the fingers.
     1) Abduction—spread the fingers and the thumb apart.   _____ _____ _____
     2) Adduction—brought the fingers and the thumb together.   _____ _____ _____
     3) Flexion—made a fist.   _____ _____ _____
     4) Extension—straightened the fingers so the fingers, hand,
        and arm were straight.   _____ _____ _____
     5) Repeated abduction, adduction, flexion, and extension
        5 times—or the number of times stated on the care plan.   _____ _____ _____
   g. Exercised the hip.
     1) Supported the leg. Placed 1 hand under the knee. Placed
        your other hand under the ankle.   _____ _____ _____
     2) Flexion—raised the leg.   _____ _____ _____
     3) Extension—straightened the leg.   _____ _____ _____
     4) Hyperextension—moved the leg behind the body.
        (Did this if the person was standing.)   _____ _____ _____
     5) Abduction—moved the leg away from the body.   _____ _____ _____
     6) Adduction—moved the leg toward the other leg.   _____ _____ _____
     7) Internal rotation—turned the leg inward.   _____ _____ _____
     8) External rotation—turned the leg outward.   _____ _____ _____
     9) Repeated flexion, extension, hyperextension, abduction,
        adduction, and internal and external rotation 5 times—or
        the number of times stated on the care plan.   _____ _____ _____
   h. Exercised the knee.
     1) Supported the knee. Placed 1 hand under the knee.
        Placed your other hand under the ankle.   _____ _____ _____
     2) Flexion—bent the knee.   _____ _____ _____
     3) Extension—straightened the knee.   _____ _____ _____
     4) Repeated flexion and extension of the knee 5 times—or the
        number of times stated on the care plan.   _____ _____ _____

Date of Satisfactory Completion _____   Instructor's Initials _____

Procedure—cont'd	S	U	Comments

i. Exercised the ankle.
   1) Supported the foot and ankle. Placed 1 hand under the foot. Placed your other hand under the ankle.
   2) Dorsiflexion—pulled the foot forward. Pushed down on the heel at the same time.
   3) Plantar flexion—turned the foot down. Or pointed the toes.
   4) Repeated dorsiflexion and plantar flexion 5 times—or the number of times stated on the care plan.

j. Exercised the foot.
   1) Continued to support the foot and ankle.
   2) Pronation—turned the outside of the foot up and the inside down.
   3) Supination—turned the inside of the foot up and the outside down.
   4) Repeated pronation and supination 5 times—or the number of times stated on the care plan.

k. Exercised the toes.
   1) Flexion—curled the toes.
   2) Extension—straightened the toes.
   3) Abduction—spread the toes apart.
   4) Adduction—pulled the toes together.
   5) Repeated flexion, extension, abduction, and adduction 5 times—or the number of times stated on the care plan.

Post-Procedure

25. Provided for comfort.
26. Covered the person with the top linens. Removed the bath blanket.
27. Placed the call light and other needed items within reach.
28. Lowered the bed to a safe and comfortable level for the person. Followed the care plan.
29. Raised or lowered bed rails. Followed the care plan.
30. Folded and returned the bath blanket to its proper place.
31. Unscreened the person.
32. Completed a safety check of the room.
33. Practiced hand hygiene.
34. Reported and recorded your observations.

Date of Satisfactory Completion _____   Instructor's Initials _____

Helping the Person Walk

Name: _____   Date: _____

	S	U	Comments

Quality of Life
- Knocked before entering the person's room.
- Addressed the person by name.
- Introduced yourself by name and title.
- Explained the procedure before starting and during the procedure.
- Protected the person's rights during the procedure.
- Handled the person gently during the procedure.

Pre-Procedure
1. Followed *Delegation Guidelines: Ambulation.*
   Saw *Promoting Safety and Comfort: Ambulation.*
2. Practiced hand hygiene.
3. Collected the following:
   - Robe and non-skid footwear
   - Paper or sheet to protect bottom linens
   - Gait (transfer) belt
4. Identified the person. Checked the ID (identification) bracelet against the assignment sheet. Used 2 identifiers. Also called the person by name.
5. Provided for privacy.

Procedure
6. Lowered the bed to a safe and comfortable level for the person. Locked (braked) the bed wheels. Lowered the bed rail near you if up.
7. Fan-folded top linens to the foot of the bed.
8. Placed the paper or sheet under the person's feet. Put the shoes on the person. Fastened the shoes.
9. Helped the person sit on the side of the bed.
10. Made sure the person's feet were flat on the floor.
11. Helped the person put on the robe.
12. Applied the gait belt at the waist over the clothing.
13. Positioned the walker (if used) in front of the person. Or had the person hold the cane (if used) on his or her strong side.
14. Helped the person stand. Grasped the gait belt at each side.
15. Stood at the person's weak side while he or she gained balance. Held the belt at the side and back.
16. Encouraged the person to stand erect with the head up and back straight.
17. *If using a walker or cane:*
    a. Walker—the walker was 6 to 8 inches in front of the person.
    b. Cane—the cane was held on the strong side.
       1) The cane tip was 6 to 10 inches to the side of the strong foot.
       2) The cane tip was 6 to 10 inches in front of the strong foot.
18. Helped the person walk. Walked to the side and slightly behind the person on the person's weak side. Provided support with the gait belt. Encouraged the person to use the hand rail on his or her strong side (unless using a walker or cane).
19. *If using a walker or cane:*
    a. Walker—with both hands, the person pushed the walker 6 to 8 inches in front of the feet.
    b. Cane:
       1) The cane was moved forward 6 to 10 inches.
       2) The weak leg (opposite the cane) was moved forward even with the cane.
       3) The strong leg was moved forward and ahead of the cane and the weak leg.

Date of Satisfactory Completion _____   Instructor's Initials _____

Procedure—cont'd	S	U	Comments

20. Encouraged the person to walk normally. The heel struck the floor first. Discouraged shuffling, sliding, or walking on tip-toes. ___ ___ _____
21. Walked the required distance if the person tolerated the activity. Did not rush the person. ___ ___ _____
22. Helped the person return to bed. Removed the gait belt. ___ ___ _____
23. Lowered the head of the bed. Helped the person to the center of the bed. ___ ___ _____
24. Removed the shoes. Removed the paper or sheet over the bottom sheet. ___ ___ _____

Post-Procedure

25. Provided for comfort. ___ ___ _____
26. Placed the call light and other needed items within reach. ___ ___ _____
27. Raised or lowered bed rails. Followed the care plan. ___ ___ _____
28. Returned the robe and shoes to their proper place. ___ ___ _____
29. Unscreened the person. ___ ___ _____
30. Completed a safety check of the room. ___ ___ _____
31. Practiced hand hygiene. ___ ___ _____
32. Reported and recorded your observations. ___ ___ _____

Date of Satisfactory Completion _____ Instructor's Initials _____

Giving a Back Massage

Name: _____ Date: _____

Quality of Life	S	U	Comments
• Knocked before entering the person's room.	___	___	_____
• Addressed the person by name.	___	___	_____
• Introduced yourself by name and title.	___	___	_____
• Explained the procedure before starting and during the procedure.	___	___	_____
• Protected the person's rights during the procedure.	___	___	_____
• Handled the person gently during the procedure.	___	___	_____

Pre-Procedure

1. Followed *Delegation Guidelines: The Back Massage.* Saw *Promoting Safety and Comfort: The Back Massage.* ___ ___ _____
2. Practiced hand hygiene. ___ ___ _____
3. Identified the person. Checked the ID (identification) bracelet against the assignment sheet. Used 2 identifiers. Also called the person by name. ___ ___ _____
4. Collected the following:
   - Bath blanket ___ ___ _____
   - Bath towel ___ ___ _____
   - Lotion ___ ___ _____
5. Provided for privacy. ___ ___ _____
6. Raised the bed for body mechanics. Bed rails were up if used. ___ ___ _____

Procedure

7. Lowered the bed rail near you if up. ___ ___ _____
8. Positioned the person in the prone or side-lying position. The back was toward you. ___ ___ _____
9. Covered the person with a bath blanket. Exposed the back, shoulders, and upper arms. ___ ___ _____
10. Laid the towel on the bed along the back. Did this if the person was in a side-lying position. ___ ___ _____
11. Warmed the lotion. ___ ___ _____
12. Explained that the lotion may feel cool and wet. ___ ___ _____
13. Applied lotion to the lower back area. ___ ___ _____
14. Stroked up from the lower back to the shoulders. Then stroked down over the upper arms. Stroked up the upper arms, across the shoulders, and down the back. Used firm strokes. Kept your hands in contact with the person's skin. ___ ___ _____
15. Repeated stroking up from the lower back to the shoulders. Then stroked down over the upper arms. Stroked up the upper arms, across the shoulders, and down the back. Used firm strokes. Kept your hands in contact with the person's skin. Continued this for at least 3 minutes. ___ ___ _____
16. Kneaded the back.
    a. Grasped the skin between your thumb and fingers. ___ ___ _____
    b. Kneaded half of the back. Started at the lower back and moved up to the shoulder. Then kneaded down from the shoulder to the lower back. ___ ___ _____
    c. Repeated on the other half of the back. ___ ___ _____
17. Applied lotion to bony areas. Used circular motions with the tips of your index and middle fingers. *(Did not massage reddened bony areas.)* ___ ___ _____
18. Used fast movements to stimulate. Used slow movements to relax the person. ___ ___ _____

Date of Satisfactory Completion _____ Instructor's Initials _____

Procedure—cont'd	S	U	Comments
19. Stroked with long, firm movements to end the massage. Told the person you were finishing.	____	____	_____
20. Straightened and secured clothing or sleepwear.	____	____	_____
21. Covered the person. Removed the towel and bath blanket.	____	____	_____

Post-Procedure

	S	U	Comments
22. Provided for comfort.	____	____	_____
23. Placed the call light and other needed items within reach.	____	____	_____
24. Lowered the bed to a safe and comfortable level for the person. Followed the care plan.	____	____	_____
25. Raised or lowered bed rails. Followed the care plan.	____	____	_____
26. Returned lotion to its proper place.	____	____	_____
27. Unscreened the person.	____	____	_____
28. Completed a safety check of the room.	____	____	_____
29. Followed agency policy for used linens.	____	____	_____
30. Practiced hand hygiene.	____	____	_____
31. Reported and recorded your observations.	____	____	_____

Date of Satisfactory Completion _____   Instructor's Initials _____

Preparing the Person's Room

Name: _____   Date: _____

Procedure	S	U	Comments
1. Followed *Delegation Guidelines: Admissions, Transfers, and Discharges.*	_____	_____	_____
2. Practiced hand hygiene.	_____	_____	_____
3. Collected the following:			
• Admission kit—wash basin, soap, toothpaste, toothbrush, water mug, and so on.	_____	_____	_____
• Bedpan and urinal (for a man)	_____	_____	_____
• Admission form	_____	_____	_____
• Thermometer	_____	_____	_____
• Sphygmomanometer	_____	_____	_____
• Stethoscope	_____	_____	_____
• Patient gown or pajamas (if needed)	_____	_____	_____
• Towels and washcloth	_____	_____	_____
• IV (intravenous) pole (if needed)	_____	_____	_____
• Other items requested by the nurse	_____	_____	_____
4. Placed the following on the over-bed table.			
• Thermometer	_____	_____	_____
• Sphygmomanometer	_____	_____	_____
• Stethoscope	_____	_____	_____
• Admission form	_____	_____	_____
5. Placed the water mug on the bedside stand or over-bed table.			
6. Placed the following in the bedside stand.			
• Admission kit	_____	_____	_____
• Bedpan and urinal	_____	_____	_____
• Patient gown or pajamas	_____	_____	_____
• Towels and washcloth	_____	_____	_____
7. *If the person arrived by stretcher:*			
a. Made a surgical bed.	_____	_____	_____
b. Raised the bed for a transfer from a stretcher.	_____	_____	_____
8. *If the person was ambulatory or arrived by wheelchair:*			
a. Left the bed closed.	_____	_____	_____
b. Lowered the bed to a safe and comfortable level as directed by the nurse.	_____	_____	_____
9. Attached the call light to the bed linens.	_____	_____	_____
10. Practiced hand hygiene.	_____	_____	_____

Date of Satisfactory Completion _____   Instructor's Initials _____

Admitting the Person

Name: _____   Date: _____

	S	U	Comments

Quality of Life
- Knocked before entering the person's room.
- Addressed the person by name.
- Introduced yourself by name and title.
- Explained the procedure before starting and during the procedure.
- Protected the person's rights during the procedure.
- Handled the person gently during the procedure.

Pre-Procedure
1. Followed *Delegation Guidelines: Admissions, Transfers, and Discharges.* Saw *Promoting Safety and Comfort: Admissions, Transfers, and Discharges.*
2. Practiced hand hygiene.
3. Prepared the room.

Procedure
4. Identified the person. Used 2 identifiers. Checked the information on the admission form and ID (identification) bracelet.
5. Greeted the person by name. Asked if he or she preferred a certain name.
6. Introduced yourself to the person and others present. Gave your name and title. Explained that you assist the nurse in giving care.
7. Introduced the roommate.
8. Provided for privacy. Asked family or friends to leave the room. Told them how much time you needed and directed them to the waiting area. Allowed a family member or friend to stay if the person preferred.
9. Allowed the person to stay dressed if his or her condition permitted. Or helped the person change into a patient gown or pajamas.
10. Provided for comfort. The person was in bed or in a chair as directed by the nurse.
11. Assisted the nurse with assessment.
    a. Measured vital signs.
    b. Measured weight and height.
    c. Collected information for the admission form as requested by the nurse.
12. Explained ordered activity limits.
13. Oriented the person to the area.
    a. Gave names of the nurses and nursing assistants.
    b. Identified items in the bedside stand. Explained the purpose of each.
    c. Explained how to use the over-bed table.
    d. Showed how to use the call light.
    e. Showed how to use the bed, TV, and light controls.
    f. Explained how to make phone calls. Placed the phone within reach.
    g. Showed the person the bathroom. Also showed how to use the call light in the bathroom.
    h. Explained visiting hours and policies.
    i. Explained where to find the nurses' station, lounge, chapel, dining room, and other areas.
    j. Identified staff—housekeeping, dietary, physical therapy, and others. Also identified students in the agency.
    k. Explained when meals and snacks are served.

Date of Satisfactory Completion _____   Instructor's Initials _____

Procedure—cont'd

	S	U	Comments
14. Filled the water mug if oral fluids were allowed.	___	___	_____
15. Placed the call light within reach.	___	___	_____
16. Placed other controls and needed items within reach.	___	___	_____
17. Provided a denture container if needed. Labeled it with the person's name, room, and bed number.	___	___	_____
18. Labeled the person's property and personal care items with his or her name (if not completed by the family). Followed agency policy for how to label items.	___	___	_____
19. Completed a clothing and personal belongings list. Followed agency policy for how to label clothing.	___	___	_____
20. Helped the person put away clothes and personal items. Put them in the closet, drawers, and bedside stand. (The family may have helped with this step.)	___	___	_____

Post-Procedure

	S	U	Comments
21. Provided for comfort.	___	___	_____
22. Lowered the bed to a safe and comfortable level for the person. Followed the nurse's direction.	___	___	_____
23. Raised or lowered bed rails as directed by the nurse.	___	___	_____
24. Completed a safety check of the room.	___	___	_____
25. Practiced hand hygiene.	___	___	_____
26. Reported and recorded your observations.	___	___	_____

Date of Satisfactory Completion _____   Instructor's Initials _____

Measuring Weight and Height

Name: _____   Date: _____

Quality of Life	S	U	Comments

Quality of Life
- Knocked before entering the person's room.
- Addressed the person by name.
- Introduced yourself by name and title.
- Explained the procedure before starting and during the procedure.
- Protected the person's rights during the procedure.
- Handled the person gently during the procedure.

Pre-Procedure
1. Followed *Delegation Guidelines: Weight and Height.* Saw *Promoting Safety and Comfort: Weight and Height.*
2. Asked the person to void.
3. Practiced hand hygiene.
4. Brought the scale and paper towels (for a standing scale) to the person's room.
5. Practiced hand hygiene.
6. Identified the person. Checked the ID (identification) bracelet against the assignment sheet. Used 2 identifiers. Also called the person by name.
7. Provided for privacy.

Procedure
8. Placed the paper towels on the scale platform.
9. Raised the height rod.
10. Moved the weights to zero (0). The pointer was in the middle.
11. Had the person remove the robe and footwear. Assisted as needed. (NOTE: For some state competency tests, shoes were worn.)
12. Helped the person stand on the scale. The person stood in the center of the scale. Arms were at the sides. The person did not hold on to anyone or anything.
13. Moved the lower and upper weights until the balance pointer was in the middle.
14. Noted the weight on your note pad or assignment sheet.
15. Asked the person to stand very straight.
16. Lowered the height rod until it rested on the person's head.
17. Read the height at the movable part of the height rod. Recorded the height in inches (or in feet and inches) to the nearest ¼ inch.
18. Noted the height on your note pad or assignment sheet.
19. Raised the height rod. Helped the person step off of the scale.
20. Helped the person put on a robe and non-skid footwear if he or she would be up. Or helped the person back to bed.
21. Lowered the height rod. Adjusted the weights to zero (0) if this was your agency policy.

Post-Procedure
22. Provided for comfort.
23. Placed the call light and other needed items within reach.
24. Raised or lowered bed rails. Followed the care plan.
25. Unscreened the person.
26. Completed a safety check of the room.
27. Discarded the paper towels.
28. Returned the scale to its proper place.
29. Practiced hand hygiene.
30. Reported and recorded the measurements.

Date of Satisfactory Completion _____   Instructor's Initials _____

Measuring Height—The Person Is in Bed

Name: _____   Date: _____

	S	U	Comments
Quality of Life			
• Knocked before entering the person's room.	___	___	_____
• Addressed the person by name.	___	___	_____
• Introduced yourself by name and title.	___	___	_____
• Explained the procedure before starting and during the procedure.	___	___	_____
• Protected the person's rights during the procedure.	___	___	_____
• Handled the person gently during the procedure.	___	___	_____

Pre-Procedure

	S	U	Comments
1. Followed *Delegation Guidelines: Weight and Height.* Saw *Promoting Safety and Comfort: Weight and Height.*	___	___	_____
2. Practiced hand hygiene.	___	___	_____
3. Asked a co-worker to help you.	___	___	_____
4. Collected a measuring tape and ruler.	___	___	_____
5. Practiced hand hygiene.	___	___	_____
6. Identified the person. Checked the ID (identification) bracelet against the assignment sheet. Used 2 identifiers. Also called the person by name.	___	___	_____
7. Provided for privacy.	___	___	_____
8. Raised the bed for body mechanics. Bed rails were up if used.	___	___	_____

Procedure

	S	U	Comments
9. Lowered the bed rails (if up).	___	___	_____
10. Positioned the person supine if the position was allowed.	___	___	_____
11. Had your co-worker place and hold the beginning of the tape measure at the person's heel.	___	___	_____
12. Pulled the other end of the tape measure along the person's body. Pulled it until it extended past the head.	___	___	_____
13. Placed the ruler flat across the top of the person's head. The ruler extended from the person's head to over the tape measure. Made sure the ruler was level.	___	___	_____
14. Read the height measurement. This was the point where the lower edge of the ruler touched the tape measure.	___	___	_____
15. Noted the height on your note pad or assignment sheet.	___	___	_____

Post-Procedure

	S	U	Comments
16. Provided for comfort.	___	___	_____
17. Placed the call light and other needed items within reach.	___	___	_____
18. Lowered the bed to a safe and comfortable level for the person. Followed the care plan.	___	___	_____
19. Raised or lowered bed rails. Followed the care plan.	___	___	_____
20. Completed a safety check of the room.	___	___	_____
21. Returned equipment to its proper place.	___	___	_____
22. Practiced hand hygiene.	___	___	_____
23. Reported and recorded the height.	___	___	_____

Date of Satisfactory Completion _____   Instructor's Initials _____

Moving the Person to a New Room

Name: _____   Date: _____

	S	U	Comments

Quality of Life
- Knocked before entering the person's room.
- Addressed the person by name.
- Introduced yourself by name and title.
- Explained the procedure before starting and during the procedure.
- Protected the person's rights during the procedure.
- Handled the person gently during the procedure.

Pre-Procedure
1. Followed *Delegation Guidelines: Admissions, Transfers, and Discharges.* Saw *Promoting Safety and Comfort: Admissions, Transfers, and Discharges.*
2. Asked a co-worker to help you.
3. Practiced hand hygiene.
4. Collected the following:
   - Wheelchair or stretcher
   - Utility cart
   - Bath blanket
5. Practiced hand hygiene.
6. Identified the person. Checked the ID (identification) bracelet against the assignment sheet. Used 2 identifiers. Also called the person by name.
7. Provided for privacy.

Procedure
8. Collected the person's belongings and care equipment. Placed them on the cart.
9. Transferred the person to a wheelchair or a stretcher. Covered him or her with the bath blanket.
10. Transported the person to the new room. Your co-worker brought the cart.
11. Helped transfer the person to the bed or chair. Helped position the person.
12. Helped arrange the person's belongings and equipment.
13. Reported the following to the receiving nurse.
    a. How the person tolerated the transfer
    b. Any observations made during the transfer
    c. That the nurse will bring the person's drugs and written documents—medical record, care plan, Kardex, and so on

Post-Procedure
14. Returned the wheelchair or stretcher and the cart to the storage area.
15. Practiced hand hygiene.
16. Reported and recorded the following:
    - The time of the transfer
    - Who helped you with the transfer
    - Where the person was taken
    - How the person was transferred (bed, wheelchair, or stretcher)
    - How the person tolerated the transfer
    - Who received the person
    - Any other observations
17. Stripped the bed and cleaned the unit. Practiced hand hygiene and put on gloves for this step. (The housekeeping staff may have done this step.)
18. Removed the gloves. Practiced hand hygiene.
19. Followed agency policy for used linens.
20. Made a closed bed.
21. Practiced hand hygiene.

Date of Satisfactory Completion _____   Instructor's Initials _____

Transferring or Discharging the Person

Name: _____   Date: _____

	S	U	Comments
Quality of Life			
• Knocked before entering the person's room.			
• Addressed the person by name.			
• Introduced yourself by name and title.			
• Explained the procedure before starting and during the procedure.			
• Protected the person's rights during the procedure.			
• Handled the person gently during the procedure.			

Pre-Procedure

1. Followed *Delegation Guidelines: Admissions, Transfers, and Discharges.*
   Saw *Promoting Safety and Comfort: Admissions, Transfers, and Discharges.*
2. Asked a co-worker to help you.
3. Practiced hand hygiene.
4. Identified the person. Checked the ID (identification) bracelet against the assignment sheet. Used 2 identifiers. Also called the person by name.
5. Provided for privacy.

Procedure

6. Helped the person dress as needed.
7. Helped the person pack. Checked the bathroom and all drawers and closets. Made sure all items were collected.
8. Checked off the clothing list and personal belongings. Gave the lists to the nurse.
9. Told the nurse that the person was ready for the final visit. The nurse:
   a. Gave prescriptions written by the doctor.
   b. Provided discharge instructions.
   c. Retrieved valuables from the safe.
   d. Had the person sign the clothing and personal belongings lists.
10. *If the person left by wheelchair:*
    a. Got a wheelchair and a utility cart for the person's items. Asked a co-worker to help you.
    b. Helped the person into the wheelchair.
    c. Took the person to the exit area.
    d. Locked (braked) the wheelchair wheels.
    e. Helped the person out of the wheelchair and into the car.
    f. Helped put the person's items into the car.
11. *If the person left by ambulance:*
    a. Raised the bed rails.
    b. Placed the call light within reach.
    c. Waited for the ambulance attendants.
    d. Raised the bed for a transfer to the stretcher when the ambulance attendants arrived.

Post-Procedure

12. Returned the wheelchair and cart to the storage area.
13. Practiced hand hygiene.
14. Reported and recorded the following:
    • The time of the discharge
    • Who helped you with the procedure
    • How the person was transported
    • Who was with the person
    • The person's destination
    • Any other observations

Date of Satisfactory Completion _____   Instructor's Initials _____

Post-Procedure—cont'd   S   U   Comments

15. Stripped the bed and cleaned the unit. Practiced hand hygiene
    and put on gloves for this step. (The housekeeping staff may
    have done this step.)   _____   _____   _____
16. Removed the gloves. Practiced hand hygiene.   _____   _____   _____
17. Followed agency policy for used linens.   _____   _____   _____
18. Made a closed bed.   _____   _____   _____
19. Practiced hand hygiene.   _____   _____   _____

Date of Satisfactory Completion _____   Instructor's Initials _____

Preparing the Person for an Examination

Name: _____   Date: _____

	S	U	Comments
Quality of Life			
• Knocked before entering the person's room.	___	___	_____
• Addressed the person by name.	___	___	_____
• Introduced yourself by name and title.	___	___	_____
• Explained the procedure before starting and during the procedure.	___	___	_____
• Protected the person's rights during the procedure.	___	___	_____
• Handled the person gently during the procedure.	___	___	_____

Pre-Procedure

1. Followed *Delegation Guidelines: Preparing the Person.* Saw *Promoting Safety and Comfort: Preparing the Person.* ___ ___ _____
2. Practiced hand hygiene. ___ ___ _____
3. Collected the following:
   - Exam form ___ ___ _____
   - Flashlight ___ ___ _____
   - Blood pressure equipment ___ ___ _____
   - Stethoscope ___ ___ _____
   - Thermometer ___ ___ _____
   - Pulse oximeter ___ ___ _____
   - Scale ___ ___ _____
   - Tongue depressors (blades) ___ ___ _____
   - Laryngeal mirror ___ ___ _____
   - Ophthalmoscope ___ ___ _____
   - Otoscope ___ ___ _____
   - Nasal speculum ___ ___ _____
   - Percussion (reflex) hammer ___ ___ _____
   - Tuning fork ___ ___ _____
   - Vaginal speculum ___ ___ _____
   - Tape measure ___ ___ _____
   - Gloves ___ ___ _____
   - Water-soluble lubricant ___ ___ _____
   - Cotton-tipped applicators ___ ___ _____
   - Specimen containers and labels ___ ___ _____
   - Disposable bag ___ ___ _____
   - Kidney basin ___ ___ _____
   - Towel ___ ___ _____
   - Bath blanket ___ ___ _____
   - Tissues ___ ___ _____
   - Drape (sheet, bath blanket, drawsheet, or paper drape) ___ ___ _____
   - Paper towels ___ ___ _____
   - Cotton balls ___ ___ _____
   - Waterproof pad ___ ___ _____
   - Eye chart (Snellen chart) ___ ___ _____
   - Slides ___ ___ _____
   - Patient gown ___ ___ _____
   - Alcohol wipes ___ ___ _____
   - Wastebasket ___ ___ _____
   - Container for soiled instruments ___ ___ _____
   - Marking pencils or pens ___ ___ _____
4. Practiced hand hygiene. ___ ___ _____
5. Identified the person. Checked the ID (identification) bracelet against the assignment sheet. Used 2 identifiers. Also called the person by name. ___ ___ _____
6. Provided for privacy. ___ ___ _____

Date of Satisfactory Completion _____   Instructor's Initials _____

Procedure   S   U   **Comments**

7. Had the person put on the gown. Told him or her what
    clothes to remove. Assisted as needed.   _____   _____   _____

8. Asked the person to void. Collected a urine specimen, if needed.
    Provided for privacy.   _____   _____   _____

9. Transported the person to the exam room. (Omitted this step
    when exam was in the person's room.)   _____   _____   _____

10. Measured weight and height. Recorded the measurements on
    the exam form.   _____   _____   _____

11. Helped the person onto the exam table. Provided a step stool if
    necessary. (Omitted this step for an exam in the person's room.)   _____   _____   _____

12. Raised the far bed rail (if used). Raised the bed to a safe and
    comfortable working height. (Omitted this step if an exam
    table was used.)   _____   _____   _____

13. Measured vital signs and oxygen concentration. Recorded them
    on the exam form.   _____   _____   _____

14. Positioned the person as directed.   _____   _____   _____

15. Draped the person.   _____   _____   _____

16. Placed a waterproof pad under the buttocks.   _____   _____   _____

17. Raised the bed rail near you if used.   _____   _____   _____

18. Provided adequate lighting.   _____   _____   _____

19. Put the call light on for the examiner. Did not leave
    the person alone.   _____   _____   _____

Date of Satisfactory Completion _____   Instructor's Initials _____

Collecting a Random Urine Specimen

Name: _____   Date: _____

	S	U	Comments

Quality of Life
- Knocked before entering the person's room.
- Addressed the person by name.
- Introduced yourself by name and title.
- Explained the procedure before starting and during the procedure.
- Protected the person's rights during the procedure.
- Handled the person gently during the procedure.

Pre-Procedure
1. Followed *Delegation Guidelines: Urine Specimens*.
   Saw *Promoting Safety and Comfort:*
   a. *Collecting and Testing Specimens*
   b. *Urine Specimens*
2. Practiced hand hygiene.
3. Collected the following before going to the person's room.
   - Laboratory requisition slip
   - Specimen container and lid
   - Voiding device—bedpan and cover, urinal, commode, or specimen pan
   - Specimen label
   - Plastic bag
   - *BIOHAZARD* label (if needed)
   - Gloves
4. Arranged collected items in the person's bathroom.
5. Practiced hand hygiene.
6. Identified the person. Checked the ID (identification) bracelet against the requisition slip. Compared all information. Also called the person by name. Asked the person to state his or her first and last name and state his or her birth date.
7. Labeled the container in the person's presence.
8. Put on gloves.
9. Collected a graduate to measure output.
10. Provided for privacy.

Procedure
11. Asked the person to void into the device. Reminded the person to put toilet tissue into the wastebasket or toilet. Toilet tissue was not put in the bedpan or specimen pan.
12. Took the voiding device to the bathroom.
13. Poured about 120 mL (milliliters) (4 oz [ounces]) into the specimen container.
14. Placed the lid on the specimen container. Put the container in the plastic bag. Did not let the container touch the outside of the bag. Applied a *BIOHAZARD* label.
15. Measured urine if intake and output (I&O) was ordered. Included the specimen amount.
16. Emptied, rinsed, cleaned, disinfected, and dried equipment. Returned equipment to its proper place.
17. Removed and discarded the gloves. Practiced hand hygiene. Put on clean gloves.
18. Assisted with hand-washing.
19. Removed and discarded the gloves. Practiced hand hygiene.

Post-Procedure
20. Provided for comfort.
21. Placed the call light and other needed items within reach.

Date of Satisfactory Completion _____   Instructor's Initials _____

Post-Procedure—cont'd   S   U   **Comments**

22. Raised or lowered bed rails. Followed the care plan.
23. Unscreened the person.
24. Completed a safety check of the room.
25. Practiced hand hygiene.
26. Took the specimen and the requisition slip to the laboratory or storage area. Wore gloves if that was agency policy.
27. Removed and discarded the gloves. Practiced hand hygiene.
28. Reported and recorded your observations.

Date of Satisfactory Completion _____   Instructor's Initials _____

Collecting a Midstream Specimen

Name: _____   Date: _____

	S	U	Comments

Quality of Life
- Knocked before entering the person's room.
- Addressed the person by name.
- Introduced yourself by name and title.
- Explained the procedure before starting and during the procedure.
- Protected the person's rights during the procedure.
- Handled the person gently during the procedure.

Pre-Procedure
1. Followed *Delegation Guidelines: Urine Specimens.*
   Saw *Promoting Safety and Comfort:*
   a. *Collecting and Testing Specimens*
   b. *Urine Specimens*
   c. *The Midstream Specimen*
2. Practiced hand hygiene.
3. Collected the following:
   - Laboratory requisition slip
   - Midstream specimen kit—specimen container, label, towelettes, sterile gloves
   - Plastic bag
   - Sterile gloves (if not part of kit)
   - Disposable gloves
   - *BIOHAZARD* label (if needed)
4. Arranged your work area.
5. Practiced hand hygiene.
6. Identified the person. Checked the ID (identification) bracelet against the requisition slip. Compared all information. Also called the person by name. Asked the person to state his or her first and last name and state his or her birth date.
7. Put on disposable gloves.
8. Collected the following:
   - Voiding device—bedpan and cover, urinal, commode, or specimen pan if needed
   - Supplies for perineal care
   - Graduate to measure output
   - Paper towel
9. Provided for privacy.

Procedure
10. Provided perineal care. Wore gloves for this step. Practiced hand hygiene after removing and discarding gloves.
11. Opened the sterile kit.
12. Put on the sterile gloves.
13. Opened the packet of towelettes.
14. Opened the sterile specimen container. Did not touch the inside of the container or the lid. Sat the lid down so the inside was up.
15. *For a female*—cleaned the perineal area with the towelettes.
    a. Spread the labia with your thumb and index finger. Used your non-dominant hand. (This hand was contaminated and did not touch anything sterile.)
    b. Cleaned down the urethral area from front to back (top to bottom). Used a clean towelette for each stroke.
    c. Kept the labia separated to collect the urine specimen.

Date of Satisfactory Completion _____   Instructor's Initials _____

Procedure—cont'd   S   U   Comments

16. *For a male*—cleaned the penis with towelettes.
   a. Held the penis with your non-dominant hand. (This hand
      was contaminated and did not touch anything.)
   b. Cleaned the penis starting at the meatus. (Retracted the
      foreskin of the uncircumcised male.) Cleaned in a circular
      motion. Started at the center and worked outward.
   c. Held the penis (kept the foreskin retracted in the
      uncircumcised male) until the specimen was collected.
17. Asked the person to void into a device.
18. Passed the specimen container into the urine stream. (Kept the
    labia separated, if female.)
19. Collected about 30 to 60 milliliters (1 to 2 ounces) of urine.
20. Removed the specimen container before the person stopped
    voiding. Released the foreskin of the uncircumcised male.
21. Released the labia or penis. Allowed the person to finish
    voiding into the device.
22. Put the lid on the specimen container. Touched only the outside
    of the container and lid. Wiped the outside of the container.
    Sat the container on a paper towel.
23. Provided toilet tissue after the person was done voiding.
24. Took the voiding device to the bathroom.
25. Measured urine if intake and output (I&O) was ordered.
    Included the specimen amount.
26. Emptied, rinsed, cleaned, disinfected, and dried equipment.
    Returned equipment to its proper place.
27. Removed and discarded the gloves. Practiced hand hygiene.
    Put on clean disposable gloves.
28. Labeled the specimen container in the person's presence. Placed
    the container in the plastic bag. Did not let the container touch
    the outside of the bag. Applied a *BIOHAZARD* label.
29. Assisted with hand-washing.
30. Removed and discarded the gloves. Practiced hand hygiene.

Post-Procedure
31. Provided for comfort.
32. Placed the call light and other needed items within reach.
33. Raised or lowered bed rails. Followed the care plan.
34. Unscreened the person.
35. Completed a safety check of the room.
36. Practiced hand hygiene.
37. Took the specimen and the requisition slip to the laboratory or
    storage area. Wore gloves if that was agency policy.
38. Removed and discarded the gloves. Practiced hand hygiene.
39. Reported and recorded your observations.

Date of Satisfactory Completion _____   Instructor's Initials _____

Collecting a 24-Hour Urine Specimen

VIDEO   VIDEO CLIP

Name: _____   Date: _____

	S	U	Comments
Quality of Life			
• Knocked before entering the person's room.	___	___	_____
• Addressed the person by name.	___	___	_____
• Introduced yourself by name and title.	___	___	_____
• Explained the procedure before starting and during the procedure.	___	___	_____
• Protected the person's rights during the procedure.	___	___	_____
• Handled the person gently during the procedure.	___	___	_____
Pre-Procedure			
1. Followed *Delegation Guidelines: Urine Specimens.* Saw *Promoting Safety and Comfort:*			
a. *Collecting and Testing Specimens*	___	___	_____
b. *Urine Specimens*	___	___	_____
c. *The 24-Hour Urine Specimen*	___	___	_____
2. Practiced hand hygiene.	___	___	_____
3. Collected the following:			
• Laboratory requisition slip	___	___	_____
• Urine container for a 24-hour collection	___	___	_____
• Specimen label	___	___	_____
• Preservative if needed	___	___	_____
• Bucket with ice if needed	___	___	_____
• Two 24-HOUR URINE labels	___	___	_____
• Funnel	___	___	_____
• BIOHAZARD label	___	___	_____
• Gloves	___	___	_____
4. Arranged collected items in the person's bathroom.	___	___	_____
5. Placed one 24-HOUR URINE label in the bathroom. Placed the other near the bed.	___	___	_____
6. Practiced hand hygiene.	___	___	_____
7. Identified the person. Checked the ID (identification) bracelet against the requisition slip. Compared all information. Also called the person by name. Asked the person to state his or her first and last name and state his or her birth date.	___	___	_____
8. Labeled the urine container in the person's presence. Applied the BIOHAZARD label. Placed the labeled container in the bathroom.	___	___	_____
9. Put on gloves.	___	___	_____
10. Collected the following:			
• Voiding device—bedpan and cover, urinal, commode, or specimen pan	___	___	_____
• Graduate to measure output	___	___	_____
11. Provided for privacy.	___	___	_____
Procedure			
12. Asked the person to void. Provided a voiding device.	___	___	_____
13. Measured and discarded the urine. Noted the time. This started the 24-hour collection period.	___	___	_____
14. Marked the time on the urine container.	___	___	_____
15. Emptied, rinsed, cleaned, disinfected, and dried equipment. Returned equipment to its proper place.	___	___	_____
16. Removed and discarded the gloves. Practiced hand hygiene. Put on gloves.	___	___	_____
17. Assisted with hand-washing.	___	___	_____
18. Removed and discarded the gloves. Practiced hand hygiene.	___	___	_____
19. Marked the time the test began and the time it will end on the room and bathroom labels.	___	___	_____

Date of Satisfactory Completion _____   Instructor's Initials _____

Procedure—cont'd   **S**   **U**   **Comments**

20. Reminded the person to:
    a. Use the voiding device during the next 24 hours.
    b. Not have a bowel movement (BM) when voiding.
    c. Put toilet tissue in the toilet or wastebasket.
    d. Put on the call light after voiding.
21. Returned to the room when the person signaled for you. Knocked before entering the room.
22. Did the following after every voiding.
    a. Practiced hand hygiene. Put on gloves.
    b. Measured urine if intake and output (I&O) was ordered.
    c. Used the funnel to pour urine into the container. Did not spill any urine. Re-started the test if you spilled or discarded the urine.
    d. Emptied, rinsed, cleaned, disinfected, and dried equipment. Returned equipment to its proper place.
    e. Removed and discarded the gloves. Practiced hand hygiene. Put on clean gloves.
    f. Assisted with hand-washing.
    g. Removed and discarded the gloves. Practiced hand hygiene.
23. Asked the person to void at the end of the 24-hour period. Did the following:
    a. Decontaminated your hands. Put on gloves.
    b. Measured urine if I&O was ordered.
    c. Poured urine into the container using the funnel. Did not spill any urine. Re-started the test if you spilled or discarded the urine.
    d. Emptied, cleaned, and disinfected equipment. Returned equipment to its proper place.
    e. Removed the gloves and practiced hand hygiene. Put on clean gloves.
    f. Assisted with hand-washing.
    g. Removed the gloves. Practiced hand hygiene.
    h. Did the following:
      1) Provided for comfort.
      2) Placed the call light and other needed items within reach.
      3) Raised or lowered bed rails. Followed the care plan.
      4) Put on gloves.
      5) Cleaned, rinsed, dried, and returned equipment to its proper place. Discarded disposable items.
      6) Removed and discarded the gloves. Practiced hand hygiene.
      7) Unscreened the person.
      8) Completed a safety check of the room.
      9) Reported and recorded your observations.

Post-Procedure
24. Provided for comfort.
25. Placed the call light and other needed items within reach.
26. Raised or lowered bed rails. Followed the care plan.
27. Put on gloves.
28. Removed the labels from the room and bathroom.
29. Cleaned, rinsed, dried, and returned equipment to its proper place. Discarded disposable items.
30. Removed and discarded the gloves. Practiced hand hygiene.
31. Unscreened the person.
32. Completed a safety check of the room.
33. Took the specimen (labeled urine container) and the requisition slip to the laboratory or storage area. Wore gloves if that was agency policy.
34. Removed and discarded the gloves. Practiced hand hygiene.
35. Reported and recorded your observations.

Date of Satisfactory Completion _____   Instructor's Initials _____

Collecting a Urine Specimen From an Infant or Child

Name: _____   Date: _____

Quality of Life	S	U	Comments
• Knocked before entering the child's room.			
• Addressed the child by name.			
• Introduced yourself by name and title.			
• Explained the procedure to the child and parents before starting and during the procedure.			
• Protected the child's rights during the procedure.			
• Handled the child gently during the procedure.			

Pre-Procedure

1. Followed *Delegation Guidelines: Urine Specimens.*
   Saw *Promoting Safety and Comfort:*
   a. *Collecting and Testing Specimens*
   b. *Urine Specimens*
2. Practiced hand hygiene.
3. Collected the following before going to the child's room.
   • Laboratory requisition slip
   • Collection bag ("wee bag")
   • BIOHAZARD label (if needed)
   • Specimen container
   • Plastic bag
   • Scissors
   • Wash basin
   • Bath towel
   • 2 diapers
   • Gloves
4. Arranged your work area.
5. Practiced hand hygiene.
6. Identified the child. Checked the ID (identification) bracelet against the requisition slip. Compared all information. Also called the child by name. Asked the parent to state the child's first and last name and state the child's birth date.
7. Provided for privacy.

Procedure

8. Practiced hand hygiene. Put on gloves.
9. Positioned the child on his or her back.
10. Removed and set aside the diaper.
11. Cleaned the perineal area with cotton balls. Used a new cotton ball for each stroke. Rinsed and dried the area.
12. Removed and discarded the gloves. Practiced hand hygiene.
13. Put on clean gloves.
14. Flexed the child's knees. Spread the legs.
15. Removed the adhesive backing from the collection bag.
16. Applied the bag to the perineum.
17. Cut a slit in the bottom of a new diaper.
18. Diapered the child.
19. Pulled the collection bag through the slit in the diaper.
20. Removed and discarded the gloves. Practiced hand hygiene.
21. Raised the head of the crib if allowed. This helped urine collect in the bottom of the bag.
22. Checked for crib safety. Medical crib rails were raised and locked before leaving the bedside.
23. Unscreened the child.
24. Disposed of the removed diaper. Followed agency policy. Wore gloves for this step.

Date of Satisfactory Completion _____   Instructor's Initials _____

Procedure—cont'd

	S	U	Comments
25. Practiced hand hygiene.			
26. Checked the child often.			
a. Checked the bag for urine.			
b. Provided for privacy.			
c. Wore gloves.			
27. Did the following if the child voided.			
a. Provided for privacy.			
b. Practiced hand hygiene. Put on clean gloves.			
c. Removed the diaper.			
d. Removed the collection bag gently.			
e. Pressed the adhesive surfaces of the bag together. Made sure the seal was tight and there were no leaks. Or transferred the urine to the specimen container using the drainage tab.			
f. Cleaned the perineal area. Rinsed and dried well.			
g. Diapered the child.			
h. Removed and discarded the gloves. Practiced hand hygiene.			
28. Put on clean gloves.			
29. Labeled the collection bag or specimen container in the child's presence. Then placed it in the plastic bag. Applied the BIOHAZARD label (if needed).			

Post-Procedure

	S	U	Comments
30. Provided for comfort.			
31. Checked for crib safety. Medical crib rails were raised and locked before leaving the bedside.			
32. Made sure the call light and other needed items were within reach for the parent.			
33. Unscreened the child.			
34. Cleaned, rinsed, dried, and returned equipment to its proper place. Discarded disposable items. Wore gloves for this step.			
35. Completed a safety check of the room.			
36. Removed and discarded the gloves. Practiced hand hygiene.			
37. Took the specimen and requisition slip to the laboratory or storage area. Wore gloves if that was agency policy.			
38. Removed and discarded the gloves. Practiced hand hygiene.			
39. Reported and recorded your observations.			

Date of Satisfactory Completion _____   Instructor's Initials _____

Testing Urine With Reagent Strips

Name: _____   Date: _____

	S	U	Comments

Quality of Life
- Knocked before entering the person's room.
- Addressed the person by name.
- Introduced yourself by name and title.
- Explained the procedure before starting and during the procedure.
- Protected the person's rights during the procedure.
- Handled the person gently during the procedure.

Pre-Procedure
1. Followed *Delegation Guidelines: Testing Urine.*
   Saw *Promoting Safety and Comfort:*
   a. *Collecting and Testing Specimens*
   b. *Testing Urine*
2. Practiced hand hygiene.
3. Collected gloves and the reagent (test) strips ordered.
4. Practiced hand hygiene.
5. Identified the person. Checked the ID (identification) bracelet against the assignment sheet. Used 2 identifiers. Also called the person by name. Asked the person to state his or her first and last name and state his or her birth date.
6. Put on gloves.
7. Collected equipment for the urine specimen.
8. Provided for privacy.

Procedure
9. Collected the urine specimen.
10. Removed the strip from the bottle. Put the cap on the bottle at once. It was on tight.
11. Dip the test strip areas into the urine.
12. Removed the strip after the correct amount of time. Saw the manufacturer's instructions.
13. Tapped the strip gently against the container. This removed excess urine.
14. Waited the required amount of time. Saw the manufacturer's instructions.
15. Compared the strip with the color chart on the bottle. Read the results.
16. Discarded disposable items and the specimen.
17. Emptied, rinsed, cleaned, disinfected, and dried equipment. Returned equipment to its proper place.
18. Removed and discarded the gloves. Practiced hand hygiene.

Post-Procedure
19. Provided for comfort.
20. Placed the call light and other needed items within reach.
21. Raised or lowered bed rails. Followed the care plan.
22. Unscreened the person.
23. Completed a safety check of the room.
24. Practiced hand hygiene.
25. Reported and recorded the results and any other observations.

Date of Satisfactory Completion _____   Instructor's Initials _____

Straining Urine

Name: _____   Date: _____

	S	U	Comments

Quality of Life
- Knocked before entering the person's room.
- Addressed the person by name.
- Introduced yourself by name and title.
- Explained the procedure before starting and during the procedure.
- Protected the person's rights during the procedure.
- Handled the person gently during the procedure.

Pre-Procedure
1. Followed *Delegation Guidelines: Urine Specimens*.
   Saw *Promoting Safety and Comfort:*
   a. *Collecting and Testing Specimens*
   b. *Urine Specimens*
2. Practiced hand hygiene.
3. Collected the following before going to the person's room.
   - Laboratory requisition slip
   - Urine strainer
   - Specimen container
   - Specimen label
   - 2 STRAIN ALL URINE labels
   - Plastic bag
   - BIOHAZARD label (if needed)
   - Gloves
4. Arranged collected items in the person's bathroom.
5. Placed 1 STRAIN ALL URINE label in the bathroom. Placed the other near the bed.
6. Practiced hand hygiene.
7. Identified the person. Checked the ID (identification) bracelet against the requisition slip. Compared all information. Also called the person by name. Asked the person to state his or her first and last name and state his or her birth date.
8. Labeled the specimen container in the person's presence.
9. Put on gloves.
10. Collected the following:
    - Voiding device—bedpan and cover, urinal, commode, or specimen pan
    - Graduate
11. Provided for privacy.

Procedure
12. Asked the person to use the voiding device for urinating. Asked the person to put on the call light after voiding.
13. Removed and discarded the gloves. Practiced hand hygiene.
14. Returned to the room when the person signaled for you. Knocked before entering the room.
15. Practiced hand hygiene. Put on clean gloves.
16. Placed the gauze or strainer into the graduate.
17. Poured urine into the graduate. Urine passed through the strainer.
18. Placed the strainer in the specimen container if any crystals, stones, or particles appeared.
19. Placed the specimen container in the plastic bag. Did not let the container touch the outside of the bag. Applied a BIOHAZARD label.
20. Measured urine if intake and output (I&O) was ordered.
21. Emptied, rinsed, cleaned, disinfected, and dried equipment. Returned equipment to its proper place.

Date of Satisfactory Completion _____   Instructor's Initials _____

Procedure—cont'd	S	U	Comments
22. Removed and discarded the gloves. Practiced hand hygiene. Put on clean gloves.	___	___	_____
23. Assisted with hand-washing.	___	___	_____
24. Removed and discarded the gloves. Practiced hand hygiene.	___	___	_____

Post-Procedure

	S	U	Comments
25. Provided for comfort.	___	___	_____
26. Placed the call light and other needed items within reach.	___	___	_____
27. Raised or lowered bed rails. Followed the care plan.	___	___	_____
28. Unscreened the person.	___	___	_____
29. Completed a safety check of the room.	___	___	_____
30. Practiced hand hygiene.	___	___	_____
31. Took the specimen container and requisition slip to the laboratory or storage area. Wore gloves if agency policy.	___	___	_____
32. Reported and recorded your observations.	___	___	_____

Date of Satisfactory Completion _____   Instructor's Initials _____

Collecting and Testing a Stool Specimen

Name: _____   Date: _____

	S	U	Comments

Quality of Life
- Knocked before entering the person's room.
- Addressed the person by name.
- Introduced yourself by name and title.
- Explained the procedure before starting and during the procedure.
- Protected the person's rights during the procedure.
- Handled the person gently during the procedure.

Pre-Procedure
1. Followed *Delegation Guidelines: Stool Specimens.*
   Saw *Promoting Safety and Comfort:*
   a. *Collecting and Testing Specimens*
   b. *Stool Specimens*
2. Practiced hand hygiene.
3. Collected the following before going to the person's room:
   - Laboratory requisition slip
   - Occult blood test kit (if needed)
   - Specimen pan for the toilet
   - Specimen container and lid
   - Specimen label
   - Tongue blade (if needed)
   - Disposable bag
   - Plastic bag
   - *BIOHAZARD* label (if needed)
   - Gloves
4. Arranged collected items in the person's bathroom.
5. Practiced hand hygiene.
6. Identified the person. Checked the ID (identification) bracelet against the requisition slip. Compared all information. Also called the person by name. Asked the person to state his or her first and last name and state his or her birth date.
7. Labeled the specimen container in the person's presence.
8. Put on gloves.
9. Collected the following:
   - Device for voiding—bedpan and cover, urinal, commode, or specimen pan
   - Toilet tissue
10. Provided for privacy.

Procedure
11. Asked the person to void. Provided the voiding device if the person did not use the bathroom. Emptied, rinsed, cleaned, disinfected, and dried the device. Returned it to its proper place.
12. Put the specimen pan on the toilet if the person used the bathroom. Placed it at the back of the toilet. Or provided a bedpan or commode.
13. Asked the person not to put toilet tissue into the bedpan, commode, or specimen pan. Provided a bag for toilet tissue.
14. Placed the call light and toilet tissue within reach. Raised or lowered bed rails. Followed the care plan.
15. Removed and discarded the gloves. Practiced hand hygiene. Left the room if the person could be left alone.
16. Returned when the person signaled. Or checked on the person every 5 minutes. Knocked before entering.

Date of Satisfactory Completion _____   Instructor's Initials _____

Procedure—cont'd	S	U	Comments
17. Practiced hand hygiene. Put on clean gloves.	___	___	_____
18. Lowered the bed rail near you if up.			
Removed the bedpan (if used). Or assisted the person off the toilet or commode (if used). Provided perineal care if needed.	___	___	_____
19. Noted the color, amount, consistency, and odor of stools.	___	___	_____
20. Collected the specimen.			
a. Used the spoon attached to the lid to pick up several spoonfuls of stool. Or used a tongue blade to take about 2 tablespoons of stool to the specimen container. Took the sample from:			
1) The middle of a formed stool	___	___	_____
2) Areas of pus, mucus, or blood and watery areas	___	___	_____
3) The middle and both ends of a hard stool	___	___	_____
b. Put the lid on the specimen container.	___	___	_____
c. Placed the container in the plastic bag. Did not let the container touch the outside of the bag. Applied a BIOHAZARD label according to agency policy.	___	___	_____
d. Wrapped the tongue blade in toilet tissue. Discarded it into the disposable bag.	___	___	_____
21. Removed and discarded the gloves. Practiced hand hygiene. Put on clean gloves.	___	___	_____
22. Tested the specimen (if needed).			
a. Opened the test kit.	___	___	_____
b. Used a tongue blade to obtain a small amount of stool.	___	___	_____
c. Applied a thin smear of stool on box A on the test paper.	___	___	_____
d. Used another tongue blade to obtain stool from another part of the specimen.	___	___	_____
e. Applied a thin smear of stool on box B on the test paper.	___	___	_____
f. Closed the packet.	___	___	_____
g. Turned the test packet to the other side. Opened the flap. Applied developer (from the kit) to boxes A and B. Followed the manufacturer's instructions.	___	___	_____
h. Waited 10 to 60 seconds as required by the manufacturer.	___	___	_____
i. Noted the color changes on your assignment sheet.	___	___	_____
j. Disposed of the test packet.	___	___	_____
k. Wrapped the tongue blades with toilet tissue. Then discarded them.	___	___	_____
23. Emptied, rinsed, cleaned, disinfected, and dried equipment. Returned equipment to its proper place.	___	___	_____
24. Removed and discarded the gloves. Practiced hand hygiene. Put on clean gloves.	___	___	_____
25. Assisted with hand-washing.	___	___	_____
26. Removed and discarded the gloves. Practiced hand hygiene.	___	___	_____

Post-Procedure

	S	U	Comments
27. Provided for comfort.	___	___	_____
28. Placed the call light and other needed items within reach.	___	___	_____
29. Raised or lowered bed rails. Followed the care plan.	___	___	_____
30. Unscreened the person.	___	___	_____
31. Completed a safety check of the room.	___	___	_____
32. Delivered the specimen and requisition slip to the laboratory or storage area. Followed agency policy. Wore gloves if that was the agency policy.	___	___	_____
33. Removed and discarded the gloves. Practiced hand hygiene.	___	___	_____
34. Reported and recorded your observations and the test results.	___	___	_____

Date of Satisfactory Completion _____   Instructor's Initials _____

Collecting a Sputum Specimen

Name: _____   Date: _____

Quality of Life	S	U	Comments
• Knocked before entering the person's room.	_____	_____	_____
• Addressed the person by name.	_____	_____	_____
• Introduced yourself by name and title.	_____	_____	_____
• Explained the procedure before starting and during the procedure.	_____	_____	_____
• Protected the person's rights during the procedure.	_____	_____	_____
• Handled the person gently during the procedure.	_____	_____	_____

Pre-Procedure
1. Followed *Delegation Guidelines: Sputum Specimens*.
   Saw *Promoting Safety and Comfort*:
   a. *Collecting and Testing Specimens*
   b. *Sputum Specimens*
2. Practiced hand hygiene.
3. Collected the following before going to the person's room:
   • Laboratory requisition slip
   • Sputum specimen container and lid
   • Specimen label
   • Plastic bag
   • BIOHAZARD label (if needed)
4. Arranged collected items in the person's bathroom.
5. Practiced hand hygiene.
6. Identified the person. Checked the ID (identification) bracelet against the assignment sheet. Compared all information. Also called the person by name. Asked the person to state his or her first and last name and state his or her birth date.
7. Labeled the specimen container in the person's presence.
8. Collected gloves and tissues.
9. Provided for privacy. If able, the person used the bathroom for this procedure.

Procedure
10. Put on gloves.
11. Asked the person to rinse the mouth out with clear water.
12. Had the person hold the container. Only the outside was touched.
13. Asked the person to cover the mouth and nose with tissues when coughing. Followed center policy for used tissues.
14. Asked the person to take 2 or 3 deep breaths and cough up sputum.
15. Had the person expectorate directly into the container. Sputum did not touch the outside of the container.
16. Collected 1 to 2 tablespoons of sputum unless told to collect more.
17. Put the lid on the container.
18. Placed the container in the plastic bag. Did not let the container touch the outside of the bag. Applied a BIOHAZARD label according to center policy.
19. Removed and discarded the gloves. Practiced hand hygiene. Put on clean gloves.
20. Assisted with hand-washing.
21. Removed and discarded the gloves. Practiced hand hygiene.

Post-Procedure
22. Provided for comfort.
23. Placed the call light and other needed items within reach.
24. Raised or lowered bed rails. Followed the care plan.
25. Unscreened the person.

Date of Satisfactory Completion _____   Instructor's Initials _____

Post-Procedure—cont'd	S	U	Comments
26. Completed a safety check of the room.	_____	_____	_____
27. Practiced hand hygiene.	_____	_____	_____
28. Delivered the specimen and requisition slip to the laboratory or storage area. Followed center policy. Wore gloves if that was agency policy.	_____	_____	_____
29. Removed and discarded the gloves. Practiced hand hygiene.	_____	_____	_____
30. Reported and recorded your observations.	_____	_____	_____

Date of Satisfactory Completion _____   Instructor's Initials _____

VIDEO   VIDEO CLIP

Measuring Blood Glucose

Name: _____   Date: _____

Quality of Life	S	U	Comments

Quality of Life
- Knocked before entering the person's room.
- Addressed the person by name.
- Introduced yourself by name and title.
- Explained the procedure before starting and during the procedure.
- Protected the person's rights during the procedure.
- Handled the person gently during the procedure.

Pre-Procedure
1. Followed *Delegation Guidelines: Blood Glucose Testing*.
   Saw *Promoting Safety and Comfort:*
   a. *Collecting and Testing Specimens*
   b. *Blood Glucose Testing*
2. Practiced hand hygiene.
3. Collected the following:
   - Sterile lancet
   - Lancing device (if used)
   - Antiseptic wipes
   - Gloves
   - 2 × 2 gauze squares
   - Glucometer
   - Reagent (test) strips (Used correct ones for the glucometer. Checked expiration date.)
   - Disinfectant
   - Paper towels
   - Warm washcloth
4. Read the manufacturer's instructions for the lancet and glucometer.
5. Disinfected the glucometer. Followed the manufacturer's instructions for the disinfectant.
6. Arranged your work area.
7. Identified the person. Checked the ID (identification) bracelet against the assignment sheet. Used 2 identifiers. Also called the person by name. Asked the person to state his or her first and last name and state his or her birth date.
8. Provided for privacy.
9. Raised the bed for body mechanics. The far bed rail was up if used.

Procedure
10. Helped the person to a comfortable position.
11. Put on gloves.
12. Prepared the supplies.
    a. Opened the antiseptic wipes.
    b. Prepared the lancet. If a lancing device was used, followed the manufacturer's instructions.
    c. Turned on the glucometer.
    d. Followed the prompts. You may have needed to enter a user-ID and the person's ID number. Scanned the bar code on the bottle of test strips if needed. Or compared the code on the bottle of regent strips to the code on the glucometer.
    e. Removed a test strip from the bottle. Closed the cap tightly.
    f. Inserted a test strip into the glucometer.

Date of Satisfactory Completion _____   Instructor's Initials _____

	S	U	Comments
Procedure—cont'd			
13. Performed a skin puncture to obtain a drop of blood.			
a. Inspected the person's finger. Selected a puncture site.	___	___	_____
b. Did the following to increase blood flow to the puncture side.			
1) Warmed the finger. Rubbed it gently or applied a warm washcloth.	___	___	_____
2) Massaged the hand and finger toward the puncture site.	___	___	_____
3) Lowered the finger below the person's waist.	___	___	_____
c. Held the finger with thumb and index finger. Used your non-dominant hand. Held the finger until the specimen was collected.	___	___	_____
d. Cleaned the site with antiseptic wipe. *Did not touch the site after cleaning.*	___	___	_____
e. Allowed the site to dry.	___	___	_____
f. Placed the lancet or lancing device against the puncture site.	___	___	_____
g. Pushed the button on the lancet to puncture the skin. (Followed the manufacturer's instructions.)			
h. Applied gentle pressure below the puncture site.	___	___	_____
i. Allowed a large drop of blood to form.	___	___	_____
14. Collected and tested the specimen. Followed the manufacturer's instructions and agency policy for the glucometer used.			
a. Held the test strip to the drop of blood. The glucometer tested the sample when enough blood was applied.	___	___	_____
b. Applied pressure to the puncture site until the bleeding stopped. Used a gauze square. If able, allowed the person to apply pressure to the site.	___		_____
c. Read the results on the display. Noted the results on your note pad or assignment sheet. Told the person the results.	___	___	_____
d. Turned off the glucometer.	___	___	_____
15. Discarded the lancet into the sharps container.	___	___	_____
16. Discarded the gauze square and test strip. Followed agency policy.	___	___	_____
17. Removed and discarded gloves. Practiced hand hygiene.	___	___	_____
Post-Procedure			
18. Provided for comfort.	___	___	_____
19. Placed the call light and other needed items within reach.	___	___	_____
20. Lowered the bed to a safe and comfortable level for the person. Followed the care plan.	___	___	_____
21. Raised or lowered bed rails. Followed the care plan.	___	___	_____
22. Unscreened the person.	___	___	_____
23. Discarded used supplies.	___	___	_____
24. Completed a safety check of the room.	___	___	_____
25. Followed agency policy for used linens.	___	___	_____
26. Disinfected the glucometer. (Wore gloves.) Followed the manufacturer's instructions. Returned the device to its proper place.	___	___	_____
27. Removed and discarded the gloves. Practiced hand hygiene.	___	___	_____
28. Reported and recorded the test results and your observations.	___	___	_____

Date of Satisfactory Completion _____   Instructor's Initials _____

The Surgical Skin Prep—Shaving the Skin

Name: _____   Date: _____

	S	U	Comments

Quality of Life
- Knocked before entering the person's room.
- Addressed the person by name.
- Introduced yourself by name and title.
- Explained the procedure before starting and during the procedure.
- Protected the person's rights during the procedure.
- Handled the person gently during the procedure.

Pre-Procedure
1. Followed *Delegation Guidelines: Skin Preparation.* Saw *Promoting Safety and Comfort: Skin Preparation.*
2. Practiced hand hygiene.
3. Collected the following:
   - Skin prep kit
   - Bath blanket
   - Warm water
   - Gloves
   - Waterproof pad
   - Bath towel
4. Identified the person. Checked the ID (identification) bracelet against the assignment sheet. Used 2 identifiers. Also called the person by name.
5. Provided for privacy.

Procedure
6. Provided for good lighting.
7. Raised the bed for body mechanics. Lowered the bed rail near you (if up).
8. Covered the person with a bath blanket. Fan-folded top linens to the foot of the bed.
9. Positioned the person for the skin prep.
10. Placed the waterproof pad under the area you would shave.
11. Opened the skin prep kit.
12. Draped him or her with the drape.
13. Added warm water to the basin. Bed rails (if used) were up before you left the bedside.
14. Put on the gloves.
15. Lathered the skin with the sponge.
16. Held the skin taut. Shaved in the direction of hair growth.
17. Shaved outward from the center with short strokes.
18. Rinsed the razor often.
19. Made sure the entire area was free of hair. Checked for cuts, scratches, or nicks.
20. Rinsed the skin thoroughly. Patted dry.
21. Removed the drape and waterproof pad.
22. Removed and discarded the gloves. Practiced hand hygiene.
23. Returned top linens. Removed the bath blanket.

Post-Procedure
24. Provided for comfort.
25. Placed the call light and other needed items within reach.
26. Lowered the bed to a safe and comfortable level for the person. Followed the care plan. Locked (braked) the bed wheels.
27. Raised or lowered bed rails. Followed the care plan.
28. Unscreened the person.
29. Returned equipment to its proper place.

Date of Satisfactory Completion _____   Instructor's Initials _____

Post-Procedure—cont'd   **S**   **U**   **Comments**

30. Discarded supplies.   ——— ——— ————————
31. Completed a safety check of the room.   ——— ——— ————————
32. Followed agency policy for used linens.   ——— ——— ————————
33. Practiced hand hygiene.   ——— ——— ————————
34. Told the nurse that the skin prep was done. Reported your observations.   ——— ——— ————————

Date of Satisfactory Completion —————————————   Instructor's Initials ——————————

Applying Elastic Stockings

Name: _____   Date: _____

	S	U	Comments

Quality of Life
- Knocked before entering the person's room.   ___ ___ _____
- Addressed the person by name.   ___ ___ _____
- Introduced yourself by name and title.   ___ ___ _____
- Explained the procedure before starting and during the procedure.   ___ ___ _____
- Protected the person's rights during the procedure.   ___ ___ _____
- Handled the person gently during the procedure.   ___ ___ _____

Pre-Procedure
1. Followed *Delegation Guidelines: Elastic Stockings.* Saw *Promoting Safety and Comfort: Elastic Stockings.*   ___ ___ _____
2. Practiced hand hygiene.   ___ ___ _____
3. Obtained elastic stockings in the correct size and length. Noted the location of the toe opening.   ___ ___ _____
4. Identified the person. Checked the ID (identification) bracelet against the assignment sheet. Used 2 identifiers. Also called the person by name.   ___ ___ _____
5. Provided for privacy.   ___ ___ _____
6. Raised the bed for body mechanics. Bed rails were up if used.   ___ ___ _____

Procedure
7. Lowered the bed rail near you.   ___ ___ _____
8. Positioned the person supine.   ___ ___ _____
9. Exposed 1 leg. Fan-folded top linens toward the other leg.   ___ ___ _____
10. Gathered or turned the stocking inside out down to the heel.   ___ ___ _____
11. Slipped the foot of the stocking over the toes, foot, and heel. Made sure the stocking heel pocket was properly positioned on the person's heel. The toe opening was over or under the toes.   ___ ___ _____
12. Grasped the stocking top. Rolled or pulled the stocking up the leg. It turned right side out as it was rolled or pulled up.   ___ ___ _____
13. Made sure the stocking did not cause pressure on the toes. Adjusted the stocking as needed.   ___ ___ _____
14. Removed twists, creases, or wrinkles. Made sure the stocking was even, snug, smooth, and wrinkle-free.   ___ ___ _____
15. Covered the leg. Repeated for the other leg.
    a. Exposed the other leg. Fan-folded top linens toward the covered leg.   ___ ___ _____
    b. Gathered or turned the stocking inside out down to the heel.   ___ ___ _____
    c. Slipped the foot of the stocking over the toes, foot, and heel. Made sure the heel pocket was properly positioned on the person's heel. The toe opening was over or under the toes.   ___ ___ _____
    d. Grasped the stocking top. Rolled or pulled the stocking up the leg. It turned right side out as it rolled or pulled up.   ___ ___ _____
    e. Made sure the stocking did not cause pressure on the toes. Adjusted the stocking as needed.   ___ ___ _____
    f. Removed twists, creases, or wrinkles. Made sure the stocking was even, snug, smooth, and wrinkle-free.   ___ ___ _____
16. Covered the person.   ___ ___ _____

Post-Procedure
17. Provided for comfort.   ___ ___ _____
18. Placed the call light and other needed items within reach.   ___ ___ _____
19. Lowered the bed to a safe and comfortable level for the person. Followed the care plan.   ___ ___ _____

Date of Satisfactory Completion _____   Instructor's Initials _____

Post-Procedure—cont'd   S   U   **Comments**

20. Raised or lowered bed rails. Followed the care plan.
21. Unscreened the person.
22. Completed a safety check of the room.
23. Practiced hand hygiene.
24. Reported and recorded your observations.

Date of Satisfactory Completion _____   Instructor's Initials _____

Applying an Elastic Bandage

Name: _____   Date: _____

	S	U	Comments

Quality of Life
- Knocked before entering the person's room.
- Addressed the person by name.
- Introduced yourself by name and title.
- Explained the procedure before starting and during the procedure.
- Protected the person's rights during the procedure.
- Handled the person gently during the procedure.

Pre-Procedure
1. Followed *Delegation Guidelines: Elastic Bandages.* Saw *Promoting Safety and Comfort: Elastic Bandages.*
2. Practiced hand hygiene.
3. Collected the following:
   - Elastic bandage as directed by the nurse
   - Tape or clips (unless the bandage was Velcro)
4. Identified the person. Checked the ID (identification) bracelet against the assignment sheet. Used 2 identifiers. Also called the person by name.
5. Provided for privacy.
6. Raised the bed for body mechanics. Bed rails were up if used.

Procedure
7. Lowered the bed rail near you if up.
8. Helped the person to a comfortable position. Exposed the part you would bandage.
9. Made sure the area was clean and dry.
10. Held the bandage so the roll was up. The loose end was on the bottom.
11. Applied the bandage to the smallest part of the wrist, foot, ankle, or knee.
12. Made 2 circular turns around the part.
13. Made over-lapping spiral turns in an upward direction. Each turn over-lapped about ½ to ¾ of the previous turn. Each over-lap was equal.
14. Applied the bandage smoothly with firm, even pressure. It was not tight.
15. Ended the bandage with 2 circular turns.
16. Secured the bandage in place with Velcro, tape, or clips. The clips were not under any body part.
17. Checked the fingers or toes for coldness or cyanosis (bluish color). Asked about pain, itching, numbness, or tingling. Removed the bandage if any were noted. Reported your observations.

Post-Procedure
18. Provided for comfort.
19. Placed the call light and other needed items within reach.
20. Lowered the bed to a safe and comfortable level for the person. Followed the care plan.
21. Raised or lowered bed rails. Followed the care plan.
22. Unscreened the person.
23. Completed a safety check of the room.
24. Practiced hand hygiene.
25. Reported and recorded your observations.

Date of Satisfactory Completion _____   Instructor's Initials _____

Applying a Dry, Non-Sterile Dressing

Name: _____   Date: _____

Quality of Life	S	U	Comments
• Knocked before entering the person's room.	___	___	_____
• Addressed the person by name.	___	___	_____
• Introduced yourself by name and title.	___	___	_____
• Explained the procedure before starting and during the procedure.	___	___	_____
• Protected the person's rights during the procedure.	___	___	_____
• Handled the person gently during the procedure.	___	___	_____

Pre-Procedure

1. Followed *Delegation Guidelines: Applying Dressings.*
   Saw *Promoting Safety and Comfort:*
   a. *Wound Care*
   b. *Applying Dressings*
2. Practiced hand hygiene.
3. Collected the following:
   - Gloves
   - PPE (personal protective equipment) as needed
   - Tape or Montgomery ties
   - Dressings as directed by the nurse 4 × 4 gauze
   - Saline solution as directed by the nurse
   - Cleansing solution as directed by the nurse
   - Adhesive remover
   - Dressing set with scissors and forceps
   - Plastic bag
   - Bath blanket
4. Practiced hand hygiene.
5. Identified the person. Checked the ID (identification) bracelet against the assignment sheet. Used 2 identifiers. Also called the person by name.
6. Provided for privacy.
7. Arranged your work area. You did not have to reach over or turn your back on your work area.
8. Raised the bed for body mechanics. Bed rails were up if used.

Procedure

9. Lowered the bed rail near you if up.
10. Helped the person to a comfortable position.
11. Covered the person with a bath blanket. Fan-folded top linens to the foot of the bed.
12. Exposed the affected body part.
13. Made a cuff on the plastic bag. Placed it within reach.
14. Practiced hand hygiene.
15. Put on needed PPE. Put on gloves.
16. Removed tape or undid Montgomery ties.
    a. *Tape:* held the skin down. Gently pulled the tape toward the wound.
    b. *Montgomery ties:* folded ties away from the wound.
17. Removed any adhesive from the skin. Wet a 4 × 4 gauze dressing with adhesive remover. Picked up a gauze square with the forceps. Cleaned away from the wound.
18. Removed gauze dressings. Started with the top dressing and removed each layer. Kept the soiled side from the person's sight. Put dressings in the plastic bag. They did not touch the outside of the bag.
19. Removed the dressing over the wound very gently. Moistened the dressing with saline if it stuck to the wound.

Date of Satisfactory Completion _____   Instructor's Initials _____

Procedure—cont'd

	S	U	Comments
20. Observed the wound, drain site, and wound drainage.			
21. Removed the gloves and put them in a plastic bag. Practiced hand hygiene.			
22. Opened the new dressings.			
23. Cut the length of tape needed.			
24. Put on clean gloves.			
25. Cleaned the wound with saline as directed by the nurse.			
26. Applied dressings as directed by the nurse.			
27. Secured the dressings. Used tape or Montgomery ties.			
28. Removed the gloves. Put them in the bag.			
29. Removed and discarded PPE.			
30. Practiced hand hygiene.			
31. Covered the person. Removed the bath blanket.			

Post-Procedure

	S	U	Comments
32. Provided for comfort.			
33. Placed the call light and other needed items within reach.			
34. Lowered the bed to a safe and comfortable level for the person. Followed the care plan.			
35. Raised or lowered bed rails. Followed the care plan.			
36. Returned equipment and supplies to the proper place. Left extra dressings and tape in the room.			
37. Discarded used supplies in the bag. Tied the bag closed. Discarded the bag following agency policy. Wore gloves for this step.			
38. Cleaned your work area. Followed the Bloodborne Pathogen Standard.			
39. Unscreened the person.			
40. Completed a safety check of the room.			
41. Removed and discarded the gloves. Practiced hand hygiene.			
42. Reported and recorded your observations.			

Date of Satisfactory Completion _____   Instructor's Initials _____

Applying Heat and Cold Applications

Name: _____   Date: _____

	S	U	Comments

Quality of Life
- Knocked before entering the person's room.
- Addressed the person by name.
- Introduced yourself by name and title.
- Explained the procedure before starting and during the procedure.
- Protected the person's rights during the procedure.
- Handled the person gently during the procedure.

Pre-Procedure
1. Followed *Delegation Guidelines: Warm and Cold Applications.*
   Saw *Promoting Safety and Comfort: Warm and Cold Applications.*
2. Practiced hand hygiene.
3. Collected the following:
   a. *For a hot compress:*
      - Basin
      - Bath thermometer
      - Small towel, washcloth, or gauze squares
      - Plastic wrap or aquathermia pad
      - Ties, tape, or rolled gauze
      - Bath towel
      - Waterproof pad
   b. *For a hot soak:*
      - Water basin or arm or foot bath
      - Bath thermometer
      - Waterproof pad
      - Bath blanket
      - Towel
   c. *For a sitz bath:*
      - Disposable sitz bath
      - Bath thermometer
      - 2 bath blankets, bath towels, and a clean gown
   d. *For a hot or cold pack:*
      - Commercial pack
      - Pack cover
      - Ties, tape, or rolled gauze (if needed)
      - Waterproof pad
   e. *For an aquathermia pad:*
      - Aquathermia pad and heating unit
      - Distilled water
      - Flannel cover or other cover as directed
      - Ties, tape, or rolled gauze
   f. *For an ice bag, ice collar, ice glove, or dry cold pack:*
      - Ice bag, collar, glove, or cold pack
      - Crushed ice (except for cold pack)
      - Flannel cover or other cover as directed
      - Paper towels
   g. *For a cold compress:*
      - Large basin with ice
      - Small basin with cold water
      - Gauze squares, washcloths, or small towels
      - Waterproof pad
4. Identified the person. Checked the ID (identification) bracelet against the assignment sheet. Used 2 identifiers. Also called the person by name.

Date of Satisfactory Completion _____   Instructor's Initials _____

Procedure	S	U	Comments
5. Provided for privacy.	___	___	_____
6. Positioned the person for the procedure.	___	___	_____
7. Placed the waterproof pad (if needed) under the body part.	___	___	_____
8. *For a hot compress:*			
a. Filled the basin ½ to ⅔ full with hot water as directed. Measured water temperature.	___	___	_____
b. Placed the compress in the water.	___	___	_____
c. Wrung out the compress.	___	___	_____
d. Applied the compress over the area. Noted the time.	___	___	_____
e. Covered the compress as directed. Did 1 of the following:			
1) Applied plastic wrap and then a bath towel. Secured the towel in place with ties, tape, or rolled gauze.	___	___	_____
2) Applied an aquathermia pad.	___	___	_____
9. *For a hot soak:*			
a. Filled a container ½ full with hot water. Measured water temperature.	___	___	_____
b. Placed the part into the water. Padded the edge of the container with a towel. Noted the time.	___	___	_____
c. Covered the person with a bath blanket for warmth.	___	___	_____
10. *For a sitz bath:*			
a. Placed the disposable sitz bath on the toilet seat.	___	___	_____
b. Filled the sitz bath ⅔ full with water. Measured water temperature.	___	___	_____
c. Secured the gown above the waist.	___	___	_____
d. Helped the person sit on the sitz bath. Noted the time.	___	___	_____
e. Provided for warmth. Placed a bath blanket around the shoulders. Placed another over the legs.	___	___	_____
f. Stayed with the person if he or she was weak or unsteady.	___	___	_____
11. *For an aquathermia pad:*			
a. Filled the heating unit to the fill line with distilled water.	___	___	_____
b. Removed the bubbles. Placed the pad and tubing below the heating unit. Tilted the heating unit from side to side.	___	___	_____
c. Set the temperature as the nurse directed (usually 105°F [40.5°C]). Removed the key.	___	___	_____
d. Placed the pad in the cover.	___	___	_____
e. Plugged in the unit. Allowed water to warm to the desired temperature.	___	___	_____
f. Set the heating unit on the bedside stand. Kept the pad and connecting hoses level with the unit. Hoses did not have kinks.	___	___	_____
g. Applied the pad to the part. Noted the time.	___	___	_____
h. Secured the pad in place with ties, tape, or rolled gauze. Did not use pins.	___	___	_____
12. *For a hot or cold pack:*			
a. Squeezed, kneaded, or struck the pack as directed by the manufacturer.	___	___	_____
b. Placed the pack in the cover.	___	___	_____
c. Applied the pack. Noted the time.	___	___	_____
d. Secured the pack in place with ties, tape, or rolled gauze. Some packs are secured with Velcro straps.	___	___	_____
13. *For an ice bag, collar, or glove:*			
a. Filled the device with water. Put in the stopper. Turned the device upside down to check for leaks.	___	___	_____
b. Emptied the device.	___	___	_____
c. Filled the device ½ to ⅔ full with crushed ice or ice chips.	___	___	_____
d. Removed excess air. Bent, twisted, or squeezed the device. Or pressed it against a firm surface.	___	___	_____
e. Placed the cap or stopper on securely.	___	___	_____
f. Dried the device with paper towels.	___	___	_____

Date of Satisfactory Completion _____   Instructor's Initials _____

Procedure—cont'd	S	U	Comments
g. Placed the device in the cover.	___	___	_____
h. Applied the device. Noted the time.	___	___	_____
i. Secured the device in place with ties, tape, or rolled gauze.	___	___	_____
14. *For a cold compress:*			
a. Placed the small basin with cold water into the large basin with ice.	___	___	_____
b. Placed the compress into the cold water.	___	___	_____
c. Wrung out the compress.	___	___	_____
d. Applied the compress to the part. Noted the time.	___	___	_____
15. Placed the call light and other needed items within reach. Unscreened the person if appropriate.	___	___	_____
16. Raised or lowered bed rails. Followed the care plan.	___	___	_____
17. Did the following every 5 minutes:			
a. Checked the person for signs and symptoms of complications. Removed the application if complications occurred. Told the nurse at once.	___	___	_____
b. Checked the application for cooling (hot application) or warming (cold application).			
18. Removed the application at the specified time. Heat and cold applications are usually left on for 15 to 20 minutes.	___	___	_____

Post-Procedure

	S	U	Comments
19. Provided for comfort.	___	___	_____
20. Placed the call light and other needed items within reach.	___	___	_____
21. Raised or lowered bed rails. Followed the care plan.	___	___	_____
22. Unscreened the person.	___	___	_____
23. Cleaned, rinsed, dried, and returned re-usable items to the proper place. Followed agency policy for used linens. Wore gloves for this step.	___	___	_____
24. Completed a safety check of the room.	___	___	_____
25. Removed and discarded the gloves. Practiced hand hygiene.	___	___	_____
26. Reported and recorded your observations.	___	___	_____

Date of Satisfactory Completion _____   Instructor's Initials _____

Using a Pulse Oximeter

Name: _____ Date: _____

	S	U	Comments

Quality of Life
- Knocked before entering the person's room.
- Addressed the person by name.
- Introduced yourself by name and title.
- Explained the procedure before starting and during the procedure.
- Protected the person's rights during the procedure.
- Handled the person gently during the procedure.

Pre-Procedure
1. Followed *Delegation Guidelines: Pulse Oximetry.* Saw *Promoting Safety and Comfort: Pulse Oximetry.*
2. Practiced hand hygiene.
3. Collected the following before going to the person's room:
   - Oximeter
   - Tape
   - Towel
4. Arranged your work area.
5. Practiced hand hygiene.
6. Identified the person. Checked the ID (identification) bracelet against the assignment sheet. Used 2 identifiers. Also called the person by name.
7. Provided for privacy.

Procedure
8. Provided for comfort.
9. Dried the site with a towel.
10. Clipped or taped the sensor to the site.
11. Turned on the oximeter.
12. *For continuous monitoring:*
   a. Set the high and low alarm limits for SpO_2 (saturation of peripheral oxygen) and pulse rate.
   b. Turned on audio and visual alarms.
13. Checked the person's pulse (apical or radial) with the pulse on the display. The pulses should have been about the same. Noted both pulses on your assignment sheet.
14. Read the SpO_2 on the display. Noted the value on the flow sheet and your assignment sheet.
15. Left the sensor in place for continuous monitoring. Otherwise, turned off the device and removed the sensor.

Post-Procedure
16. Provided for comfort.
17. Placed the call light and other needed items within reach.
18. Unscreened the person.
19. Completed a safety check of the room.
20. Returned the device to its proper place (unless monitoring was continuous).
21. Practiced hand hygiene.
22. Reported and recorded the SpO_2, the pulse rate, and your other observations.

Date of Satisfactory Completion _____ Instructor's Initials _____

Assisting With Deep-Breathing and Coughing Exercises

Name: _____   Date: _____

Quality of Life	S	U	Comments
• Knocked before entering the person's room.	___	___	_____
• Addressed the person by name.	___	___	_____
• Introduced yourself by name and title.	___	___	_____
• Explained the procedure before starting and during the procedure.	___	___	_____
• Protected the person's rights during the procedure.	___	___	_____
• Handled the person gently during the procedure.	___	___	_____

Pre-Procedure

1. Followed *Delegation Guidelines: Deep Breathing and Coughing.* Saw *Promoting Safety and Comfort: Deep Breathing and Coughing.*   ___ ___ _____
2. Practiced hand hygiene.   ___ ___ _____
3. Identified the person. Checked the ID (identification) bracelet against the assignment sheet. Used 2 identifiers. Also called the person by name.   ___ ___ _____
4. Provided for privacy.   ___ ___ _____

Procedure

5. Lowered the bed rail if up.   ___ ___ _____
6. Helped the person to a comfortable sitting position.
   - Sitting on the side of the bed   ___ ___ _____
   - Semi-Fowler's   ___ ___ _____
   - Fowler's   ___ ___ _____
7. Had the person deep breathe.
   a. Had the person place the hands over the rib cage.   ___ ___ _____
   b. Had the person breathe as deeply as possible. Reminded the person to inhale through the nose.   ___ ___ _____
   c. Asked the person to hold the breath for 2 to 3 seconds.   ___ ___ _____
   d. Asked the person to exhale slowly through pursed lips. Asked the person to exhale until the ribs moved as far down as possible.   ___ ___ _____
   e. Repeated 4 more times. Had the person:
      1) Deep breathe in through the nose.   ___ ___ _____
      2) Hold the breath for 2 to 3 seconds.   ___ ___ _____
      3) Exhale slowly with pursed lips until the ribs moved as far down as possible.   ___ ___ _____
8. Asked the person to cough.
   a. Had the person place both hands over the incision. One hand was on top of the other. The person could have held a pillow or folded towel over the incision. If the person covered the nose and mouth for respiratory etiquette, you supported the incision with your hands or a pillow. Wore gloves.   ___ ___ _____
   b. Had the person take a deep breath through the nose.   ___ ___ _____
   c. Asked the person to cough strongly 2 times with the mouth open.   ___ ___ _____

Post-Procedure

9. Provided for comfort.   ___ ___ _____
10. Placed the call light and other needed items within reach.   ___ ___ _____
11. Raised or lowered bed rails. Followed the care plan.   ___ ___ _____
12. Unscreened the person.   ___ ___ _____
13. Completed a safety check of the room.   ___ ___ _____
14. Practiced hand hygiene.   ___ ___ _____
15. Reported and recorded your observations.   ___ ___ _____

Date of Satisfactory Completion _____   Instructor's Initials _____

Setting Up Oxygen

Name: _____   Date: _____

	S	U	Comments

Quality of Life
- Knocked before entering the person's room.
- Addressed the person by name.
- Introduced yourself by name and title.
- Explained the procedure before starting and during the procedure.
- Protected the person's rights during the procedure.
- Handled the person gently during the procedure.

Pre-Procedure
1. Followed *Delegation Guidelines: Oxygen Set-Up.* Saw *Promoting Safety and Comfort: Oxygen Set-Up.*
2. Practiced hand hygiene.
3. Collected the following before going to the person's room:
   - Oxygen (O_2) device with connecting tubing
   - Flowmeter
   - Humidifier (if ordered)
   - Distilled water (if used humidifier)
4. Arranged your work area.
5. Practiced hand hygiene.
6. Identified the person. Checked the ID (identification) bracelet against the assignment sheet. Used 2 identifiers. Also called the person by name.

Procedure
7. Made sure the flowmeter was in the OFF position.
8. Attached the flowmeter to the wall outlet or to the tank.
9. Filled the humidifier with distilled water.
10. Attached the humidifier to the bottom of the flowmeter.
11. Attached the O_2 device and connecting tubing to the humidifier. *Did not set the flowmeter. Did not apply the O_2 device on the person.*
12. Placed the cap securely on the distilled water. Stored the water according to agency policy.
13. Discarded the packaging from the O_2 device and connecting tubing.

Post-Procedure
14. Provided for comfort.
15. Placed the call light and other needed items within reach.
16. Completed a safety check of the room.
17. Practiced hand hygiene.
18. Told the nurse when you were done. The nurse would then:
    - Turn on the O_2 and set the flow rate.
    - Apply the O_2 device on the person.

Date of Satisfactory Completion _____   Instructor's Initials _____

Caring for Eyeglasses

Name: _____   Date: _____

	S	U	Comments
Quality of Life			
• Knocked before entering the person's room.	___	___	_____
• Addressed the person by name.	___	___	_____
• Introduced yourself by name and title.	___	___	_____
• Explained the procedure before starting and during the procedure.	___	___	_____
• Protected the person's rights during the procedure.	___	___	_____
• Handled the person gently during the procedure.	___	___	_____

Pre-Procedure

1. Followed *Delegation Guidelines: Eyeglasses.*
   Saw *Promoting Safety and Comfort: Corrective Lenses.*   ___ ___ _____
2. Practiced hand hygiene.   ___ ___ _____
3. Collected the following:
   - Eyeglass case   ___ ___ _____
   - Cleaning solution or warm water   ___ ___ _____
   - Disposable lens cloth or cotton cloth   ___ ___ _____

Procedure

4. Removed the eyeglasses.
   a. Held the frames in front of the ears.   ___ ___ _____
   b. Lifted the frames from the ears. Brought the eyeglasses
      down away from the face.   ___ ___ _____
5. Cleaned the lenses with cleaning solution or warm water.
   Cleaned in a circular motion. Dried the lenses with the cloth.   ___ ___ _____
6. *If the person did not wear the glasses:*
   a. Opened the eyeglass case.   ___ ___ _____
   b. Folded the glasses. Put them in the case. Did not touch
      the clean lenses.   ___ ___ _____
   c. Placed the eyeglass case in the top drawer of the bedside stand.   ___ ___ _____
7. *If the person wore the eyeglasses:*
   a. Held the frames at each side. Placed them over the ears.   ___ ___ _____
   b. Adjusted the eyeglasses so the nose-piece rested on the nose.   ___ ___ _____
   c. Returned the eyeglass case to the top drawer in
      the bedside stand.   ___ ___ _____

Post-Procedure

8. Provided for comfort.   ___ ___ _____
9. Placed the call light and other needed items within reach.   ___ ___ _____
10. Returned the cleaning solution to its proper place.   ___ ___ _____
11. Discarded the disposable cloth.   ___ ___ _____
12. Completed a safety check of the room.   ___ ___ _____
13. Practiced hand hygiene.   ___ ___ _____
14. Reported and recorded your observations.   ___ ___ _____

Date of Satisfactory Completion _____   Instructor's Initials _____

Cleaning Baby Bottles

Name: _____   Date: _____

Pre-Procedure	S	U	Comments
1. See *Promoting Safety and Comfort: Cleaning Baby Bottles.*	___	___	_____
2. Practiced hand hygiene.	___	___	_____
3. Collected the following:			
• Bottles, nipples, and caps	___	___	_____
• Funnel	___	___	_____
• Can opener	___	___	_____
• Bottle brush	___	___	_____
• Dishwashing soap	___	___	_____
• Other items used to prepare formula	___	___	_____
• Towel	___	___	_____

Procedure	S	U	Comments
4. Washed the bottles, nipples, caps, funnel, and can opener in hot, soapy water. Washed other items used to prepare formula.	___	___	_____
5. Cleaned inside baby bottles with the bottle brush.	___	___	_____
6. Squeezed hot, soapy water through the nipples. This removed formula.	___	___	_____
7. Rinsed all items thoroughly in hot water. Squeezed hot water through the nipples to remove soap.	___	___	_____
8. Laid a clean towel on the counter.	___	___	_____
9. Stood bottles upside down to drain. Placed nipples, caps, and other items on the towel. Let the items dry.	___	___	_____

Date of Satisfactory Completion _____   Instructor's Initials _____

Diapering a Baby

Name: _____   Date: _____

	S	U	Comments

Quality of Life
- Knocked before entering the baby's room.
- Addressed the baby and parents by name.
- Introduced yourself by name and title.
- Explained the procedure to the parents before starting and during the procedure.
- Protected the baby's rights during the procedure.
- Handled the baby gently during the procedure.

Pre-Procedure
1. Followed *Delegation Guidelines: Diapering a Baby.* Saw *Promoting Safety and Comfort: Diapering a Baby.*
2. Practiced hand hygiene.
3. Collected the following:
   - Gloves
   - Clean diaper
   - Waterproof changing pad
   - Washcloth
   - Disposable wipes or cotton balls
   - Basin of warm water
   - Baby soap
   - Baby lotion or cream

Procedure
4. Put on the gloves.
5. Placed the changing pad under the baby.
6. Unfastened the dirty diaper. Placed diaper pins out of the baby's reach.
7. Wiped the genital area with the front of the diaper. Wiped from the front to the back (top to bottom).
8. Noted the color and amount of urine and feces. Folded the diaper so urine and feces were inside. Set the diaper aside.
9. Cleaned the genital area from front to back (top to bottom). Used a wet washcloth, disposable wipes, or cotton balls. Washed with mild soap and water for a large amount of feces or if the baby had a rash. Rinsed thoroughly and patted the area dry.
10. Cleaned the circumcision. Gave cord care.
11. Applied cream or lotion to the genital area and buttocks. Did not use too much. Avoided caking lotion.
12. Raised the baby's legs. Slid a clean diaper under the buttocks.
13. Folded a cloth diaper as follows:
    a. *For a boy:* the extra thickness was in the front.
    b. *For a girl:* the extra thickness was in the back.
    c. Brought the diaper between the baby's legs.
14. Made sure the diaper was snug around the hips and abdomen.
    a. It was loose near the penis if the circumcision had not healed.
    b. It was below the umbilicus if the cord stump had not healed.
15. Secured the diaper in place. Used the tape strips or Velcro on the disposable diapers. Made sure the tabs stuck in place. Used baby pins or Velcro for cloth diapers. Pins pointed away from the abdomen.
16. Applied a diaper cover or plastic pants if cloth diapers were worn.
17. Placed the baby in the crib, infant seat, or other safe place.

Date of Satisfactory Completion _____   Instructor's Initials _____

Post-Procedure

	S	U	Comments
18. Rinsed feces from the cloth diaper into the toilet and flushed.	___	___	_____
19. Stored used cloth diapers in a covered pail. Placed a disposable diaper and paper tabs in the trash.	___	___	_____
20. Removed and discarded the gloves. Practiced hand hygiene.	___	___	_____
21. Put on clean gloves.	___	___	_____
22. Cleaned, rinsed, dried, and returned other items to their proper place.	___	___	_____
23. Removed and discarded the gloves. Practiced hand hygiene.	___	___	_____
24. Reported and recorded your observations.	___	___	_____

Date of Satisfactory Completion _____   Instructor's Initials _____

Giving a Baby a Sponge Bath

Name: _____   Date: _____

	S	U	Comments

Quality of Life
- Knocked before entering the baby's room.
- Addressed the baby and parents by name.
- Introduced yourself by name and title.
- Explained the procedure to the parents before starting and during the procedure.
- Protected the baby's rights during the procedure.
- Handled the baby gently during the procedure.

Pre-Procedure
1. Followed *Delegation Guidelines: Bathing an Infant.* Saw *Promoting Safety and Comfort: Bathing an Infant.*
2. Practiced hand hygiene.
3. Placed the following items in your work area.
   - Bath basin
   - Bath thermometer
   - Bath towel
   - 2 hand towels
   - Receiving blanket
   - Washcloth
   - Clean diaper
   - Clean clothing for the baby
   - Cotton balls
   - Baby soap (if needed)
   - Baby shampoo
   - Baby lotion
   - Gloves
4. Identified the baby. Checked the ID (identification) bracelet against the assignment sheet. Used 2 identifiers. Followed agency policy.
5. Provided for privacy.

Procedure
6. Filled the bath basin with warm water. Water temperature was 100°F to 103°F (37.7°C to 40.5°C). Measured water temperature with the bath thermometer or used the inside of your wrist. The water felt warm and comfortable.
7. Put on gloves.
8. Undressed the baby. Left the diaper on.
9. Washed the baby's eye lids.
   a. Dipped a cotton ball into the water.
   b. Squeezed out excess water.
   c. Washed 1 eye lid from the inner part to the outer part.
   d. Repeated for the other eye with a new cotton ball.
10. Moistened the washcloth and made a mitt. Cleaned the outside of the ear and then behind the ear. Repeated for the other ear. Was gentle.
11. Rinsed and squeezed out the washcloth. Made a mitt with the washcloth.
12. Washed the baby's face. Cleaned inside the nostrils with the washcloth. *Did not use cotton swabs to clean inside the nose.* Patted the face dry.
13. Picked up the baby. Held the baby over the bath basin using the football hold. Supported the baby's head and neck with your wrist and hand.

Date of Satisfactory Completion _____   Instructor's Initials _____

Procedure—cont'd	S	U	Comments
14. Washed the baby's head.			
a. Squeezed a small amount of water from the washcloth onto the baby's head. Or brought water to the baby's head using a cupped hand.	___	___	_____
b. Applied a small amount of baby shampoo to the head.	___	___	_____
c. Washed the head with circular motions.	___	___	_____
d. Rinsed the head by squeezing water from a washcloth over the baby's head. Or brought water to the baby's head using a cupped hand. Rinsed thoroughly. Did not get soap in the baby's eyes.	___	___	_____
e. Used a small hand towel to dry the head.	___	___	_____
15. Laid the baby on the table.	___	___	_____
16. Removed the diaper.	___	___	_____
17. Washed the front of the body with a washcloth or your hands. Did not get the cord wet. Also washed the arms, hands, fingers, legs, feet, and toes. Washed the genital area. Rinsed thoroughly. Patted dry. Was sure to wash and dry all creases and folds.	___	___	_____
18. Gave cord care. Cleaned the circumcision.	___	___	_____
19. Turned the baby to the prone position. Washed the back and buttocks. Used a washcloth or your hands. Rinsed thoroughly. Patted dry.	___	___	_____
20. Applied baby lotion as directed by the nurse.	___	___	_____
21. Removed and discarded the gloves. Practiced hand hygiene.	___	___	_____
22. Put a clean diaper and clean clothes on the baby.	___	___	_____
23. Wrapped the baby in the receiving blanket. Put the baby in the crib or other safe area.	___	___	_____

Post-Procedure

	S	U	Comments
24. Practiced hand hygiene. Put on gloves.	___	___	_____
25. Cleaned, rinsed, dried, and returned equipment and supplies to the proper place. Did this when the baby was settled.	___	___	_____
26. Removed and discarded the gloves. Practiced hand hygiene.	___	___	_____
27. Completed a safety check of the room.	___	___	_____
28. Reported and recorded your observations.	___	___	_____

Date of Satisfactory Completion _____   Instructor's Initials _____

Giving a Baby a Tub Bath

Name: _____   Date: _____

	S	U	Comments

Quality of Life
- Knocked before entering the baby's room.
- Addressed the baby and parents by name.
- Introduced yourself by name and title.
- Explained the procedure to the parents before starting and during the procedure.
- Protected the baby's rights during the procedure.
- Handled the baby gently during the procedure.

Procedure
1. Did the following:
   a. Followed *Delegation Guidelines: Bathing an Infant*.
      Saw *Promoting Safety and Comfort: Bathing an Infant*.
   b. Practiced hand hygiene.
   c. Placed the following items in your work area.
      - Bath basin
      - Bath thermometer
      - Bath towel
      - 2 hand towels
      - Receiving blanket
      - Washcloth
      - Clean diaper
      - Clean clothing for the baby
      - Cotton balls
      - Baby soap (if needed)
      - Baby shampoo
      - Baby lotion
      - Gloves
   d. Identified the baby. Checked the ID (identification) bracelet against the assignment sheet. Used 2 identifiers. Followed agency policy.
   e. Provided for privacy.
   f. Filled the bath basin with warm water. Water temperature was 100°F to 103°F (37.7°C to 40.5°C). Measured water temperature with the bath thermometer or used the inside of your wrist. The water felt warm and comfortable.
   g. Put on gloves.
   h. Undressed the baby. Left the diaper on.
   i. Washed the baby's eye lids.
      1) Dipped a cotton ball into the water.
      2) Squeezed out excess water.
      3) Washed 1 eye lid from the inner part to the outer part.
      4) Repeated for the other eye with a new cotton ball.
   j. Moistened the washcloth and made a mitt. Cleaned the outside of the ear and then behind the ear. Repeated for the other ear. Was gentle.
   k. Rinsed and squeezed out the washcloth. Made a mitt with the washcloth.
   l. Washed the baby's face. Cleaned inside the nostrils with the washcloth. *Did not use cotton swabs to clean inside the nose.* Patted the face dry.
   m. Picked up the baby. Held the baby over the bath basin using the football hold. Supported the baby's head and neck with your wrist and hand.

Date of Satisfactory Completion _____   Instructor's Initials _____

Procedure—cont'd   S   U   Comments

   n. Washed the baby's head.
      1) Squeezed a small amount of water from the washcloth
         onto the baby's head. Or brought water to the baby's
         head using a cupped hand.   _____ _____ _____
      2) Applied a small amount of baby shampoo to the head.   _____ _____ _____
      3) Washed the head with circular motions.   _____ _____ _____
      4) Rinsed the head by squeezing water from a washcloth over
         the baby's head. Or brought water to the baby's head using
         a cupped hand. Rinsed thoroughly. Did not get soap in the
         baby's eyes.   _____ _____ _____
      5) Used a small hand towel to dry the head.   _____ _____ _____
   o. Laid the baby on the table.   _____ _____ _____
   p. Removed the diaper.   _____ _____ _____
 2. Held the baby.
   a. Placed 1 hand under the baby's shoulders. Your thumb was
     over the baby's shoulder. Your fingers were under the arm.   _____ _____ _____
   b. Supported the buttocks with your other hand. Slid your hand
     under the thighs. Held the far thigh with your other hand.   _____ _____ _____
 3. Lowered the baby into the water feet first.
 4. Washed the front of the baby's body. Also washed the arms, hands,
   fingers, legs, feet, and toes. Washed the genital area. Gently washed
   all creases and folds.   _____ _____ _____
 5. Reversed your hold. Used your other hand to hold the baby.   _____ _____ _____
 6. Washed the baby's back and buttocks. Rinsed thoroughly.   _____ _____ _____
 7. Reversed your hold again. Held the baby with your other hand.   _____ _____ _____
 8. Lifted the baby out of the water and onto a towel.   _____ _____ _____
 9. Wrapped the baby in the towel. Also covered the baby's head.   _____ _____ _____
10. Patted the baby dry. Dried all folds and creases.   _____ _____ _____
11. Did the following:
   a. Applied baby lotion as directed by the nurse.   _____ _____ _____
   b. Removed and discarded the gloves. Practiced hand hygiene.   _____ _____ _____
   c. Put a clean diaper and clean clothes on the baby.   _____ _____ _____
   d. Wrapped the baby in the receiving blanket. Put the baby in the
     crib or other safe area.   _____ _____ _____
   e. Practiced hand hygiene. Put on gloves.   _____ _____ _____
   f. Cleaned, rinsed, dried, and returned equipment and supplies
     to the proper place. Did this when the baby was settled.   _____ _____ _____
   g. Removed and discarded the gloves. Practiced hand hygiene.   _____ _____ _____
   h. Completed a safety check of the room.   _____ _____ _____
   i. Reported and recorded your observations.   _____ _____ _____

Date of Satisfactory Completion _____   Instructor's Initials _____

Weighing an Infant

Name: _____ Date: _____

	S	U	Comments

Quality of Life
- Knocked before entering the baby's room.
- Addressed the baby and parents by name.
- Introduced yourself by name and title.
- Explained the procedure to the parents before starting and during the procedure.
- Protected the baby's rights during the procedure.
- Handled the baby gently during the procedure.

Pre-Procedure
1. Followed *Delegation Guidelines: Weighing Infants*. Saw *Promoting Safety and Comfort: Weighing Infants*.
2. Practiced hand hygiene.
3. Collected the following:
   - Baby scale
   - Paper for the scale
   - Items for diaper changing
   - Gloves
4. Identified the baby. Checked the ID (identification) bracelet against the assignment sheet. Used 2 identifiers. Followed agency policy.

Procedure
5. Placed the paper on the scale. Adjusted the scale to zero (0).
6. Put on gloves.
7. Undressed the baby and removed the diaper. Cleaned the genital area.
8. Removed and discarded the gloves and practiced hand hygiene. Put on clean gloves.
9. Laid the baby on the scale. Kept 1 hand over the baby to prevent falling.
10. Read the digital display or moved the weights until the scale was balanced.
11. Noted the measurement.
12. Took the baby off of the scale.
13. Diapered and dressed the baby. Laid the baby in the crib.
14. Discarded the paper and soiled diaper.
15. Disinfected the scale; followed agency policy.
16. Removed and discarded the gloves. Practiced hand hygiene.

Post-Procedure
17. Returned the scale to its proper place.
18. Practiced hand hygiene.
19. Reported and recorded your observations.

Date of Satisfactory Completion _____ Instructor's Initials _____

Adult CPR—1 Rescuer

Name: _____   Date: _____

Procedure	S	U	Comments
1. Made sure the scene was safe.			
2. Checked for a response. Tapped or gently shook the person. Called the person by name, if known. Shouted: "Are you okay?"			
3. Shouted for nearby help if the person did not respond.			
4. Activated the EMS system or the agency's RRT (MET).			
a. If alone with a mobile phone, used it while continuing to give care.			
b. If alone without a mobile phone, left the person to activate the EMS system before started CPR.			
c. If help arrived, sent him or her to activate the EMS system.			
5. Got an AED and emergency equipment.			
a. If alone, got the AED and emergency equipment before started CPR.			
b. If help arrived, asked him or her to get the AED and emergency equipment.			
6. Checked for breathing and a pulse.			
7. Positioned the person for CPR if not already done. The person was supine on a hard, flat surface. Logrolled the person so there was no twisting of the spine. Placed the arms alongside the body.			
8. Exposed the person's chest.			
9. Gave CPR.			
a. Placed 2 hands on the lower half of the sternum. Gave chest compressions at a rate of 100 to 120 per minute. Established a regular rhythm. Counted out loud. Pressed down at least 2 inches but no more that 2.4 inches. Allowed the chest to recoil between compressions. Did not lean on the chest after each compression. Gave 30 chest compressions.			
b. Opened the airway. Used the head tilt-chin lift method.			
c. Gave 2 breaths. Each breath should have taken only 1 second. The chest rose. If the first breath did not make the chest rise:			
i) Opened the airway again. Used the head tilt-chin lift method.			
ii) Gave another breath.			
10. Continued the cycle of 30 chest compressions followed by 2 breaths. Limited interruptions in compressions to less than 10 seconds. Used the AED as soon as it arrived.			
11. Continued until help took over or the person began to move. If movement occurred, placed the person in the recovery position.			

Date of Satisfactory Completion _____   Instructor's Initials _____

Adult CPR With AED—2 Rescuers

Name: _____   Date: _____

Procedure	S	U	Comments
1. Made sure the scene was safe.			
2. *Rescuer 1:*			
a. Checked for a response. Tapped or gently shook the person. Called the person by name, if known. Shouted: "Are you okay?"			
b. Shouted for nearby help if the person did not respond.			
3. *Rescuer 2:*			
a. Activated the EMS system or agency's RRT (MET) using a mobile phone (if available) or left to do so.			
b. Got an AED and emergency equipment.			
4. *Rescuer 1:*			
a. Checked for breathing and a pulse. Looked for no breathing or only gasping. At the same time, checked for a carotid pulse. CPR was done if there was no breathing (or only gasping) and you did not definitely feel a pulse within 10 seconds.			
b. Positioned the person for CPR if not already done. The person was supine on a hard, flat surface. Logrolled the person so there was no twisting of the spine. Placed the arms alongside the body.			
c. Exposed the person's chest.			
d. Placed 2 hands on the lower half of the sternum. Gave chest compressions at a rate of 100 to 120 per minute. Established a regular rhythm. Counted out load. Pressed down at least 2 inches but no more than 2.4 inches. Allowed the chest to recoil between compressions. Did not lean on the chest after each compression. Gave 30 chest compressions.			
e. Opened the airway. Used the head tilt-chin lift method.			
f. Gave 2 breaths. Each breath should have taken only 1 second. The chest rose. If the first breath did not make the chest rise:			
i) Opened the airway again. Used the head tilt-chin lift method.			
ii) Gave another breath.			
g. Continued the cycle of 30 compressions followed by 2 breaths. Limited interruptions to less than 10 seconds.			
5. *Rescuer 2:*			
a. Opened the case with the AED.			
b. Turned on the AED.			
c. Applied the electrode pads to the person's chest. Followed the instructions and diagram provided with the AED.			
d. Attached the connecting cables to the AED.			
e. Cleared away from the person. Made sure no one was touching the person.			
f. Allowed the AED to check the person's heart rhythm.			
g. Made sure everyone was clear of the person if the AED advised a "shock." Loudly instructed others not to touch the person. Said: "I am clear, you are clear, everyone is clear!" Looked to make sure no one was touching the person.			
h. Pressed the SHOCK button if the AED advised a "shock."			
6. *Rescuers 1 and 2*—Performed 2-rescuer CPR.			
a. Began with compressions. One rescuer gave 30 chest compressions. The rescuer paused to allow the other rescuer to give 2 breaths.			
b. The other rescuer gave 2 breaths after every 30 chest compressions.			

Date of Satisfactory Completion _____   Instructor's Initials _____

Procedure—cont'd   S   U   **Comments**

7. Paused to allow a rhythm check when prompted by
   the AED (after about 2 minutes of CPR). Repeated: _____   _____   _____
     i. Cleared away from the person. Made sure no
        one was touching the person.   _____   _____   _____
    ii. Allowed the AED to check the person's heart rhythm. _____   _____   _____
   iii. Made sure everyone was clear of the person if the AED
        advised a "shock". Loudly instructed others not to
        touch the perosn. Said, "I am clear, you are clear,
        everyone is clear!". Looked to make sure no
        one was touching the person.   _____   _____   _____
    iv. Pressed the SHOCK button if the AED advised a "shock". _____   _____   _____
   Changed positions and continued CPR beginning
   with compressions.   _____   _____   _____
8. Continued CPR and used the AED until help took over or
   the person began to move. If movement occurred,
   placed the person in the recovery position.   _____   _____   _____

Date of Satisfactory Completion _____   Instructor's Initials _____

Child CPR—1 Rescuer

Name: _____   Date: _____

Procedure	S	U	Comments
1. Made sure the scene was safe.			
2. Checked for a response. Tapped or gently shook the child. Called the child by name, if known. Shouted "Are you okay?"			
3. Shouted for nearby help if the child did not respond.			
4. Activated the EMS system or the agency's RRT (MET). Got an AED and emergency equipment.			
a. If the collapse was sudden and witnessed – did the following:			
i. If alone with a mobile phone, used it while continuing to give care.			
ii. If alone without a mobile phone, left the child to activate the EMS system before starting CPR.			
iii. If help arrived, sent him or her to activate the EMS system.			
iv. If alone, got the AED and emergency equipment before starting CPR.			
v. If help arrived, asked him or her to get the AED and emergency equipment.			
b. If the collapse was unwitnessed – gave 2 minutes of CPR before leaving the child to activate the EMS system or RRT (MET) and got the AED.			
5. Checked for breathing and a pulse. Looked for no breathing or only gasping. At the same time, checked for a carotid pulse. CPR was done if there was no breathing (or only gasping) and you did not definitely feel a pulse within 10 seconds. (NOTE: CPR was done if the child's pulse was 60 or less with signs of poor circulation.)			
6. Positioned the child for CPR if not already done. The child was supine on a hard, flat surface. Logrolled the child so there was no twisting of the spine. Placed the arms alongside the body.			
7. Exposed the child's chest.			
8. Gave CPR.			
a. Placed 2 hands on the lower half of the sternum. (Used 1 or 2 hands for a very small child.) Gave chest compressions at a rate of 100 to 120 per minute. Established a regular rhythm. Counted out loud. Pressed down at least ⅓ the depth of the chest (about 2 inches). Allowed the chest to recoil between compressions. Did not lean on the chest after each compression. Gave 30 chest compressions.			
b. Opened the airway. Used the head tilt-chin lift method.			
c. Gave 2 breaths. Each breath should take only 1 second. The chest rose. If the first breath did not make the chest rise:			
i. Opened the airway again. Used the head tilt-chin lift method.			
ii. Gave another breath.			
9. Continued the cycle of 30 chest compressions followed by 2 breaths. Limited interruptions in compressions to less than 10 seconds.			
10. Did the following after about 2 minutes of CPR if not already done.			
a. Activated the EMS system or the agency's RRT (MET).			
b. Got an AED.			

Date of Satisfactory Completion _____   Instructor's Initials _____

Procedure—cont'd	S	U	Comments
11. Used the AED:			
a. Opened the case with the AED.	___	___	_____
b. Turned on the AED.	___	___	_____
c. Applied child electrode pads if available. Or used the key or switch to change to the child settings. The pads did not touch or overlap. Followed the instructions and diagram provided with the AED.	___	___	_____
d. Attached the connecting cables to the AED.	___	___	_____
e. Cleared away from the child. Made sure no one was touching the child.	___	___	_____
f. Allowed the AED to check the child's heart rhythm.	___	___	_____
g. Made sure everyone was clear of the child if the AED advised a "shock." Loudly instructed others not to touch the child. Said: "I am clear, you are clear, everyone is clear!" Looked to make sure no one was touching the child.	___	___	_____
h. Pressed the SHOCK button if the AED advised a "shock."			
i. Gave 1 shock if advised. Then started CPR beginning with compressions.	___	___	_____
j. If the rhythm was not shockable, started CPR beginning with compressions.	___	___	_____
12. Paused to allow a rhythm check when prompted by the AED (after about 2 minutes of CPR).	___	___	_____
13. Continued CPR and use of the AED until help arrived or the child started to move.	___	___	_____

Date of Satisfactory Completion _____   Instructor's Initials _____

Child CPR With AED—2 Rescuers

Name: _____   Date: _____

Procedure	S	U	Comments
1. Made sure the scene was safe.	___	___	_____
2. *Rescuer 1:*			
a. Checked for a response. Tapped or gently shook the child. Called the child by name if known. Shouted "Are you okay?"	___	___	_____
b. Shouted for nearby help if the child did not respond.	___	___	_____
3. *Rescuer 2:*			
a. Activated the EMS system or the agency's RRT (MET); used a mobile phone (if available) or left to do so.	___	___	_____
b. Got an AED and emergency equipment.	___	___	_____
4. *Rescuer 1:*			
a. Checked for breathing and a pulse. Looked for no breathing or only gasping. At the same time, checked for a carotid pulse. CPR was done if there was no breathing (or only gasping) and you did not definitely feel a pulse within 10 seconds. (NOTE: CPR was done if the child's pulse was 60 or less with signs of poor circulation.)	___	___	_____
b. Positioned the child for CPR if not already done. The child was supine on a hard, flat surface. Logrolled the child so there was no twisting of the spine. Placed the arms alongside the body.	___	___	_____
c. Exposed the child's chest.	___	___	_____
d. Began 1-rescuer CPR until the AED was ready for use.	___	___	_____
5. *Rescuer 2:*			
a. Opened the case with the AED.	___	___	_____
b. Turned on the AED.	___	___	_____
c. Applied child electrode pads if available. Or used the key or switch to change to the child setting. If neither was available, used the adult pads and settings. The pads did not touch or overlap. Followed the instructions and diagram provided with the AED.	___	___	_____
d. Attached the connecting cables to the AED.	___	___	_____
e. Cleared away from the child. Made sure no one was touching the child.	___	___	_____
f. Allowed the AED to check the child's heart rhythm.	___	___	_____
g. Made sure everyone was clear of the child if the AED advised a "shock." Loudly instructed others not to touch the child. Said: "I am clear, you are clear, everyone is clear!" Looked to make sure no one was touching the child.	___	___	_____
h. Pressed the SHOCK button if the AED advised a "shock."	___	___	_____
6. *Rescuers 1 and 2*—Performed 2-rescuer CPR.			
a. Began with chest compressions. One rescuer placed 2 hands on the lower half of the sternum. (Used 1 or 2 hands for a very small child.) Gave chest compressions at a rate of 100 to 120 per minute. Established a regular rhythm. Counted out loud. Pressed down at least ⅓ the depth of the chest (about 2 inches). Allowed the chest to recoil between compressions. Did not lean on the chest after each compression. Gave 15 chest compressions. Paused to allow the other rescuer to give 2 breaths.	___	___	_____
b. The other rescuer gave 2 breaths after every 15 chest compressions.	___	___	_____

Date of Satisfactory Completion _____   Instructor's Initials _____

Procedure—cont'd   S   U   **Comments**

7. Paused to allow a rhythm check when prompted by the AED
   (after about 2 minutes of CPR). Repeated the following:
   a. Cleared away from the child. Made sure no one was
      touching the child.   _____ _____ _____
   b. Allowed the AED to check the child's heart rhythm.   _____ _____ _____
   c. Made sure everyone was clear of the child if the AED advised
      a "shock." Loudly instructed others not to touch the child.
      Said: "I am clear, you are clear, everyone is clear!" Looked to
      make sure no one was touching the child.   _____ _____ _____
   d. Pressed the SHOCK button if the AED advised a "shock." _____ _____ _____
   e. Changed positions and continued CPR beginning
      with compressions.   _____ _____ _____
8. Continued CPR and use of the AED until help took over or the
   child began to move.   _____ _____ _____

Date of Satisfactory Completion _____   Instructor's Initials _____

Infant CPR—1 Rescuer

Name: _____ Date: _____

Procedure	S	U	Comments
1. Made sure the scene was safe.	___	___	___
2. Checked for a response. Tapped the infant's foot. Shouted, "Are you okay?" (NOTE: Infants cannot answer you. Shouting startled the responsive infant.)	___	___	___
3. Shouted for nearby help if the infant did not respond.			
4. Activated the EMS system or the agency's RRT (MET). Got an AED and emergency equipment.	___	___	___
a. If the collapse was sudden and witnessed:	___	___	___
i. If alone with a mobile phone, used it while continued to give care and got the AED and emergency equipment before starting CPR.	___	___	___
ii. If alone without a mobile phone, left the infant to activate the EMS system before starting CPR.	___	___	___
iii. If help arrived, sent him or her to activate the EMS system and get the AED and emergency equipment	___	___	___
b. If the collapse was unwitnessed – gave about 2 minutes of CPR before leaving the infant to activate the EMS or RRT (MET) and got the AED.	___	___	___
5. Checked for breathing and a pulse. Looked for no breathing or only gasping. At that time checked for a brachial pulse. CPR was done if there was no breathing (or only gasping) and you did not definitely feel a pulse within 10 seconds. (NOTE: CPR is done if the infant's pulse was 60 or less with signs of poor circulation.)	___	___	___
6. Positioned the infant supine on a hard, flat surface if not done.	___	___	___
7. Exposed the infant's chest.	___	___	___
8. Gave CPR.			
a. Placed 2 fingers on the sternum just below the nipple line. Gave chest compressions at a rate of at least 100–120 per minute. Counted out loud. Pressed down at least ⅓ the depth of the chest (about 1½ inches). Allowed the chest to recoil between compressions. Did not lean on the chest after each compression. Gave 30 chest compressions.	___	___	___
b. Opened the airway. Used the head tilt–chin lift method. The head was in a neutral ("sniffing") position.	___	___	___
c. Gave 2 breaths. Each breath took only 1 second. The chest rose. If the first breath did not make the chest rise:			
i. Opened the airway again. Used the head tilt–chin lift method.	___	___	___
ii. Gave another breath.	___	___	___
9. Continued the cycle of 30 chest compressions followed by 2 breaths. Limited interruptions in compressions to less than 10 seconds.	___	___	___
10. Did the following after 2 minutes of CPR if not already done.			
a. Activated the EMS system or agency's RRT (MET).	___	___	___
b. Got a defibrillator (AED).	___	___	___
11. Used the AED:			
• Opened the case with the AED.	___	___	___
• Turned on the AED.	___	___	___
• Applied child electrode pads if available. Or used the key or switch to change to the child setting. If neither were available, used the adult pads and settings. The pads did not touch or overlap. Followed the instructions and diagram provided with the AED.	___	___	___
• Attached the connecting cables to the AED.	___	___	___
• Cleared away from the infant. Made sure no one was touching the infant.	___	___	___

Date of Satisfactory Completion _____   Instructor's Initials _____

Procedure—cont'd   S   U   **Comments**

- Allowed the AED to check for the infant's heart rhythm.   _____   _____   _____
- Made sure everyone was clear of the infant if the AED advised
  a "shock." Loudly instructed others not to touch the infant. Said:
  "I am clear, you are clear, everyone is clear!" Looked to make
  sure no one was touching the infant.   _____   _____   _____
- Pressed the SHOCK button if the AED advised a "shock."   _____   _____   _____
  a. Gave 1 shock if advised. Then started CPR beginning
     with compressions.   _____   _____   _____
  b. If the rhythm was not shockable, started CPR beginning
     with compressions.   _____   _____   _____
12. Paused to allow a rhythm check when prompted by the AED
    (after about 2 minutes of CPR).   _____   _____   _____
13. Continued CPR and use of the AED until help arrived or the
    infant began to move.   _____   _____   _____

Date of Satisfactory Completion _____   Instructor's Initials _____

Infant CPR With AED—2 Rescuers

Name: _____   Date: _____

Procedure	S	U	Comments
1. Made sure the scene was safe.	_____	_____	_____
2. *Rescuer 1:*			
a. Checked for a response. Tapped the infant's foot. Shouted: "Are you okay?" (NOTE: Infants cannot answer you. However, shouting startles the responsive infant.)	_____	_____	_____
b. Shouted for nearby help if the infant did not respond.	_____	_____	_____
3. *Rescuer 2:*			
a. Activated the EMS system or agency's RRT (MET); used a mobile phone if available or left to do so.	_____	_____	_____
b. Got a defibrillator (AED) and emergency equipment.	_____	_____	_____
4. *Rescuer 1:*			
a. Checked for breathing and a pulse. Looked for no breathing or only gasping. At the same time, checked for a brachial pulse. CPR was done if there was no breathing (or only gasping) and you did not definitely feel a pulse within 10 seconds. (NOTE: CPR was done if the infant's pulse was 60 or less with signs of poor circulation.)	_____	_____	_____
b. Positioned the infant supine on a hard, flat surface if not done.	_____	_____	_____
c. Exposed the infant's chest.	_____	_____	_____
d. Began 1-rescuer CPR until the AED was ready for use.	_____	_____	_____
5. *Rescuer 2:*			
a. Opened the case with the AED.	_____	_____	_____
b. Turned on the AED.	_____	_____	_____
c. Applied child electrode pads if available. Or used the key or switch to change to the child setting. If neither was available, used the adult pads and settings. The pads did not touch or overlap. Followed the instructions and diagram provided with the AED.	_____	_____	_____
d. Attached the connecting cables to the AED.	_____	_____	_____
e. Cleared away from the infant. Made sure no one was touching the infant.	_____	_____	_____
f. Allowed the AED to check the infant's heart rhythm.	_____	_____	_____
g. Made sure everyone was clear of the infant if the AED advised a "shock." Loudly instructed others not to touch the infant. Said: "I am clear, you are clear, everyone is clear!" Looked to make sure no one was touching the infant.	_____	_____	_____
h. Pressed the SHOCK button if the AED advised a "shock."	_____	_____	_____
6. *Rescuers 1 and 2*—Performed 2-rescuer CPR.			
a. Began with compressions. One rescuer used the 2 thumb-encircling hands method to give compressions at a rate of at least 100 to 120 per minute. Established a regular rhythm. Counted out loud. Allowed the chest to recoil between compressions. Gave 15 chest compressions. Paused to allow the other rescuer to give 2 breaths.	_____	_____	_____
b. The other rescuer gave 2 breaths after every 15 chest compressions.	_____	_____	_____
7. Paused to allow a rhythm check when prompted by the AED (after about 2 minutes of CPR). Repeated the following and then changed positions and continued CPR beginning with compressions.	_____	_____	_____
• Cleared away from the infant. Made sure no one was touching the infant.	_____	_____	_____
• Allowed the AED to check the infant's heart rhythm.	_____	_____	_____
• Made sure everyone was clear of the infant if the AED advised a "shock." Loudly instructed others not to touch the infant. Said:			

Date of Satisfactory Completion _____   Instructor's Initials _____

Procedure—cont'd   S   U   Comments

"I am clear, you are clear, everyone is clear!" Looked to make
sure no one was touching the infant.   _____   _____   _____

- Pressed the SHOCK button if the AED advised a "shock."   _____   _____   _____

8. Continued CPR and use of the AED until help arrived or the
infant began to move.   _____   _____   _____

Date of Satisfactory Completion _____   Instructor's Initials _____

Assisting With Post-Mortem Care

Name: _____   Date: _____

Pre-Procedure	S	U	Comments

1. Followed *Delegation Guidelines: Care of the Body After Death.*
   Saw *Promoting Safety and Comfort: Care of the Body After Death.*
2. Practiced hand hygiene.
3. Collected the following:
   - Post-mortem kit (shroud or body bag, gown,
     ID [identification] tags, gauze squares, safety pins)
   - Bed protectors
   - Wash basin
   - Bath towel and washcloths
   - Denture cup
   - Items for shaving facial hair
   - Tape
   - Dressings
   - Gloves
   - Cotton balls
   - Valuables envelope
4. Provided for privacy.
5. Raised the bed for body mechanics.
6. Made sure the bed was flat.

Procedure

7. Put on gloves.
8. Positioned the body supine. Arms and legs were straight.
   A pillow was under the head and shoulders. Or raised the
   head of the bed 15 to 20 degrees, if agency policy.
9. Closed the eyes. Gently pulled the eyelids over the eyes.
   Applied moist cotton balls gently over the eyelids if the eyes
   did not stay closed.
10. Inserted dentures if it is agency policy to do so. If not, placed
    them in a labeled denture cup.
11. Closed the mouth. If necessary, placed a rolled towel under the
    chin to keep the mouth closed.
12. Followed agency policy for jewelry. Removed all jewelry, except
    for wedding rings if this was agency policy. Listed the jewelry
    that you removed. Placed the jewelry and the list in a
    valuables envelope.
13. Placed cotton balls over the rings. Taped them in place.
14. Removed drainage containers.
15. Removed tubes and catheters. Used the gauze squares as needed.
16. Shaved facial hair if this was agency policy or desired by the family.
17. Bathed soiled areas with plain water. Dried thoroughly.
18. Placed a bed protector under the buttocks.
19. Removed soiled dressings. Replaced them with clean ones.
20. Put a clean gown on the body. Positioned the body supine.
    Arms and legs were straight. A pillow was under the head and
    shoulders. Or the head of the bed was raised 15 to 20 degrees
    if center policy.
21. Brushed and combed the hair if necessary.
22. Covered the body to the shoulders with a sheet if the family
    viewed the body.
23. Gathered the person's belongings. Put them in a bag labeled
    with the person's name. Made sure you included eyeglasses,
    hearing aids, and other valuables.
24. Removed supplies, equipment, and linens. Straightened
    the room. Provided soft lighting.
25. Removed and discarded the gloves. Practiced hand hygiene.

Date of Satisfactory Completion _____   Instructor's Initials _____

Procedure—cont'd	**S**	**U**	**Comments**
26. Let the family view the body. Provided for privacy. Returned to the room after they left.	_____	_____	_____
27. Practiced hand hygiene. Put on gloves.	_____	_____	_____
28. Filled out the ID tags. Tied 1 to the ankle or to the right big toe.	_____	_____	_____
29. Placed the body in the body bag or covered it with a sheet. Or applied the shroud.			
a. Positioned the shroud under the body.	_____	_____	_____
b. Brought the top down over the head.	_____	_____	_____
c. Folded the bottom up over the feet.	_____	_____	_____
d. Folded the sides over the body.	_____	_____	_____
e. Pinned or taped the shroud in place.	_____	_____	_____
30. Attached the second ID tag to the shroud, sheet, or body bag.	_____	_____	_____
31. Left the denture cup with the body.	_____	_____	_____
32. Pulled the privacy curtain around the bed. Or closed the door.	_____	_____	_____

Post-Procedure

	S	**U**	**Comments**
33. Removed and discarded the gloves. Practiced hand hygiene.	_____	_____	_____
34. Stripped the unit after the body had been removed. Wore gloves.	_____	_____	_____
35. Removed and discarded the gloves. Practiced hand hygiene.	_____	_____	_____
36. Reported the following:			
• The time the body was taken by the funeral director	_____	_____	_____
• What was done with jewelry, other valuables, and personal items	_____	_____	_____
• What was done with dentures	_____	_____	_____

Date of Satisfactory Completion _____   Instructor's Initials _____

Competency Evaluation Review

Preparing for the Competency Evaluation

After completing your state's training program, you need to pass the competency evaluation. The purpose of the competency evaluation is to make sure you can do your job safely. This section will help you prepare for the test.

Competency Evaluation

The competency evaluation has a written test and a skills test. The number of questions varies with each state. Each question has 4 answer choices. Although some questions may appear to have more than one possible answer, there is only 1 best answer. You will have about 1 minute to read and answer each question. Some questions take less time to read and answer. Other questions take longer. You should have enough time to take the test without feeling rushed.

The content of the written test varies depending on your state. Content may include:
- Activities of Daily Living—hygiene, dressing and grooming, nutrition and hydration, elimination, rest/sleep/comfort
- Basic Nursing Skills—infection control, safety/emergency, therapeutic/technical procedures (e.g., vital signs, bedmaking), data collection and reporting
- Restorative Skills—prevention, self-care/independence
- Emotional and Mental Health Needs
- Spiritual and Cultural Needs
- The Person's Rights
- Legal and Ethical Behavior
- Being a Member of the Health Care Team
- Communication

The written test is given as a paper and pencil test in most states. Some test sites may use computers. You do not need computer experience to take the test on the computer. If you have difficulty reading English, you may request to take an oral test. Talk with your instructor or employer about details for computer testing or oral testing.

The skills test involves performing 5 nursing skills that you learned in your training program. These skills are chosen randomly. You do not select the skills. You are allowed about 30 minutes to do the skills. See p. 503 for more information about the skills test.

Taking the Competency Evaluation

To register for the test, you need to complete an application. Your instructor or employer tells you when and where the tests are given. There is a fee for the evaluation. If you work in a nursing center, the employer may pay this fee. If you pay the fee, you may need to purchase a money order or certified check. Make sure your name is on the money order or certified check. Cash and personal checks may not be accepted.

Plan to arrive at the test site about 15 to 30 minutes before the evaluation begins. Most centers do not admit you if you are late. Know the exact location of the test site and room. Actually drive or take transportation to the test site a few days or a week before the test. Making a "dry run" lets you know how much time you need to travel, park, and get to the test site. It will also help decrease your anxiety level on the test day.

To be admitted to the test, you need two pieces of identification (ID). The first form of ID is a government-issued document such as a driver's license or passport. It must have a current photo and your signature. The name on the ID must be the same as the name on your application form. If your name has changed and you have not been able to have the name changed on your identification documents, ask your instructor or employer what to do. The second form of ID must include your name and signature. Examples include a library card, hunting license, or credit card.

Take several sharpened Number 2 pencils to the test. For the skills test you will need a watch with a second hand. You may need a person to play the role of the patient or resident. Ask your instructor or employer how this is done in your state.

Taking the written test and skills test may take several hours. You may want to bring snacks or lunch and a beverage to the testing site. Eating and drinking are not allowed during the test. However, you may be told where you can eat while waiting for the test.

You cannot bring textbooks, study notes, or other materials into the testing room. The only exception may be a language translation dictionary that you show to the proctor (a person who monitors the test) before the test begins. Cellphones, pagers, calculators, or other electronic devices are not permitted during testing. Children and pets are not allowed in the testing areas.

Studying for the Competency Evaluation

You began to prepare for the written test and skills test during your training program. You learned the basic nursing content and skills needed to provide safe, quality care. The following suggestions can help you study for the competency evaluation.
- Begin to study at least 2 to 3 weeks before the test. Plan to study for 1 to 2 hours each day.
- Decide on a specific time to study. Choose a study time that is best for you. This may be early in the morning before others are awake. It may be in the evening after others go to sleep. Try to choose a time when you are mentally alert.
- Choose a specific area to study in. This area should be quiet, well lit, and comfortable. You should have enough room to write and to spread out your books, notes, and other study aids. The area does not need to be noise-free. The testing site is not absolutely quiet. You want to concentrate and not be distracted by the noise around you.

- Collect everything you need before settling down to study. This includes your textbook, notes, paper, highlighters, and pens or pencils.
- Take short breaks when you need them. Take a break when your mind begins to wander or if you feel sleepy.
- Develop a study plan. Write your plan down so you can refer to it. Study 1 content area before going on to the next. For example, study personal hygiene before going on to vital signs. Do not jump from 1 subject to another.
- Use a variety of ways to study.
  - Use index cards to help you review abbreviations and terminology. Put the abbreviation or term on the front of the card and place the meaning on the back. Take the cards with you and review them whenever you have a break or are waiting.
  - Record key points. You can listen to the recording while cooking or while riding in the car.
  Study groups are another way to prepare for a test. Group members can quiz each other.
- To remember what you are learning, try these ideas.
  - Relax when you study. When relaxed, you learn information quickly and recall it with greater ease.
  - Repeat what you are learning. Say it out loud. This helps you remember the idea.
  - Make the information you are learning meaningful. Think about how the information will help you be a good nursing assistant.
  - Write down what you are learning. Writing helps you remember information. Prepare study sheets.
  - Be positive about what you are learning. You remember what you find interesting.
- Suggestions for studying if you have children:
  - When you first come home from work or school, spend time with your children. Then plan study time.
  - Select educational programs on TV that your children can watch as you study.
  - When you take your study breaks, spend time with your children.
  - Ask other adults to take care of the children while you study.
- Take the two 75-question practice tests in this section. Each question has the correct answer and the reason why an answer is correct or incorrect. If you practice taking tests, you are more likely to pass them. Take the practice tests under conditions similar to the real test. Work within time limits.
- If your state has a practice test and a candidate handbook, study the content. Some states have practice tests on-line.

Managing Anxiety

Almost everyone dreads taking tests. It is common and normal to experience anxiety before taking a test. If used wisely, anxiety can actually help you do well. When you are anxious, that means you are concerned. You may be concerned about how prepared you are to take the test. Or you may be concerned about how you will feel about yourself if you do not pass the test. Being concerned

usually results in some action. To overcome anxiety before the test:
- Study and prepare for the test. That helps increase your confidence as you recall or clarify what you have learned. Anxiety decreases as confidence increases. When you think you know the information, keep studying. This reinforces your learning.
- Develop a positive mental attitude. You can pass this test. You took tests in your training program and passed them. Praise yourself. Talk to yourself in a positive way. If a negative thought enters your mind, stop it at once. Challenge the mental thought and tell yourself you will pass the test.
- Visualize success. Think about how wonderful you will feel when you are notified that you have passed the test.
- Perform breathing exercises. Breathe slowly and deeply.
- Perform regular exercise. Exercise helps you stay physically fit. It also helps keep you calm.
- Good nourishment helps you think clearly. Eat a nourishing meal before the test. Do not skip breakfast. Vitamin C helps fight short-term stress. Protein and calcium help overcome the effects of long-term stress. Complex carbohydrates (pasta, nuts, yogurt) can help settle your nerves. Eat familiar foods the day before and the day of the test. Do not eat foods that could cause stomach or intestinal upset.
- Maintain a normal routine the day before the test.
- Get a good night's sleep before the test. Go to bed early enough so you do not oversleep or are too tired to get up. Set your alarm clock properly. You may want to set two alarm clocks.
- Do not "cram" the evening before or the day of the test. Last-minute cramming increases your anxiety. Do something relaxing with family and friends.
- Avoid drinking large amounts of coffee, colas, water, or other beverages. You do not want to be uncomfortable with a full bladder when you take the test.
- Wear comfortable clothes. Dress in layers so that you are prepared for a cold or warm room.
- If you are a woman, remember that worry and anxiety can affect your menstrual cycle. Wear a panty liner, sanitary napkin, or tampon if you think your period may start. This eliminates worry about soiling your clothing during the test.
- Allow plenty of time for travel, traffic, and parking.
- Arrive early enough to use the restroom before the test begins.
- Do not talk about the test with others. Their panic or anxiety may affect your self-confidence.

Taking the Test

Follow these guidelines for taking the test.
- Listen carefully and follow the instructions given by the proctor (person administering the test).
- When you receive the test, make certain you have all the test pages.
- Read and follow all directions carefully.
- You are not allowed to ask questions about the content of the test questions.

- Do deep-breathing and muscle-relaxation exercises as needed.
- Cheating of any kind is not allowed. If the proctor sees you giving or receiving any type of assistance, your test booklet is taken and you must leave the testing site.
- If using a computer answer sheet, completely fill in the bubble.
- If you make a mistake, erase the wrong answer completely. Do not make any stray marks on the paper. Not erasing completely or leaving stray marks could cause the computer to misread your answer.
- Do not worry or get anxious if people finish the test before you do. Persons who finish a test early do not necessarily have a better score than those who finish later.
- You cannot take any evaluation materials or notes out of the testing room.

Answering Multiple-Choice Questions

Pace yourself during the test. First, answer all the questions that you know. Then go back and answer skipped questions. Sometimes you will remember the answer later. Or another test question may give you a clue to the one you skipped. Spending too much time on a question can cost you valuable time later. To help you answer the questions or statements:

- Always read the questions or statements carefully. Do not scan or glance at questions. Scanning or glancing can cause you to miss important key words. Read each word of the question.
- Before reading the answers, decide what the answer is in your own words. Then read all 4 answers to the question. Select the 1 best answer.
- Do not read into a question. Take the question as it is asked. Do not add your own thoughts and ideas to the question. Do not assume or suppose "what if." Just respond to the information provided.
- Trust your common sense. If unsure of an answer, select your first choice. Do not change your answer unless you are absolutely sure of the correct answer. Your first reaction is usually correct.

- Look for key words in every question. Sometimes key words are in italics, highlighted, or underlined. Common key words are *always*, *never*, *first*, *except*, *best*, *not*, *correct*, *incorrect*, *true*, and *false*.
- Know which words can make a statement correct (e.g., *may*, *can*, *usually*, *most*, *at least*, *sometimes*). The word "except" can make a question a false statement.
- Be careful of answers with these key words or phrases: *always*, *never*, *every*, *only*, *all*, *none*, *at all times*, or *at no time*. These words and phrases do not allow for exceptions. In nursing, exceptions are generally present. However, sometimes answers containing these words are correct. For example, which of the following is correct and which are incorrect?
  a. Always use a turning sheet.
  b. Never shake linens.
  c. Soap is used for all baths.
  d. The call light must always be attached to the bed.
  The correct answer is b. Incorrect answers are a, c, and d.
- Omit answers that are obviously wrong. Then choose the best of the remaining answers.
- Go back to the questions you skipped. Answer all questions by eliminating or narrowing your choices. Always mark an answer even if you are not sure.
- Review the test a second time for completeness and accuracy before turning it in.
- Make sure you have answered each question. Also check that you have given only 1 answer for each question.
- Remember, the test is not designed to trick or confuse you. The written competency evaluation tests what you know, not what you do not know. You know more than you are asked.

On-Line Testing

The test may be given by computer at the test site. Ask your instructor what computer skills you will need. You usually do not need keyboard or typing skills. You will use a computer mouse to select answers. Also, you will usually receive instruction before the test begins. This will let you practice using the computer before starting the test.

NOTE: This review covers selected chapters only based on Competency Evaluation requirements.

CHAPTER 1 INTRODUCTION TO HEALTH CARE AGENCIES

Health Care Agency Purposes

- Health promotion
- Disease prevention
- Detection and treatment of disease
- Rehabilitation and restorative care

Hospitals

- Hospitals provide emergency care, surgery, nursing care, x-ray procedures and treatments, and laboratory testing.
- Hospitals also provide respiratory, physical, occupational, speech, and other therapies.
- Persons cared for in hospitals are called *patients*. Hospital patients have acute, chronic, or terminal illnesses.

Rehabilitation and Sub-Acute Care Agencies

- Provide medical and nursing care for people who do not need hospital care but are too sick to go home.

Long-Term Care Centers

- Provide care for people who do not need hospital care but cannot care for themselves at home.
- Provide medical and nursing, dietary, recreational, rehabilitative, and social services. Housekeeping and laundry services are also provided.
- Residents are older or disabled.
- Skilled nursing facilities provide more complex care.
- Some residents are recovering from illness, injury, or surgery.
- Some residents return home when well enough. Some residents need nursing care until death.

Assisted Living Facilities

- Provide housing, personal care, support services, health care, and social activities in a home-like setting for persons needing help with daily activities.

Other Health Agencies

- Other health agencies include mental health centers, home care, hospice, and health care systems.

The Health Team

- Involves many health care workers whose skills and knowledge focus on total care.
- Works together to provide coordinated care to meet each person's needs.
- Follows the direction of the registered nurse (RN) leading the team.

The Nursing Team

- Provides quality care to people.
- Care is coordinated by an RN.

Nursing Assistants

- Report to the nurse supervising their work.
- Perform delegated tasks under the supervision of a licensed nurse.
- Have passed a nursing assistant training and competency evaluation program.

Meeting Standards

Survey Process

- Surveys are done to see if agencies meet standards for licensure, certification, and accreditation.
- A license is issued by the state. A center must have a license to operate and provide care.
- Certification is required to receive Medicare and Medicaid funds.
- Accreditation is voluntary. It signals quality and excellence.

Your Role

- Provide quality care.
- Protect the person's rights.
- Provide for the person's and your own safety.
- Help keep the center clean and safe.
- Conduct yourself in a professional manner.
- Have good work ethics.
- Follow agency policies and procedures.
- Answer questions honestly and completely.

CHAPTER 1 REVIEW QUESTIONS

Circle the BEST answer.

1. Nursing assistants do all of the following *except*
   a. Provide quality care
   b. Follow agency policies and procedures
   c. Conduct themselves in an unprofessional manner
   d. Help keep the agency clean and safe
2. Nursing assistants report to
   a. Other nursing assistants
   b. Licensed nurses
   c. The administrator
   d. The medical director
3. All the following are true about the health team *except*
   a. Involves many health care workers
   b. Follows the direction of the physician
   c. Works together to provide coordinated care
   d. Follows the direction of the RN

Answers to these questions are on p. 516.

CHAPTER 2 THE PERSON'S RIGHTS

- Centers must protect and promote residents' rights. Residents must be free to exercise their rights without interference. If residents are not able to exercise their rights, legal representatives do so for them.

The Omnibus Budget Reconciliation Act of 1987 (OBRA)

- OBRA is a federal law.
- OBRA requires that nursing centers provide care in a manner and in a setting that maintains or improves each person's quality of life, health, and safety.
- OBRA requires nursing assistant training and competency evaluation.
- Resident rights are a major part of OBRA.

Information

- The right to information includes:
  - Access to all records about the person, including medical records, incident reports, contracts, and financial records
  - Information about the person's health condition
  - Information about the person's doctor, including name, specialty, and contact information
- Report any request for information to the nurse.

Refusing Treatment

- The person has the right to refuse treatment.
- A person who does not give consent or refuses treatment cannot be treated against his or her wishes.
- The center must find out what the person is refusing and why.
- Advance directives are part of the right to refuse treatment.
- Report any treatment refusal to the nurse.

Privacy and Confidentiality

- Residents have the right to:
  - Personal privacy. The person's body is not exposed unnecessarily. Only staff directly involved in care and treatments are present. The person must give consent for others to be present. A person has the right to use the bathroom in private. Privacy is maintained for all personal care measures.
  - Visit with others in private—in areas where others cannot see or hear them. This includes phone calls.
  - Send and receive mail without others interfering. No one can open mail the person sends or receives without his or her consent. Unopened mail is given to the person within 24 hours of delivery to the center.
- Information about the person's care, treatment, and condition is kept confidential. So are medical and financial records. Consent is needed to release information to other agencies or persons.

Personal Choice

- Residents have the right to make their own choices. They can:
  - Choose their own doctors.
  - Take part in planning and deciding their care and treatment.
  - Choose activities, schedules, and care based on their preferences.
  - Choose when to get up and go to bed, what to wear, how to spend their time, and what to eat.
  - Choose friends and visitors inside and outside the center.

Grievances

- Residents have the right to voice concerns, questions, and complaints about treatment or care.
- The center must try to correct the matter promptly.
- No one can punish the person in any way for voicing the grievance.

Work

- The person is not required to work or perform services for the center.
- The person has the right to work or perform services if he or she wants to.
- Residents volunteer or are paid for their services.

Taking Part in Resident Groups

- The person has the right to:
  - Form and take part in resident and family groups.
  - Take part in social, cultural, religious, and community events. The resident has the right to help in getting to and from events of their choice.

Personal Items

- The resident has the right to:
  - Keep and use personal items, such as clothing and some furnishings.
  - Have his or her property treated with care and respect. Items are labeled with the person's name.
- Protect yourself and the center from being accused of stealing a person's property. Do not go through a person's closet, drawers, purse, or other space without the person's knowledge and consent. If you have to inspect closets and drawers, follow center policy for reporting and recording the inspection.

Freedom From Abuse, Mistreatment, and Neglect

- Residents have the right to be free from:
  - Verbal, sexual, physical, or mental abuse
  - Involuntary seclusion—separating a person from others against his or her will, confining a person to a certain area, or keeping the person away from his or her room without consent
- No one can abuse, neglect, or mistreat a resident. This includes center staff, volunteers, staff from other agencies or groups, other residents, family members, friends, visitors, and legal representatives.
- Nursing centers must investigate suspected or reported cases of abuse.

Freedom From Restraint

- Residents have the right to not have body movements restricted by restraints or drugs.
- Restraints are used only if required to treat the person's medical symptoms or if necessary to protect the person or others from harm. If a restraint is required, a doctor's order is needed.

Quality of Life

- Residents must be cared for in a manner that promotes dignity and self-esteem. Physical, psychological, and mental well-being must be promoted. Review Box 2-3, OBRA-Required Actions to Promote Dignity and Privacy, in the Textbook.
- Centers must provide activity programs that promote physical, intellectual, social, spiritual, and emotional well-being.
- Residents have the right to a safe, clean, comfortable, and home-like setting. The center must provide a setting and services that meet the person's needs and preferences. The setting and staff must promote the person's independence, dignity, and well-being.

Ombudsman Program

- The Older Americans Act requires a long-term care ombudsman program in every state.
- Ombudsmen are employed by a state agency. They are not nursing center employees. Some are volunteers.
- Ombudsmen protect the health, safety, welfare, and rights of residents. They also may investigate and resolve complaints, provide support to resident and family groups, and help the center manage difficult problems.
- OBRA requires that nursing centers post the names, addresses, and phone numbers of local and state ombudsmen where the residents can easily see it.
- Because a family member or resident may share a concern with you, you must know the state and center policies and procedures for contacting an ombudsman.

CHAPTER 2 REVIEW QUESTIONS

Circle the BEST answer.

1. Residents have all the following rights *except*
   a. Refusing a treatment
   b. Making a telephone call in private
   c. Choosing activities to attend
   d. Being punished for voicing a grievance
2. OBRA does not require nursing assistant training and competency evaluation.
   a. True
   b. False
3. The person has a right to take part in planning and deciding their care and treatment.
   a. True
   b. False
4. The person is required to work for the center.
   a. True
   b. False

Answers to these questions are on p. 516.

CHAPTER 3 THE NURSING ASSISTANT

Federal and State Laws

Nurse Practice Acts

- Each state has a nurse practice act. It regulates nursing practice in that state.

Nursing Assistants

- A state's nurse practice act is used to decide what nursing assistants can do. Some nurse practice acts also regulate nursing assistant roles, functions, education, and certification requirements. Some states have separate laws for nursing assistants.
- Nursing assistants must be able to function with skill and safety. They can have their certification, license, or registration denied, revoked, or suspended.

The Omnibus Budget Reconciliation Act of 1987 (OBRA)

- The purpose of OBRA, a federal law, is to improve the quality of life of nursing center residents.
- OBRA sets minimum training and competency evaluation requirements for nursing assistants. Each state must have a nursing assistant training and competency evaluation program (NATCEP). A nursing assistant must successfully complete a NATCEP to work in a nursing center, hospital, long-term care unit, or home care agency receiving Medicare funds.
- OBRA requires at least 75 hours of instruction. Some states have more hours. At least 16 hours of supervised training in a laboratory or clinical setting are required.
  - The competency evaluation has a written test and a skills test.
  - The written test has multiple-choice questions.
  - The number of questions varies from state to state.
  - The skills test involves performing certain skills learned in your training program.
- OBRA requires a nursing assistant registry in each state. It is an official record that lists persons who have successfully completed the NATCEP.
- Re-training and a new competency evaluation program are required for nursing assistants who have not worked for 24 months. To work in another state, nursing assistants must meet that state's NATCEP.
- Each state's NATCEP must meet OBRA requirements.

Roles and Responsibilities

- Nurse practice acts, OBRA, state laws, and legal and advisory opinions direct what nursing assistants can do.
- The range of functions for nursing assistants varies among states and agencies. Before performing a nursing task make sure that:
  - The state allows nursing assistants to do that task.
  - It is in the job description.
  - You have the necessary education and training.
  - A nurse is available to answer questions and to supervise the task.
- Rules for nursing assistants to follow are in Box 3-2 in the Textbook.
  - You are an assistant to the nurse.
  - A nurse assigns and supervises your work.
  - You report observations about the person's physical and mental status to the nurse. Report changes in the person's condition or behavior at once.

- ○ The nurse decides what should be done for a person. You do not make these decisions.
  - ○ Review directions and the care plan with the nurse before going to the person.
  - ○ Perform only those nursing tasks that you are trained to do.
  - ○ Ask a nurse to supervise you if you are not comfortable performing a nursing task.
  - ○ Perform only the nursing tasks that your state and job description allow.
- State laws and rules limit nursing assistant functions. State laws differ. Know what you can do in the state in which you are working.
- Role limits for nursing assistants are in Box 3-3 in the Textbook.
  - ○ Never give drugs.
  - ○ Never insert tubes or objects into body openings. Do not remove tubes from the body.
  - ○ Never take oral or telephone orders from doctors.
  - ○ Never perform procedures that require sterile technique.
  - ○ Never tell the person or family the person's diagnosis or treatment plans.
  - ○ Never diagnose or prescribe treatments or drugs for anyone.
  - ○ Never supervise others, including other nursing assistants.
  - ○ Never ignore an order or request to do something. This includes nursing tasks that you can do, those you cannot do, and those that are beyond your legal limits.

Nursing Assistant Standards
- OBRA defines the basic range of functions for nursing assistants.
- All NATCEPs include those functions. Some states allow other functions.
- Review Box 3-4, Nursing Assistant Standards, in the Textbook.

Job Description and Job Titles
- Always obtain a written job description when you apply for a job. Do not take a job that requires you to:
  - ○ Act beyond the legal limits of your role.
  - ○ Function beyond your training limits.
  - ○ Perform acts that are against your morals or religion.
- For job purposes, agencies often use other titles for nursing assistants who have completed a NATCEP and are on a state registry. Your job title depends on the setting and your roles and functions in the agency.

CHAPTER 3 REVIEW QUESTIONS
Circle the BEST answer.
1. Nursing assistants perform nursing tasks delegated to them by a registered nurse (RN) or licensed practical nurse/licensed vocational nurse (LPN/LVN).
   a. True
   b. False

2. A resident asks you about his or her medical condition. You
   a. Tell the nurse about the resident's request
   b. Tell the resident what is in his or her medical record
   c. Ignore the question
   d. Tell another nursing assistant about the resident's request
3. You answer the telephone. The doctor starts to give you an order. You
   a. Take the order from the doctor
   b. Politely give your name and title, ask the doctor to wait for the nurse, and promptly find the nurse
   c. Politely ask the doctor to call back later
   d. Ask the doctor if the nurse may call him or her back
4. When should you refuse a task?
   a. The task is not in your job description.
   b. The task is within the legal limits of your role.
   c. The directions for the task are clear.
   d. A nurse is available for questions and supervision.
Answers to these questions are on p. 516.

CHAPTER 4 DELEGATION
Who Can Delegate
- Registered nurses (RNs) can delegate tasks to nursing assistants. In some states, licensed practical nurses/licensed vocational nurses (LPNs/LVNs) can delegate tasks to nursing assistants.
- The delegating nurse is legally responsible for his or her actions and the actions of others who performed the delegated tasks.
- Nursing assistants cannot delegate. You cannot delegate any task to other nursing assistants or to any other worker.

The Delegation Process
- Delegation decisions must protect the person's health and safety.
- If you perform a task that places the person at risk, you may face serious legal problems.
- Step 1—Assessment and Planning. The nurse assesses the person's needs and then decides if it is safe to delegate the task.
- Step 2—Communication. The nurse must give clear and complete directions about the task and you must understand the directions to give safe care. After the task, you report and record the care that was given.
- Step 3—Surveillance and Supervision. The nurse observes the care you give and makes sure you complete the task correctly. The nurse must follow up on problems or concerns if you did not perform the task according to expectations or there is a change in the person's condition.
- Step 4—Evaluation and Feedback. The nurse decides if the delegation was successful by observing if the task was done correctly and the outcome and the person's response were as expected. The nurse should provide feedback to the nursing assistant about what was done correctly and what errors should be corrected.

The Five Rights of Delegation

- *The right task*. Can the task be delegated and is the nurse allowed to delegate the task? Is the task in your job description?
- *The right circumstances*. What are the person's physical, mental, emotional, and spiritual needs at the time?
- *The right person*. Do you have the training and experience to perform the task safely?
- *The right directions and communication*. The nurse gives clear directions and instructions. The nurse allows questions and helps you set priorities.
- *The right supervision*. The nurse guides, directs, and evaluates the care you give. The nurse demonstrates tasks as needed and is available for questions. The nurse assesses how the task affected the person and how well you performed the task and tells you what you did well and how to improve your work.

Your Role in Delegation

- When you agree to perform a delegated task on a person, you must protect the person from harm. You are responsible for your own actions. You must complete the task safely. You must ask for help if you have questions or are unsure. Report to the nurse what you did and the observations you made.
- You should refuse to perform a task when:
  - The task is beyond the legal limits of your role.
  - The task is not in your job description.
  - You were not trained to perform the task.
  - The task could harm the person.
  - The person's condition has changed.
  - You do not know how to use the supplies or equipment.
  - Directions are not ethical or legal.
  - Directions are against agency policies.
  - Directions are unclear or incomplete.
  - A nurse is not available for supervision.
- Never ignore an order or refuse a task because you do not like it or do not want to do it. Tell the nurse about your concerns.

CHAPTER 4 REVIEW QUESTIONS

Circle the BEST answer.

1. A nurse delegates a task that you did not learn in your training. The task is in your job description. What is your appropriate response to the nurse?
   a. "I cannot do that task."
   b. "I did not learn that task in my training. Can you show me how to do it?"
   c. "I will ask the other nursing assistant to watch me do the task."
   d. "I will ask the other nursing assistant to do the task for me."
2. You are busy with a new resident. It is time for another resident's bath. You may delegate the bath to another nursing assistant.
   a. True
   b. False

3. You may perform a task that is not in your job description as long as a nurse has delegated the task.
   a. True
   b. False

Answers to these questions are on p. 516.

CHAPTER 5 ETHICS AND LAWS

Ethical Aspects

- Ethics is the knowledge of what is right conduct and wrong conduct. It also deals with choices or judgments about what should or should not be done. An ethical person does not cause a person harm.
- Ethical behavior involves not being prejudiced or biased. To be prejudiced or biased means to make judgments and have views before knowing the facts. You should not judge a person by your values and standards. Also, do not avoid persons whose standards and values differ from your own.
- Ethical problems involve making choices. You must decide what is the right thing to do.

Codes of Ethics

- Professional groups have codes of ethics. A **code of ethics** has rules, or standards of conduct, for group members to follow.
- Rules of conduct for nursing assistants can be found in Box 5-1 in the Textbook.

Boundaries

- **Professional boundaries** separate helpful behaviors from behaviors that are not helpful.
- A **boundary crossing** is a brief act of over-involvement with the person in order to meet the person's needs, such as giving a crying patient a hug.
- A **boundary violation** is an act or behavior that meets your needs, not the person's. The act or behavior is unethical. Boundary violations include abuse, keeping secrets with a person, or giving a lot of personal information about yourself to another.
- **Professional sexual misconduct** is an act, behavior, or comment that is sexual in nature. It is sexual misconduct even if the person consents or makes the first move.
- To maintain professional boundaries, review Box 5-2, Rules for Maintaining Professional Boundaries. Be alert to **boundary signs** (acts, behaviors, or thoughts that warn of a boundary crossing or violation).

Legal Aspects

- Ethics is about what you *should or should not do*. Laws tell you what you *can and cannot do*.
- **Negligence** is an unintentional wrong. The negligent person did not act in a reasonable and careful manner. As a result, the person or person's property was harmed. The person causing harm did not mean to cause harm.
- **Malpractice** is negligence by a professional person.

- You are legally responsible (liable) for your own actions. The nurse is liable as your supervisor.
- **Defamation** is injuring a person's name and reputation by making false statements to a third person. **Libel** is making false statements in print, writing (including e-mails and texts), or through pictures or drawings. **Slander** is making false statements orally. Never make false statements about a patient, resident, family member, co-worker, or any other person.
- **False imprisonment** is the unlawful restraint or restriction of a person's freedom of movement. It involves threatening to restrain a person, restraining a person, and preventing a person from leaving the agency.
- **Invasion of privacy** is violating a person's right not to have his or her name, photo, or private affairs exposed or made public without giving consent. Review Box 5-4, Protecting the Right to Privacy, in the Textbook.
- The Health Insurance Portability and Accountability Act (HIPAA) of 1996 protects the privacy and security of a person's health information. **Protected health information** refers to identifying information and information about the person's health care that is maintained or sent in any form (paper, electronic, oral). Direct any questions about the person or the person's care to the nurse.
- **Fraud** is saying or doing something to trick, fool, or deceive a person. The act is fraud if it does or could cause harm to a person or the person's property.
- **Assault** is intentionally attempting or threatening to touch a person's body without the person's consent. The person fears bodily harm.
- **Battery** is touching a person's body without his or her consent. Protect yourself from being accused of assault and battery. Explain to the person what you are going to do and get the person's consent.

Wrongful Use of Electronic Communication

- Electronic communications include e-mail, text messages, faxes, websites, video sites, and social media sites. Video and social media sites include Facebook, Twitter, LinkedIn, YouTube, Instagram, Pinterest, Tumblr, blogs and comments to blog postings, chat rooms, bulletin boards, and so on.
- Wrongful use of electronic communications can result in job loss and loss of your certification (license, registration) for:
  - Defamation
  - Invasion of privacy
  - HIPAA violations
  - Violating the right to confidentiality
  - Patient or resident abuse
  - Unprofessional or unethical conduct

Informed Consent

- A person has the right to decide what will be done to his or her body and who can touch his or her body. Consent is informed when the person clearly understands all aspects of treatment.

- Persons who cannot give consent are persons who are under the legal age or are mentally incompetent. Unconscious, sedated, or confused persons cannot give consent. Informed consent is given by a responsible party—wife, husband, daughter, son, or legal representative.
- You are never responsible for obtaining written consent.

Reporting Abuse

- **Abuse** is
  - The willful infliction of injury, unreasonable confinement, intimidation, or punishment that results in physical harm, pain, or mental anguish. Intimidation means to make afraid with threats of force or violence.
  - Depriving the person (or the person's caregiver) of the goods or services needed to attain or maintain well-being.
- Abuse also includes involuntary seclusion.
- **Vulnerable adults** are persons 18 years old or older who have disabilities or conditions that make them at risk to be wounded, attacked, or damaged. They have problems caring for or protecting themselves due to:
  - A mental, emotional, physical, or developmental disability
  - Brain damage
  - Changes from aging
- All residents are vulnerable. Older persons and children are at risk for abuse.
- **Elder abuse** is any knowing, intentional, or negligent act by a caregiver or another person to an older adult. It may include physical abuse, neglect, verbal abuse, involuntary seclusion, financial exploitation or misappropriation, emotional or mental abuse, sexual abuse, or abandonment. Review Box 5-7, Signs of Elder Abuse, in the Textbook.
- Federal and state laws require the reporting of elder abuse.
- If you suspect a person is being abused, report your observations to the nurse.

CHAPTER 5 REVIEW QUESTIONS

Circle the BEST answer.
1. A resident offers you a gift certificate for being kind to her. You should
   a. Say "thank you" and accept the gift
   b. Accept the gift and give it to charity
   c. Thank the resident for thinking of you and then explain it is against policy for you to accept the gift
   d. Accept the gift and give it to your daughter
2. To protect a person's privacy, you should do the following *except*
   a. Keep all information about the person confidential
   b. Discuss the person's treatment or diagnosis with the nurse supervising your work
   c. Open the person's mail
   d. Allow the person to visit with others in private

3. What should you do if you suspect an older person is being abused?
    a. Report the situation to the health department.
    b. Notify the nurse and discuss the observations with him or her.
    c. Notify the doctor about the suspected abuse.
    d. Ask the family why they are abusing the person.
4. A resident needs help going to the bathroom. You do not answer her call light promptly. She gets up without help, falls, and breaks a leg. This is an example of
    a. Negligence
    b. Defamation
    c. False imprisonment
    d. Slander
5. Examples of defamation include all the following *except*
    a. Implying or suggesting that a person uses drugs
    b. Saying that a person is insane or mentally ill
    c. Implying that a person steals money from staff
    d. Burning a resident with water that is too hot
6. Which statement about ethics is *false*?
    a. An ethical person does not judge others by his or her values and standards.
    b. An ethical person avoids persons whose standards and values differ from his or her own.
    c. An ethical person is not prejudiced or biased.
    d. An ethical person does not cause harm to another person.
7. Examples of false imprisonment include all of the following *except*
    a. Threatening to restrain a resident
    b. Restraining a resident without a doctor's order
    c. Treating the resident with respect
    d. Preventing a resident from leaving the agency
8. To protect yourself from being accused of assault and battery, you should explain to the resident what you plan to do before touching him or her and get consent.
    a. True
    b. False

Answers to these questions are on p. 516.

CHAPTER 6 STUDENT AND WORK ETHICS

- **Professionalism** involves following laws, being ethical, having good work ethics, and having the skills to do your work.
- **Work ethics** deals with behavior in the workplace. Work ethics also applies to students in nursing assistant training and competency evaluation programs (NATCEPs).
- To be a successful student, practice good work ethics in the classroom and clinical setting and in your relationships with instructors and fellow students.

Health, Hygiene, and Appearance

- To give safe and effective care, you must be physically and mentally healthy. You need a balanced diet, sleep and rest, good body mechanics, and exercise on a regular basis. Smoking, drugs, and alcohol can affect performance and safety.

- Personal hygiene needs careful attention. Bathe daily, use deodorant or antiperspirant, and brush your teeth often. Shampoo often. Keep fingernails clean, short, and neatly shaped.
- Review Box 6-2, Practices for a Professional Appearance, in the Textbook.

Teamwork

- Practice good work ethics—work when scheduled, be cheerful and friendly, perform delegated tasks, be kind to others, and be available to help others.
- Be ready to work when your shift starts. Arrive on your nursing unit a few minutes early. Stay the entire shift. When it is time to leave, report off duty to the nurse.
- A good attitude is needed. Review Box 6-1, Qualities and Traits for Good Work Ethics, in the Textbook.
- Gossiping is unprofessional and hurtful. To avoid being a part of gossip:
    ○ Remove yourself from a group or setting where people are gossiping.
    ○ Do not make or repeat any comment that can hurt another person or the agency.
    ○ Do not make or repeat any comment that you do not know is true.
    ○ Do not talk about residents, family members, patients, visitors, co-workers, or the agency at home or in social settings.
- **Confidentiality** means trusting others with personal and private information. The person's information is shared only among staff involved in his or her care. Agency, family, and co-worker information also is confidential.
- Your speech and language must be professional.
    ○ Do not swear or use foul, vulgar, or abusive language.
    ○ Do not use slang.
    ○ Speak softly, gently, and clearly.
    ○ Do not shout or yell.
    ○ Do not fight or argue with a person, family member, visitor, or co-worker.
- A courtesy is a polite, considerate, or helpful comment or act.
    ○ Address others by Miss, Mrs., Ms., Mr., or Doctor. Use a first name only if the person asks you to do so.
    ○ Say "please" and "thank you." Say "I'm sorry" when you make a mistake or hurt someone.
    ○ Let residents, families, and visitors enter elevators first.
    ○ Be thoughtful—compliment others, give praise.
    ○ Wish the person and family well when they leave the center.
    ○ Hold doors open for others.
    ○ Help others willingly when asked.
    ○ Do not take credit for another person's deeds. Give the person credit for the action.
- Keep personal matters out of the workplace.
    ○ Make personal phone calls during meals and breaks.
    ○ Do not let family and friends visit you on the unit.
    ○ Do not use the agency's computers and other equipment for personal use.

- Do not take agency supplies for personal use.
- Do not discuss personal problems at work.
- Control your emotions.
- Do not borrow money from or lend money to co-workers.
- Do not sell things or engage in fund-raising at work.
- Do not have wireless phones or personal pagers on while at work.
- Do not text message.
- Leave for and return from breaks and meals on time. Tell the nurse when you leave and return to the unit.
- Protect yourself and others from harm.
  - Understand the roles, functions, and responsibilities in your job description.
  - Follow agency rules, policies, and procedures in the employee handbook or policy and procedure manual.
  - Know what is right and wrong conduct and what you can and cannot do.
  - Follow the nurse's directions and instructions and question unclear directions and things you do not understand. Ask for any training you might need.
  - Help others willingly when asked.
  - Report accurately. This includes measurements, observations, the care given, the person's complaints, and any errors.
  - Accept responsibility for your actions. Admit when you are wrong or make mistakes. Do not blame others. Do not make excuses for your actions. Learn what you did wrong and why. Always try to learn from your mistakes.
  - Handle the person's property carefully and prevent damage.
  - Always follow safety measures.
- Planning your work involves setting priorities. Decide:
  - Which person has the greatest or most life-threatening needs.
  - What task the nurse or person needs done first.
  - What tasks need to be done at a certain time.
  - What tasks need to be done when your shift starts.
  - What tasks need to be done at the end of your shift.
  - How much time it takes to complete a task.
  - How much help you need to complete a task.
  - Who can help you and when.
- Priorities change as the person's needs change.

Managing Stress
- These guidelines can help you reduce or cope with stress.
  - Exercise regularly.
  - Get enough sleep or rest.
  - Eat healthy.
  - Plan personal and quiet time for yourself.
  - Use common sense about what you can do.
  - Do 1 thing at a time.
  - Do not judge yourself harshly.
  - Give yourself praise.
  - Have a sense of humor.
  - Talk to the nurse if your work or a person is causing too much stress.
- Conflict in the workplace can cause stress and care can suffer. Resolving conflict involves defining and collecting information about the problem, identifying possible solutions, carrying out the best solution, and evaluating the results.
- Communication and good work ethics help prevent and resolve conflicts.
- **Burnout** is a job stress resulting in physical or mental exhaustion and doubts about your abilities or the value of your work. Managing stress can prevent burnout.

Harassment
- **Harassment** means to trouble, torment, offend, or worry a person by one's behavior or comments.
- Harassment can be sexual or it can involve age, race, ethnic background, religion, or disability.
- You must respect others. Do not offend others by your gestures, remarks, or use of touch. Do not offend others with jokes, photos, or other pictures.

CHAPTER 6 REVIEW QUESTIONS
Circle the BEST answer.
1. You believe you have good work ethics. This means you do the following *except*
   a. Work when scheduled
   b. Act cheerful and friendly
   c. Refuse to help others
   d. Perform tasks assigned by the nurse
2. A nursing assistant is gossiping about a co-worker. You should
   a. Stay with the group and listen to what is being said
   b. Repeat the comment to your family
   c. Remove yourself from the group where gossip is occurring
   d. Repeat the comment to another co-worker
3. You want to maintain confidentiality about others. You do the following *except*
   a. Share information about a resident with a nurse who is on another unit
   b. Avoid talking about a resident in the elevator, hallway, or dining area
   c. Avoid talking about co-workers and residents when others are present
   d. Avoid eavesdropping
4. When you are at work, you should do which of the following?
   a. Swear and use foul language.
   b. Use slang.
   c. Argue with a visitor.
   d. Speak clearly and softly.
5. To give safe and effective care, you do all of the following *except*
   a. Eat a balanced diet
   b. Get enough sleep and rest
   c. Exercise on a regular basis
   d. Drink too much alcohol
6. While at work, you should do all of the following *except*
   a. Be courteous to others
   b. Make personal phone calls
   c. Admit when you are wrong or make mistakes
   d. Respect others
Answers to these questions are on p. 516.

CHAPTER 7 COMMUNICATING WITH THE HEALTH TEAM

Communication

- For good communication:
  - Use words that mean the same thing to you and the receiver of the message.
  - Use familiar words.
  - Be brief and concise.
  - Give information in a logical and orderly manner.
  - Give facts and be specific.

The Medical Record

- The **medical record, chart, or clinical record** is the permanent, legal account of the person's condition and response to treatment and care. Medical records can be written or stored electronically. The electronic health record (EHR) or electronic medical record (EMR) is the electronic version of the person's medical record. It is a permanent legal document.
- The medical record is a way for the health team to share information about the person. Agencies have policies about medical records and who can see them. Some agencies allow nursing assistants to read and/or record observations in medical records. Follow your agency's policies.
- Medical records can include the person's admission record, health history, graphic and flow sheets for recording measurements and observations, and progress reports.
- The Kardex or care summary is a summary of the person's medical record. The summary can be in a type of card file or computers organize the record in an electronic summary.

Reporting and Recording

- The health team communicates by reporting and recording.

Reporting

- You report care and observations to the nurse. Report to the nurse:
  - Whenever there is a change from normal or a change in the person's condition. Report these changes at once.
  - When the nurse asks you to do so.
  - When you leave the unit for meals, breaks, or other reasons.
  - Before the end-of-shift report.
- Follow the rules of reporting.
  - Be prompt, thorough, and accurate.
  - Give the person's name and room and bed numbers.
  - Give the time your observations were made or the care was given.
  - Report only what you observed or did yourself.
  - Report care measures that you expect the person to need.
  - Report expected changes in the person's condition.
  - Give reports as often as the person's condition requires or when the nurse asks you to.
  - Report any changes from normal or changes in the person's condition at once.
  - Use your written notes to give a specific, concise, and clear report.

Recording

- When recording or documenting, communicate clearly and thoroughly what you observed, what you did, and the person's response.
- The general rules for recording are:
  - Always use ink. Use the color required by the center.
  - Include the date and time for every recording.
  - Make sure writing is readable and neat.
  - Use only agency-approved abbreviations.
  - Use correct spelling, grammar, and punctuation.
  - Do not use ditto marks.
  - Never erase or use correction fluid. Follow agency procedure for correcting errors.
  - Sign all entries with your name and title as required by agency policy.
  - Do not skip lines.
  - Make sure each form has the person's name and other identifying information.
  - Record only what you observed and did yourself.
  - Never chart a procedure, treatment, or care measure until after it is completed.
  - Be accurate, concise, and factual. Do not record judgments or interpretations.
  - Record in a logical and sequential manner.
  - Be descriptive. Avoid terms with more than one meaning.
  - Use the person's exact words whenever possible. Use quotation marks to show that the statement is a direct quote.
  - Chart any changes from normal or changes in the person's condition. Also chart that you informed the nurse (include the nurse's name), what you told the nurse, and the time you made the report.
  - Do not omit information.
  - Record safety measures. Example: Reminding a person not to get out of bed.
- Review the 24-hour clock, Figure 7-6, and Box 7-1 in the Textbook.
- Review Box 7-3 for recording rules on paper and on computer.

Computers and Other Electronic Devices

- Computers contain vast amounts of information about a person. Therefore the right to privacy must be protected. If allowed access, you must follow the agency's policies.
- Review Box 7-4, Computers and Other Electronic Devices, in the Textbook.

Phone Communications

- Guidelines for answering phones:
  - Answer the call after the first ring if possible.
  - Do not answer the phone in a rushed or hasty manner.

○ Give a courteous greeting. Identify the nursing unit and your name and title.

○ When taking a message, write down the caller's name, phone number, date and time, and message.

○ Repeat the message and phone number back to the caller.

○ Ask the caller to "Please hold" if necessary.

○ Do not lay the phone down or cover the receiver with your hand when not speaking to the caller. The caller may hear confidential information.

○ Return to a caller on hold within 30 seconds.

○ Do not give confidential information to any caller.

○ Transfer a call if appropriate. Tell the caller you are going to transfer the call. Give the name and phone number in case the call gets disconnected or the line is busy.

○ End the conversation politely.

○ Give the message to the appropriate person.

Medical Terminology and Abbreviations

- Medical terminology and abbreviations are used in health care. Someone may use a word or phrase that you do not understand. If so, ask the nurse to explain its meaning.
- Review Box 7-6, Medical Terminology, and Box 7-7, Common Health Care Terms and Phrases, in the Textbook.
- Use only the abbreviations accepted by the center. If you are not sure that an abbreviation is acceptable, write the term out in full. See the inside back cover of the Textbook for common abbreviations.

CHAPTER 7 REVIEW QUESTIONS

Circle the BEST answer.

1. For good communication, you should do the following *except*
   a. Use words with more than 1 meaning
   b. Use words familiar to the person or family
   c. Give facts in a brief and concise manner
   d. Give information in a logical and orderly manner

2. When you record in a person's chart, you do the following *except*
   a. Record what you observed and did
   b. Record the person's response to the treatment or procedure
   c. Use abbreviations that are not on the accepted list for the center
   d. Record the time the observation was made or the treatment performed

3. When reporting care and observations to the nurse, you do the following *except*
   a. Give the person's name and room and bed numbers
   b. Report only what you observed or did yourself
   c. Report any changes from normal or changes in the person's condition at once
   d. Report any changes from normal or changes in the person's condition at the end of the shift

Answers to these questions are on p. 516.

CHAPTER 8 ASSISTING WITH THE NURSING PROCESS

- The **nursing process** is the method nurses use to plan and deliver nursing care. It has 5 steps: assessment, nursing diagnosis, planning, implementation, and evaluation.
- **Assessment** involves collecting information about the person. A health history is taken. A registered nurse (RN) assesses the person's body systems and mental systems. Although the nursing assistant does not assess, you play a key role in assessment. You make many observations as you give care and talk to the person.
- **Observation** is using the senses of sight, hearing, touch, and smell to collect information.
- Basic observations are outlined in Box 8-2 in the Textbook. Observations you need to report to the nurse at once are (see Box 8-1 in the Textbook):
  ○ A change in the person's ability to respond
  ○ A change in the person's mobility
  ○ Complaints of sudden, severe pain
  ○ A sore or reddened area on the person's skin
  ○ Complaints of a sudden change in vision
  ○ Complaints of pain or difficulty breathing
  ○ Abnormal respirations
  ○ Complaints of or signs of difficulty swallowing
  ○ Vomiting
  ○ Bleeding
  ○ Vital signs outside their normal ranges
- **Objective data (signs)** are seen, heard, felt, or smelled by an observer. For example, you can feel a pulse.
- **Subjective data (symptoms)** are things a person tells you about that you cannot observe through your senses. For example, you cannot see the person's nausea.
- The nurse uses assessment data to form a **nursing diagnosis,** or a health problem that can be treated by nursing measures.
- The nurse will then conduct **planning** to set priorities and goals for the person's care.
- **Nursing interventions** or **implementations** are the actions taken by the nursing team to help the person reach a goal.
- The nursing diagnoses, goals, and actions for each goal are recorded in the **nursing care plan.** The care plan is a communication tool. Each agency has a care plan tool.
- The RN may conduct a care conference with the health care team to share information and ideas about the person's care.
- The nurse will **evaluate** the planning and implementation based on the person's progress toward the stated goal.
- The nurse may delegate tasks to the nursing assistant via the assignment sheet during any step of the nursing process.

CHAPTER 8 REVIEW QUESTIONS
Circle the BEST answer.

1. Which statement about observations is *false?*
   a. You make observations as you care for and talk with people.
   b. Observation uses the senses of smell, sight, touch, and hearing.
   c. A reddened area on the person's skin is reported to the nurse at once.
   d. You report observations to the doctor.
2. Objective data include all the following *except*
   a. The person has pain in his abdomen
   b. The person's pulse is 76
   c. The person's urine is dark amber
   d. The person's breath has an odor

Answers to these questions are on p. 516.

CHAPTER 9 UNDERSTANDING THE PERSON
Caring for the Person
- The whole person needs to be considered when you provide care—physical, social, psychological, and spiritual parts. These parts are woven together and cannot be separated.
- Follow these rules to address persons with dignity and respect.
  - Call persons by their titles—Mrs. Dennison, Mr. Smith, Miss Turner, or Dr. Gonzalez.
  - Do not call persons by their first names unless they ask you to.
  - Do not call persons by any other name unless they ask you to.
  - Do not call persons Grandma, Papa, Sweetheart, Honey, or other names.

Basic Needs
- A **need** is something necessary or desired for maintaining life and mental well-being.
- According to Maslow, basic needs must be met for a person to survive and function. Needs are arranged in order of importance, lower level to higher level.
  - *Physiological or physical needs*—are required for life. They are oxygen, food, water, elimination, rest, and shelter.
  - *Safety and security needs*—relate to feeling safe from harm, danger, and fear.
  - *Love and belonging needs*—relate to love, closeness, affection, and meaningful relationships with others. Family, friends, and the health team can meet love and belonging needs.
  - *Self-esteem needs*—relate to thinking well of oneself and to seeing oneself as useful and having value. People often lack self-esteem when ill, injured, older, or disabled.
  - *The need for self-actualization*—involves learning, understanding, and creating to the limit of a person's capacity. Rarely, if ever, is it totally met.

Culture and Religion
- **Culture** is the characteristics of a group of people. People come from many cultures, races, and nationalities. Family practices, food choices, hygiene habits, clothing styles, and language are part of their culture. The person's culture also influences health beliefs and practices.
- **Religion** relates to spiritual beliefs, needs, and practices. A person's religion influences health and illness practices. Many may want to pray and observe religious practices. Assist residents to attend religious services as needed. If a person wants to see a spiritual leader or adviser, tell the nurse. Provide privacy during the visit.
- A person may not follow all the beliefs and practices of his or her culture or religion. Some people do not practice a religion.
- Respect and accept the person's culture and religion. Learn about practices and beliefs different from your own. Do not judge a person by your standards.

Communicating With the Person
- For effective communication between you and the person, you must:
  - Follow the rules of communication in Chapter 7 in the Textbook.
  - Understand and respect the patient or resident as a person.
  - View the person as a physical, psychological, social, and spiritual human being.
  - Appreciate the person's problems and frustrations.
  - Respect the person's rights.
  - Respect the person's religion and culture.
  - Give the person time to understand the information that you give.
  - Repeat information as often as needed.
  - Ask questions to see if the person understood you.
  - Be patient. People with memory problems may ask the same question many times.
  - Include the person in conversations when others are present.

Verbal Communication
- When talking with a person, follow these rules.
  - Face the person. Look directly at the person.
  - Position yourself at the person's eye level.
  - Control the loudness and tone of your voice.
  - Speak clearly, slowly, and distinctly.
  - Do not use slang or vulgar words.
  - Repeat information as needed.
  - Ask 1 question at a time and wait for an answer.
  - Do not shout, whisper, or mumble.
  - Be kind, courteous, and friendly.
- Use written words if the person cannot speak or hear but can read. Keep written messages brief and concise. Use a black felt pen on white paper and print in large letters.
- Some persons cannot speak or read. Ask questions that have "yes" or "no" answers. A picture board may be helpful.

Nonverbal Communication

- Messages are sent with gestures, facial expressions, posture, body movements, touch, and smell. Nonverbal messages more accurately reflect a person's feelings than words do. A person may say one thing but act another way. Watch the person's eyes, hand movements, gestures, posture, and other actions.
- Touch conveys comfort, caring, love, affection, interest, trust, concern, and reassurance. Touch should be gentle. Touch means different things to different people. Some people do not like to be touched. To use touch, follow the care plan. Maintain professional boundaries.
- People send messages through their **body language**— facial expressions, gestures, posture, hand and body movements, gait, eye contact, and appearance. Your body language should show interest, enthusiasm, caring, and respect for the person. Often you need to control your body language. Control reactions to odors from body fluids, secretions, or excretions.

Communication Methods

- *Listening* means to focus on verbal and nonverbal communication. You use sight, hearing, touch, and smell. To be a good listener:
  - Face the person.
  - Have good eye contact with the person.
  - Lean toward the person. Do not sit back with your arms crossed.
  - Respond to the person. Nod your head and ask questions.
  - Avoid communication barriers.
- *Paraphrasing* is re-stating the person's message in your own words.
- *Direct questions* focus on certain information. You ask the person something you need to know.
- *Open-ended questions* lead or invite the person to share thoughts, feelings, or ideas. The person chooses what to talk about.
- *Clarifying* lets you make sure that you understand the message. You can ask the person to repeat the message, say you do not understand, or re-state the message.
- *Focusing* deals with a certain topic. It is useful when a person wanders in thought.
- *Silence* is a very powerful way to communicate. Silence gives time to think, organize thoughts, choose words, make decisions, and gain control. Silence on your part shows caring and respect for the person's situation and feelings.

Communication Barriers

- *Language.* You and the person must use and understand the same language.
- *Cultural differences.* A person from another country may attach different meanings to verbal and nonverbal communication than what you intended.
- *Changing the subject.* Avoid changing the subject whenever possible.
- *Giving your opinions.* Opinions involve judging values, behaviors, or feelings. Let others express feelings and concerns without adding your opinion. Do not make judgments or jump to conclusions.

- *Talking a lot when others are silent.* Talking too much is usually because of nervousness and discomfort with silence.
- *Failure to listen.* Do not pretend to listen. It shows lack of caring and interest. You may miss complaints of pain, discomfort, or other symptoms that you must report to the nurse.
- *Pat answers.* "Don't worry." "Everything will be okay." These make the person feel that you do not care about his or her concerns, feelings, and fears.
- *Illness and disability.* Speech, hearing, vision, cognitive function, and body movements may be affected. Verbal and nonverbal communication is affected.
- *Age.* Values and communication styles vary among age-groups.

Persons With Special Needs

- Common courtesies and manners apply to any person with a disability. Review Box 9-1, Disability Etiquette, in the Textbook.
- The person who is comatose is unconscious and cannot respond to others. Often the person can hear and feel touch and pain. Assume that the person hears and understands you. Use touch and give care gently. Practice these measures.
  - Knock before entering the person's room.
  - Tell the person your name, the time, and the place every time you enter the room.
  - Give care on the same schedule every day.
  - Explain what you are going to do.
  - Tell the person when you are finishing care.
  - Use touch to communicate care, concern, and comfort.
  - Tell the person what time you will be back to check on him or her.
  - Tell the person when you are leaving the room.

Family and Friends

- If you need to give care when visitors are there, protect the person's right to privacy. Politely ask the visitors to leave the room when you give care. A partner or family member may help you if the patient or resident consents.
- Treat family and visitors with courtesy and respect.
- Do not discuss the person's condition with family and friends. Refer questions to the nurse. A visitor may upset or tire a person. Report your observations to the nurse.

Behavior Issues

- Many people do not adjust well to illness, injury, and disability. They have some of the following behaviors.
  - *Anger.* Anger may be communicated verbally and nonverbally. Verbal outbursts, shouting, and rapid speech are common. Some people are silent. Others are uncooperative and may refuse to answer questions. Nonverbal signs include rapid movements, pacing, clenched fists, and a red face. Glaring and getting close to you when speaking are other signs. Violent behaviors can occur.

○ *Demanding behavior.* Nothing seems to please the person. The person is critical of others.

○ *Self-centered behavior.* The person cares only about his or her own needs. The needs of others are ignored. The person becomes impatient if needs are not met.

○ *Aggressive behavior.* The person may swear, bite, hit, pinch, scratch, or kick. Protect the person, others, and yourself from harm.

○ *Withdrawal.* The person has little or no contact with family, friends, and staff. Some people are generally not social and prefer to be alone.

○ *Inappropriate sexual behavior.* Some people make inappropriate sexual remarks or touch others in the wrong way. These behaviors may be on purpose. Or they are caused by disease, confusion, dementia, or drug side effects.

• You cannot avoid persons with unpleasant behaviors or lose control. Review Box 9-2, Dealing With Behavior Issues, in the Textbook.

CHAPTER 9 REVIEW QUESTIONS

Circle the BEST answer.

1. While caring for a person, you need to
   a. Consider only the person's physical and social needs
   b. Consider the person's physical, social, psychological, and spiritual needs
   c. Consider only the person's cultural needs
   d. Ignore the person's spiritual needs

2. When referring to residents, you should
   a. Refer to them by their room number
   b. Call them "Honey"
   c. Call them by their first name
   d. Call them by their name and title

3. Based on Maslow's theory of basic needs, which person's needs must be met first?
   a. The person who wants to talk about her granddaughter's wedding
   b. The person who is uncomfortable in the dining room
   c. The person who wants mail opened
   d. The person who asks for more water

4. Which statement about culture is *false?*
   a. A person's culture influences health beliefs and practices.
   b. You must respect a person's culture.
   c. You should ignore the person's culture while you give his or her care.
   d. You should learn about another person's culture that is different from yours.

5. Which statement about religion and spiritual beliefs is *false?*
   a. A person's religion influences health and illness practices.
   b. You should assist a person to attend services in the nursing center.
   c. Many people find comfort and strength from religion during illness.
   d. A person must follow all beliefs of his or her religion.

6. A person is angry and is shouting at you. You should do the following *except*
   a. Stay calm and professional
   b. Yell so the person will listen to you
   c. Listen to what the person is saying
   d. Report the person's behavior to the nurse

7. A person tries to scratch and kick you. You should
   a. Protect yourself from harm
   b. Argue with the person
   c. Become angry with the person
   d. Refuse to care for the person

8. When speaking with another person, you do the following *except*
   a. Position yourself at the person's eye level
   b. Speak slowly, clearly, and distinctly
   c. Shout, mumble, and whisper
   d. Ask 1 question at a time

9. Which statement about listening is *false?*
   a. You use sight, hearing, touch, and smell when you listen.
   b. You observe nonverbal cues.
   c. You have good eye contact with the person.
   d. You sit back with your arms crossed.

10. Which statement about silence is *false?*
    a. Silence is a powerful way to communicate.
    b. Silence gives people time to think.
    c. You should talk a lot when the other person is silent.
    d. Silence helps when the person is upset and needs to gain control.

11. A person speaks a foreign language. You should do the following *except*
    a. Keep messages short and simple
    b. Use gestures and pictures
    c. Shout or speak loudly
    d. Repeat the message in other words

12. When caring for a person who is comatose, you do the following *except*
    a. Tell the person your name when you enter the room
    b. Explain what you are doing
    c. Use touch to communicate care and comfort
    d. Make jokes about how sick the person is

13. A person is in a wheelchair. You should do all of the following *except*
    a. Lean on a person's wheelchair
    b. Sit or squat to talk to a person in a wheelchair or chair
    c. Think about obstacles before giving directions to a person in a wheelchair
    d. Extend the same courtesies to the person as you would to anyone else

14. A person's daughter is visiting and you need to provide care to the person. You
    a. Expose the person's body in front of the visitor
    b. Politely ask the visitor to leave the room
    c. Decide to not provide the care at all
    d. Discuss the person's condition with the visitor

Answers to these questions are on p. 516.

CHAPTER 11 GROWTH AND DEVELOPMENT

- **Growth** is the physical changes that are measured and that occur in a steady and orderly manner.
- **Development** relates to changes in mental, emotional, and social function.
- Growth and development occur in a sequence, order, and pattern. Review the stages of growth and development detailed in the Textbook.
- Middle adulthood (40 to 65 years old). At this stage, developmental tasks are adjusting to physical changes, having grown children, developing leisure-time activities, and adjusting to aging parents.
- Late adulthood (65 years and older). At this stage, developmental tasks are adjusting to decreased strength and loss of health, adjusting to retirement and reduced income, coping with a partner's death, developing new friends and relationships, and preparing for one's own death.

CHAPTER 11 REVIEW QUESTIONS

Circle the BEST answer.

1. Growth and development occur in a sequence, order, and pattern.
   a. True
   b. False
2. Growth relates to changes in mental, emotional, and social function.
   a. True
   b. False
3. Which is a developmental task of late adulthood?
   a. Accepting changes in appearance
   b. Adjusting to decreased strength
   c. Developing a satisfactory sex life
   d. Performing self-care

Answers to these questions are on p. 516.

CHAPTER 12 CARE OF THE OLDER PERSON

- Aging is normal. It is not a disease. Normal changes occur in body structure and function. Psychological and social changes also occur.

Psychological and Social Changes

- Physical reminders of growing old affect self-esteem and may threaten self-image, feelings of self-worth, and independence.
- People cope with aging in their own way. How they cope depends on their health status, life experiences, finances, education, and social support systems.
- *Retirement.* Many people enjoy retirement. Others are in poor health and have medical bills that can make retirement hard.
- *Reduced income.* Retirement usually means reduced income. The retired person still has expenses. Reduced income may force life-style changes. One example is the person avoids health care or needed drugs.
- *Social relationships.* Social relationships change throughout life. Family time helps prevent loneliness.

So do hobbies, religious and community events, and new friends.

- *Children as caregivers.* Some older persons feel more secure when children care for them. Others feel unwanted and useless. Some lose dignity and self-respect. Tensions may occur among the child, parent, and other household members.
- *Death and grieving.* Death of an adult child or a partner can cause immense grief. Emotional needs will be great. The person may be left with few family and friends to provide support.

Physical Changes

- Body processes slow down. Energy level and body efficiency decline.
- *The integumentary system.* The skin loses its elasticity, strength, and fatty tissue layer. Wrinkles appear. Dry skin occurs and may cause itching. The skin is fragile and easily injured. The person is more sensitive to cold. Nails become thick and tough. Feet may have poor circulation. White or gray hair is common. Hair thins. Facial hair may occur in women. Hair is drier. The risk of skin cancer increases.
- *The musculo-skeletal system.* Muscle and bone strength are lost. Bones become brittle and break easily. Vertebrae shorten. Joints become stiff and painful. Mobility decreases. There is a gradual loss of height.
- *The nervous system.* Confusion, dizziness, and fatigue may occur. Responses are slower. The risk for falls increases. Forgetfulness increases. Memory is shorter. Events from long ago are remembered better than recent ones. Older persons have a harder time falling asleep. Sleep periods are shorter. Older persons wake often during the night and have less deep sleep. Less sleep is needed. They may rest or nap during the day. They may go to bed early and get up early.
- *The senses.* Hearing and vision losses occur. Taste and smell dull. Appetite decreases. Touch and sensitivity to pain, pressure, hot, and cold are reduced.
- *The circulatory system.* The heart muscle weakens. Arteries narrow and are less elastic. Poor circulation occurs in many body parts.
- *The respiratory system.* Respiratory muscles weaken. Lung tissue becomes less elastic. Difficult, labored, or painful breathing may occur with activity. The person may lack strength to cough and clear the airway of secretions. Respiratory infections and diseases may develop.
- *The digestive system.* Less saliva is produced. The person may have difficulty swallowing (dysphagia). Indigestion may occur. Loss of teeth and ill-fitting dentures cause chewing problems and digestion problems. Flatulence and constipation can occur. Fewer calories are needed as energy and activity levels decline. More fluids are needed.
- *The urinary system.* Urine is more concentrated. Bladder muscles weaken. Bladder size decreases. Urinary frequency or urgency may occur. Urinary tract infections are risks. Many older persons have to urinate at night. Urinary incontinence may occur. In men, the prostate gland enlarges. This may cause difficulty urinating or frequent urination.

- *The reproductive system.* In men, testosterone decreases. An erection takes longer. Orgasm is less forceful. Women experience menopause. Female hormones of estrogen and progesterone decrease. The uterus, vagina, and genitalia shrink (atrophy). Vaginal walls thin. There is vaginal dryness. Arousal takes longer. Orgasm is less intense.

Housing Options

- A person's home is more than a place to live. It holds memories, is a link to neighbors and communities, and brings pride and self-esteem. Aging can lead to changes in a person's home setting.
- Most older people live in their own homes. Others need help from family or community agencies. Review Box 12-3, In-Home and Community-Based Services, in the Textbook.

Nursing Centers

- The person needing nursing center care may suffer some or all of these losses.
  - Loss of identity as a productive member of a family and community
  - Loss of possessions—home, household items, car, and so on
  - Loss of independence
  - Loss of real-world experiences—shopping, traveling, cooking, driving, hobbies
  - Loss of health and mobility
- The person may feel useless, powerless, and hopeless. The health team helps the person cope with loss and improve quality of life. Treat the person with dignity and respect. Also practice good communication skills. Follow the care plan.

CHAPTER 12 REVIEW QUESTIONS

Circle the BEST answer.
1. Which statement is *false*?
   a. Physical changes occur with aging.
   b. Energy level and body efficiency decline with age.
   c. Some people age faster than others.
   d. Normal aging means loss of health.
2. As a person ages, the integumentary system changes. Which statement is *false*?
   a. Dry skin and itching occur.
   b. Nails become thick and tough.
   c. The person is less sensitive to cold.
   d. Skin is injured more easily.
3. Which statement is *false* about the musculo-skeletal system and aging?
   a. Strength decreases.
   b. Vertebrae shorten.
   c. Mobility increases.
   d. Bone mass decreases.
4. Which statement about the nervous system and aging is *false*?
   a. Reflexes slow.
   b. Memory may be shorter.
   c. Sleep patterns change.
   d. Forgetfulness decreases.

5. Which statement about the digestive system and aging is *false*?
   a. Appetite decreases.
   b. Less saliva is produced.
   c. Flatulence and constipation may decrease.
   d. Teeth may be lost.
6. Which statement about the urinary system and aging is *false*?
   a. Urine becomes more concentrated.
   b. Urinary frequency may occur.
   c. Urinary urgency may occur.
   d. Bladder muscles become stronger.

Answers to these questions are on p. 516.

CHAPTER 13 SAFETY

Accident Risk Factors

- *Age.* Older persons are at risk for falls and other injuries.
- *Awareness of surroundings.* People need to know their surroundings to protect themselves from injury.
- *Agitated and aggressive behaviors.* Pain, confusion, fear, and decreased awareness of surroundings can cause these behaviors.
- *Vision loss.* Persons can fall or trip over items. Some have problems reading labels on containers.
- *Hearing loss.* Persons have problems hearing explanations and instructions. They may not hear warning signals or fire alarms. They do not know to move to safety.
- *Impaired smell and touch.* Illness and aging affect smell and touch. The person may not detect smoke or gas or may be unaware of injury. Burns are a risk.
- *Impaired mobility.* Some diseases and injuries affect mobility. A person may know there is danger but cannot move to safety. Some persons are paralyzed. Some persons cannot walk or propel wheelchairs.
- *Drugs.* Drugs have side effects. Reduced awareness, confusion, and disorientation can occur. Report behavior changes and the person's complaints.

Identifying the Person

- You must give the right care to the right person. To identify the person:
  - Compare identifying information on the assignment sheet or treatment card with that on the identification (ID) bracelet.
  - Call the person by name when checking the ID bracelet. Just calling the person by name is not enough to identify him or her. Confused, disoriented, drowsy, hard-of-hearing, or distracted persons may answer to any name.
- Use at least 2 identifiers. Agencies have different requirements. Some may require the person to state and spell his or her name and give a birth date. Others require using the person's ID number. Always follow agency policy.

Preventing Burns

- Smoking, spilled hot liquids, very hot water, and electrical devices are common causes of burns. See Box 13-1 in the Textbook for safety measures to prevent burns.

Preventing Poisoning

- Drugs and household products are common poisons. Poisoning in adults may be from carelessness, confusion, or poor vision when reading labels. To prevent poisoning:
  - Make sure patients and residents cannot reach hazardous materials.
  - Follow agency policy for storing personal care items.
- See Box 13-2 in the Textbook for safety measures to prevent poisoning.

Preventing Suffocation

- **Suffocation** is when breathing stops from the lack of oxygen. Death occurs if the person does not start breathing.
- To prevent suffocation, review Box 13-5, Preventing Suffocation, in the Textbook.

Choking

- Choking or foreign-body airway obstruction (FBAO) occurs when a foreign body obstructs the airway. Air cannot pass through the air passages into the lungs. The body does not get enough oxygen. This can lead to cardiac arrest.
- Choking often occurs during eating. A large, poorly chewed piece of meat is the most common cause. Other common causes include laughing and talking while eating.
- With *mild airway obstruction*, some air moves in and out of the lungs. The person is conscious. Usually the person can speak. Often, forceful coughing can remove the object.
- With *severe airway obstruction*, the conscious person clutches at the throat—the "universal sign of choking." The person has difficulty breathing. Some persons cannot breathe, speak, or cough. The person appears pale and cyanotic (bluish color). Air does not move in and out of the lungs. If the obstruction is not removed, the person will die. Severe airway obstruction is an emergency.
- Use abdominal thrusts to relieve severe choking. Chest thrusts are used for very obese persons and pregnant women.
- Call for help when a person has an obstructed airway. Report and record what happened, what you did, and the person's response.

Preventing Equipment Accidents

- All equipment is unsafe if broken, not used correctly, or not working properly. Inspect all equipment before use. Review Box 13-7, Preventing Equipment Accidents, in the Textbook.

Hazardous Chemicals

- A hazardous substance is any chemical in the workplace that can cause harm. Hazardous substances include oxygen, mercury, disinfectants, and cleaning agents.
- Hazardous substance containers must have a warning label. If a label is removed or damaged, do not use the substance. Take the container to the nurse. Do not leave the container unattended.

- Check the material safety data sheet (MSDS) before using a hazardous substance, cleaning up a leak or spill, or disposing of the substance. Tell the nurse about a leak or spill right away. Do not leave a leak or spill unattended. Review Box 13-8 in the Textbook.

Disasters

- A **disaster** is a sudden catastrophic event. The agency has procedures for disasters that could occur in your area. Follow them to keep patients, residents, visitors, staff, and yourself safe.
- Natural disasters include tornadoes, hurricanes, blizzards, earthquakes, volcanic eruptions, floods, and some fires.
- Human-made disasters include auto, bus, train, and airplane accidents. They also include fires, bombings, nuclear power plant accidents, gas or chemical leaks, explosions, and wars.
- Follow agency protocol for a bomb threat or if you find an item that looks or sounds strange.

Fire Safety

- Faulty electrical equipment and wiring, over-loaded electrical circuits, and smoking are major causes of fires.
- Safety measures are needed where oxygen is used and stored.
- Review Box 13-9, Fire Prevention Measures, in the Textbook.
- Know your center's policies and procedures for fire emergencies. Know where to find fire alarms, fire extinguishers, and emergency exits. Remember the word *RACE*.
  - **R**—*rescue.* Rescue persons in immediate danger. Move them to a safe place.
  - **A**—*alarm.* Sound the nearest fire alarm. Notify the telephone operator.
  - **C**—*confine.* Close doors and windows. Turn off oxygen or electrical items.
  - **E**—*extinguish.* Use a fire extinguisher on a small fire.
- Remember the word *PASS* for using a fire extinguisher.
  - **P**—*pull* the safety pin.
  - **A**—*aim* low. Aim at the base of the fire.
  - **S**—*squeeze* the lever. This starts the stream of water.
  - **S**—*sweep* back and forth. Sweep side to side at the base of the fire.
- Do not use elevators during a fire.

Elopement

- Elopement is when a resident leaves the agency without staff knowledge. The Centers for Medicare & Medicaid Services (CMS) requires that an agency's disaster plan address elopement.
- The agency must:
  - Identify persons at risk for elopement.
  - Monitor and supervise persons at risk.
  - Address elopement in the person's care plan.
  - Have a plan to find a missing patient or resident.

Workplace Violence

- **Workplace violence** is violent acts (including assault or threat of assault) directed toward persons at work or while on duty. Review Box 13-10, Workplace Violence—Safety Measures, in the Textbook.

CHAPTER 13 REVIEW QUESTIONS
Circle the BEST answer.

1. You see a water spill in the hallway. What will you do?
   a. Ask housekeeping to wipe up the spill right away.
   b. Wipe up the spill right away.
   c. Report the spill to the nurse.
   d. Ask the resident to walk around the spill.

2. An electrical outlet in a person's room does not work. What will you do?
   a. Tell the administrator about the problem.
   b. Tell another nursing assistant about the problem.
   c. Try to repair the electrical outlet.
   d. Follow the center's policy for reporting the problem.

3. Accident risk factors include all of the following *except*
   a. Walking without difficulty
   b. Hearing problems
   c. Dulled sense of smell
   d. Poor vision

4. To prevent a person from being burned, you should do the following *except*
   a. Supervise the smoking of persons who are confused
   b. Turn cold water on first; turn hot water off first
   c. Do not let the person sleep with a heating pad
   d. Allow smoking in bed

5. To prevent suffocation, you should do the following *except*
   a. Make sure dentures fit properly
   b. Check the care plan for swallowing problems before serving food or liquids
   c. Leave a person alone in a bathtub or shower
   d. Position the person in bed properly

6. Which statement about mild airway obstruction is *false?*
   a. Some air moves in and out of the lungs.
   b. The person is conscious.
   c. Usually the person cannot speak.
   d. Forceful coughing will often remove the object.

7. The "universal sign of choking" is
   a. Clutching at the chest
   b. Clutching at the throat
   c. Not being able to talk
   d. Not being able to breathe

8. Which of the following is *not* a safety measure with oxygen?
   a. NO SMOKING signs are placed on the resident's door and near the bed.
   b. Lit candles and other open flames are permitted in the room.
   c. Electrical items are turned off before being unplugged.
   d. The person wears a cotton gown or pajamas.

9. You have discovered a fire in the nursing center. You should do the following *except*
   a. Rescue persons in immediate danger
   b. Sound the nearest fire alarm
   c. Open doors and windows and keep oxygen on
   d. Use a fire extinguisher on a small fire that has not spread to a larger area

10. When using a fire extinguisher, you do the following *except*
    a. Pull the safety pin on the fire extinguisher
    b. Aim at the top of the flames
    c. Squeeze the lever to start the stream
    d. Sweep the stream back and forth

Answers to these questions are on p. 516.

CHAPTER 14 FALL PREVENTION
- Falls are a leading cause of injuries and deaths among older persons. A history of falls increases the risk of falling again.
- Most falls occur in resident rooms and bathrooms.
- Causes for falls are poor lighting, cluttered floors, throw rugs, needing to use the bathroom, out-of-place furniture, wet and slippery floors, bathtubs, and showers. Review Box 14-1, Fall Risk Factors, in the Textbook.
- Agencies have fall prevention programs. Review Box 14-2, Safety Measures to Prevent Falls, in the Textbook. The person's care plan also lists measures specific for the person.
- Bed and chair alarms alert staff when the person is moving from the bed or chair.

Bed Rails
- A **bed rail** (*side rail*) is a device that serves as a guard or barrier along the side of the bed.
- The nurse and care plan tell you when to raise bed rails. They are needed by persons who are unconscious or sedated with drugs. Some confused and disoriented people need them. If a person needs bed rails, keep them up at all times except when giving bedside nursing care.
- Bed rails present hazards. The person can fall when trying to get out of bed. Or the person can get caught, trapped, entangled, or strangled.
- Bed rails are considered restraints if the person cannot get out of bed or lower them without help.
- Accrediting agency standards and state and federal laws affect bed rail use. They are allowed when the person's condition requires them. The need for bed rails is carefully noted in the person's medical record and the care plan. If a person uses bed rails, check the person often. Record when you checked the person and your observations.
- To prevent falls:
  o Never leave the person alone when the bed is raised.
  o Always lower the bed to its lowest position when you are done giving care.
  o If a person does not use bed rails and you need to raise the bed, ask a co-worker to stand on the far side of the bed to protect the person from falling.
  o If you raise the bed to give care, always raise the far bed rail if you are working alone.
  o Be sure the person who uses raised bed rails has access to items on the bedside stand and over-bed table. The call light, water pitcher and cup, tissues, phone, and TV and light controls should be within the person's reach.

Hand Rails and Grab Bars

- Hand rails give support to persons who are weak or unsteady when walking.
- Grab bars provide support for sitting down or getting up from a toilet. They also are used for getting in and out of the shower or tub.

Wheel Locks

- Bed wheels are locked at all times except when moving the bed.
- Wheelchair and stretcher wheels are locked when transferring a person.

Transfer/Gait Belts

- Use a **transfer belt (gait belt)** to support a person who is unsteady or disabled. Always follow the manufacturer's instructions. Apply the belt over clothing and under the breasts. The belt buckle is never positioned over the person's spine. Tighten the belt so it is snug. You should be able to slide your open, flat hand under the belt. Tuck the excess strap under the belt. Remove the belt after the procedure.
- Check with the nurse and care plan before using a transfer/gait belt if the person has:
  - A colostomy, ileostomy, gastrostomy, or urostomy
  - A gastric tube
  - Chronic obstructive pulmonary disease
  - An abdominal wound, incision, or drainage tube
  - A chest wound, incision, or drainage tube
  - Monitoring equipment
  - A hernia
  - Other conditions or care equipment involving the chest or abdomen

The Falling Person

- If a person starts to fall, do not try to prevent the fall. You could injure yourself and the person. Ease the person to the floor and protect the person's head.
- Do not let the person get up before the nurse checks for injuries. An incident report is completed after all falls.

CHAPTER 14 REVIEW QUESTIONS

Circle the BEST answer.

1. Most falls occur in
   a. Resident rooms and bathrooms
   b. Dining rooms
   c. Hallways
   d. Activity rooms
2. Which statement about falls is *false?*
   a. Poor lighting, cluttered floors, and throw rugs may cause falls.
   b. Improper shoes and needing to use the bathroom may cause falls.
   c. Most falls occur between 4:00 PM and 8:00 PM.
   d. Falls are less likely to occur during shift changes.
3. You note the following after a person got dressed. Which is unsafe?
   a. Non-skid footwear is worn.
   b. Pant cuffs are dragging on the floor.
   c. Clothing fits properly.
   d. The belt is fastened.

4. Which statement about bed rails is *false?*
   a. The nurse and care plan tell you when to raise bed rails.
   b. Bed rails are considered restraints.
   c. You may leave a person alone when the bed is raised and the bed rails are down.
   d. Bed rails can present hazards because people try to climb over them.
5. Which statement about transfer/gait belts is *false?*
   a. To use the belt safely, follow the manufacturer's instructions.
   b. Always apply the belt over clothing.
   c. Tighten the belt so it is very snug and breathing is impaired.
   d. Place the belt buckle off-center so it is not over the spine.
6. A person becomes faint in the hallway and begins to fall. You should do the following *except*
   a. Ease the person to the floor
   b. Protect the person's head
   c. Let the person get up before the nurse checks him or her
   d. Help the nurse complete the incident report

Answers to these questions are on p. 516.

CHAPTER 15 RESTRAINT ALTERNATIVES AND SAFE RESTRAINT USE

- The Centers for Medicare & Medicaid Services (CMS) has rules for using restraints. These rules protect the person's rights and safety.
- Restraints may be used only to treat a medical symptom or for the immediate physical safety of the person or others. Restraints may be used only when less restrictive measures fail to protect the person or others. They must be discontinued at the earliest possible time.
- The CMS uses these to define restraints.
  - A **physical restraint** is any manual method or physical or mechanical device, material, or equipment attached to or near the person's body that he or she cannot remove easily and that restricts freedom of movement or normal access to one's body.
  - A **chemical restraint** is a drug that is used for discipline or convenience and not required to treat medical symptoms. The drug or dosage is not a standard treatment for the person's condition.
  - **Freedom of movement** is any change in place or position of the body or any part of the body that the person is able to control.
  - **Remove easily** is the manual method, device, material, or equipment used to restrain the person that can be removed intentionally by the person in the same manner it was applied by staff.
  - **Convenience** is any action taken to control or manage a person's behavior that requires less effort by the staff; the action is not in the person's best interest.
  - **Discipline** is any action taken by the agency to punish or penalize a patient or resident.
- Federal, state, and accrediting agencies have guidelines about restraint use. They do not forbid restraint use. They require considering or trying all other appropriate alternatives first.

- Every agency has policies and procedures about restraints. They include identifying persons at risk for harm, harmful behaviors, restraint alternatives, and proper restraint use. Staff training is required.

Restraint Alternatives

- Knowing and treating the cause for harmful behaviors can prevent restraint use. There are many alternatives to restraints, such as answering the call light promptly. For other alternatives see Box 15-1, Restraint Alternatives.

Safe Restraint Use

- Restraints are used only when necessary to treat a person's medical symptoms—physical, emotional, or behavioral problems. Sometimes restraints are needed to protect the person or others.

Physical and Chemical Restraints

- *Physical restraints* are applied to the chest, waist, elbows, wrists, hands, or ankles. They confine the person to a bed or chair. Or they prevent movement of a body part. Some furniture or barriers prevent free movement.
- Drugs or drug dosages are *chemical restraints* if they:
  - Control behavior or restrict movement.
  - Are not standard treatment for the person's condition.

Risks From Restraints

- Restraints can cause many complications. Injuries occur as the person tries to get free of the restraint. Injuries also occur from using the wrong restraint, applying it wrong, or keeping it on too long. Cuts, bruises, and fractures are common. The most serious risk is death from strangulation. Review Box 15-2, Risks From Restraint Use, in the Textbook.

Legal Aspects

- *Restraints must protect the person.* A restraint is used only when it is the best safety measure for the person.
- *A doctor's order is required.* The doctor gives the reason for the restraint, what body part to restrain, what to use, and how long to use it.
- *The least restrictive method is used.* It allows the greatest amount of movement or body access possible.
- *Restraints are used only after other measures fail to protect the person.* Box 15-1 in the Textbook lists alternatives to restraint use.
- *Unnecessary restraint is false imprisonment.* If you apply an unneeded restraint, you could face false imprisonment charges.
- *Informed consent is required.* The person must understand the reason for the restraint. If the person cannot give consent, his or her legal representative must give consent before a restraint can be used. The doctor or nurse provides the necessary information and obtains the consent.

Safety Guidelines

- Review Box 15-3, Safety Measures for Using Restraints, in the Textbook.

- *Observe for increased confusion and agitation.* Restraints can increase confusion and agitation. Restrained persons need repeated explanations and re-assurance. Spending time with them has a calming effect.
- *Protect the person's quality of life.* Restraints are used for as short a time as possible. You must meet the person's physical, emotional, and social needs.
- *Follow the manufacturer's instructions.* The restraint must be snug and firm but not tight. You could be negligent if you do not apply or secure a restraint properly.
- *Apply restraints with enough help to protect the person and staff from injury.*
- *Observe the person at least every 15 minutes or more often as noted in the care plan.* Injuries and deaths can result from improper restraint use and poor observation.
- *Remove or release the restraint, re-position the person, and meet basic needs at least every 2 hours or as often as noted in the care plan.* The restraint is removed for at least 10 minutes. Provide for food, fluid, comfort, safety, hygiene, and elimination needs and give skin care. Perform range-of-motion exercises or help the person walk.

Reporting and Recording

- Report and record the following:
  - Type of restraint applied
  - Body part or parts restrained
  - Reason for the application
  - Safety measures taken
  - Time you applied the restraint
  - Time you removed or released the restraint
  - Care given when restraint was removed
  - Person's vital signs
  - Skin color and condition
  - Condition of the limbs
  - Pulse felt in the restrained part
  - Changes in the person's behavior
- Report these complaints to the nurse at once: complaints of discomfort; a tight restraint; difficulty breathing; or pain, numbness, or tingling in the restrained part.

CHAPTER 15 REVIEW QUESTIONS

Circle the BEST answer.

1. A geriatric chair or a bed rail may be considered a restraint if free movement is restricted.
   a. True
   b. False
2. Restraints can be used for staff convenience.
   a. True
   b. False
3. Restraints can increase a person's confusion and agitation.
   a. True
   b. False
4. The person with a restraint should be observed at least every
   a. 15 minutes
   b. 30 minutes
   c. Hour
   d. 2 hours

5. Restraints need to be removed at least every
   a. Hour
   b. 2 hours
   c. 3 hours
   d. 4 hours
6. You should record all the following *except*
   a. The type of restraint used
   b. The consent for the restraint
   c. The time you removed the restraint
   d. The care you gave when the restraint was removed

Answers to these questions are on p. 516.

CHAPTER 16 PREVENTING INFECTION

- An **infection** is a disease state resulting from the invasion and growth of microbes in the body. Infection is a major safety hazard.
- The health team follows certain practices and procedures to prevent the spread of infection (**infection control**).

Microorganisms

- A **microorganism (microbe)** is a small (*micro*) living plant or animal (*organism*).
- Some microbes are harmful and can cause infections (**pathogens**). Others do not usually cause infection (**non-pathogens**).

Multidrug-Resistant Organisms

- *Multidrug-resistant organisms (MDROs) can resist the effects of antibiotics. Such organisms are able to change their structures to survive in the presence of antibiotics. The infections they cause are harder to treat.*
- MDROs are caused by prescribing antibiotics when they are not needed (over-prescribing). Not taking antibiotics for the prescribed length of time is also a cause.
- Two common types of MDROs are resistant to many antibiotics.
  - *Methicillin-resistant Staphylococcus aureus (MRSA)*
  - *Vancomycin-resistant Enterococcus (VRE)*

Infection

- **A local infection** is in a body part.
- **A systemic infection** involves the whole body.
- Older persons may not show the normal signs and symptoms of infection. The person may have only a slight fever or no fever at all. Redness and swelling may be very slight. The person may not complain of pain. Confusion and delirium may occur.
- Infections can become life-threatening before the older person has obvious signs and symptoms. Be alert to minor changes in the person's behavior or condition.
- Report any concerns to the nurse at once. Review Box 16-1, Signs and Symptoms of Infection, in the Textbook.

Healthcare-Associated Infection

- A **healthcare-associated infection (HAI)** is an infection that develops in a person cared for in any setting where health care is given. Review Box 16-2 in the Textbook. The infection is related to receiving health care. Hospitals, nursing centers, clinics, and home care settings are examples. HAIs also are called *nosocomial infections*.
- The health team must prevent the spread of HAIs by:
  - Medical asepsis. This includes hand hygiene.
  - Surgical asepsis.
  - Standard Precautions and Transmission-Based Precautions.
  - The Bloodborne Pathogen Standard.

Medical Asepsis

- **Asepsis** is being free of disease-producing microbes.
- **Medical asepsis (clean technique)** refers to the practices used to:
  - Remove or destroy pathogens.
  - Prevent pathogens from spreading from 1 person or place to another person or place.

Common Aseptic Practices

- To prevent the spread of microbes, wash your hands:
  - After urinating or having a bowel movement.
  - After changing tampons or sanitary pads.
  - After contact with your own or another person's blood, body fluids, secretions, or excretions. This includes saliva, vomitus, urine, feces, vaginal discharge, mucus, semen, wound drainage, pus, and respiratory secretions.
  - After coughing, sneezing, or blowing your nose.
  - Before and after handling, preparing, or eating food.
  - After smoking.
- Also do the following:
  - Provide all persons with their own linens and personal care items.
  - Cover your nose and mouth when coughing, sneezing, or blowing your nose.
  - Bathe, wash hair, and brush your teeth regularly.
  - Wash fruits and raw vegetables before eating or serving them.
  - Wash cooking and eating utensils with soap and water after use.

Hand Hygiene

- *Hand hygiene is the easiest and most important way to prevent the spread of infection.* Practice hand hygiene before and after giving care. Review Box 16-3, Rules of Hand Hygiene, in the Textbook.

Supplies and Equipment

- Most health care equipment is disposable. Bedpans, urinals, wash basins, water pitchers, and drinking cups are multi-use items. Do not "borrow" them for another person.
- Non-disposable items are cleaned and then disinfected. Then they are sterilized.

Other Aseptic Measures

- Review Box 16-4, Aseptic Measures, in the Textbook.

Isolation Precautions

- Isolation precautions prevent the spread of **communicable diseases (contagious diseases).** They are diseases caused by pathogens that spread easily.
- The Centers for Disease and Control and Prevention's (CDC's) isolation precautions guideline has 2 tiers of precautions.

○ Standard Precautions
○ Transmission-Based Precautions

Standard Precautions

- Standard Precautions reduce the risk of spreading pathogens and known and unknown infections. Standard Precautions are used for all persons whenever care is given. They prevent the spread of infection from:
  ○ Blood.
  ○ All body fluids, secretions, and excretions even if blood is not visible. Sweat is not known to spread infections.
  ○ Non-intact skin (skin with open breaks).
  ○ Mucous membranes.
- Review Box 16-5, Standard Precautions, in the Textbook.

Transmission-Based Precautions

- Some infections require Transmission-Based Precautions. Review Box 16-6, Transmission-Based Precautions, in the Textbook.
- Agency policies may differ from those in the Textbook. The rules in Box 16-7, Rules for Isolation Precautions, in the Textbook are a guide for giving safe care.

Personal Protective Equipment (PPE)

- The PPE needed —gloves, a gown, a mask, and goggles or a face shield—depends on the task, the procedures, care measures, and the type of Transmission-Based Precautions used. The nurse will tell you what equipment is needed.
- Gowns must completely cover you from your neck to your knees. The gown front and sleeves are considered contaminated. A wet gown is contaminated. Gowns are used once. When removing a gown, roll it away from you. Keep it inside out.
- Masks are disposable. A wet or moist mask is contaminated. When removing a mask, touch only the ties or elastic bands. The front of the mask is contaminated.
- The front of goggles or a face shield is contaminated. Use the device's ties, headband, or ear-pieces to remove the device.

Gloves

- Wear gloves whenever contact with blood, body fluids, secretions, excretions, mucous membranes, and non-intact skin is likely. Wearing gloves is the most common protective measure used with Standard Precautions and Transmission-Based Precautions. Remember the following when using gloves.
  ○ The outside of gloves is contaminated.
  ○ Gloves are easier to put on when your hands are dry.
  ○ Do not tear gloves when putting them on.
  ○ You need a new pair for every person.
  ○ Remove and discard torn, cut, or punctured gloves at once. Practice hand hygiene. Then put on a new pair.
  ○ Apply a new pair for every person.
  ○ Wear gloves once. Discard them after use.
  ○ Put on clean gloves just before touching mucous membranes or non-intact skin.
  ○ Put on new gloves whenever gloves become contaminated with blood, body fluids, secretions, or excretions. A task may require more than 1 pair of gloves.

○ Change gloves whenever moving from a contaminated body site to a clean body site.
○ Change gloves if interacting with the person involves touching portable computer keyboards or other mobile equipment that is transported from room to room.
○ Put on gloves last when worn with other PPE.
○ Make sure gloves cover your wrists. If you wear a gown, gloves cover the cuffs.
○ Remove gloves so the inside part is on the outside. The inside is clean.
○ Practice hand hygiene after removing gloves.
- Latex allergies are common and can cause skin rashes. Asthma and shock are more serious problems. Report skin rashes and breathing problems at once. If you or a resident has a latex allergy, wear latex-free gloves.

Donning and Removing PPE

- According to the CDC, PPE is donned in the following order.
  ○ Gown
  ○ Mask or respirator
  ○ Eyewear (goggles or face shield)
  ○ Gloves
- Removing PPE (removed at the doorway before leaving the person's room):
  ○ *Method 1*
    1. Gloves
    2. Eyewear (goggles or face shield)
    3. Gown
    4. Mask or respirator (respirator is removed after leaving the person's room and closing the door)
  ○ *Method 2*
    1. Gown and gloves
    2. Eyewear (goggles or face shield)
    3. Mask or respirator (respirator is removed after leaving the person's room and closing the door)
- Review Figure 16-18 Donning and Removing PPE, in the Textbook.
- Practice hand hygiene after removing PPE. Practice hand hygiene between steps if your hands become contaminated. Then practice hand hygiene again after removing all PPE.
- NOTE: Some state competency tests require hand hygiene after removing each PPE item. And some states use a different order for donning and removing PPE. Follow the procedures used in your state and agency.
- Some infections such as Ebola are very severe and deadly. Such infections require additional PPE.

Bagging Items

- Contaminated items, linens, and trash are bagged to remove them from the person's room. Leak-proof plastic bags are used. They have the BIOHAZARD symbol. Double-bagging is not needed unless the outside of the bag is wet, soiled, or may be contaminated.

Bloodborne Pathogen Standard

- The health team is at risk for exposure to human immunodeficiency virus (HIV) and the hepatitis B virus (HBV). HIV and HBV are bloodborne pathogens found in the blood.

- The Bloodborne Pathogen Standard is intended to protect you from exposure.
- Staff at risk for exposure to HIV and HBV receive free training.
- *Hepatitis B vaccination.* You can receive the hepatitis B vaccination within 10 working days of being hired. The agency pays for it. If you refuse the vaccination, you must sign a statement. You can have the vaccination at a later date.

Work Practice Controls

- *Work practice controls* reduce employee exposure in the workplace. All tasks involving blood or other potentially infectious materials (OPIM) are done in ways to limit splatters, splashes, and sprays. The Occupational Safety and Health Administration (OSHA) requires these work practice controls.
  - Do not eat, drink, smoke, apply cosmetics or lip balm, or handle contact lenses in areas of occupational exposure.
  - Do not store food or drinks where blood or OPIM are kept.
  - Practice hand hygiene after removing gloves.
  - Wash hands as soon as possible after skin contact with blood or OPIM.
  - Never re-cap, bend, or remove needles by hand.
  - Never shear or break needles.
  - Discard needles and sharp instruments (razors) in containers that are closable, puncture-resistant, and leak-proof. Containers are color-coded in red and have the BIOHAZARD symbol.

Personal Protective Equipment (PPE)

- This includes gloves, goggles, face shields, masks, laboratory coats, gowns, shoe covers, and surgical caps. OSHA requires these measures for PPE.
  - Remove PPE before leaving the work area.
  - Remove PPE when a garment becomes contaminated.
  - Place used PPE in marked areas or containers when being stored, washed, decontaminated, or discarded.
  - Wear gloves when you expect contact with blood or OPIM.
  - Wear gloves when handling or touching contaminated items or surfaces.
  - Replace worn, punctured, or contaminated gloves.
  - Never wash or decontaminate disposable gloves for re-use.
  - Discard utility gloves that show signs of cracking, peeling, tearing, or puncturing. Utility gloves are decontaminated for re-use if the process will not ruin them.

Equipment

- Contaminated equipment is cleaned and decontaminated. Decontaminate work surfaces with a proper disinfectant:
  - Upon completing tasks
  - At once when there is obvious contamination
  - After any spill of blood or OPIM
  - At the end of the work shift when surfaces become contaminated since the last cleaning

Laundry

- OSHA requires these measures for contaminated laundry.
  - Handle it as little as possible.
  - Wear gloves or other needed PPE.
  - Bag contaminated laundry where it is used.
  - Mark laundry bags or containers with the BIOHAZARD symbol for laundry sent off-site.
  - Place wet, contaminated laundry in leak-proof containers before transport. The containers are color-coded in red or have the BIOHAZARD symbol.

Exposure Incidents

- An **exposure incident** is any eye, mouth, other mucous membrane, non-intact skin, or parenteral contact with blood or OPIM (other potentially infectious materials).
- Report exposure incidents at once. Medical evaluation, follow-up, and required tests are free. Your blood is tested for HIV and HBV. Confidentiality is important.

CHAPTER 16 REVIEW QUESTIONS

Circle the BEST answer.

1. A healthcare-associated infection (nosocomial infection) is
   a. An infection free of disease-producing microbes
   b. An infection that develops in a person cared for in any setting where health care is given
   c. An infection acquired by health care workers
   d. An infection acquired only by older persons
2. Which statement about hand hygiene is *false?*
   a. Hand hygiene is the easiest way to prevent the spread of infection.
   b. Hand hygiene is the most important way to prevent the spread of infection.
   c. Hand hygiene is practiced before and after giving care to a person.
   d. If hands are visibly soiled, hand hygiene can be done with an alcohol-based hand rub.
3. When washing your hands, you should do the following *except*
   a. Stand away from the sink so your clothes do not touch the sink
   b. Keep your hands lower than your elbows
   c. Wash your hands for at least 15 seconds
   d. Dry your arms from the forearms to the fingertips
4. Which statement about wearing gloves is *false?*
   a. The insides of gloves are contaminated.
   b. You need a new pair of gloves for each person you care for.
   c. Change gloves when moving from a contaminated body site to a clean body site.
   d. Gloves need to cover your wrists.
5. Which statement is *false?*
   a. Gowns must cover you from your neck to your waist.
   b. A moist mask is contaminated.
   c. The outside of goggles is contaminated.
   d. You should wash your hands after removing a gown, mask, or goggles.

6. Which statement about PPE is *false?*
   a. Remove PPE when a garment becomes contaminated.
   b. Wear gloves when handling or touching contaminated items or surfaces.
   c. Wash or decontaminate disposable gloves for re-use.
   d. Remove PPE before leaving the work area.

Answers to these questions are on p. 516.

CHAPTER 17 BODY MECHANICS
Principles of Body Mechanics
- Your strongest and largest muscles are in the shoulders, upper arms, hips, and thighs. Use these muscles to lift and move persons and heavy objects.
- For good body mechanics:
  ○ Bend your knees and squat to lift a heavy object. Do not bend from your waist.
  ○ Hold items close to your body and base of support.
- Review Box 17-1, Rules for Body Mechanics, in the Textbook.

Work-Related Injuries
- **Work-related musculo-skeletal disorders (MSDs)** are injuries and disorders of the muscles, tendons, ligaments, joints, and cartilage.
- The Occupational Safety and Health Administration (OSHA) identifies MSD risk factors as:
  ○ Force: the amount of physical effort needed to perform a task.
  ○ Repeating action: doing the same motions or series of motions continually or frequently.
  ○ Awkward postures: assuming positions that place stress on the body.
  ○ Heavy lifting: manually lifting people who cannot lift themselves.
- According to the U.S. Department of Labor, nursing assistants are at the greatest risk of MSDs.
- Always report a work-related injury as soon as possible. Early attention can help prevent the problem from becoming worse. Review Box 17-2, Preventing Work-Related Injuries, in the Textbook.

Positioning the Person
- The person must be properly positioned at all times. Regular position changes and good alignment promote comfort and well-being. Breathing is easier. Circulation is promoted. Pressure ulcers and contractures are prevented.
- Whether in bed or in a chair, the person is re-positioned at least every 2 hours. To safely position a person:
  ○ Use good body mechanics.
  ○ Ask a co-worker to help you if needed.
  ○ Explain the procedure to the person.
  ○ Be gentle when moving the person.
  ○ Provide for privacy.
  ○ Use pillows as directed by the nurse for support and alignment.
  ○ Provide for comfort after positioning.
  ○ Place the call light within reach after positioning.
  ○ Complete a safety check before leaving the room.
- **Fowler's position** is a semi-sitting position. In **semi-Fowler's** position, the head of the bed is raised 30 degrees but some agencies define semi-Fowler's position as raising the head of the bed 30 degrees and the knee portion 15 degrees. In **high-Fowler's** position, the head of the bed is raised between 60 and 90 degrees.
- The **supine position (dorsal recumbent position)** is the back-lying position.
- A person in the **prone position** lies on the abdomen with the head turned to 1 side.
- A person in the **lateral position (side-lying position)** lies on 1 side or the other.
- The **Sims' position (semi-prone side position)** is a left side-lying position. The upper (right) leg is sharply flexed so it is not on the lower (left) leg. The lower (left) arm is behind the person.
- Persons who sit in chairs must hold their upper bodies and heads erect. For good alignment:
  ○ The person's back and buttocks are against the back of the chair.
  ○ Feet are flat on the floor or wheelchair footplates. Never leave feet unsupported.
  ○ Backs of the knees and calves are slightly away from the edge of the seat.

CHAPTER 17 REVIEW QUESTIONS
Circle the BEST answer.
1. To lift and move residents and heavy objects you should
   a. Use the muscles in your lower arms
   b. Use the muscles in your legs
   c. Use the muscles in your shoulders, upper arms, hips, and thighs
   d. Use the muscles in your abdomen
2. For good body mechanics, you should do all of the following *except*
   a. Bend your knees and squat to lift a heavy object
   b. Bend from your waist to lift a heavy object
   c. Hold items close to your body and base of support
   d. Bend your legs; do not bend your back
3. Which statement is *false?*
   a. A person must be properly positioned at all times.
   b. Regular position changes and good alignment promote comfort and well-being.
   c. Regular position changes and good alignment promote pressure ulcers and contractures.
   d. When a person is in good alignment, breathing is easier and circulation is promoted.
4. In high-Fowler's position
   a. The head of the bed is raised to 30 degrees
   b. The head of the bed is raised between 30 and 45 degrees
   c. The head of the bed is raised between 45 and 60 degrees
   d. The head of the bed is raised between 60 and 90 degrees

Answers to these questions are on p. 516.

CHAPTER 18 SAFELY MOVING THE PERSON

Preventing Work-Related Injuries

- Good body mechanics alone will not prevent injury. The Occupational Safety and Health Administration (OSHA) recommends
  - Minimizing manual lifting in all cases.
  - Eliminating manual lifting whenever possible.
  - Getting help from other staff.
- Careful planning is needed to move the person safely. You must know the person's functional status, the number of staff needed, what procedure to use, and the equipment needed.

Protecting the Skin

- Protect the person's skin from friction and shearing. Both cause infection and pressure ulcers. To reduce friction and shearing:
  - Roll the person.
  - Use friction-reducing devices such as a lift sheet (turning sheet), turning pads, and slide sheets.

Moving Persons in Bed

- Know how much help and what equipment or friction-reducing devices are needed.
- Review Box 18-2, Guidelines for Moving Persons in Bed, in the Textbook.

Raising the Person's Head and Shoulders

- You can raise the person's head and shoulders easily and safely by locking arms with the person (do not pull on the person's arm or shoulder).
- Have help with older persons and with those who are heavy or hard to move.

Moving the Person Up in Bed

- You can sometimes move light-weight adults up in bed alone if they can assist using a trapeze.
- Two or more staff members are needed to move heavy, weak, and very old persons up in bed. Always protect the person and yourself from injury.

Moving the Person Up in Bed With an Assist Device

- Assist devices are used to reduce shearing and friction. Such assist devices include a drawsheet (lift sheet), flat sheet folded in half, turning pad, slide sheet, and large incontinence product.
- Assist devices are used to move most patients and residents and at least 2 staff members are needed to position and use the assist device.
- Moving the person to the side of the bed can be done alone if the person is small enough. You move the person in segments by placing your hands and arms underneath the person. Move the upper body first (while supporting the person's neck), then the lower body, and finally the legs and feet.

Turning Persons

- Turning persons onto their sides helps prevent complications from bedrest. Certain procedures and care measures also require the side-lying position. After the person is turned, position him or her in good alignment. Use pillows as directed to support the person in the side-lying position.
- **Logrolling** is turning the person as a unit, in alignment, with 1 motion. The spine is kept straight.

Sitting on the Side of the Bed (Dangling)

- Many persons become dizzy or faint when getting out of bed too fast. They may need to sit on the side of the bed for 1 to 5 minutes before walking or transferring. Some persons increase activity in stages—bedrest, to sitting on the side of the bed, to sitting in a chair, to walking.
- While dangling, the person coughs and deep breathes. He or she moves the legs back and forth in circles to stimulate circulation. Provide for warmth during dangling.
- If dizziness or faintness occurs, lay the person down.

Re-Positioning in a Chair or Wheelchair

- Some persons slide down into the chair. For good alignment and safety, the person's back and buttocks must be against the back of the chair.
- Follow the nurse's directions and the care plan for the best way to re-position a person in a chair or wheelchair. Do not pull the person from behind the chair or wheelchair.
- If the chair reclines, have a co-worker assist, recline the chair, put an assist device under the person, and use the assist device to move the person up.
- If the person is in a wheelchair and has strength to assist, lock the wheels of the wheelchair and move the foot rests to the sides. Position a transfer belt around the person, stand in front of the person, and grasp the transfer belt with both hands. Ask the person to push with his or her feet and arms on the count of 3 and move the person back into the wheelchair while the person pushes with his or her feet and arms.

CHAPTER 18 REVIEW QUESTIONS

Circle the BEST answer.

1. Friction and shearing are reduced by doing all the following *except*
   a. Rolling the person
   b. Using a lift sheet or turning pad
   c. Using a pillow
   d. Using a slide board or slide sheet
2. After a person is turned, you must position him or her in good alignment.
   a. True
   b. False
3. Which statement about dangling is *false*?
   a. Many older persons become dizzy or faint when they first dangle.
   b. The person should cough and deep breathe while dangling.

c. The person moves his or her legs before dangling.
d. You should cover the person's shoulders with a robe or blanket while dangling.

Answers to these questions are on p. 516.

CHAPTER 19 SAFELY TRANSFERRING THE PERSON

- A transfer is how a person safely moves to and from surfaces—bed, chair, wheelchair, toilet, or standing position.
- The amount of help needed and the method used vary with the person's ability.

Wheelchair and Stretcher Safety

- Wheelchairs are used for persons who cannot walk or who have severe problems walking. Stretchers are used to transfer persons who are seriously ill, cannot sit up, or must stay in a lying position from 1 area to another.
- Review Box 19-2, Wheelchair and Stretcher Safety, in the Textbook.

Stand and Pivot Transfers

- Some persons are able to stand and pivot (move one's body from a set standing position). Use this transfer if the person's legs are strong enough to bear weight and the person is cooperative and can follow directions and assist in the transfer.
- Transfer belts (gait belts) are used to support persons during transfers and to re-position persons in chairs and wheelchairs.
- Arrange the room so there is enough space for a safe transfer. Correct placement of the chair, wheelchair, or other device also is needed for a safe transfer.
- Have the person wear non-skid footwear for transfers.
- Lock the wheels of the bed, wheelchair, stretcher, or other assist device.
- The person must not put his or her arms around your neck when assisting the person to stand.
- After the transfer, position the person in good alignment.
- For bed to chair or wheelchair transfers, the strong side moves first. Help the person out of bed on his or her strong side. When transferring the person from the chair or wheelchair back to bed, the same rules apply. Help the person from the wheelchair to the bed on his or her strong side. If the person is weak on 1 side, position the chair or wheelchair so that the person's strong side is nearest the bed. The strong side moves first.
- Transferring the person to and from the toilet is often hard because bathrooms are small. If the wheelchair can fit in the bathroom, place it at a 90-degree angle to the toilet and use a sliding board or the stand and pivot transfer from the wheelchair to the toilet.

Lateral Transfers

- A lateral transfer moves a person between 2 horizontal surfaces, such as from a bed to a stretcher. The person slides from 1 surface to the other.
- Use friction-reducing devices to protect the skin from friction and shearing during lateral transfers.
- When moving a person from a bed to a stretcher, use a friction-reducing device and at least 2 or 3 staff members to assist. If the person weighs more than 200 pounds, a mechanical lift with supine sling, mechanical lateral device, or inflatable device is used.
- Persons who cannot help themselves are transferred with mechanical lifts. So are persons who are too heavy for the staff to transfer.
- Before using a mechanical lift, you must be trained in its use. The sling, straps, hooks, and chains must be in good repair. The person's weight must not exceed the lift's capacity. At least 2 staff members are needed. Always follow the manufacturer's instructions for using the lift.
- Falling from the lift is a common fear. To promote the person's mental comfort, always explain the procedure before you begin. Also show the person how the lift works.

CHAPTER 19 REVIEW QUESTIONS

Circle the BEST answer.

1. You are transferring a person from the bed to a wheelchair. Which statement is *false?*
   a. The person should wear non-skid footwear.
   b. The person may put his or her arms around your neck.
   c. You should use a gait/transfer belt.
   d. You should lock the wheelchair wheels.
2. A person has a weak left side and a strong right side. In transferring the person from the bed to the wheelchair, his or her strong (right) side moves first.
   a. True
   b. False
3. Before using a mechanical lift, you do all of the following *except*
   a. Check the sling, straps, and chains to ensure good repair
   b. Check the person's weight to be sure it does not exceed the lift's capacity
   c. Follow the manufacturer's instructions for using the lift
   d. Operate the lift without a co-worker

Answers to these questions are on p. 516.

CHAPTER 20 THE PERSON'S UNIT

- A person's unit is the personal space, furniture, and equipment provided for the person by the agency. The Omnibus Budget Reconciliation Act of 1987 (OBRA) requires that resident units be as personal and home-like as possible.
- Keep the person's room clean, neat, safe, and comfortable. Follow the rules in Box 20-1, Maintaining the Person's Unit, and Box 20-2, OBRA and CMS Requirements for Resident Rooms, in the Textbook.

Comfort

- Age, illness, and activity are factors that affect comfort.
- Temperature, ventilation, noise, odors, and lighting are factors that are controlled to meet the person's needs.

Temperature and Ventilation

- Older persons and those who are ill may need higher temperatures for comfort. Ventilation systems provide fresh air and move air within the room.
- To protect older and ill persons from drafts, make sure the person wears enough clothing, offer lap robes to cover the legs, provide blankets, cover the person with a bath blanket when providing care, and move the person from drafty areas.

Odors

- To reduce odors in nursing centers:
  - Empty, clean, and disinfect bedpans, urinals, commodes, and kidney basins promptly.
  - Check to make sure toilets are flushed.
  - Check incontinent people often.
  - Clean persons who are wet or soiled from urine, feces, vomitus, or wound drainage.
  - Change wet or soiled linens and clothing promptly.
  - Keep laundry containers closed.
  - Follow agency policy for wet or soiled linens and clothing.
  - Dispose of incontinence and ostomy products promptly.
  - Provide good hygiene to prevent body and breath odors.
  - Use room deodorizers as needed and as allowed by agency policy.
- If you smoke, practice hand-washing after handling smoking materials and before giving care. Give careful attention to your uniforms, hair, and breath because of smoke odors.

Noise

- To decrease noise:
  - Control your voice.
  - Handle equipment carefully.
  - Keep equipment in good working order.
  - Answer phones, call lights, and intercoms promptly.

Lighting

- Adjust lighting to meet the person's needs. Glares, shadows, and dull lighting can cause falls, headaches, and eyestrain. A bright room is cheerful. Dim light is better for relaxing and rest. Persons with poor vision need bright light. Always keep light controls within the person's reach.

Room Furniture and Equipment

- Rooms are furnished and equipped to meet basic needs.

The Bed

- Beds are raised horizontally to give care. This reduces bending and reaching.
- Bed wheels are locked at all times except when moving the bed.
- Use bed rails as the nurse and care plan direct.
- Basic bed positions:
  - *Flat*—the usual sleeping position.
  - *Fowler's position*—a semi-sitting position. The head of the bed is raised between 45 and 60 degrees.
  - *High-Fowler's position*—a semi-sitting position. The head of the bed is raised 60 to 90 degrees.
  - *Semi-Fowler's position*—the head of the bed is raised 30 degrees. Some agencies define semi-Fowler's position as when the head of the bed is raised 30 degrees and the knee portion is raised 15 degrees. Know the definition used by your agency.
  - *Trendelenburg's position*—the head of the bed is lowered and the foot of the bed is raised. A doctor orders the position.
  - *Reverse Trendelenburg's position*—the head of the bed is raised and the foot of the bed is lowered. A doctor orders the position.

Bed Safety

- *Entrapment* means the person can get caught, trapped, or entangled in spaces created by bed rails, the mattress, the bed frame, or the head-board and foot-board. Serious injuries and deaths have occurred from entrapment. If a person is at risk for entrapment, report your concerns to the nurse at once. If a person is caught, trapped, or entangled, try to release the person. Call for the nurse at once.

The Over-Bed Table

- Only clean and sterile items are placed on the table. Never place bedpans, urinals, or soiled linens on the over-bed table or on top of the bedside stand.
- Clean the table and bedside stand after using them for a work surface and before serving meal trays.

Privacy Curtains

- Always pull the curtain completely around the bed before giving care. Privacy curtains do not block sound or conversations.

The Call System

- The call light must always be kept within the person's reach—in the room, bathroom, and shower or tub room. You must:
  - Place the call light on the person's strong side.
  - Remind the person to signal when help is needed.
  - Answer call lights promptly.
  - Answer bathroom and shower or tub room call lights at once.
- Persons with limited hand mobility may need special communication measures.
- Be careful when using the intercom. Remember confidentiality. Persons nearby can hear what you and the person say.

The Bathroom

- Grab bars are by the toilet so persons can use them to get on and off the toilet.
- Some toilet seats are raised to make transfers easier and for persons with joint problems.
- A call light or button is within reach of the toilet if the person needs assistance.

Closet and Drawer Space

- The person must have free access to the closet and its contents. You must have the person's permission to open or search closets or drawers.
- Agency staff can inspect a person's closet or drawers if hoarding is suspected. The person is informed of the inspection and is present when it takes place. Have a co-worker present when you inspect a person's closet.

CHAPTER 20 REVIEW QUESTIONS

Circle the BEST answer.

1. Serious injuries and death have occurred from entrapment.
    a. True
    b. False
2. You should never place bedpans, urinals, or soiled linens on the over-bed table.
    a. True
    b. False
3. You should clean the bedside stand if you use it for a work surface.
    a. True
    b. False
4. The following protect a person from drafts *except*
    a. Wearing enough clothing
    b. Lap robes
    c. Using a sheet when giving care
    d. Providing blankets
5. To reduce odors, you do the following *except*
    a. Empty bedpans and commodes promptly
    b. Keep laundry containers open
    c. Check to make sure toilets are flushed
    d. Clean persons who are wet or soiled from urine or feces
6. Which statement about the call light is *false?*
    a. The call light must always be within the person's reach.
    b. Place the call light on the person's strong side.
    c. You have to answer the call lights only for residents assigned to you.
    d. Answer call lights promptly.
7. You suspect a person is hoarding food in her closet. Before you inspect the closet, what do you do?
    a. Tell another nursing assistant what you suspect.
    b. Inspect the closet without telling the resident.
    c. Tell the family.
    d. Ask the resident if you can inspect the closet.

Answers to these questions are on p. 516.

CHAPTER 21 BEDMAKING

- Clean, dry, and wrinkle-free linens promote comfort. Skin breakdown and pressure ulcers are prevented.
- To keep beds neat and clean:
    ○ Change linens whenever they become wet, soiled, or damp.
    ○ Straighten linens whenever loose or wrinkled and at bedtime.
    ○ Check for and remove food and crumbs after meals and snacks.
    ○ Check linens for dentures, eyeglasses, hearing aids, sharp objects, and other items.
    ○ Follow Standard Precautions and the Bloodborne Pathogen Standard.

Types of Beds

- Beds are made in these ways.
    ○ A closed bed is not in use or the bed is ready for a new resident. Top linens are not folded back.
    ○ An open bed is in use. Top linens are fan-folded back so the person can get into bed. A closed bed becomes an open bed by fan-folding back the top linens.
    ○ An occupied bed is made with the person in it.
    ○ A surgical bed is made to transfer a person from a stretcher. This bed is also made for persons who arrive by ambulance.

Linens

- When handling linens and making beds:
    ○ Practice medical asepsis.
    ○ Always hold linens away from your body and uniform. Your uniform is considered dirty.
    ○ Never shake linens.
    ○ Place clean linens on a clean surface.
    ○ Never put clean or used linens on the floor.
- Collect enough linens. Do not bring unneeded linens to the person's room. Once in the room, extra linens are considered contaminated. They cannot be used for another person.
- Roll each piece of used linens away from you. The side that touched the person is inside the roll and away from you.

Making Beds

- When making beds, safety and medical asepsis are important. Use good body mechanics. Follow the rules for safe resident handling, moving, and transfers. Practice hand hygiene before handling clean linens and after handling used linens. To save time and energy, make beds with a co-worker.
- Review Box 21-1, Rules for Bedmaking, in the Textbook.
- Closed beds are made for nursing center residents who are up and away from the bed for all or most of the day. Change linens as needed. For beds awaiting new residents or patients, the entire bed requires clean linens after the bed system has been cleaned and disinfected.
- The closed bed becomes an open bed by fan-folding back the top linens so the person can get into bed with ease.
- An occupied bed is made while the person stays in bed. Keep the person in good alignment. Follow restrictions or limits in the person's movement or position. Explain each procedure step to the person before it is done. This is important even if the person cannot respond to you.

CHAPTER 21 REVIEW QUESTIONS

Circle the BEST answer.

1. Once in the person's room, extra linens are considered contaminated. They can be used for another person.
    a. True
    b. False
2. Roll each piece of used linens away from you. The side that touched the person is inside the roll.
    a. True
    b. False
3. Wear gloves when removing linens from the person's bed.
    a. True
    b. False

4. To keep beds neat and clean, do the following *except*
   a. Straighten linens whenever loose or wrinkled
   b. Check for and remove food and crumbs after meals
   c. Check linens for dentures, eyeglasses, and hearing aids
   d. Change linens monthly
5. Which statement is *false*?
   a. Practice medical asepsis when handling linens.
   b. Always hold linens away from your body and uniform.
   c. Shake linens to remove crumbs.
   d. Put used linens in the used laundry bin.

Answers to these questions are on p. 516.

CHAPTER 22 PERSONAL HYGIENE
- Besides cleansing, good hygiene prevents body and breath odors. It is relaxing and increases circulation.
- Culture and personal choice affect hygiene.

Daily Care
- Most people have hygiene routines and habits. Hygiene measures are often done before and after meals and at bedtime. You assist with hygiene whenever it is needed. Protect the person's right to privacy and to personal choice.

Oral Hygiene
- Oral hygiene keeps the mouth and teeth clean. It prevents mouth odors and infections, increases comfort, and makes food taste better. Mouth care also reduces the risk for cavities and periodontal disease.
- Assist with oral hygiene after sleep, after meals, and at bedtime. Follow the care plan.
- Follow Standard Precautions and the Bloodborne Pathogen Standard.
- Report and record:
  - Dry, cracked, swollen, or blistered lips
  - Mouth or breath odor
  - Redness, swelling, irritation, sores, or white patches in the mouth or on the tongue
  - Bleeding, swelling, or redness of the gums
  - Loose teeth
  - Rough, sharp, or chipped areas on dentures

Brushing and Flossing Teeth
- Flossing removes plaque and tartar from the teeth as well as food from between the teeth. Flossing is usually done after brushing. If done once a day, bedtime is the best time to floss.
- Some persons need help gathering and setting up equipment for oral hygiene. You may have to perform oral care for persons who are weak, cannot move their arms, or are too confused to brush their teeth.

Mouth Care for the Unconscious Person
- Unconscious persons have dry mouths and crusting on the tongue and mucous membranes. Oral hygiene keeps the mouth clean and moist. It also helps prevent infection.

- Use sponge swabs to apply the cleaning agent. To prevent cracking of the lips, apply a lubricant to the lips. Check the care plan.
- To prevent aspiration on the unconscious person:
  - Position the person on 1 side with the head turned well to the side.
  - Use only a small amount of fluid to clean the mouth.
  - Do not insert dentures. Dentures are not worn when the person is unconscious.
- When giving oral hygiene, keep the person's mouth open with a padded tongue blade.
- Mouth care is given at least every 2 hours. Follow the nurse's direction and the care plan.

Denture Care
- Mouth care is given and dentures are cleaned as often as natural teeth. Dentures are usually removed at bedtime. Some persons remove dentures at meal time. Remind people not to wrap dentures in tissues or napkins at meal time, as they could be discarded accidentally.
- Dentures are slippery when wet. Hold them firmly. During cleaning, hold them over a basin of water lined with a towel. Use a cleaning agent and follow the manufacturer's instructions.
- Hot water causes dentures to lose their shape. If dentures are not worn after cleaning, store them in a container with cool water or a denture soaking solution.
- Label the denture cup with the person's name, room number, and bed number. Report lost or damaged dentures to the nurse at once. Losing or damaging dentures is negligent conduct.
- Many people do not like being seen without their dentures. Privacy is important. If you clean dentures, return them to the person as quickly as possible.
- Persons with partial dentures have some natural teeth. They need to brush and floss the natural teeth.

Bathing
- Bathing cleans the skin. The mucous membranes of the genital and anal areas are cleaned as well. A bath is refreshing and relaxing. Circulation is stimulated and body parts exercised. You have time to talk to the person and make observations.
- Review Box 22-2, Rules for Bathing, in the Textbook.
- Soap dries the skin. Therefore older persons usually need a complete bath or shower twice a week. Partial baths are taken the other days. Some bathe daily but not with soap. Thorough rinsing is needed when using soap. Lotions and oils keep the skin soft.
- Water temperature for complete bed baths and partial bed baths is between 110°F and 115°F. Older persons have fragile skin and need lower water temperatures. Measure water temperature according to agency policy.
- Report and record:
  - The color of the skin, lips, nail beds, and sclera (whites of the eyes)
  - If the skin appears pale, grayish, yellow (jaundice), or bluish (cyanotic)
  - The location and description of rashes
  - Skin texture—smooth, rough, scaly, flaky, dry, moist

- ○ Diaphoresis—profuse (excessive) sweating
- ○ Bruises or open areas
- ○ Pale or reddened areas, particularly over bony parts
- ○ Drainage or bleeding from wounds or body openings
- ○ Swelling of the feet and legs
- ○ Corns or calluses on the feet
- ○ Skin temperature
- ○ Complaints of pain or discomfort
- Use caution when applying powders. Do not use powders near persons with respiratory disorders. Do not sprinkle or shake powder onto the person. To safely apply powder:
  - ○ Turn away from the person.
  - ○ Sprinkle a small amount onto your hands or a cloth.
  - ○ Apply the powder in a thin layer.
  - ○ Make sure powder does not get on the floor. Powder is slippery and can cause falls.

The Complete Bed Bath

- The complete bed bath involves washing the person's entire body in bed. Wash around the person's eyes with water. Do not use soap. Gently wipe from the inner to the outer aspect of the eye. Use a clean part of the washcloth for each stroke. Ask the person if you should use soap to wash the face. Let the person wash the genital area if he or she is able.
- Give a back massage after the bath. Apply deodorant or antiperspirant, lotion, and powder as requested. Comb and brush the hair. Empty and clean the wash basin.

The Partial Bath

- The partial bath involves bathing the face, hands, axillae (underarms), back, buttocks, and perineal area. You assist the person as needed. Most need help washing the back.

Tub Baths and Showers

- Falls, burns, and chilling from water are risks. Review Box 22-2, Rules for Bathing, and 22-3, Tub Bath and Shower Safety, in the Textbook.
- A tub bath can cause a person to feel faint, weak, or tired. The person may need a transfer bench, a tub with a side entry door, a wheelchair or stretcher lift, or a mechanical lift to get in and out of the tub.
- Some people can use a regular shower. Have the person use the grab bars for support during the shower. Use a bath mat if the shower does not have non-skid surfaces. Never let weak or unsteady persons stand in the shower. They may need to use shower chairs, shower stalls or cabinets, or shower trolleys. Some shower rooms have 2 or more stations. Protect the person's privacy. Properly screen and cover the person.
- Water temperature for tub baths and showers is usually 105°F. Report and record dizziness and light-headedness.
- Clean and disinfect the tub or shower before and after use.

Perineal Care

- Perineal care involves cleaning the genital and anal areas. It is done daily during the bath and whenever the area is soiled with urine or feces. The person does perineal care if able.
- *Perineal* and *perineum* are not common terms. Most people understand *privates*, *private parts*, *crotch*, *genitals*, or *the area between the legs*. Use terms the person understands.
- Standard Precautions, medical asepsis, and the Bloodborne Pathogen Standard are followed.
- Work from the cleanest area to the dirtiest—commonly called cleaning from "front to back." On a woman, clean from the urethra (cleanest) to the anal (dirtiest) area. On a male, start at the meatus of the urethra and work outward.
- Use warm water. Use washcloths, towelettes, cotton balls, or swabs according to agency policy. Rinse thoroughly. Pat dry. Water temperature is usually 105°F to 109°F.
- Report and record:
  - ○ Bleeding, redness, swelling, irritation, discharge
  - ○ Complaints of pain, burning, or other discomfort
  - ○ Signs of urinary or fecal incontinence
  - ○ Signs of skin breakdown
  - ○ Odors

CHAPTER 22 REVIEW QUESTIONS

Circle the BEST answer.

1. Oral hygiene does the following *except*
   a. Keep the mouth and teeth clean
   b. Prevent mouth odors and infections
   c. Decrease comfort
   d. Make food taste better
2. When giving oral hygiene, you should report and record the following *except*
   a. Dry, cracked, swollen, or blistered lips
   b. Redness, sores, or white patches in the mouth
   c. Bleeding, swelling, or redness of the gums
   d. The number of fillings a person has
3. A person is unconscious. When you do mouth care, you do the following *except*
   a. Use only a small amount of fluid to clean the mouth
   b. Use your fingers to keep the mouth open
   c. Explain what you are doing
   d. Give mouth care at least every 2 hours
4. Which statement about dentures is *false?*
   a. Dentures are slippery when wet.
   b. During cleaning, hold dentures over a basin of water lined with a towel.
   c. Store dentures in cool water.
   d. Remind people to wrap their dentures in tissues or napkins.
5. Bathing does the following *except*
   a. Cleanses the skin
   b. Stimulates circulation
   c. Makes a person tense
   d. Permits you to observe the person's skin
6. The water temperature for a complete bed bath is
   a. 102°F to 108°F
   b. 110°F to 115°F
   c. 115°F to 120°F
   d. 120°F to 125°F

7. Which statement is *false*?
   a. Use powder near persons with respiratory disorders.
   b. Before applying powder, check with the nurse and the care plan.
   c. Before applying powder, sprinkle a small amount of powder onto your hands.
   d. Apply powder in a thin layer.
8. When washing a person's eyes, you should do the following *except*
   a. Use only water
   b. Gently wipe from the inner to the outer aspect of the eye
   c. Gently wipe from the outer to the inner aspect of the eye
   d. Use a clean part of the washcloth for each stroke
9. When giving female perineal care, you should work from the urethra to the anal area.
   a. True
   b. False
10. When giving male perineal care, start at the meatus and work outward.
    a. True
    b. False

Answers to these questions are on p. 516.

CHAPTER 23 GROOMING
- Hair care, shaving, nail and foot care, and clean garments prevent infection and promote comfort. They also affect love, belonging, and self-esteem needs.

Hair Care
- You assist patients and residents with brushing and combing hair and with shampooing as needed and according to the care plan. The nursing process reflects the person's culture, personal choice, skin and scalp condition, health history, and self-care ability.

Brushing and Combing Hair
- Encourage residents to brush and comb their own hair but assist as needed.
- Daily brushing and combing prevent tangled and matted hair.
- When brushing and combing hair, start at the scalp and brush or comb to the hair ends.
- Never cut hair for any reason.
- Special measures are needed for curly, coarse, and dry hair. Check the care plan.
- When giving hair care, place a towel across the person's back and shoulders to protect garments from falling hair. If the person is in bed, give hair care before changing the linens and pillowcase.

Shampooing
- Shampooing frequency depends on the person's needs and preferences.
- Keep shampoo away from and out of eyes. Have the person hold a washcloth over the eyes.
- Wear gloves if the person has scalp sores.
- Follow Standard Precautions and the Bloodborne Pathogen Standard.
- Water temperature is usually 105°F.
- Hair is dried and styled as soon as possible after the shampooing.
- During shampooing, report and record:
  - Scalp sores
  - Flaking
  - Itching
  - Presence of nits or lice
  - Patches of hair loss
  - Hair falling out in patches
  - Very dry or very oily hair
  - Matted or tangled hair
  - How the person tolerated the procedure

Shaving
- Many men shave for comfort and well-being. Many women shave their underarms and legs.
- Electric shaver or safety razors are used. Some persons have their own shavers. Do not use safety razors on persons with healing problems or persons taking anticoagulant drugs. Older persons with wrinkled skin are at risk for nicks and cuts. Safety razors are not used to shave them or persons with dementia.
- Wash and comb mustaches and beards daily and as needed. Ask the person how to groom his mustache or beard. Never trim a mustache or beard without the person's consent.
- Many women shave their legs and underarms. This practice varies among cultures. Legs and underarms are shaved after bathing when the skin is soft.
- Review Box 23-1, Rules for Shaving, in the Textbook.

Nail and Foot Care
- Nail and foot care prevent infection, injury, and odors.
- Nails are easier to trim and clean right after soaking or bathing.
- Use nail clippers to cut fingernails. Never use scissors. Use extreme caution to prevent damage to nearby tissues.
- Some agencies do not let nursing assistants cut or trim toenails. Follow agency policy.
- Follow Standard Precautions and the Bloodborne Pathogen Standard.
- Report and record:
  - Dry, reddened, irritated, or callused areas
  - Breaks in the skin
  - Corns on top of and between the toes
  - Blisters
  - Very thick nails
  - Loose nails
- You do not cut or trim toenails if a person has diabetes or poor circulation to the legs and feet or takes drugs that affect blood clotting. Also, do not cut or trim toenails if the person has very thick nails or ingrown toenails. The nurse or podiatrist cuts toenails and provides foot care for these persons.
- When doing foot care, check between the toes for cracks and sores. If left untreated, a serious infection could occur.

- The feet of persons with decreased sensation or circulatory problems may easily burn because they do not feel hot temperatures.
- After soaking, apply lotion to the feet. Because the lotion can cause slippery feet, help the person put on non-skid footwear before you transfer the person or let the person walk.

Changing Garments

- Garments are changed after the bath and whenever wet or soiled.
- When changing clothing:
  - Provide for privacy.
  - Encourage the person to do as much as possible.
  - Let the person choose what to wear. Make sure the right under-garments are chosen.
  - Make sure garments and footwear are the correct size.
  - Remove clothing from the strong or "good" (unaffected) side first.
  - Put clothing on the weak (affected) side first.
  - Support the arm or leg when removing or putting on a garment.
  - Move or handle the body gently. Do not force a joint beyond its range of motion or to the point of pain.
- When changing gowns, remove the gown from the strong arm first while supporting the weak arm. Put a clean gown on the weak arm first and then the strong arm.
- To change the gown of a person with an intravenous (IV) bag, gather the sleeve of the arm with the IV bag and slide it over the IV site and tubing. Remove the IV bag, draw it through the sleeve, and re-hang the IV bag. Gather the sleeve of the clean gown, remove the IV bag, slide the sleeve over the IV bag, then re-hang the bag. Slide the sleeve over the tubing, hand, arm, and IV site. Do not pull on the tubing.
- Have the nurse check the flow rate after changing the gown of a person with an IV. If the person is on an IV pump, do not change the gown.

CHAPTER 23 REVIEW QUESTIONS

Circle the BEST answer.

1. Hair care, shaving, and nail and foot care prevent infection and promote comfort.
   a. True
   b. False
2. If a person's hair is matted, you may cut the hair.
   a. True
   b. False
3. When giving hair care, place a towel across the person's back and shoulders to protect garments from falling hair.
   a. True
   b. False
4. You should wear gloves when shampooing a person who has scalp sores.
   a. True
   b. False

5. A person takes an anticoagulant. Therefore he shaves with a blade razor.
   a. True
   b. False
6. You should wear gloves when shaving a person with a safety razor.
   a. True
   b. False
7. Never trim a mustache or beard without the person's consent.
   a. True
   b. False
8. Mustaches and beards need daily care.
   a. True
   b. False
9. A person has diabetes. You can cut his or her toenails.
   a. True
   b. False
10. Fingernails are cut with
    a. Scissors
    b. Nail clippers
    c. An emery board
    d. A nail file
11. Which statement is *false*?
    a. Provide privacy when a person is changing clothes.
    b. Most residents wear street clothes during the day.
    c. Let the person choose what to wear.
    d. You may tear a person's clothing.

Answers to these questions are on p. 516.

CHAPTER 24 URINARY ELIMINATION

Normal Urination

- The healthy adult produces about 1500 milliliters (mL) of urine a day.
- The frequency of urination is affected by amount of fluid intake, habits, availability of toilet facilities, activity, work, and illness. People usually void at bedtime, after sleep, and before meals. Some people void every 2 to 3 hours. The need to void at night disturbs sleep. Some persons need help getting to the bathroom and others use bedpans, urinals, or commodes. Review Box 24-1, Rules for Normal Urination, in the Textbook.

Observations

- Observe urine for color, clarity, odor, amount, particles, and blood. Normal urine is pale yellow, straw-colored, or amber. It is clear with no particles. A faint odor is normal.
- Some foods and drugs affect urine color. Ask the nurse to observe urine that looks or smells abnormal.
- Report the following urinary problems.
  - **Dysuria**—painful or difficult urination
  - **Hematuria**—blood in the urine
  - **Nocturia**—frequent urination at night
  - **Oliguria**—scant amount of urine; less than 500 mL in 24 hours
  - **Polyuria**—abnormally large amounts of urine
  - **Urinary frequency**—voiding at frequent intervals

- ○ **Urinary incontinence**—involuntary loss or leakage of urine
  - ○ **Urinary urgency**—the need to void at once
- Follow Standard Precautions and the Bloodborne Pathogen Standard when handling bedpans, urinals, commodes, and their contents.
- Thoroughly clean and disinfect bedpans, urinals, and commodes after use.
- Men stand or sit at the side of the bed to use the urinal. Some men need support when standing.
- You may have to place and hold the urinal for some men. This may embarrass both the person and you. Act in a professional manner at all times.
- Remind men to hang urinals on bed rails and to signal after using them.
- Commodes are chairs or wheelchairs with an opening for a container. Persons unable to walk to the bathroom often use commodes.

Urinary Incontinence

- **Urinary incontinence** is the involuntary loss or leakage of urine.
- If urinary incontinence is a new problem, tell the nurse at once.
- Incontinence is embarrassing. Garments are wet and odors develop. Skin irritation, infection, and pressure ulcers are risks. The person's pride, dignity, and self-esteem are affected. Social isolation, loss of independence, and depression are common.
- Good skin care and dry garments and linens are essential. Promoting normal urinary elimination prevents incontinence in some people. Other people may need bladder training.
- Review Box 24-3, Nursing Measures for Urinary Incontinence, in the Textbook.
- Caring for persons with incontinence is stressful. Remember, the person does not choose to be incontinent. If you find yourself becoming short-tempered and impatient, talk to the nurse at once. Kindness, empathy, understanding, and patience are needed.

Applying Incontinence Products

- Incontinence products are used to keep the person dry. Most are disposable and only used once.
- Incontinence products include a complete incontinence brief, a pad and under-garment, pull-on underwear, or a belted under-garment. Follow the manufacturer's instructions for applying incontinence products.
- Observations to report and record:
  - ○ Complaints of pain, burning, irritation, or the need to void
  - ○ Signs and symptoms of skin breakdown, including redness, irritation, blisters, and complaints of pain, burning, itching, or tingling
  - ○ The amount of urine and urine color
  - ○ Blood in the urine
  - ○ Leakage or a poor product fit
- Review Box 24-4, Applying Incontinence Products, in the Textbook.

Bladder Training

- Bladder training helps some persons with urinary incontinence. Control of urination is the goal. Bladder control promotes comfort and quality of life. It also increases self-esteem.
- You assist with bladder training as directed by the nurse and the care plan. The care plan may include one of the following: bladder rehabilitation, prompted voiding, habit training/scheduled voiding, or catheter clamping.

CHAPTER 24 REVIEW QUESTIONS

Circle the BEST answer.
1. Which statement is *false?*
   a. Normal urine is yellow, straw-colored, or amber.
   b. Urine with a strong odor is normal.
   c. A person normally voids 1500 mL a day.
   d. Observe urine for color, clarity, odor, amount, and particles.
2. Which observation does *not* need to be reported to the nurse promptly?
   a. Complaints of urgency
   b. Burning on urination
   c. Painful or difficult urination
   d. Clear amber urine
3. Which statement is *false?*
   a. Incontinence is embarrassing.
   b. Caring for persons with incontinence may be stressful.
   c. Incontinence is a personal choice.
   d. Be kind and patient to persons who are incontinent.
4. A person with a catheter complains of pain. You should notify the nurse at once.
   a. True
   b. False
5. The goal of bladder training is to
   a. Allow the person to use the toilet
   b. Keep the catheter
   c. Gain control of urination
   d. Decrease self-esteem

Answers to these questions are on p. 516.

CHAPTER 25 URINARY CATHETERS

- A catheter is a tube used to drain or inject fluid through a body opening. A urinary catheter is inserted through the urethra into the bladder and is used to drain urine.
- The types of catheters are a **straight catheter,** which is used to drain the urine and then removed, and an **indwelling catheter (retention or Foley catheter),** which is left in the bladder and drains urine constantly into a drainage bag.

Catheter Care

- The risk of a urinary tract infection (UTI) is high. Review Box 25-1, Indwelling Catheter Care, in the Textbook.
- The catheter must not pull at the insertion site. Hold the catheter securely during catheter care. Then properly secure the catheter. Also make sure the tubing is not under the person. Besides obstructing urine flow, lying

on the tubing is uncomfortable. It can also cause skin breakdown.
- Follow Standard Precautions and the Bloodborne Pathogen Standard.
- Report and record:
  - Complaints of pain, burning, irritation, or the need to void (report at once)
  - Crusting, abnormal drainage, or secretions
  - The color, clarity, and odor of urine
  - Particles in the urine
  - Blood in the urine
  - Cloudy urine
  - Urine leaking at the insertion site
  - Drainage system leaks

Urine Drainage Systems

- A closed urinary drainage system is used for indwelling catheters. Infections can occur if microbes enter the drainage system. The two types of drainage bags are standard drainage bags and leg bags.
- The standard drainage bag hangs from the bed frame, chair, or wheelchair. It must not touch the floor. The bag is always kept lower than the person's bladder. Do not hang the drainage bag on a bed rail.
- If the drainage system is disconnected accidentally, tell the nurse at once. Do not touch the ends of the catheter or tubing. Do the following:
  - Practice hand hygiene. Put on gloves.
  - Wipe the end of the drainage tube with an antiseptic wipe.
  - Wipe the end of the catheter with another antiseptic wipe.
  - Do not put the ends down. Do not touch the ends after you clean them.
  - Connect the drainage tubing to the catheter.
  - Discard the wipes into a biohazard bag.
  - Remove the gloves. Practice hand hygiene.
- Check with the nurse and care plan about when to empty and measure the urine in the drainage bag. Follow Standard Precautions and the Bloodborne Pathogen Standard.
- A leg bag is a drainage system that attaches to the thigh or calf. Empty and measure a leg bag when it is half full.
- Report and record:
  - The amount of urine measured
  - The color, clarity, and odor of urine
  - Particles in the urine
  - Blood in the urine
  - Cloudy urine
  - Complaints of pain, burning, irritation, or the need to urinate
  - Drainage system leaks

Removing Indwelling Catheters

- Before removing an indwelling catheter, be sure that your state allows you to perform this procedure, the procedure is in your job description, you know how to use the supplies and equipment, and you review the procedure with the nurse.

- The balloon of an indwelling catheter is inflated with water injected with a syringe. A syringe is also used to remove the water. Before removing the indwelling catheter, learn the size of the balloon before deflating it. If the balloon is 5 mL in size, you must withdraw 5 mL of water with the syringe. Do not remove the catheter if water remains in the balloon. Call the nurse.
- Report and record the following observations.
  - The amount of urine in the drainage bag
  - The color, clarity, and odor of urine
  - Particles in the urine
  - Blood in the urine
  - How the person tolerated the procedure
  - Complaints of pain, burning, irritation, or the need to void

Condom Catheters

- Condom catheters are often used for incontinent men. They are also called external catheters, Texas catheters, and urinary sheaths.
- These catheters are changed daily after perineal care.
- To apply a condom catheter, follow the manufacturer's instructions. Thoroughly wash and dry the penis before applying the catheter.
- Some condom catheters are self-adhering. Other catheters are secured in place with elastic tape in a spiral manner. Never use adhesive tape to secure catheters. It does not expand. Blood flow to the penis is cut off, injuring the penis.
- When removing or applying a condom catheter, report and record the following observations.
  - Reddened or open areas on the penis
  - Swelling of the penis
  - Color, clarity, and odor of urine
  - Particles in the urine
  - Blood in the urine
  - Cloudy urine
- Do not apply a condom catheter if the penis is red, is irritated, or shows signs of skin breakdown. Report your observations to the nurse at once.

CHAPTER 25 REVIEW QUESTIONS

Circle the BEST answer.
1. Which statement is *false?*
   a. The urine drainage system should hang from the bed frame or chair.
   b. The urine drainage system should hang on a bed rail.
   c. The urine drainage system must be off the floor.
   d. The urine drainage system must be kept lower than the person's bladder.
2. If the drainage system becomes accidentally disconnected, you need to
   a. Call the nurse
   b. Put on gloves and use antiseptic wipes to clean the ends of the tubing
   c. Pub on gloves and clamp the tubing
   d. Put the ends of the tubing on paper towels

3. Before removing an indwelling catheter, what do you do first?
   a. Tug on the catheter to see if it will come out.
   b. Wipe the meatus with an antiseptic wipe.
   c. Drain the balloon with a syringe.
   d. Check the balloon size.
4. Which statement is *false*?
   a. Condom catheters are changed daily.
   b. Follow the manufacturer's instructions when applying a condom catheter.
   c. Use adhesive tape to secure a condom catheter in place.
   d. Report and record open or reddened areas on the penis at once.

Answers to these questions are on p. 516.

CHAPTER 26 BOWEL ELIMINATION
Normal Bowel Elimination

- Stools are normally brown, soft, formed, moist, and shaped like the rectum. They have a normal odor caused by bacterial action in the intestines. Certain foods and drugs cause odors.
- Carefully observe stools before disposing of them. Observe and report the color, amount, consistency, odor, and shape of stools. Also observe and report the presence of blood or mucus, the time the person had the bowel movement (BM), the frequency of BMs, and any complaints of pain or discomfort.

Factors Affecting Bowel Elimination

- *Privacy.* Bowel elimination is a private act.
- *Habits.* Many people have a BM after breakfast. Some read. Defecation is easier when a person is relaxed.
- *Diet—high-fiber foods.* Fiber helps prevent constipation.
- *Diet—other foods.* Some foods cause constipation. Other foods cause frequent stools or diarrhea.
- *Fluids.* Drinking 6 to 8 glasses of water daily promotes normal bowel elimination. Warm fluids—coffee, tea, hot cider, warm water—increase peristalsis.
- *Activity.* Exercise and activity maintain muscle tone and stimulate peristalsis.
- *Drugs.* Drugs can prevent constipation or control diarrhea. Some have diarrhea or constipation as side effects.
- *Disability.* Some people cannot control BMs. A bowel training program is needed.
- *Aging.* Older persons are at risk for constipation. Some older persons lose bowel control and have fecal incontinence.
- To provide comfort and safety during bowel elimination, review Box 26-1, Safety and Comfort During Bowel Elimination, in the Textbook. Follow Standard Precautions and the Bloodborne Pathogen Standard.

Common Problems

- Common problems include constipation, fecal impaction, diarrhea, fecal incontinence, and flatulence.
- **Constipation** is the passage of a hard, dry stool.

- Common causes of constipation are a low-fiber diet and ignoring the urge to defecate. Other causes include decreased fluid intake, inactivity, drugs, aging, and certain diseases.
- Dietary changes, fluids, and activity prevent or relieve constipation. So do stool softeners, laxatives, suppositories, and enemas.
- A **fecal impaction** is the prolonged retention and buildup of feces in the rectum.
- Fecal impaction results if constipation is not relieved. The person cannot defecate. Liquid feces pass around the hardened fecal mass in the rectum. The liquid feces seep from the anus.
- Abdominal discomfort, abdominal distention, nausea, cramping, and rectal pain are common. Older persons have poor appetite or confusion. Some persons have a fever. Report these signs and symptoms to the nurse.
- Checking for and removing a fecal impaction can be dangerous, because the vagus nerve can be stimulated, resulting in a slowing of the heart rate. Check with your state and agency policies to determine if you may perform this procedure.
- **Diarrhea** is the frequent passage of liquid stools.
- The need to have a BM is urgent. Some people cannot get to a bathroom in time. Abdominal cramping, nausea, and vomiting may occur.
- Assist with elimination needs promptly, dispose of stools promptly, and give good skin care. Liquid stools irritate the skin. So does frequent wiping with toilet paper. Skin breakdown and pressure ulcers are risks.
- Follow Standard Precautions and the Bloodborne Pathogen Standard when in contact with stools.
- Report signs of diarrhea at once. Ask the nurse to observe the stool.
- **Fecal incontinence** is the inability to control the passage of feces and gas through the anus.
- Fecal incontinence affects the person emotionally. Frustration, embarrassment, anger, and humiliation are common. The person may need:
  ○ Bowel training
  ○ Help with elimination after meals and every 2 to 3 hours
  ○ Incontinence products to keep garments and linens clean
  ○ Good skin care
- **Flatulence** is the excessive formation of gas or air in the stomach and intestines.
- Causes include swallowing air while eating and drinking and bacterial action in the intestines. Other causes may be gas-forming foods, constipation, bowel and abdominal surgeries, and drugs that decrease peristalsis.
- If flatus is not expelled, the intestines distend (swell or enlarge from the pressure of gases). Abdominal cramping or pain, shortness of breath, and a swollen abdomen occur. "Bloating" is a common complaint. Exercise, walking, moving in bed, and the left side-lying position often produce flatus. Enemas and drugs may be ordered.

Bowel Training

- Bowel training has 2 goals.
  - To gain control of BMs.
  - To develop a regular pattern of elimination. Fecal impactions, constipation, and fecal incontinence are prevented.
- Factors that promote elimination are part of the care plan and bowel training program.

Suppositories

- A suppository is a cone-shaped, solid drug that is inserted into a body opening. A rectal suppository is inserted into the rectum. Suppositories melt at body temperature.
- A BM occurs about 30 minutes after inserting a suppository.
- Check with your state and agency policies to determine if you can insert a suppository.

Enemas

- An **enema** is the introduction of fluid into the rectum and lower colon.
- Doctors order enemas to:
  - Remove feces.
  - Relieve constipation, fecal impaction, or flatulence.
  - Clean the bowel of feces before certain surgeries and diagnostic procedures.
- Review Box 26-2, Giving Enemas, in the Textbook.
- The preferred position for an enema is the Sims' or left side-lying position.
- A cleansing enema is used to clean the bowel of feces and flatus and to relieve constipation and fecal impaction. Cleansing enemas take effect in 10 to 20 minutes.
- A small-volume enema irritates the bowel and distends the rectum, causing a BM. The person should retain the enema solution until he or she needs to have a BM, which usually takes 5 to 10 minutes.
- An oil-retention enema relieves constipation and fecal impaction by softening the feces and lubricating the rectum so the feces can pass. The oil is retained for 30 minutes to 1 to 3 hours.

The Person With an Ostomy

- Sometimes part of the intestines is removed surgically. An ostomy is sometimes necessary. An **ostomy** is a surgically created opening for the elimination of body wastes. The opening is called a **stoma.** The person wears an ostomy pouch over the stoma to collect stools and flatus.
- Stools irritate the skin. Skin care prevents skin breakdown around the stoma. The skin is washed and dried. Then a skin barrier is applied around the stoma. It prevents stools from having contact with the skin. The skin barrier is part of the ostomy pouch or a separate device.
- The pouch has an adhesive backing that is applied to the skin. Sometimes pouches are secured to ostomy belts.

- The pouch is changed every 3 to 7 days and when it leaks. Frequent pouch changes can damage the skin.
- Many pouches have a drain at the bottom that closes with a clip, clamp, or wire closure. The drain is opened to empty the pouch. The drain is wiped with toilet tissue before it is closed.
- Observations to report and record include signs of skin breakdown, color, amount, consistency, and odor of stools, and complaints of pain or discomfort.

CHAPTER 26 REVIEW QUESTIONS

Circle the BEST answer.
1. Which statement is *false?*
   a. Lack of privacy can prevent defecation.
   b. Low-fiber foods promote defecation.
   c. Drinking 6 to 8 glasses of water daily promotes normal bowel elimination.
   d. Exercise stimulates peristalsis.
2. Which of the following does *not* prevent constipation?
   a. A high-fiber diet
   b. Increased fluid intake
   c. Exercise
   d. Ignoring the urge to defecate
3. A person has fecal incontinence. You should do the following *except*
   a. Be patient
   b. Help with elimination after meals
   c. Provide good skin care
   d. Scold the person for being incontinent
4. The preferred position for an enema is the
   a. Sims' position or the left side-lying position
   b. Prone position
   c. Supine position
   d. Trendelenburg's position

Answers to these questions are on p. 516.

CHAPTER 27 NUTRITION AND FLUIDS

- Food and water are necessary for life. A poor diet and poor eating habits:
  - Increase the risk for disease and infection.
  - Cause chronic illnesses to become worse.
  - Cause healing problems.
  - Increase the risk of accidents and injuries.

Basic Nutrition

- **Nutrition** is the process involved in the ingestion, digestion, absorption, and use of foods and fluids by the body. Good nutrition is needed for growth, healing, and body functions.
- A *nutrient* is a substance that is ingested, digested, absorbed, and used by the body.
- A *calorie* is the fuel or energy value of food.

Dietary Guidelines for Americans

- The Dietary Guidelines help people attain and maintain a healthy weight, reduce the risk of chronic disease, and promote overall health. The Dietary Guidelines focus on consuming fewer calories, making informed food choices, and being physically active.

MyPlate

- The MyPlate symbol, issued by the United States Department of Agriculture (USDA), helps you make wise food choices by balancing calories, increasing certain foods like fruits and vegetables, and reducing certain foods with excess salt and sugar.

Nutrients

- A well-balanced diet ensures an adequate intake of essential nutrients.
- *Protein*—is needed for tissue growth and repair. Sources include meat, fish, poultry, eggs, milk and milk products, cereals, beans, peas, and nuts.
- *Carbohydrates*—provide energy and fiber for bowel elimination. They are found in fruits, vegetables, breads, cereals, and sugar.
- *Fats*—provide energy, add flavor to food, and help the body use certain vitamins. Sources include meats, lard, butter, shortening, oils, milk, cheese, egg yolks, and nuts.
- *Vitamins*—are needed for certain body functions. The body stores vitamins A, D, E, and K. The vitamin C and the B complex vitamins are not stored and must be ingested daily.
- *Minerals*—are needed for bone and tooth formation, nerve and muscle function, fluid balance, and other body processes.
- *Water*—is needed for all body processes.
- Review Tables 27-2, Common Vitamins, and 27-3, Common Minerals, in the Textbook.

OBRA Dietary Requirements

- The Omnibus Budget Reconciliation Act of 1987 (OBRA) has requirements for food served in nursing centers.
  - Each person's nutritional and dietary needs are met.
  - The person's diet is well-balanced. It is nourishing and tastes good. Food is well-seasoned.
  - Food is appetizing. It has an appealing aroma and is attractive.
  - Hot food is served hot. Cold food is served cold.
  - Food is served promptly.
  - Food is prepared to meet each person's needs. Some people need food cut, ground, or chopped. Others have special diets ordered by the doctor.
  - Other foods are offered if the person refused the food served. Substituted food must have a similar nutritional value to the first foods served.
  - Each person receives at least 3 meals a day. A bedtime snack is offered.
  - The center provides needed adaptive equipment and utensils.

Factors Affecting Eating and Nutrition

- *Culture.* Culture influences dietary practices, food choices, and food preparation.
- *Religion.* Selecting, preparing, and eating food often involve religious practices. A person may follow all, some, or none of the dietary practices of his or her faith.
- *Finances.* People with limited incomes often buy the cheaper carbohydrate foods. Their diets often lack protein and certain vitamins and minerals.

- *Appetite.* Illness, drugs, anxiety, pain, and depression can cause loss of appetite. Unpleasant sights, thoughts, and smells are other causes.
- *Personal choice.* Food likes and dislikes are influenced by foods served in the home. Usually food likes expand with age and social experiences.
- *Body reactions.* People usually avoid foods that cause allergic reactions. They also avoid foods that cause nausea, vomiting, diarrhea, indigestion, gas, or headaches.
- *Illness.* Appetite usually decreases during illness and recovery from injuries. However, nutritional needs are increased.
- *Drugs.* Drugs can cause loss of appetite, confusion, nausea, constipation, impaired taste, or changes in gastro-intestinal (GI) function. They can cause inflammation of the mouth, throat, esophagus, and stomach.
- *Chewing problems.* Mouth, teeth, and gum problems can affect chewing. Examples include oral pain, dry or sore mouth, gum disease, and dentures that fit poorly. Broken, decayed, or missing teeth also affect chewing, especially the meat group.
- *Swallowing problems.* Many health problems can affect swallowing. They include stroke, pain, confusion, dry mouth, and diseases of the mouth, throat, and esophagus.
- *Disability.* Disease or injury can affect the hands, wrists, and arms. Adaptive equipment lets the person eat independently.
- *Impaired cognitive function.* Impaired cognitive function may affect the person's ability to use eating utensils. And it may affect eating, chewing, and swallowing.

Special Diets

The Sodium-Controlled Diet

- A sodium-controlled diet decreases the amount of sodium in the body. The diet involves:
  - Omitting high-sodium foods. Review Box 27-3, High-Sodium Foods, in the Textbook.
  - Not adding salt when eating.
  - Limiting the amount of salt used in cooking.
  - Diet planning.

Diabetes Meal Planning

- Diabetes meal planning is for people with diabetes. It involves the person's food preferences and calories needed. It also involves eating meals and snacks at regular times.
- Serve the person's meals and snacks on time to maintain a certain blood sugar level.
- Always check the tray to see what was eaten. Tell the nurse what the person did and did not eat. If not all the food was eaten, a between-meal nourishment is needed. The nurse tells you what to give. Tell the nurse about changes in the person's eating habits.

The Dysphagia Diet

- **Dysphagia** means difficulty swallowing. Food thickness is changed to meet the person's needs. Review Box 27-4, Dysphagia, in the Textbook.

- You may need to feed a person with dysphagia. To promote the person's comfort:
  - Know the signs and symptoms of dysphagia. Review Box 27-4 in the Textbook.
  - Feed the person according to the care plan.
  - Follow aspiration precautions (see Box 27-5, Aspiration Precautions, in the Textbook) and the care plan.
  - Report changes in how the person eats.
  - Report choking, coughing, or difficulty breathing during or after meals. Also report abnormal breathing or respiratory sounds. Report these observations at once.

Food Intake

- Food intake is measured in different ways. Follow agency policy for the method use.
- *Percentage of food eaten.* Some agencies measure the percent of the whole meal tray. Other agencies measure the percent of each food item eaten.
- *Calorie counts.* Note what the person ate and how much. A nurse or dietitian converts the portion amounts into calories.

Fluid Balance

- Fluid balance is needed for health. The amount of fluid taken in (**intake**) and the amount of fluid lost (**output**) must be roughly equal. If fluid intake exceeds fluid output, body tissues swell with water (**edema**).
- **Dehydration** is a decrease in the amount of water in body tissues. Fluid output exceeds intake. Review Box 27-6, Common Causes of Dehydration, in the Textbook.

Normal Fluid Requirements

- An adult needs 1500 milliliters (mL) of water daily to survive. About 2000 to 2500 mL of fluid per day is needed for normal fluid balance. Water requirements increase with hot weather, exercise, fever, illness, and excess fluid loss.
- Older persons may have a decreased sense of thirst. Their bodies need water but they may not feel thirsty. Offer fluids according to the care plan.

Special Fluid Orders

- The doctor may order the amount of fluid a person can have in 24 hours. Intake and output (I&O) measurements may be ordered by the doctor or nurse.
- *Encourage fluids.* The person drinks an increased amount of fluid.
- *Restrict fluids.* Fluids are limited to a certain amount.
- *Nothing by mouth (NPO).* The person cannot eat or drink.
- *Thickened liquids.* All liquids are thickened, including water.

Intake and Output

- All fluids taken by mouth are measured and recorded—water, milk, and so forth. So are foods that melt at room temperature—ice cream, sherbet, custard, pudding, gelatin, and Popsicles.
- Output includes urine, vomitus, diarrhea, and wound drainage.

Measuring Intake and Output (I&O)

- To measure I&O, you need to know:
  - 1 cubic centimeter (cc) equals 1 mL.
  - 1 teaspoon equals 5 mL.
  - 1 ounce (oz) equals 30 mL.
  - A pint is about 500 mL.
  - A quart is about 1000 mL.
  - The serving sizes of bowls, dishes, cups, pitchers, glasses, and other containers.
- An I&O record is kept at the bedside. Record I&O measurements in the correct column. Amounts are totaled at the end of the shift. The totals are recorded in the person's chart. They are also shared during the end-of-shift report.
- The urinal, commode, bedpan, or specimen pan is used for voiding. Remind the person not to void in the toilet. Also remind the person not to put toilet tissue into the receptacle.

Meeting Food and Fluid Needs

- Preparing residents for meals promotes their comfort.
  - Assist with elimination needs.
  - Provide oral hygiene. Make sure dentures are in place.
  - Make sure eyeglasses and hearing aids are in place.
  - Make sure incontinent persons are clean and dry.
  - Position the person in a comfortable position.
  - Assist the person with hand-washing.
- Food is served in containers that keep foods at the correct temperature. Hot food is kept hot. Cold food is kept cold.
- Prompt serving keeps food at the correct temperature.

Feeding the Person

- Serve food and fluid in the order the person prefers. Offer fluids during the meal.
- Use teaspoons to feed the person.
- Persons who need to be fed are often angry, humiliated, and embarrassed. Some are depressed or refuse to eat. Let them do as much as possible. If strong enough, let them hold milk or juice glasses. Never let them hold hot drinks.
- Tell the visually impaired person what is on the tray. Describe what you are offering. For persons who feed themselves, use the numbers on the clock for the location of foods.
- Many people pray before eating. Allow time and privacy for prayer.
- Meals provide social contact with others. Engage the person in pleasant conversations. Also sit facing the person. Allow time for chewing and swallowing. The person will eat better if not rushed. Wipe the person's hands, face, and mouth as needed during the meal.
- Report and record:
  - The amount and kind of food eaten
  - Complaints of nausea or dysphagia
  - Signs and symptoms of dysphagia
  - Signs and symptoms of aspiration
- Many special diets involve between-meal snacks. These snacks are served upon arrival on the nursing unit. Follow the same considerations and procedures for serving meal trays and feeding persons.

Providing Drinking Water

- Patients and residents need fresh drinking water each shift. Follow the agency's procedure for providing fresh water.
- Water mugs and pitchers can spread microbes. To prevent the spread of microbes:
  - Label the water mug with the person's name and room and bed number.
  - Do not touch the rim or inside of the mug or lid.
  - Do not let the ice scoop touch the mug, lid, or straw.
  - Place the ice scoop in the holder or on a towel, not in the ice container or dispenser.
  - Make sure the person's water mug is clean and free of cracks and chips. Provide a new mug as needed.

CHAPTER 27 REVIEW QUESTIONS

Circle the BEST answer.

1. A person is on a sodium-controlled diet. Which statement is *true?*
   a. High-sodium foods are allowed.
   b. Salt is added at the table.
   c. Pretzels and potato chips are a good snack.
   d. The amount of salt used in cooking is limited.
2. A person is a diabetic. You should do the following *except*
   a. Serve his meals and snacks late
   b. Always check his tray to see what he ate
   c. Tell the nurse what he ate and did not eat
   d. Provide a between-meal snack as the nurse directs
3. A person has dysphagia. You should do the following *except*
   a. Report choking and coughing during a meal at once
   b. Report difficulty in breathing during a meal at the end of the shift
   c. Report changes in how the person eats
   d. Follow aspiration precautions
4. Older persons have a decreased sense of thirst.
   a. True
   b. False
5. When feeding a person, you do the following *except*
   a. Use a teaspoon to feed the person
   b. Offer fluids during the meal
   c. Let the person do as much as possible
   d. Stand so you can feed 2 people at once
6. A person is visually impaired. You do the following *except*
   a. Tell the person what is on the tray
   b. Use the numbers on a clock to tell the person the location of food
   c. If feeding the person, describe what you are offering
   d. Let the person guess what is served
7. A person is on intake and output. He just ate ice cream. This is recorded as intake.
   a. True
   b. False
8. A person drank a pint of milk at lunch. You know she drank
   a. 250 mL of milk
   b. 350 mL of milk
   c. 500 mL of milk
   d. 750 mL of milk
9. The soup bowl holds 6 ounces. A person ate all of the soup. You record his intake as
   a. 50 mL
   b. 120 mL
   c. 180 mL
   d. 200 mL

Answers to these questions are on p. 516.

CHAPTER 29 MEASURING VITAL SIGNS

Vital Signs

- The vital signs of body function are temperature, pulse, respirations, blood pressure, and, in some agencies, pain.
- Accuracy is essential when you measure, record, and report vital signs. If unsure of your measurements, promptly ask the nurse to take them again.
- Report the following at once.
  - Any vital sign that is changed from a prior measurement
  - Vital signs above or below the normal range

Body Temperature

- Thermometers are used to measure temperature. It is measured using the Fahrenheit (F) and centigrade or Celsius (C) scales.
- Temperature sites are the mouth, rectum, axilla (underarm), tympanic membrane (ear), and temporal artery (forehead).
- Review Box 29-2, Temperature Sites, in the Textbook.
- Normal range for body temperatures depends on the site.
  - Oral: 97.6°F to 99.6°F
  - Rectal: 98.6°F to 100.6°F
  - Axillary: 96.6°F to 98.6°F
  - Tympanic membrane: 98.6°F
  - Temporal artery: 99.6°F
- Older persons have lower body temperatures than younger persons.

Thermometers

- Electronic thermometers show the temperature on the front of the device when the temperature is registered.
- Electronic thermometers include:
  - Standard electronic thermometers with a blue probe for oral and axillary temperatures and red probes for rectal temperatures. A disposable cover protects the probe.
  - Tympanic membrane thermometer, which measures body temperature at the tympanic membrane in the ear.
  - Temporal artery thermometer, which measures body temperature at the temporal artery in the forehead.
  - Digital thermometers, which measure body temperature at the oral, axillary, or rectal sites.
  - Pacifier thermometers, which look like a baby pacifier. The baby sucks on the device to record temperature.
- Other thermometers include disposable thermometers, temperature-sensitive tape, and glass thermometers.

Taking Temperatures
- *The oral site*. Place the thermometer under the person's tongue and to the side.
- *The rectal site*. Lubricate the bulb end of the rectal thermometer. Insert the probe ½ inch into the rectum. Privacy is important.
- *The axillary site*. The axilla must be dry. Place the probe in the center of the axilla and place the person's arm over the chest to hold the probe in place.
- Tympanic membrane thermometers are inserted gently into the ear. Pull the adult ear up and back to straighten the ear canal.
- Glass thermometers are rarely used in hospitals and nursing centers but may be used in the home. Review Box 29-3, Glass Thermometers.

Pulse
- The adult pulse rate is between 60 and 100 beats per minute. Report these abnormal rates to the nurse at once.
  - *Tachycardia*—the heart rate is more than 100 beats per minute.
  - *Bradycardia*—the heart rate is less than 60 beats per minute.
- The rhythm of the pulse should be regular. Report and record an irregular pulse rhythm.
- Report and record if the pulse force is strong, full, bounding, weak, thready, or feeble.

Taking Pulses
- The radial pulse is used for routine vital signs. Place the first 2 or 3 fingers against the radial pulse. Do not use your thumb to take a pulse. Count the pulse for 30 seconds and multiply by 2 if the agency policy permits. If the pulse is irregular, count it for 1 minute. Report and record if the pulse is regular or irregular, strong or weak.
- The apical pulse is on the left side of the chest slightly below the nipple. A stethoscope is used to measure the apical or the apical-radial pulse. Count the apical pulse for 1 minute.

Respirations
- The healthy adult has 12 to 20 respirations per minute. Respirations are normally quiet, effortless, and regular. Both sides of the chest rise and fall equally.
- Count respirations when the person is at rest. Count respirations right after taking a pulse.
- Count respirations for 30 seconds and multiply the number by 2 if the agency policy permits. If an abnormal pattern is noted, count the respirations for 1 minute.
- Report and record:
  - The respiratory rate
  - Equality and depth of respirations
  - If the respirations were regular or irregular
  - If the person has pain or difficulty breathing
  - Any respiratory noises
  - An abnormal respiratory pattern

Blood Pressure
Normal and Abnormal Blood Pressures
- Blood pressure has normal ranges.
  - *Systolic pressure* (upper number)—90 mm Hg and higher but lower than 120 mm Hg
  - *Diastolic pressure* (lower number)—60 mm Hg and higher but lower than 80 mm Hg
- **Hypertension**—blood pressure measurements that remain above a systolic pressure of 140 mm Hg or a diastolic pressure of 90 mm Hg. Report any systolic measurement above 120 mm Hg. Also report a diastolic pressure above 80 mm Hg.
- **Hypotension**—when the systolic blood pressure is below 90 mm Hg and the diastolic pressure is below 60 mm Hg. Report a systolic pressure below 90 mm Hg. Also report a diastolic pressure below 60 mm Hg.
- Review Box 29-6, Guidelines for Measuring Blood Pressure, in the Textbook.

CHAPTER 29 REVIEW QUESTIONS
Circle the BEST answer.
1. Which statement about taking a rectal temperature is *false*?
   a. The bulb end of the thermometer needs to be lubricated.
   b. The thermometer is inserted 1 inch into the rectum.
   c. Privacy is important.
   d. The normal range is 98.6°F to 100.6°F.
2. Which pulse rate should you report at once?
   a. A pulse rate of 52 beats per minute
   b. A pulse rate of 60 beats per minute
   c. A pulse rate of 76 beats per minute
   d. A pulse rate of 100 beats per minute
3. Which statement is *false*?
   a. An irregular pulse is counted for 1 minute.
   b. You may use your thumb to take a radial pulse rate.
   c. The radial pulse is usually used to count a pulse rate.
   d. Tachycardia is a fast pulse rate.
4. Which blood pressure should you report?
   a. 120/80 mm Hg
   b. 88/62 mm Hg
   c. 110/70 mm Hg
   d. 92/68 mm Hg

Answers to these questions are on p. 516.

CHAPTER 30 EXERCISE AND ACTIVITY
Bedrest
- The doctor may order bedrest to treat a health problem.
- Bedrest is ordered to:
  - Reduce physical activity.
  - Reduce pain.
  - Encourage rest.
  - Regain strength.
  - Promote healing.

Complications From Bedrest
- Pressure ulcers, constipation, and fecal impactions can result. Urinary tract infections and renal calculi (kidney stones) can occur. So can blood clots and pneumonia.

- The musculo-skeletal system is affected by lack of exercise and activity. These complications must be prevented to maintain normal movement.
  - A **contracture** is the lack of joint mobility caused by abnormal shortening of a muscle. Common sites are the fingers, wrists, elbows, toes, ankles, knees, and hips. The person is permanently deformed and disabled.
  - **Atrophy** is the decrease in size or the wasting away of tissue. Tissues shrink in size.
- **Orthostatic hypotension (postural hypotension)** is abnormally low blood pressure when the person stands up suddenly. The person is dizzy and weak and has spots before the eyes. Fainting can occur. To prevent orthostatic hypotension, have the person change slowly from a lying or sitting position to a standing position.

Positioning

- Supportive devices are often used to support and maintain the person in a certain position.
  - *Bed-boards*—are placed under the mattress to prevent the mattress from sagging.
  - *Foot-boards*—are placed at the foot of mattresses to prevent plantar flexion that can lead to footdrop.
  - *Trochanter rolls*—prevent the hips and legs from turning outward (external rotation).
  - *Hip abduction wedges*—keep the hips abducted (apart).
  - *Hand rolls or hand grips*—prevent contractures of the thumb, fingers, and wrist.
  - *Splints*—keep the elbows, wrists, thumbs, fingers, ankles, and knees in normal position.
  - *Bed cradles*—keep the weight of top linens off the feet and toes.

Range-of-Motion Exercises

- **Range-of-motion (ROM)** exercises involve moving the joints through their complete range of motion without causing pain. They are usually done at least 2 times a day.
  - *Active ROM*—exercises are done by the person.
  - *Passive ROM*—you move the joints through their range of motion.
  - *Active-assistive ROM*—the person does the exercises with some help.
- Review Box 30-2, Range-of-Motion Exercises, in the Textbook.
- ROM exercises can cause injury if not done properly. Practice these rules.
  - Exercise only the joints the nurse tells you to exercise.
  - Expose only the body part being exercised.
  - Use good body mechanics.
  - Support the part being exercised.
  - Move the joint slowly, smoothly, and gently.
  - Do not force a joint beyond its present range of motion.
  - Do not force a joint to the point of pain.
  - Ask the person if he or she has pain or discomfort.
  - Perform ROM exercises to the neck only if allowed by your agency and if the nurse instructs you to do so.

Ambulation

- **Ambulation** is the act of walking.
- Follow the care plan when helping a person walk. Use a gait (transfer) belt if the person is weak or unsteady. The person uses hand rails along the wall. Always check the person for orthostatic hypotension.
- When you help the person walk, walk to the side and slightly behind the person on the person's weak side. Encourage the person to use the hand rail on his or her strong side.

Walking Aids

- A cane is held on the strong side of the body. The cane tip is about 6 to 10 inches to the side of the foot. It is about 6 to 10 inches in front of the foot on the strong side. The grip is level with the hip. To walk:
  - Step A: The cane is moved forward 6 to 10 inches.
  - Step B: The weak leg (opposite the cane) is moved forward even with the cane.
  - Step C: The strong leg is moved forward and ahead of the cane and the weak leg.
- A walker gives more support than a cane. Wheeled walkers are common. They have wheels on the front legs and rubber tips on the back legs. The person pushes the walker about 6 to 8 inches in front of his or her feet.
- Braces support weak body parts, prevent or correct deformities, or prevent joint movement. A brace is applied over the ankle, knee, or back. Skin and bony points under braces are kept clean and dry. Report redness or signs of skin breakdown at once. Also report complaints of pain or discomfort. The care plan tells you when to apply and remove a brace.

CHAPTER 30 REVIEW QUESTIONS

Circle the BEST answer.

1. To prevent orthostatic hypotension, you should
   a. Move a person from the lying position to the sitting position quickly
   b. Move a person from the sitting position to the standing position quickly
   c. Move a person from the lying or sitting position to a standing position slowly
   d. Keep the person in bed
2. Exercise helps prevent contractures and muscle atrophy.
   a. True
   b. False
3. When performing ROM exercises, you should force a joint to the point of pain.
   a. True
   b. False
4. A person's left leg is weaker than his right. The person holds the cane on his right side.
   a. True
   b. False

Answers to these questions are on p. 516.

CHAPTER 31 COMFORT, REST, AND SLEEP

- Comfort is a state of well-being. Many factors affect comfort.
- Pain or discomfort means to ache, hurt, or be sore. Pain is subjective. You cannot see, hear, touch, or smell pain or discomfort. You must rely on what the person says.
- Pain is often considered the fifth vital sign. Report the person's complaints of pain and your observations to the nurse.

Factors Affecting Pain

- *Past experience.* The severity of pain, its cause, how long it lasted, and if relief occurred all affect the person's current response to pain.
- *Anxiety.* Pain and anxiety are related. Pain can cause anxiety. Anxiety increases how much pain the person feels. Reducing anxiety helps lessen pain.
- *Rest and sleep.* Pain seems worse when a person is tired or restless. Pain often seems worse at night.
- *Attention.* The more a person thinks about pain, the worse it seems.
- *Personal and family duties.* Often pain is ignored when there are children to care for. Some deny pain if a serious illness is feared.
- *The value or meaning of pain.* To some people, pain is a sign of weakness. For some persons, pain means avoiding work, daily routines, and people. Some people like doting and pampering by others. The person values pain and wants such attention.
- *Support from others.* Dealing with pain is often easier when family and friends offer comfort and support. Facing pain alone is hard for persons.
- *Culture.* Culture affects pain responses. Non–English-speaking persons may have problems describing pain.
- *Illness.* Some diseases cause decreased pain sensations.
- *Age.* Older persons may have chronic pain that masks new pain. They may deny or ignore new pain, thinking it is related to a known problem. Or they may deny or ignore pain because they are afraid of what it may mean. For persons who cannot tell you about pain, changes in usual behavior may signal pain. Loss of appetite also signals pain. Report any changes in a person's usual behavior to the nurse.

Signs and Symptoms

- You cannot see, hear, touch, or smell the person's pain. Rely on what the person tells you. Promptly report any information you collect about pain. Use the person's exact words when reporting and recording pain.
- The nurse needs the following information.
  - *Location.* Where is the pain?
  - *Onset and duration.* When did the pain start? How long has it lasted?
  - *Intensity.* Ask the person to rate the pain. Use a pain scale.
  - *Description.* Ask the person to describe the pain.
  - *Factors causing pain.* Ask what the person was doing before the pain started and when it started.
  - *Factors affecting pain.* Ask what makes the pain better and what makes it worse.
  - *Vital signs.* Increases often occur with acute pain. They may be normal with chronic pain.
  - *Other signs and symptoms.* Dizziness, nausea, vomiting, weakness, numbness, and tingling.
- Review Box 31-2, Signs and Symptoms of Pain, and Box 31-3, Comfort and Pain-Relief Measures, in the Textbook.

The Back Massage

- The back massage can promote comfort and relieve pain. It relaxes muscles and stimulates circulation.
- A good time to give a massage is after baths and showers and with evening care. Massages last 3 to 5 minutes.
- Observe the skin for breaks, bruises, reddened areas, and other signs of skin breakdown.
- Lotion reduces friction during the massage. It is warmed before applying.
- Use firm strokes. Keep your hands in contact with the person's skin.
- After the massage, apply some lotion to the elbows, knees, and heels.
- Back massages are dangerous for persons with certain heart diseases, back injuries, back and other surgeries, skin diseases, and some lung disorders. Check with the nurse and the care plan before giving back massages to persons with these conditions.
- Do not massage reddened bony areas. Reddened areas signal skin breakdown and pressure ulcers. Massage can lead to more tissue damage.
- Wear gloves if the person's skin is not intact. Always follow Standard Precautions and the Bloodborne Pathogen Standard.
- Report and record skin breakdown, redness, bruising, and breaks in the skin.

Rest

- *Rest* means to be calm, at ease, and relaxed with no anxiety or stress. Rest may involve inactivity. Or the person does things that are calming and relaxing.
- Promote rest by meeting physical, safety, and security needs.
  - Thirst, hunger, pain or discomfort, and elimination needs can affect rest. A comfortable position and good alignment are important. A quiet setting promotes rest.
  - The person must feel safe from falling or other injuries. The person is secure with the call light within reach. Understanding the reasons for care and knowing how care is given also help the person feel safe.
- Many persons have rituals or routines before resting. Follow them whenever possible.
- Love and belonging are important for rest. Visits or calls from family and friends may relax the person. Reading cards and letters may also help.
- Meet self-esteem needs.
- Some persons are refreshed after a 15- or 20-minute rest. Others need more time.

- Ill or injured persons need to rest more often. Do not push the person beyond his or her limits.

Sleep

- Sleep is a basic need. Tissue healing and repair occur during sleep. Sleep lowers stress, tension, and anxiety. It refreshes and renews the person. The person regains energy and mental alertness. The person thinks and functions better after sleep.

Factors Affecting Sleep

- *Age.* The amount of sleep needed decreases with age.
- *Illness.* Illness increases the need for sleep.
- *Nutrition.* Sleep needs increase with weight gain. Foods with caffeine prevent sleep.
- *Exercise.* People feel good after exercise. Eventually they tire, which helps people sleep well. Avoid exercise at least 2 hours before bedtime.
- *Environment.* People adjust to their usual sleep settings.
- *Drugs and other substances.* Sleeping pills promote sleep. Drugs for anxiety, depression, and pain may cause the person to sleep but may interfere with the quality of sleep.
- *Life-style changes.* Changes in daily routines may affect sleep.
- *Emotional problems.* Fear, worry, depression, and anxiety affect sleep.

Sleep Disorders

- **Insomnia** is a chronic condition in which the person cannot sleep or stay asleep all night.
- **Sleep deprivation** means that the amount and quality of sleep are decreased. Sleep is interrupted.
- **Sleepwalking** is when the person leaves the bed and walks about. If a person is sleepwalking, protect the person from injury. Guide sleepwalkers back to bed. They startle easily. Awaken them gently.

Promoting Sleep

- To promote sleep, allow a flexible bedtime, provide a comfortable room temperature, and have the person void before going to bed. Review Box 31-6, Promoting Sleep, in the Textbook for other measures.

CHAPTER 31 REVIEW QUESTIONS

Circle the BEST answer.

1. A person complains of pain. You will do the following *except*
   a. Ask where the pain is
   b. Ask when the pain started
   c. Ask what the intensity of the pain is on a scale of 1 to 10
   d. Ask why the person is complaining about pain
2. Older persons or persons who cannot communicate may not complain of pain. Which of the following might be a signal of pain?
   a. Illness
   b. Mental alertness
   c. Loss of appetite
   d. Forgetfulness
3. Which statement is *false?*
   a. A back massage relaxes and stimulates circulation.
   b. Massages are given after the bath and with evening care.
   c. You can observe the person's skin before beginning the massage.
   d. You should use cold lotion for the massage.
4. You can promote rest for a person by doing the following *except*
   a. Asking the person if he or she would like coffee or tea
   b. Placing the call light within reach
   c. Providing a quiet setting
   d. Following the person's routines and rituals before rest
5. To promote sleep for a person, you should do the following *except*
   a. Follow the person's wishes
   b. Follow the care plan
   c. Follow the person's rituals and routines before bedtime
   d. Tell the person when to go to bed

Answers to these questions are on p. 516.

CHAPTER 32 ADMISSIONS, TRANSFERS, AND DISCHARGES

- Admission is the official entry of a person into a health care setting. It can cause anxiety and fear in patients, residents, and families.
- Transfer is moving the person to another health care setting or moving the person to a new room within the agency.
- Discharge is the official departure of a person from a health care setting.
- During the admission process:
  ○ Identifying information is obtained from the person or family.
  ○ A nurse or social worker explains the resident's rights to the person and family.
  ○ The person is given an identification (ID) number and bracelet.
  ○ The person signs admitting papers and a general consent form.
- You prepare the person's room before the person arrives.

Admitting the Person

- Admission is your first chance to make a good impression. You must:
  ○ Greet the person by name and title. Use the admission form to find out the person's name.
  ○ Introduce yourself by name and title to the person, family, and friends.
  ○ Make roommate introductions.
  ○ Act in a professional manner.
  ○ Treat the person with dignity and respect.
- During the admission procedure the nurse may ask you to:
  ○ Collect some information for the admission form.
  ○ Measure the person's weight and height.
  ○ Measure the person's vital signs.
  ○ Obtain a urine specimen (if needed).

- ○ Complete a clothing and personal belongings list.
- ○ Orient the person to the room, nursing unit, and agency.

Weight and Height

- When weighing a person, follow the manufacturer's instructions and center procedures for using the scales. Follow these guidelines when measuring weight and height.
  - ○ The person wears only a gown or pajamas. No footwear is worn.
  - ○ The person voids before being weighed and a dry incontinence product is worn if needed.
  - ○ Weigh the person at the same time of day. Before breakfast is the best time.
  - ○ Use the same scale for daily, weekly, and monthly weights.
  - ○ Balance the scale at zero before weighing the person.

Moving the Person to a New Room

- Sometimes a person is moved to a new room because of a change in condition or care needs, the person requests a room change, or roommates do not get along. Support and reassure the person moving to a new room with new staff.
- The person is transported by wheelchair, stretcher, or the bed.

Transfers and Discharges

- When transferred or discharged, the person leaves the agency. He or she goes home or to another health care setting.
- Transfers and discharges are usually planned in advance by the health team.
- For discharges, the health team teaches the person and family about diet, exercise, and drugs. They also teach them about procedures and treatments and arrange for home care, equipment, and therapies as needed.
- The nurse tells you when to start the transfer or discharge procedure. The doctor must give the order before the person can leave. Usually a wheelchair is used. If leaving by ambulance, a stretcher is used.
- If a person wants to leave the agency without the doctor's permission, tell the nurse at once. The nurse or social worker handles the matter.

CHAPTER 32 REVIEW QUESTIONS

Circle the BEST answer.

1. When admitted, you explain the resident's rights to the person and family.
   a. True
   b. False
2. When a person is admitted, you do the following *except*
   a. Greet the person by name and title
   b. Treat the person with dignity and respect
   c. Introduce the person to his or her roommate
   d. Rush the admission procedure
3. Which statement is *false?*
   a. Have the person void before being weighed.

b. Weigh the person at the same time of day.
c. Balance the scale at zero before weighing the person.
d. Have the person wear shoes when being weighed.

4. A person wants to leave the nursing center without the doctor's permission. You should tell the nurse at once.
   a. True
   b. False

Answers to these questions are on p. 516.

CHAPTER 35 THE PERSON HAVING SURGERY

- Surgery may be in-patient, requiring a hospital stay, or same-day surgery, also called out-patient, 1-day, or ambulatory surgery. The person is prepared for what happens before, during, and after surgery.

Pre-Operative Care

- The person may have special tests such as chest x-ray or electrocardiogram (ECG). Nutrition and fluids may be restricted 6 to 8 hours before surgery.
- Personal care before surgery includes:
  - ○ A complete bath, shower, or tub bath and shampoo. A special soap or shampoo may be ordered to reduce the number of microbes and the risk of infection.
  - ○ Make-up, nail polish, and fake nails are removed.
  - ○ Hair accessories, wigs, and hairpieces are removed and a surgical cap keeps the hair out of the face and the operative site.
  - ○ Dentures, eyeglasses, contact lenses, hearing aids, and other prostheses are removed.
- Skin prep before surgery may include cleansing with an anti-microbial soap, clipping the hair at and around the site, or removing the hair at and around the site.
- After skin prep, report and record the following: the area prepped; any cuts, nicks, or scratches from skin shaving; bleeding; and sites of non-intact skin.

Post-Operative Care

- The person's room must be ready. Make a surgical bed, place supplies in the room, and move furniture out of the way for a stretcher.
- Your role in post-operative care depends on the person's condition. Often vital signs and pulse oximetry are taken. The nurse tells you how often to check the person. Review Box 35-2, Post-Op Complications and Observations, in the Textbook.
- The person is positioned for comfort and to prevent complications. The person is re-positioned every 1 to 2 hours to prevent respiratory and circulatory complications. Turning may be painful. Provide support and use smooth, gentle motions.
- Coughing and deep-breathing exercises help prevent respiratory complications.
- Circulation must be stimulated for blood flow in the legs. If blood flow is sluggish, blood clots may form.
- Report the following at once.
  - ○ Swollen area of a leg.

- Pain or tenderness in a leg. This may occur only when standing or walking.
- Warmth in the part of the leg that is swollen or painful.
- Red or discolored skin.

Elastic Stockings

- Elastic stockings exert pressure on the veins. The pressure promotes venous blood return to the heart. The stockings help prevent blood clots in the leg veins.
- Elastic stockings also are called AE stockings (anti-embolism or anti-embolic). They also are called TED hose. TED means thrombo-embolic disease.
- The nurse measures the person for the correct size of elastic stockings. Most stockings have an opening near the toes that is used to check circulation, skin color, and skin temperature.
- The person usually has 2 pairs of stockings. One pair is washed; the other pair is worn.
- Stockings should not have twists, creases, or wrinkles after you apply them. Twists can affect circulation. Creases and wrinkles can cause skin breakdown.
- Loose stockings do not promote venous blood return to the heart. Stockings that are too tight can affect circulation. Tell the nurse if the stockings are too loose or too tight.

CHAPTER 35 REVIEW QUESTIONS

Circle the BEST answer.

1. A person with a swollen calf with red, discolored skin is at risk for a blood clot.
   a. True
   b. False
2. Which statement about elastic stockings is *true?*
   a. Elastic stockings should be loose to promote venous blood return to the heart.
   b. Stockings should not have twists, creases, or wrinkles after you apply them.
   c. The doctor measures the person for the correct size of elastic stockings.
   d. The person should have only 1 pair of stockings.

Answers to these questions are on p. 516.

CHAPTER 36 WOUND CARE

- A **wound** is a break in the skin or mucous membrane.
- The wound is a portal of entry for microbes. Infection is a major threat. Wound care involves preventing infection and further injury to the wound and nearby tissues.

Skin Tears

- A **skin tear** is a break or rip in the skin.
- Skin tears are caused by friction, shearing, pulling, or pressure on the skin. Bumping a hand, arm, or leg on any hard surface can cause a skin tear. Beds, bed rails, chairs, wheelchair footplates, and tables are dangers. So is holding the person's arm or leg too tight, removing tape or adhesives, bathing, dressing, and other tasks. Buttons, zippers, jewelry, or long or jagged finger or toenails can also cause skin tears.

- Skin tears are painful. They are portals of entry for microbes. Wound complications can develop. Tell the nurse at once if you cause or find a skin tear.
- Review Box 36-2, Preventing Skin Tears, in the Textbook.

Circulatory Ulcers

- *Circulatory ulcers (vascular ulcers)* are open sores on the lower legs or feet. They are caused by decreased blood flow through the arteries or veins.
- Review Box 36-3, Preventing Circulatory Ulcers, in the Textbook.
- *Venous ulcers (stasis ulcers)* are open sores on the lower legs or feet. They are caused by poor blood flow through the veins. The heels and inner aspect of the ankles are common sites for venous ulcers.
- *Arterial ulcers* are open wounds on the lower legs or feet caused by poor arterial blood flow. They are found between the toes, on top of the toes, and on the outer side of the ankle.
- A *diabetic foot ulcer* is an open wound on the foot caused by complications from diabetes. When nerves are affected, the person can lose sensation in a foot or leg. The person may not feel pain, heat, or cold. Therefore the person may not feel a cut, blister, burn, or other trauma to the foot. Infection and a large sore can develop. When blood flow to the foot decreases, tissues and cells do not get needed oxygen and nutrients. A sore does not heal properly. Tissue death (gangrene) can occur. Review Box 36-4, Diabetes Foot Care, in the Textbook.

Prevention and Treatment

- Check the person's feet and legs every day. Report any sign of a problem to the nurse at once. Follow the care plan to prevent and treat circulatory ulcers.
- Some agencies let you apply simple, dry, non-sterile dressings to simple wounds. Follow the rules in Box 36-6, Applying Dressings, in the Textbook.

CHAPTER 36 REVIEW QUESTIONS

Circle the BEST answer.

1. The following can cause a skin tear *except*
   a. Friction and shearing
   b. Holding a person's arm or leg too tight
   c. Rings, watches, bracelets
   d. Trimmed, short nails
2. A person is diabetic. Which statement is *false?*
   a. The person may not feel pain in her feet.
   b. The person may not feel heat or cold in her feet.
   c. You need to check her feet weekly for foot problems.
   d. The person is at risk for diabetic foot ulcers.
3. Which statement about elastic stockings is *false?*
   a. Elastic stockings are also called anti-embolic stockings.
   b. Elastic stockings should be wrinkle-free after being applied.
   c. A person usually has 2 pairs of elastic stockings.
   d. Elastic stockings are applied after a person gets out of bed.

Answers to these questions are on p. 516.

CHAPTER 37 PRESSURE ULCERS

- A **pressure ulcer** is defined by the National Pressure Ulcer Advisory Panel as a localized injury to the skin and/or underlying tissue. The Centers for Medicare & Medicaid Services (CMS) define pressure ulcers as any lesion caused by unrelieved pressure that results in damage to underlying tissues.
- Pressure ulcers usually occur over a bony prominence—the back of the head, shoulder blades, elbows, hips, spine, sacrum, knees, ankles, heels, and toes.
- *Decubitus ulcer, bed sore,* and *pressure sore* are other terms for pressure ulcer.
- Pressure, shearing, and friction are common causes of skin breakdown and pressure ulcers. Risk factors include breaks in the skin, poor circulation to an area, moisture, dry skin, and irritation by urine and feces.

Persons at Risk
- Persons at risk for pressure ulcers are those who:
  - Are confined to a bed or chair.
  - Need some or total help in moving.
  - Are agitated or have involuntary muscle movements.
  - Have loss of bowel or bladder control.
  - Are exposed to moisture.
  - Have poor nutrition or poor fluid balance.
  - Have limited awareness.
  - Have problems sensing pain or pressure.
  - Have circulatory problems.
  - Are obese or very thin.
  - Have a medical device.
  - Have a healed pressure ulcer.

Pressure Ulcer Stages
- In persons with light skin, a reddened bony area is the first sign of a pressure ulcer. In persons with dark skin, a bony area may appear red, blue, or purple. The area may feel warm or cool. The person may complain of pain, burning, tingling, or itching in the area.
- Box 37-2 in the Textbook describes pressure ulcer stages.
- Figure 37-5 in the Textbook shows the stages of pressure ulcers.

Prevention and Treatment
- Preventing pressure ulcers is much easier than trying to heal them. Review Box 37-3, Preventing Pressure Ulcers, in the Textbook.
- The person at risk for pressure ulcers may be placed on a foam, air, alternating air, gel, or water mattress.
- Protective devices are often used to prevent and treat pressure ulcers and skin breakdown. Protective devices include:
  - Bed cradle
  - Heel and elbow protectors
  - Heel and foot elevators
  - Gel or fluid-filled pads and cushions
  - Special beds
  - Other equipment—pillows, trochanter rolls, and footboards

CHAPTER 37 REVIEW QUESTIONS
Circle the BEST answer.
1. You may expect to find a pressure ulcer at all of the following sites *except*
   a. Back of the head
   b. Ears
   c. Top of the thigh
   d. Toes
2. Which of the following is not a protective device used to prevent and treat pressure ulcers?
   a. Heel elevator
   b. Bed cradle
   c. Draw sheet
   d. Elbow protector
3. In obese people, pressure ulcers can occur between abdominal folds.
   a. True
   b. False
4. Pressure ulcers never occur over a bony prominence.
   a. True
   b. False

Answers to these questions are on p. 516.

CHAPTER 38 HEAT AND COLD APPLICATIONS

Heat Applications
- Heat relieves pain, relaxes muscles, promotes healing, reduces tissue swelling, and decreases joint stiffness.

Complications
- High temperatures can cause burns. Report pain, excessive redness, and blisters at once. Also observe for pale skin.
- Metal implants pose risks. Pacemakers and joint replacements are made of metal. Do not apply heat to an implant area.
- Heat is not applied to a pregnant woman's abdomen. The heat can affect fetal growth.

Moist and Dry Heat Applications
- In moist heat applications, water is in contact with the skin. Moist heat applications include hot compresses, hot soaks, sitz baths, and hot packs.
- Dry heat applications do not use water, allowing the application to stay at the desired temperature longer. Some hot packs and warming therapy pads are dry heat applications, as well as aquathermia pads.

Cold Applications
- Cold applications reduce pain, prevent swelling, and decrease circulation and bleeding.
- Complications include pain, burns, blisters, and poor circulation. Burns and blisters occur from intense cold. They also occur when dry cold is in direct contact with the skin.

Applying Heat and Cold

- Protect the person from injury during heat and cold applications. Review Box 38-1, Applying Heat and Cold, in the Textbook.

CHAPTER 38 REVIEW QUESTIONS

Circle the BEST answer.
1. Complications from a heat application include the following *except*
   a. Excessive redness
   b. Blisters
   c. Pale skin
   d. Cyanotic (bluish) nail beds
2. When applying heat or cold, you should do the following *except*
   a. Ask the nurse what the temperature of the application should be
   b. Cover dry heat or cold applications before applying them
   c. Observe the skin every 2 hours
   d. Know how long to leave the application in place

Answers to these questions are on p. 516.

CHAPTER 39 OXYGEN NEEDS

Altered Respiratory Function

- Hypoxia means that cells do not have enough oxygen.
- Restlessness, dizziness, and disorientation are signs of hypoxia.
- Report signs and symptoms of hypoxia to the nurse at once. Hypoxia is life-threatening.
- Review Box 39-1, Altered Respiratory Function, in the Textbook.

Abnormal Respirations

- Adults normally have 12 to 20 respirations per minute. They are quiet, effortless, and regular. Both sides of the chest rise and fall equally. Report these observations at once.
  - **Tachypnea**—rapid breathing. Respirations are 20 or more per minute.
  - **Bradypnea**—slow breathing. Respirations are fewer than 12 per minute.
  - **Apnea**—lack or absence of breathing.
  - **Hypoventilation**—respirations are slow, shallow, and sometimes irregular.
  - **Hyperventilation**—respirations are rapid and deeper than normal.
  - **Dyspnea**—difficult, labored, painful breathing.
  - **Cheyne-Stokes respirations**—respirations gradually increase in rate and depth. Then they become shallow and slow. Breathing may stop for 10 to 20 seconds.
  - **Orthopnea**—breathing deeply and comfortably only when sitting.
  - **Biot's respirations**—rapid and deep respirations followed by 10 to 30 seconds of apnea.
  - **Kussmaul respirations**—very deep and rapid respirations.

Pulse Oximetry

- Pulse oximetry measures the oxygen concentration in arterial blood.
- A sensor attaches to a finger, toe, earlobe, nose, or forehead.
- Avoid swollen sites and sites with skin breaks. Do not use a finger site if blood flow to the fingers is poor, the person has fake nails, or the person has movements from shivering, seizures, or tremors.

Promoting Oxygenation

- Breathing is usually easier in semi-Fowler's and Fowler's positions. Persons with difficulty breathing often prefer the **orthopneic position** (sitting up and leaning over a table to breathe).
- Deep breathing moves air into most parts of the lungs. Coughing removes mucus. Deep breathing and coughing are usually done every 1 to 2 hours while the person is awake. They help prevent pneumonia and atelectasis (the collapse of a portion of the lung).

Oxygen Devices

- A nasal cannula allows eating and drinking. Tight prongs can irritate the nose. Pressure on the ears and cheekbones is possible.
- A simple face mask covers the nose and mouth. Talking and eating are hard to do with a mask. Listen carefully. Moisture can build up under the mask. Keep the face clean and dry. Masks are removed for eating. Usually oxygen is given by cannula during meals.

Oxygen Flow Rates

- When giving care and checking the person, always check the flow rate. Tell the nurse at once if it is too high or too low. A nurse or respiratory therapist will adjust the flow rate.

Oxygen Safety

- You do not give oxygen. You assist the nurse in providing safe care.
- Always check the oxygen level when you are with or near persons using oxygen systems that contain a limited amount of oxygen. Oxygen tanks and liquid oxygen systems are examples. Report a low oxygen level to the nurse at once.
- Follow the rules for fire and the use of oxygen in Chapter 13 in the Textbook.
- Never remove the oxygen device. However, turn off the oxygen flow if there is a fire.
- Make sure the oxygen device is secure but not tight.
- Check for signs of irritation from the oxygen device— behind the ears, under the nose, around the face, and on the cheekbones.
- Keep the face clean and dry when a mask is used.
- Never shut off the oxygen flow.
- Do not adjust the flow rate unless allowed by your state and agency.
- Tell the nurse at once if the flow rate is too high or too low.

- Tell the nurse at once if the humidifier is not bubbling.
- Secure tubing to the person's garment. Follow agency policy.
- Make sure there are no kinks in the tubing.
- Make sure the person does not lie on any part of the tubing.
- Report signs of hypoxia, respiratory distress, or abnormal breathing to the nurse at once.
- Give oral hygiene as directed. Follow the care plan.
- Make sure the oxygen device is clean and free of mucus.
- Make sure the oxygen tank is secure in its holder.

CHAPTER 39 REVIEW QUESTIONS

Circle the BEST answer.

1. Which statement is *false?*
   a. Restlessness, dizziness, and disorientation are signs of hypoxia.
   b. Hypoxia is life-threatening.
   c. Report signs and symptoms of hypoxia at the end of the shift.
   d. Anything that affects respiratory function can cause hypoxia.
2. Adults normally have
   a. 8 to 10 respirations per minute
   b. 12 to 20 respirations per minute
   c. 10 to 12 respirations per minute
   d. 20 to 24 respirations per minute
3. Dyspnea is
   a. Difficult, labored, or painful breathing
   b. Slow breathing with fewer than 12 respirations per minute
   c. Rapid breathing with 24 or more respirations per minute
   d. Lack or absence of breathing
4. Which statement about positioning is *false?*
   a. Breathing is usually easier in semi-Fowler's or Fowler's position.
   b. Persons with difficulty breathing often prefer the orthopneic position.
   c. Position changes are needed at least every 4 hours.
   d. Follow the person's care plan for positioning preferences.
5. A person has a nasal cannula. Which statement is *false?*
   a. You will leave the nasal cannula on while the person is eating.
   b. You will watch the nose area for irritation.
   c. You will watch the ears and cheekbones for skin breakdown.
   d. You will take the nasal cannula off while the person is eating.

Answers to these questions are on p. 516.

CHAPTER 41 REHABILITATION AND RESTORATIVE NURSING CARE

- A **disability** is any lost, absent, or impaired physical or mental function.
- **Rehabilitation** is the process of restoring the person to his or her highest possible level of physical, psychological, social, and economic function. The focus is on improving abilities. This promotes function at the highest level of independence.

Rehabilitation and the Whole Person

- Rehabilitation takes longer in older persons. Changes from aging affect healing, mobility, vision, hearing, and other functions. Chronic health problems can slow recovery.

Physical Aspects

- Rehabilitation starts when the person first seeks health care. Complications, such as contractures and pressure ulcers, are prevented.
- *Elimination.* Bowel or bladder training may be needed. Fecal impaction, constipation, and fecal incontinence are prevented.
- *Self-care.* Self-care for activities of daily living (ADL) is a major goal. Self-help devices are often needed.
- *Mobility.* The person may need crutches, a walker, a cane, a brace, or a wheelchair.
- *Nutrition.* The person may need a dysphagia diet or enteral nutrition.
- *Communication.* Speech therapy and communication devices may be helpful.

Psychological and Social Aspects

- A disability can affect function and appearance. Self-esteem and relationships may suffer. The person may feel unwhole, useless, unattractive, unclean, or undesirable. The person may deny the disability. The person may expect therapy to correct the problem. He or she may be depressed, angry, and hostile.
- Successful rehabilitation depends on the person's attitude. The person must accept his or her limits and be motivated. The focus is on abilities and strengths. Despair and frustration are common. Progress may be slow. Old fears and emotions may recur.
- Remind persons of their progress. They need help accepting disabilities and limits. Give support, re-assurance, and encouragement. Spiritual support helps some people. Psychological and social needs are part of the care plan.

The Rehabilitation Team

- Rehabilitation is a team effort. The person is the key member. The health team and family help the person set goals and plan care. All help the person regain function and independence.

Your Role

- Every part of your job focuses on promoting the person's independence. Preventing decline in function also is a goal. Review Box 41-2, Assisting With Rehabilitation and Restorative Care, in the Textbook.

Quality of Life

- To promote quality of life:
  ○ *Protect the right to privacy.* The person re-learns old or practices new skills in private. Others do not need to see mistakes, falls, spills, clumsiness, anger, or tears.
  ○ *Encourage personal choice.* This gives the person control.

○ *Protect the right to be free from abuse and mistreatment.* Sometimes improvement is not seen for weeks. Repeated explanations and demonstrations may have little or no results. You and other staff and family may become upset and short-tempered. However, no one can shout, scream, or yell at the person. Nor can they call the person names or hit or strike the person. Unkind remarks are not allowed. Report signs of abuse or mistreatment.

○ *Learn to deal with your anger and frustration.* The person does not choose loss of function. If the process upsets you, discuss your feelings with the nurse.

○ *Encourage activities.* Provide support and re-assurance to the person with the disability. Remind the person that others with disabilities can give support and understanding.

○ *Provide a safe setting.* The setting must meet the person's needs. The over-bed table, bedside stand, and call light are moved to the person's strong side.

○ *Show patience, understanding, and sensitivity.* The person may be upset and discouraged. Give support, encouragement, and praise when needed. Stress the person's abilities and strengths. Do not give pity or sympathy.

CHAPTER 41 REVIEW QUESTIONS

Circle the BEST answer.

1. Successful rehabilitation depends on the person's attitude.
   a. True
   b. False
2. A person with a disability may be depressed, angry, and hostile.
   a. True
   b. False
3. A person needs rehabilitation. You should do the following *except*
   a. Let the person re-learn old skills in private
   b. Let the person practice new skills in private
   c. Encourage the person to make choices
   d. Shout at the person
4. You saw a family member hit and scream at a person. You need to report your observations to the nurse.
   a. True
   b. False
5. A person has a weak left arm. You will
   a. Place the call light on his left side
   b. Place the call light on his right side
   c. Give him sympathy
   d. Give him pity

Answers to these questions are on p. 517.

CHAPTER 42 HEARING, SPEECH, AND VISION PROBLEMS

Hearing Loss

- Hearing loss is not being able to hear the normal range of sounds associated with normal hearing. Deafness is the most severe form of hearing loss.

- Obvious signs and symptoms of hearing loss include:
  ○ Speaking too loudly
  ○ Leaning forward to hear
  ○ Turning and cupping the better ear toward the speaker
  ○ Answering questions or responding inappropriately
  ○ Asking for words to be repeated
  ○ Asking others to speak louder or to speak more slowly and clearly
  ○ Having trouble hearing over the phone
  ○ Finding it hard to follow conversations when 2 or more people are talking
  ○ Turning up the TV, radio, or music volume so loud that others complain
- Persons with hearing loss may wear hearing aids or lip-read (speech-read). They watch facial expressions, gestures, and body language. Some people learn American Sign Language (ASL). Others may have hearing assistance dogs.
- Review Box 42-3, Measures to Promote Hearing, in the Textbook.
- Hearing aids are battery-operated. If they do not seem to work properly:
  ○ Check if the hearing aid is on. It has an on and off switch.
  ○ Check the battery position.
  ○ Insert a new battery if needed.
  ○ Clean the hearing aid. Follow the nurse's direction and the manufacturer's instructions.
- Hearing aids are turned off when not in use. The battery is removed.
- Handle and care for hearing aids properly. If lost or damaged, report it to the nurse at once.

Speech Disorders

Aphasia

- **Aphasia** is the total or partial loss of the ability to use or understand language.
- *Expressive aphasia* relates to difficulty expressing or sending out thoughts. Thinking is clear. The person knows what to say but has difficulty or cannot speak the words.
- *Receptive aphasia* relates to difficulty understanding language. The person has trouble understanding what is said or read. People and common objects are not recognized.

Eye Disorders

- *Cataract.* Cataract is a clouding of the lens in the eye. Signs and symptoms include cloudy, blurry, or dimmed vision. Persons may also be sensitive to light and glares or see halos around lights. Poor vision at night and double vision in 1 eye are other symptoms. Surgery is the only treatment.
- *Age-related macular degeneration (AMD).* AMD blurs central vision needed for reading, sewing, driving, and seeing faces and fine detail. Risk factors include smoking and family history. Whites are at greater risk than any other group. Treatment may stop or slow the disease progress.

- *Diabetic retinopathy.* Diabetic retinopathy causes blood vessels in the retina to become damaged. Usually both eyes are affected. It is the leading cause of blindness. Control of diabetes, blood pressure, and cholesterol can control diabetic retinopathy.
- *Glaucoma.* Glaucoma results when fluid builds up in the eye and causes pressure on the optic nerve. The optic nerve is damaged. Vision loss with eventual blindness occurs. Drugs and surgery can control glaucoma and prevent further damage to the optic nerve. Prior damage cannot be reversed.

Impaired Vision and Blindness
- Birth defects, injuries, accidents, and eye diseases are among the many causes of impaired vision and blindness. They also are complications of some diseases.
- Review Box 42-6, Caring for Blind and Visually Impaired Persons, in the Textbook.

Corrective Lenses
- Clean eyeglasses daily and as needed.
- Protect eyeglasses from loss or damage. When not worn, put them in their case.
- Contact lenses are cleaned, removed, and stored according to the manufacturer's instructions.

CHAPTER 42 REVIEW QUESTIONS
Circle the BEST answer.
1. A person is hard-of-hearing. You do the following *except*
   a. Face the person when speaking
   b. Speak clearly, distinctly, and slowly
   c. Use facial expressions and gestures to give clues
   d. Use long sentences
2. A person has taken his hearing aid out for the evening. You do the following *except*
   a. Make sure the hearing aid is turned off
   b. Keep the battery in the hearing aid
   c. Place the hearing aid in a safe place
   d. Handle the hearing aid carefully
3. A person is blind. You do the following *except*
   a. Identify yourself when you enter her room
   b. Describe people, places, and things thoroughly
   c. Re-arrange her furniture without telling her
   d. Encourage her to do as much for herself as possible
4. Fluid buildup in the eye that causes pressure on the optic nerve is
   a. Cataract
   b. Cerumen
   c. Glaucoma
   d. Tinnitus
Answers to these questions are on p. 517.

CHAPTER 43 CANCER, IMMUNE SYSTEM, AND SKIN DISORDERS
Cancer
- Cancer is the second leading cause of death in the United States.
- Review Box 43-1, Cancer: Signs and Symptoms, in the Textbook.

- Surgery, radiation therapy, and chemotherapy are the most common treatments.
- Persons with cancer have many needs. They include:
  - Pain relief or control
  - Rest and exercise
  - Fluids and nutrition
  - Preventing skin breakdown
  - Preventing bowel problems (constipation, diarrhea)
  - Dealing with treatment side effects
  - Psychological and social needs
  - Spiritual needs
  - Sexual needs
- Anger, fear, and depression are common. Some surgeries are disfiguring. The person may feel unwhole, unattractive, or unclean. The person and family need support.
- Talk to the person. Do not avoid the person because you are uncomfortable. Use touch and listening to show that you care.
- Spiritual needs are important. A spiritual leader may provide comfort.

Immune System Disorders
- The immune system protects the body from microbes, cancer cells, and other harmful substances. It defends against threats inside and outside the body.

HIV/AIDS
- Acquired immunodeficiency syndrome (AIDS) is caused by the human immunodeficiency virus (HIV). The virus is spread through body fluids—blood, semen, vaginal secretions, rectal fluids, and breast-milk. HIV is not spread by air, saliva, tears, sweat, sneezing, coughing, insects, casual contact, closed mouth or social kissing, or toilet seats.
- Persons with AIDS are at risk for pneumonia, tuberculosis, Kaposi's sarcoma (a cancer), nervous system disorders, mental health disorders, and dementia.
- To protect yourself and others from HIV, follow Standard Precautions and the Bloodborne Pathogen Standard.
- Review Box 43-4, Caring for the Person With AIDS, in the Textbook.
- Older persons also get AIDS. They get and spread HIV through sexual contact and intravenous (IV) drug use. Aging and some diseases can mask the signs and symptoms of AIDS. Older persons are less likely to be tested for HIV/AIDS.

Skin Disorders—Shingles
- Shingles is caused by the same virus that causes chicken pox. A rash or blisters can occur. Pain is mild to intense and itching is a common complaint.
- Shingles is most common in persons over 50 years of age. Persons at risk are those who have had chicken pox as children and who have weakened immune systems. Shingles lesions are infectious until they crust over.
- Treatments include anti-viral and pain-relief drugs. A vaccine is not available.

CHAPTER 43 REVIEW QUESTIONS

Circle the BEST answer.

1. A person with cancer may need all the following *except*
   a. Pain relief or control
   b. Avoidance by you
   c. Fluids and nutrition
   d. Psychological support
2. Which statement about HIV is *false?*
   a. HIV is spread through body fluids.
   b. Standard Precautions and the Bloodborne Pathogen Standard are followed.
   c. Older persons cannot get and spread HIV.
   d. Older persons are less likely to be tested for HIV / AIDS.
3. The immune system defends against threats inside and outside the body.
   a. True
   b. False
4. Shingles lesions are not infectious.
   a. True
   b. False

Answers to these questions are on p. 517.

CHAPTER 44 NERVOUS SYSTEM AND MUSCULO-SKELETAL DISORDERS

Nervous System Disorders

Stroke

- Stroke is also called a brain attack or cerebrovascular accident (CVA). It is the third leading cause of death in the United States. Review Box 44-1, Stroke: Warning Signs, in the Textbook.
- The effects of stroke include:
  - Loss of face, hand, arm, leg, or body control
  - **Hemiplegia**—paralysis on 1 side of the body
  - Changing emotions (crying easily or mood swings, sometimes for no reason)
  - Difficulty swallowing (dysphagia)
  - Aphasia or slowed or slurred speech
  - Changes in sight, touch, movement, and thought
  - Impaired memory
  - Urinary frequency, urgency, or incontinence
  - Loss of bowel control or constipation
  - Depression and frustration
  - Behavior changes
- The health team helps the person regain the highest possible level of function. Review Box 44-2, Stroke Care Measures, in the Textbook.

Parkinson's Disease

- Parkinson's disease is a slow, progressive disorder with no cure. Persons over the age of 50 are at risk. Signs and symptoms become worse over time. They include:
  - *Tremors*—often start in 1 finger and spread to the whole arm. Pill-rolling movements—rubbing the thumb and index finger—may occur. The person may have trembling in the hands, arms, legs, jaw, and face.
  - *Rigid, stiff muscles*—in the arms, legs, neck, and trunk.
  - *Slow movements*—the person has a slow, shuffling gait.
  - *Stooped posture and impaired balance*—it is hard to walk. Falls are a risk.
  - *Mask-like expression*—the person cannot blink and smile. A fixed stare is common.
- Other signs and symptoms that develop over time include swallowing and chewing problems, constipation, and bladder problems. Sleep problems, depression, and emotional changes (fear, insecurity) can occur. So can memory loss and slow thinking. The person may have slurred, monotone, and soft speech. Some people talk too fast or repeat what they say.
- Drugs are ordered to treat and control the disease. Exercise and physical therapy improve strength, posture, balance, and mobility. Therapy is needed for speech and swallowing problems. The person may need help with eating and self-care. Safety measures are needed to prevent falls and injury.

Multiple Sclerosis

- Multiple sclerosis (MS) is a chronic disease. The myelin (which covers nerve fibers) in the brain and spinal cord is destroyed. Nerve impulses are not sent to and from the brain in a normal manner. Functions are impaired or lost. There is no cure.
- Symptoms usually start between the ages of 20 and 40. Signs and symptoms depend on the damaged area. They may include vision problems, muscle weakness in the arms and legs, and balance problems that affect standing and walking. Tingling, prickling, or numb sensations may occur. Also, partial or complete paralysis and pain may occur.
- Persons with MS are kept active as long as possible and as independent as possible. Skin care, hygiene, and range-of-motion (ROM) exercises are important. So are turning, positioning, and deep breathing and coughing. Bowel and bladder elimination is promoted. Injuries and complications from bedrest are prevented.

Head Injuries

- Traumatic brain injury (TBI) occurs from violent injury to the brain. Common causes include falls, traffic accidents, violence, sports, explosive blasts, and combat injuries. Review Box 44-3, Traumatic Brain Injury: Signs and Symptoms, in the Textbook.
- Disabilities from TBI include cognitive problems, sensory problems, communications problems, and emotional problems.

Spinal Cord Injury

- Spinal cord injuries can permanently damage the nervous system. Common causes are motor vehicle crashes, falls, violence, sports injuries, alcohol use, and cancer and other diseases.
- The higher the level of injury, the more functions lost.
  - Lumbar injuries—sensory and muscle function in the legs is lost. The person has **paraplegia**—paralysis and loss of sensory function in the legs and lower trunk.
  - Thoracic injuries—sensory and muscle function below the chest is lost. The person has paraplegia.

- Cervical injuries—sensory and muscle function of the arms, legs, and trunk is lost. Paralysis in the arms, legs, and trunk is called **quadriplegia** or **tetraplegia.**
- Review Box 44-4, Care of Persons With Paralysis, in the Textbook.

Musculo-Skeletal Disorders

Arthritis

- Arthritis means joint inflammation.
- *Osteoarthritis (degenerative joint disease).* The fingers, spine (neck and lower back), and weight-bearing joints (hips, knees, and feet) are often affected. Treatment involves pain relief, heat applications, exercise, rest and joint care, weight control, and a healthy life-style. Falls are prevented. Help is given with activities of daily living (ADL) as needed. Toilet seat risers are helpful when hips and knees are affected. So are chairs with higher seats and armrests. Some people need joint replacement surgery.
- *Rheumatoid arthritis.* Rheumatoid arthritis (RA) causes joint pain, swelling, stiffness, and loss of function. Joints are tender, warm, and swollen. Fatigue and fever are common. The person does not feel well. The person's care plan may include rest balanced with exercise, proper positioning, joint care, weight control, measures to reduce stress, and measures to prevent falls. Drugs are ordered for pain relief and to reduce inflammation. Heat and cold applications may be ordered. Some persons need joint replacement surgery. Emotional support is needed. Persons with RA need to stay as active as possible. Give encouragement and praise. Listen when the person needs to talk.

CHAPTER 44 REVIEW QUESTIONS

Circle the BEST answer.

1. The person had a stroke. Care includes all the following *except*
   a. Place the call light on the person's strong side
   b. Re-position the person every 2 hours
   c. Perform ROM exercises as ordered
   d. Place objects on the affected side
2. The person with hemiplegia
   a. Is paralyzed on 1 side of the body
   b. Has both arms paralyzed
   c. Has both legs paralyzed
   d. Has all extremities paralyzed
3. The person with multiple sclerosis should be kept active as long as possible.
   a. True
   b. False
4. The person has paralysis in the legs and lower trunk. This is called
   a. Quadriplegia
   b. Paraplegia
   c. Hemiplegia
   d. Tetraplegia
5. Fever is a common symptom of osteoarthritis.
   a. True
   b. False

Answers to these questions are on p. 517.

CHAPTER 45 CARDIOVASCULAR, RESPIRATORY, AND LYMPHATIC DISORDERS

Cardiovascular Disorders

- *Hypertension.* Hypertension (high blood pressure) occurs when the systolic pressure is 140 mm Hg or higher or the diastolic pressure is 90 mm Hg or higher. Narrowed blood vessels are a common cause. Review Box 45-1, Cardiovascular Disorders: Risk Factors, in the Textbook.
- *Coronary artery disease (CAD).* In CAD, the coronary artery become hardened and narrow and the heart muscle gets less blood and oxygen. The most common cause is atherosclerosis, or plaque buildup on artery walls. Complications of CAD are heart attack, irregular heartbeats, and sudden death. CAD complications may require cardiac rehabilitation, which consists of exercise training and education, counseling, and training for life-style changes.
- *Angina.* Angina is chest pain. It is caused by reduced blood flow to part of the heart muscle. Chest pain is described as tightness, pressure, squeezing, or burning in the chest. Pain can occur in the shoulders, arms, neck, jaw, or back. The person may be pale, feel faint, and perspire. Dyspnea is common. Nausea, fatigue, and weakness may occur. Some persons complain of "gas" or indigestion. Rest often relieves symptoms in 3 to 15 minutes. Chest pain lasting longer than a few minutes and not relieved by rest and nitroglycerin may signal heart attack. The person needs emergency care.
- *Myocardial infarction (MI).* MI also is called *heart attack, acute myocardial infarction (AMI),* and *acute coronary syndrome (ACS).* Blood flow to the heart muscle is suddenly blocked. Part of the heart muscle dies. MI is an emergency. Sudden cardiac death *(sudden cardiac arrest)* can occur. Review Box 45-2, Myocardial Infarction: Signs and Symptoms, in the Textbook.
- *Heart failure.* Heart failure or congestive heart failure (CHF) occurs when the heart is weakened and cannot pump normally. Blood backs up. Tissue congestion occurs. Drugs are given to strengthen the heart. They also reduce the amount of fluid in the body. A sodium-controlled diet is ordered. Oxygen is given. Semi-Fowler's position is preferred for breathing. Intake and output (I&O), daily weight, elastic stockings, and range-of-motion (ROM) exercises are part of the care plan.
- *Dysrhythmias.* Dysrhythmias are abnormal heart rhythms. Rhythms may be too fast, too slow, or irregular. Dysrhythmias are caused by changes in the heart's electrical system. Some abnormal rhythms are treated with a pacemaker.
- *Viral hemorrhagic fevers (VHFs).* VHFs are a group of illnesses caused by viruses. *Ebola* is a severe and deadly VHF caused by the *Ebolavirus.* Signs and symptoms can appear 2 to 21 days after exposure and include fever greater than 101.5°F, severe headache, muscle pain, weakness, diarrhea and vomiting, abdominal pain, and hemorrhage. The virus is contagious and is spread through direct contact with blood or body fluids, contaminated objects, and infected animals. The health team must prevent the spread of infection.

Hand hygiene, Standard Precautions, Transmission-Based Precautions, and the Bloodborne Pathogen Standard are followed. Special training is needed to care for such patients and for donning and removing personal protective equipment (PPE).

Respiratory Disorders

Chronic Obstructive Pulmonary Disease

- Two disorders are grouped under chronic obstructive pulmonary disease (COPD). They are chronic bronchitis and emphysema. These disorders obstruct airflow. Lung function is gradually lost.
- *Chronic bronchitis.* Bronchitis means inflammation of the bronchi. Chronic bronchitis occurs after repeated episodes of bronchitis. Smoking is the major cause. Smoker's cough in the morning is often the first symptom of chronic bronchitis. Over time, the cough becomes more frequent. The person has difficulty breathing and tires easily. The person must stop smoking. Oxygen therapy and breathing exercises are often ordered. If a respiratory tract infection occurs, the person needs prompt treatment.
- *Emphysema.* In emphysema, the alveoli enlarge and become less elastic. They do not expand and shrink normally when breathing in and out. Air becomes trapped when exhaling. Smoking is the most common cause. The person has shortness of breath and a cough. Sputum may contain pus. Fatigue is common. The person works hard to breathe in and out. Breathing is easier when the person sits upright and slightly forward. The person must stop smoking. Respiratory therapy, breathing exercises, oxygen, and drug therapy are ordered.

Asthma

- In asthma, the airway becomes inflamed and narrow. Extra mucus is produced. Dyspnea results. Wheezing and coughing are common. So are pain and tightening in the chest. Asthma usually is triggered by allergies. Other triggers include air pollutants and irritants, smoking and second-hand smoke, respiratory tract infections, exertion, and cold air. Asthma is treated with drugs. Severe attacks may require emergency care.

Pneumonia

- Pneumonia is an inflammation and infection of lung tissue. Bacteria, viruses, and other microbes are causes.
- High fever, chills, painful cough, chest pain on breathing, and rapid pulse occur. Shortness of breath and rapid breathing also occur. Cyanosis may be present. Sputum is thick and white, green, yellow, or rust-colored. Other signs and symptoms are nausea, vomiting, headache, tiredness, and muscle aches.
- Drugs are ordered for infection and pain. Fluid intake is increased. Intravenous (IV) therapy and oxygen may be needed. The semi-Fowler's position eases breathing. Rest is important. Standard Precautions are followed. Isolation precautions are used depending on the cause.

Tuberculosis

- Tuberculosis (TB) is a bacterial infection in the lungs. TB is spread by airborne droplets with coughing, sneezing,

speaking, singing, or laughing. Those who have close, frequent contact with an infected person are at risk. TB is more likely to occur in close, crowded areas. Age, poor nutrition, and human immunodeficiency virus (HIV) infection are other risk factors.
- Signs and symptoms are tiredness, loss of appetite, weight loss, fever, and night sweats. Cough and sputum production increase over time. Sputum may contain blood. Chest pain occurs.
- Drugs for TB are given. Standard Precautions and isolation precautions are needed. The person must cover the mouth and nose with tissues when sneezing, coughing, or producing sputum. Tissues are flushed down the toilet, placed in a BIOHAZARD bag, or placed in a paper bag and burned. Hand-washing after contact with sputum is essential.

CHAPTER 45 REVIEW QUESTIONS

Circle the BEST answer.
1. Which statement about angina is *false?*
   a. Angina is chest pain.
   b. The person may be pale and perspire.
   c. Rest often relieves the symptoms.
   d. You do not report angina to the nurse.
2. A person has heart failure. You do all of the following *except*
   a. Measure intake and output
   b. Measure weight daily
   c. Promote a diet that is high in salt
   d. Restrict fluids as ordered
3. Which position is usually best for the person with pneumonia?
   a. Semi-Fowler's
   b. Prone
   c. Supine
   d. Trendelenburg's
4. A bacterial infection in the lungs is
   a. Asthma
   b. Bronchitis
   c. Tuberculosis
   d. Emphysema

Answers to these questions are on p. 517.

CHAPTER 46 DIGESTIVE AND ENDOCRINE DISORDERS

Digestive Disorders

Gastro-Esophageal Reflux Disease (GERD)

- GERD occurs when stomach contents flow back up into the esophagus. Drugs to prevent stomach acid production or to promote stomach emptying may be ordered. Life-style changes include limiting smoking and alcohol, losing weight, eating small meals, wearing loose belts and clothing, and sitting upright for 3 hours after meals.

Vomiting

- These measures are needed.
  ○ Follow Standard Precautions and the Bloodborne Pathogen Standard.

○ Turn the person's head well to 1 side. This prevents aspiration.
○ Place a kidney basin under the person's chin.
○ Move vomitus away from the person.
○ Provide oral hygiene.
○ Observe vomitus for color, odor, and undigested food. If it looks like coffee grounds, it contains undigested blood. This signals bleeding. Report your observations.
○ Measure, report, and record the amount of vomitus. Also record the amount on the intake and output (I&O) record.
○ Save a specimen for laboratory study.
○ Dispose of vomitus after the nurse observes it.
○ Eliminate odors.
○ Provide for comfort.

Hepatitis

- Hepatitis is an inflammation of the liver. It can be mild or cause death. Signs and symptoms are listed in Box 46-1, Hepatitis, in the Textbook. Some people do not have symptoms.
- Protect yourself and others. Follow Standard Precautions and the Bloodborne Pathogen Standard. Isolation precautions are ordered as necessary. Assist the person with hygiene and hand-washing as needed.

Endocrine Disorders

Diabetes

- In this disorder the body cannot produce or use insulin properly. Insulin is needed for glucose to move from the blood into the cells. Sugar builds up in the blood. Cells do not have enough sugar for energy and cannot function.
- Diabetes must be controlled to prevent complications. Complications include blindness, renal failure, nerve damage, and damage to the gums and teeth. Heart and blood vessel diseases are other problems. They can lead to stroke, heart attack, and slow healing. Foot and leg wounds and ulcers are very serious.
- Good foot care is needed. Corns, blisters, calluses, and other foot problems can lead to an infection and amputation.
- Blood glucose is monitored for:
  ○ *Hypoglycemia*—low sugar in the blood.
  ○ *Hyperglycemia*—high sugar in the blood.
- Review Table 46-1 in the Textbook for the causes, signs, and symptoms of hypoglycemia and hyperglycemia. Both can lead to death if not corrected. You must call for the nurse at once.

CHAPTER 46 REVIEW QUESTIONS

Circle the BEST answer.

1. A person is vomiting. You should do all of the following *except*
   a. Follow Standard Precautions and the Bloodborne Pathogen Standard
   b. Keep the person supine
   c. Provide oral hygiene
   d. Observe the vomitus for color, odor, and undigested food

2. A person with diabetes is trembling, sweating, and feels faint. You
   a. Tell the nurse immediately
   b. Tell the nurse at the end of the shift
   c. Tell another nursing assistant
   d. Ignore the symptoms
3. All of the following are signs and symptoms of hepatitis *except*
   a. Itching
   b. Diarrhea
   c. Skin rash
   d. Increased appetite

Answers to these questions are on p. 517.

CHAPTER 47 URINARY AND REPRODUCTIVE DISORDERS

Urinary System Disorders

Urinary Tract Infections (UTIs)
- UTIs are common. Catheters, poor perineal hygiene, immobility, and poor fluid intake are common causes.

Prostate Enlargement
- The prostate grows larger as a man grows older. This is called benign prostatic hyperplasia (BPH). The enlarged prostate presses against the urethra. This obstructs urine flow through the urethra. Bladder function is gradually lost. Most men in their 60s and older have some symptoms of BPH.

Kidney Stones
- Kidney stones (calculi) are most common in white men 40 years of age and older. Bedrest, immobility, and poor fluid intake are risk factors. Review the list of symptoms on p. 752 in the Textbook.
- Stones vary in size from grains of sand to golf ball–sized.

Kidney Failure
- In kidney failure (renal failure) the kidneys do not function or are severely impaired. Waste products are not removed from the blood. Fluid is retained.
- Acute kidney failure is sudden. Blood flow to the kidneys is severely decreased. Causes include severe injury or bleeding, heart attack, heart failure, burns, infection, and severe allergic reactions.
- With chronic kidney failure the kidneys cannot meet the body's needs. Hypertension and diabetes are common causes. Infections, urinary tract obstructions, and tumors are other causes. Review Box 47-3, Chronic Kidney Disease: Signs and Symptoms, in the Textbook.

Reproductive Disorders

Sexually Transmitted Diseases
- A sexually transmitted disease (STD) is spread by oral, vaginal, or anal sex. Some people do not have signs and symptoms or are not aware of an infection. Others know but do not seek treatment because of embarrassment. Standard Precautions and the Bloodborne Pathogen Standard are followed.

CHAPTER 47 REVIEW QUESTIONS

Circle the BEST answer.
1. Which statement is *false*?
    a. Older persons are at high risk for urinary tract infections.
    b. Skin irritation and infection can occur if urine leaks onto the skin.
    c. Benign prostatic hypertrophy may cause urinary problems in women.
    d. Some people may not be aware of having a sexually transmitted disease.
2. An STD is spread by oral, vaginal, or anal sex.
    a. True
    b. False
3. A person with an STD always has signs and symptoms.
    a. True
    b. False

Answers to these questions are on p. 517.

CHAPTER 48 MENTAL HEALTH DISORDERS

- The whole person has physical, social, psychological, and spiritual parts. Each part affects the other.
- **Stress** is the response or change in the body caused by any emotional, physical, social, or economic factor.
- **Mental health** means the person copes with and adjusts to every-day stresses in ways accepted by society.
- **Mental disorder** is a disturbance in the ability to cope with or adjust to stress. Behavior and function are impaired. *Mental illness, emotional illness,* and *psychiatric disorder* also mean mental disorder.

Anxiety Disorders

- **Anxiety** is a vague, uneasy feeling in response to stress. The person may not know the cause. The person senses danger or harm—real or imagined. Some anxiety is normal. Review Box 48-1, Anxiety: Signs and Symptoms, in the Textbook.
- Coping and defense mechanisms are used to relieve anxiety. Review Box 48-2, Defense Mechanisms, in the Textbook.
- Some common anxiety disorders are panic disorder, phobias, obsessive-compulsive disorder, and post-traumatic stress disorder.
- *Panic disorder.* **Panic** is an intense and sudden feeling of fear, anxiety, terror, or dread. Onset is sudden with no obvious reason. The person cannot function. Signs and symptoms of anxiety are severe.
- *Phobias.* **Phobia** means an intense fear. The person has an intense fear of an object, situation, or activity that has little or no actual danger. The person avoids what is feared. When faced with the fear, the person has high anxiety and cannot function.
- *Obsessive-compulsive disorder (OCD).* An **obsession** is a recurrent, unwanted thought, idea, or image. **Compulsion** is repeating an act over and over again. The act may not make sense but the person has much anxiety if the act is not done. Some persons with OCD also have depression, eating disorders, substance abuse, and other anxiety disorders.

- *Post-traumatic stress disorder (PTSD).* PTSD occurs after a terrifying ordeal. The ordeal involved physical harm or the threat of physical harm. Review Box 48-3, Post-Traumatic Stress Disorder: Signs and Symptoms, in the Textbook. Flashbacks are common. A **flashback** is reliving the trauma in thoughts during the day and in nightmares during sleep. He or she may believe that the trauma is happening all over again. Signs and symptoms usually develop about 3 months after the harmful event. Or they may emerge years later. PTSD can develop at any age.

Schizophrenia

- **Schizophrenia** means split mind. It is a severe, chronic, disabling brain disorder that involves:
    - *Psychosis*—a state of severe mental impairment. The person does not view the real or unreal correctly.
    - *Hallucinations*—seeing, hearing, smelling, or feeling something that is not real.
    - *Delusion*—a false belief.
    - *Delusion of grandeur*—an exaggerated belief about one's importance, wealth, power, or talents.
    - *Delusion of persecution*—the false belief that one is being mistreated, abused, or harassed.
    - *Thought disorders*—trouble organizing thoughts or connecting thoughts logically.
    - *Movement disorders*—include agitated body movements; repeating motions over and over; and sitting for hours without moving, speaking, or responding.
    - *Emotional and behavioral problems*—normal functions are impaired or absent, including losing motivation or interest in daily activities, being unable to plan, lacking emotions, neglecting personal hygiene, and withdrawing socially.
    - *Cognitive problems*—trouble paying attention, understanding, or remembering information.
- The person with schizophrenia has problems relating to others. He or she may be paranoid. The person may have difficulty organizing thoughts. Responses are inappropriate. Communication is disturbed. The person may withdraw. Some people regress to an earlier time or condition. Some persons with schizophrenia attempt suicide.

Bipolar Disorder

- The person with bipolar disorder has severe extremes in mood, energy, and ability to function. There are emotional lows (depression) and emotional highs (mania). This disorder is also called manic-depressive illness. This disorder must be managed throughout life. Review Box 48-4, Bipolar Disorder: Signs and Symptoms, in the Textbook. Bipolar disorder can damage relationships and affect school or work performance. Some people are suicidal.

Depression

- Depression involves the body, mood, and thoughts. Symptoms affect work, study, sleep, eating, and other activities. The person is very sad.

- Depression is common in older persons. They have many losses—death of family and friends, loss of health, loss of body functions, and loss of independence. Loneliness and the side effects of some drugs also are causes. Review Box 48-5, Depression in Older Persons: Signs and Symptoms, in the Textbook. Depression in older persons is often overlooked or a wrong diagnosis is made.

Substance Abuse Disorder
Alcoholism
- Alcohol affects alertness, judgment, coordination, and reaction time. Over time, heavy drinking damages the brain, central nervous system, liver, kidneys, heart, blood vessels, and stomach. It also can cause forgetfulness and confusion. Alcoholism is a chronic disease. Alcoholism can be treated but not cured. Alcohol recovery, support programs, and drugs are used to help the person stop drinking. The person must avoid all alcohol to avoid a relapse.
- Alcohol effects vary with age. Even small amounts can make older persons feel "high." Older persons are at risk for falls, vehicle crashes, and other injuries from drinking. Mixing alcohol with some drugs can be harmful or fatal. Alcohol also makes some health problems worse.

Suicide
- **Suicide** means to kill oneself.
- Suicide is most often linked to depression, alcohol or substance abuse, or stressful events. Review Box 48-7, Suicide Risk Factors, in the Textbook.
- If a person mentions or talks about suicide, take the person seriously. Call for the nurse at once. Do not leave the person alone.

Care and Treatment
- Treatment of mental health disorders involves having the person explore his or her thoughts and feelings. This is done through psychotherapy and behavior, group, occupational, art, and family therapies. Often drugs are ordered.
- The care plan reflects the person's needs. The physical, safety and security, and emotional needs of the person must be met.
- Communication is important. Be alert to nonverbal communication.

CHAPTER 48 REVIEW QUESTIONS
Circle the BEST answer.
1. A person may not know why anxiety occurs.
   a. True
   b. False
2. Panic is an intense and sudden feeling of fear, anxiety, terror, or dread.
   a. True
   b. False
3. A person with an obsessive-compulsive disorder has a ritual that is repeated over and over again.
   a. True
   b. False

4. A person talks about suicide. You must do the following *except*
   a. Call the nurse at once
   b. Stay with the person
   c. Leave the person alone
   d. Take the person seriously
5. Which statement about depression in older persons is *false*?
   a. Depression is often overlooked in older persons.
   b. Depression rarely occurs in older persons.
   c. Loneliness may be a cause of depression in older persons.
   d. Side effects of some drugs may cause depression in older persons.
6. Which statement is *false*?
   a. Communication is important when caring for a person with a mental health disorder.
   b. You should be alert to nonverbal communication when caring for a person with a mental health disorder.
   c. The care plan reflects the needs of the person.
   d. The focus is only on the person's emotional needs.
Answers to these questions are on p. 517.

CHAPTER 49 CONFUSION AND DEMENTIA
- Changes in the brain and nervous system occur with aging. Review Box 49-1, Nervous System Changes From Aging, in the Textbook.
- Changes in the brain can affect **cognitive function**—memory, thinking, reasoning, ability to understand, judgment, and behavior.

Confusion
- Confusion has many causes. Diseases, infections, hearing and vision loss, brain injury, and drug side effects are some causes.
- When caring for the confused person:
  - Follow the person's care plan.
  - Provide for safety.
  - Face the person and speak clearly.
  - Call the person by name every time you are in contact with him or her.
  - State your name. Show your name tag.
  - Give the date and time each morning. Repeat as needed during the day and evening.
  - Explain what you are going to do and why.
  - Give clear, simple directions and answers to questions.
  - Break tasks into small steps.
  - Ask clear, simple questions. Allow time to respond.
  - Keep calendars and clocks with large numbers in the person's room. Remind the person of holidays, birthdays, and other events.
  - Have the person wear eyeglasses and hearing aids as needed.
  - Use touch to communicate.
  - Place familiar objects and pictures within the person's view.
  - Provide newspapers, magazines, TV, and radio. Read to the person if appropriate.

○ Discuss current events with the person.
○ Maintain the day-night cycle.
○ Provide a calm, relaxed, and peaceful setting.
○ Follow the person's routine.
○ Do not re-arrange furniture or the person's belongings.
○ Encourage the person to take part in self-care.
○ Be consistent.

Dementia

* **Dementia** is the loss of cognitive function that interferes with routine personal, social, and occupational activities.
* Dementia is not a normal part of aging. Most older people do not have dementia.
* Some early warning signs include problems with language, dressing, cooking, personality changes, poor or decreased judgment, and driving as well as getting lost in familiar places and misplacing items.
* Alzheimer's disease is the most common type of permanent dementia.

Alzheimer's Disease

* Alzheimer's disease (AD) is a brain disease. Memory, thinking, reasoning, judgment, language, behavior, mood, and personality are affected.

Signs of AD

* The classic sign of AD is gradual loss of short-term memory. Warning signs include:
  ○ Asking the same questions over and over again.
  ○ Repeating the same story—word for word, again and again.
  ○ Forgetting activities that were once done regularly with ease.
  ○ Losing the ability to pay bills or balance a checkbook.
  ○ Getting lost in familiar places. Or misplacing household objects.
  ○ Neglecting to bathe or wearing the same clothes over and over again. Meanwhile, the person insists that a bath was taken or that clothes were changed.
  ○ Relying on someone else to make decisions or answer questions that the person would have handled.
* Review Box 49-5, Signs of Alzheimer's Disease, in the Textbook for other signs of AD.

Behaviors

* The following behaviors are common with AD.
  ○ *Wandering.* Persons with AD are not oriented to person, place, and time. They may wander away from home and not find their way back. The person cannot tell what is safe or dangerous.
  ○ *Sundowning.* With sundowning, signs, symptoms, and behaviors of AD increase during hours of darkness. As daylight ends, confusion, restlessness, anxiety, agitation, and other symptoms increase.
  ○ *Hallucinations.* The person with AD may see, hear, or feel things that are not real.
  ○ *Delusions.* People with AD may think they are some other person. A person may believe that the caregiver is someone else.
  ○ *Paranoia.* The person has false beliefs and suspicion about a person or situation.
  ○ *Catastrophic reactions.* The person reacts as if there is a disaster or tragedy.
  ○ *Agitation and aggression.* The person may pace, hit, or yell.
  ○ *Communication changes.* The person has trouble expressing thoughts and emotions.
  ○ *Screaming.* Persons with AD may scream to communicate.
  ○ *Repetitive behaviors.* Persons with AD repeat the same motions over and over again.
  ○ *Rummaging and hiding things.* The person may search for things by moving things around, turning things over, or looking through something such as a drawer or closet. The person may hide things, throw things away, or lose something.
  ○ *Changes in intimacy and sexuality.* The person with AD may depend on and cling to his or her partner or may not remember life with or feelings for his or her partner. Sexual behaviors may involve the wrong person, the wrong time, and the wrong place. Persons with AD cannot control behavior.

Care of Persons With AD and Other Dementias

* People with AD do not choose to be forgetful, incontinent, agitated, or rude. Nor do they choose to have other behaviors, signs, and symptoms of the disease. The disease causes the behaviors.
* Safety, hygiene, nutrition and fluids, elimination, and activity needs must be met. So must comfort and sleep needs. Review Box 49-10, Care of Persons With AD and Other Dementias, in the Textbook.
* The person can have other health problems and injuries. However, the person may not recognize pain, fever, constipation, incontinence, or other signs and symptoms. Carefully observe the person. Report any change in the person's usual behavior to the nurse.
* Infection is a risk. Provide good skin care, oral hygiene, and perineal care after bowel and bladder elimination.
* Supervised activities meet the person's needs and cognitive abilities.
* Impaired communication is a common problem. Avoid giving orders, wanting the truth, and correcting the person's errors.
* Always look for dangers in the person's room and in the hallways, lounges, dining areas, and other areas on the nursing unit. Remove the danger if you can.
* Every staff member must be alert to persons who wander. Such persons are allowed to wander in safe areas.

The Family

* The family may have physical, emotional, social, and financial stresses. The family often feels hopeless. No matter what is done, the person only gets worse. Anger and resentment may result. Guilt feelings are common.
* The family is an important part of the health team. They may help plan the person's care. For many persons, family members provide comfort. The family also needs support and understanding from the health team.

CHAPTER 49 REVIEW QUESTIONS

Circle the BEST answer.

1. Cognitive function involves all of the following *except*
   a. Memory and thinking
   b. Reasoning and understanding
   c. Personality and mood
   d. Judgment and behavior
2. When caring for a confused person, you do the following *except*
   a. Provide for safety
   b. Maintain the day-night schedule
   c. Keep calendars and clocks in the person's room
   d. Ask difficult-to-understand questions and give complex directions
3. Which statement about dementia is *false*?
   a. Dementia is a normal part of aging.
   b. The person may have changes in personality.
   c. Alzheimer's disease is the most common type of dementia.
   d. The person may have changes in behavior.
4. When caring for persons with AD, you do the following *except*
   a. Provide good skin care
   b. Talk to them in a calm voice
   c. Observe them closely for unusual behavior
   d. Allow personal choice in wandering

Answers to these questions are on p. 517.

CHAPTER 51 SEXUALITY

Sex and Sexuality

- Sexuality involves the whole person. Illness, injury, and aging can affect sexuality.

Sexuality and Older Persons

- Love, affection, and intimacy are needed throughout life. Older persons love, fall in love, hold hands, and embrace. Many have intercourse.
- Reproductive organs change with aging. Frequency of sex decreases for many older persons.
- Sexual partners are lost through death, divorce, and relationship break-ups. Or a partner needs hospital or nursing center care.

Meeting Sexual Needs

- The nursing team promotes the meeting of sexual needs.
- Review Box 51-1, Promoting Sexuality, in the Textbook.

The Sexually Aggressive Person

- Some persons want the health team to meet their sexual needs. They flirt or make sexual advances or comments. Some expose themselves, masturbate, or touch the staff. This can anger and embarrass the staff member. These reactions are normal.
- Touch may have a sexual purpose. You must be professional about the matter.
  - Ask the person not to touch you. State the places where you were touched.

- Tell the person that you will not do what he or she wants.
- Tell the person what behaviors make you uncomfortable. Politely ask the person not to act that way.
- Allow privacy if the person is becoming aroused.
- Discuss the matter with the nurse. The nurse can help you understand the behavior.
- Follow the care plan. It has measures to deal with sexually aggressive behaviors. They are based on the cause of the behavior.

Protecting the Person

- The person must be protected from unwanted sexual comments and advances. This is sexual abuse (see Chapter 5 in the Textbook). Tell the nurse right away.
- No one should be allowed to sexually abuse another person. This includes staff members, patients, residents, family members or other visitors, and volunteers.

CHAPTER 51 REVIEW QUESTIONS

Circle the BEST answer.

1. A resident touches you in a sexual way. You should do the following *except*
   a. Ask the person not to touch you
   b. Discuss the matter with the nurse
   c. Tell the person what behaviors make you uncomfortable
   d. Yell at the person immediately
2. Unwanted sexual comments and advances are forms of sexual abuse.
   a. True
   b. False

Answers to these questions are on p. 517.

CHAPTER 54 BASIC EMERGENCY CARE

Emergency Care

- Rules for emergency care include:
  - Know your limits. Do not do more than you are able.
  - Stay calm.
  - Know where to find emergency supplies.
  - Follow Standard Precautions and the Bloodborne Pathogen Standard to the extent possible.
  - Check for life-threatening problems. Check for breathing, a pulse, and bleeding.
  - Keep the person lying down or as you found him or her.
  - Move the person only if the setting is unsafe. If the scene is not safe enough for you to approach, wait for help to arrive.
  - Perform necessary emergency measures.
  - Call for help.
  - Do not remove clothes unless necessary.
  - Keep the person warm. Cover the person with a blanket, coat, or sweater.
  - Re-assure the person. Explain what is happening and that help was called.
  - Do not give the person food or fluids.
  - Keep on-lookers away. They invade privacy.
- Review Box 54-1, Emergency Care Rules, in the Textbook for more information.

Basic Life Support for Adults

- Cardiopulmonary resuscitation (CPR) supports breathing and circulation. It provides blood and oxygen to the heart, brain, and other organs until advanced emergency care is given. CPR is done if the person does not respond, is not breathing, and has no pulse.
- CPR involves:
  - *Chest compressions*—the heart, brain, and other organs must receive blood. Chest compressions force blood through the circulatory system.
  - *Airway*—the airway must be open and clear of obstructions. The head tilt–chin lift method opens the airway.
  - *Breathing*—air is not inhaled when breathing stops. The person must get oxygen. The person is given breaths by a rescuer inflating the person's lungs.
  - *Defibrillation*—ventricular fibrillation (VF, V-fib) is an abnormal heart rhythm. Rather than beating in a regular rhythm, the heart shakes and quivers. The heart does not pump blood. The heart, brain, and other organs do not receive blood and oxygen. A *defibrillator* is used to deliver a shock to the heart. This allows the return of a regular heart rhythm. Defibrillation as soon as possible after the onset of VF (V-fib) increases the person's chance of survival.

Hemorrhage

- Hemorrhage is the excessive loss of blood in a short time. It can be internal or external.
- Internal bleeding cannot be seen but can cause pain, shock, vomiting of blood, coughing up blood, cold and moist skin, and loss of consciousness. Follow the Emergency Care Rules in Box 54-1 in the Textbook; this includes activating the Emergency Medical Services (EMS) system; keeping the person warm, flat, and quiet until help arrives; and not giving fluids.
- To control external bleeding:
  - Follow the Emergency Care Rules in Box 54-1 in the Textbook. This includes activating the EMS system.
  - Do not remove any objects that have pierced or stabbed the person.
  - Place a sterile dressing directly over the wound. Or use any clean material.
  - Apply firm pressure directly over the bleeding site. Do not release pressure or remove the dressing.
  - Bind the wound when bleeding stops.

Fainting

- **Fainting** is the sudden loss of consciousness from an inadequate blood supply to the brain.
- Warning signals are dizziness, perspiration, and blackness before the eyes. The person looks pale. The pulse is weak. Respirations are shallow if consciousness is lost. Emergency care includes:
  - Have the person sit or lie down before fainting occurs.
  - If sitting, the person bends forward and places the head between the knees.
  - If the person is lying down, raise the legs.
  - Loosen tight clothing.
  - Keep the person lying down if fainting has occurred. Raise the legs.
  - Do not let the person get up quickly.
  - Help the person to a sitting position after recovery from fainting.
- Provide Basic Life Support (BLS) if there is no response or breathing.

Seizures

- You cannot stop a seizure. However, you can protect the person from injury.
  - Follow the Emergency Care Rules in Box 54-1 in the Textbook.
  - Do not leave the person alone.
  - Lower the person to the floor.
  - Note the time the seizure started.
  - Place something soft under the person's head.
  - Loosen tight jewelry and clothing around the person's neck.
  - Turn the person onto his or her side. Make sure the head is turned to the side.
  - Do not put any object or your fingers between the person's teeth.
  - Do not try to stop the seizure or control the person's movements.
  - Move furniture, equipment, and sharp objects away from the person.
  - Note the time when the seizure ends.
  - Make sure the mouth is clear of food, fluids, and saliva after the seizure.
  - Provide BLS if the person is not breathing after the seizure.

Concussion

- Head injuries can be minor or serious and life-threatening. A concussion results from a bump or blow to the head or jolt to the head or body. The head and brain move quickly back and forth.
- Symptoms can last for days, weeks, or longer. Symptoms include difficulty thinking and concentrating, headaches, fuzzy or blurred vision, nausea and vomiting, sensitivity to noise or light, feelings of tiredness or low energy, irritability and sadness, mood swings, and more or less sleep than usual.
- The following danger signs signal the need for emergency care:
  - Headache that gets worse or does not go away
  - Stiff neck
  - Weakness, numbness, or decreased coordination
  - Nausea or vomiting more than once
  - Slurred speech
  - Very sleepy; drowsy; cannot be awakened
  - One eye pupil is larger than the other
  - Convulsions or seizures
  - Cannot recognize people, places, or things
  - Increased confusion, restlessness, or agitation
  - Unusual behavior
  - Loss of consciousness
- Follow the Emergency Care Rules in Box 54-1 in your Textbook. This includes activating the EMS system.

CHAPTER 54 REVIEW QUESTIONS

Circle the BEST answer.

1. During an emergency, you do all of the following *except*
   a. Perform only procedures you have been trained to do
   b. Keep the person lying down or as you found him or her
   c. Let the person become cold
   d. Re-assure the person and explain what is happening
2. During an emergency, you keep on-lookers away.
   a. True
   b. False
3. Which statement about fainting is *false*?
   a. If standing, have the person sit down before fainting.
   b. If sitting, have the person bend forward and place his head between his knees before fainting occurs.
   c. Tighten the person's clothing.
   d. Raise the legs if the person is lying down.
4. During a seizure, you do the following *except*
   a. Turn the person's body to the side
   b. Place your fingers in the person's mouth
   c. Note the time the seizure started and ended
   d. Turn the person's head to the side
5. The symptoms of a concussion are gone within 24 hours.
   a. True
   b. False

Answers to these questions are on p. 517.

CHAPTER 55 END-OF-LIFE CARE

Attitudes About Death

- Attitudes about death often change as a person grows older and with changing circumstances.

Culture and Spiritual Needs

- Practices and attitudes about death differ among cultures.
- Attitudes about death are closely related to religion. Many religions practice rites and rituals during the dying process and at the time of death.

Age

- Adults fear pain and suffering, dying alone, and the invasion of privacy. They also fear loneliness and separation from loved ones. Adults often resent death because it affects plans, hopes, dreams, and ambitions.
- Older persons usually have fewer fears than younger adults. Some welcome death as freedom from pain, suffering, and disability. Death also means reunion with those who have died. Like younger adults, they often fear dying alone.

The Stages of Dying

- Dr. Kübler-Ross described 5 stages of dying. They are:
  ○ *Stage 1: Denial.* The person refuses to believe he or she is going to die.
  ○ *Stage 2: Anger.* There is anger and rage, often at family, friends, and the health team.
  ○ *Stage 3: Bargaining.* Often the person bargains with God or a higher power for more time.
  ○ *Stage 4: Depression.* The person is sad and mourns things that were lost.
  ○ *Stage 5: Acceptance.* The person is calm and at peace. The person accepts death.
- Dying persons do not always pass through all 5 stages. A person may never get beyond a certain stage. Some move back and forth between stages.

Comfort Needs

- Comfort is a basic part of end-of-life care. It involves physical, mental and emotional, and spiritual needs. Comfort goals are to:
  ○ Prevent or relieve suffering to the extent possible.
  ○ Respect and follow end-of-life wishes.
- Dying persons may want to talk about their fears, worries, and anxieties. You need to listen and use touch.
  ○ *Listening.* Let the person express feelings and emotions in his or her own way. Do not worry about saying the wrong thing or finding the right words. You do not need to say anything.
  ○ *Touch.* Touch shows caring and concern. Sometimes the person does not want to talk but needs you nearby. Silence, along with touch, is a meaningful way to communicate.
- Some people may want to see a spiritual leader. Or they may want to take part in religious practices.

Physical Needs

- As the person weakens, basic needs are met. The person may depend on others for basic needs and activities of daily living (ADL). Every effort is made to promote physical and psychological comfort. The person is allowed to die in peace and with dignity.

Pain

- Some dying persons do not have pain. Others may have severe pain. Always report signs and symptoms of pain at once. Pain management is important. The nurse can give pain-relief drugs. Preventing and controlling pain is easier than relieving pain.

Breathing Problems

- Shortness of breath and difficulty breathing (dyspnea) are common end-of-life problems. The semi-Fowler's position and oxygen are helpful.
- Noisy breathing (death rattle) is common as death nears. This is due to mucus collecting in the airway. The side-lying position, suctioning by the nurse, and drugs to reduce the amount of mucus may help.

Vision, Hearing, and Speech

- Vision blurs and gradually fails. Explain what you are doing to the person or in the room. Provide good eye care.
- Hearing is one of the last functions lost. Always assume that the person can hear.
- Speech becomes difficult. Anticipate the person's needs. Do not ask questions that need long answers.

Mouth, Nose, and Skin
- Frequent oral hygiene is given as death nears.
- Crusting and irritation of the nostrils can occur. Carefully clean the nose.
- Skin care, bathing, and preventing pressure ulcers are necessary. Change linens and gowns whenever needed.

Nutrition
- Nausea, vomiting, and loss of appetite are common at the end of life. The doctor can order drugs for nausea and vomiting.
- Some persons are too tired or too weak to eat. You may need to feed them.
- As death nears, loss of appetite is common. The person may choose not to eat or drink. Do not force the person to eat or drink. Report refusal to eat or drink to the nurse.

Elimination
- Urinary and fecal incontinence may occur. Give perineal care as needed.

The Person's Room
- The person's room should be comfortable and pleasant. It should be well lit and well ventilated. Remove unnecessary equipment.
- Mementos, pictures, cards, flowers, and religious items provide comfort. The person and family arrange the room as they wish.

The Family
- This is a hard time for family. The family goes through stages like the dying person. Be available, courteous, and considerate.
- The person and family need time together. However, you cannot neglect care because the family is present. Most agencies let family members help give care.

Legal Issues
- *Advance directives.* Advance directives give persons rights to accept or refuse treatment. The advance directive is a document stating a person's wishes about health care when that person cannot make his or her own decisions.
- *Living wills.* A living will is a document about measures that support or maintain life when death is likely. A living will may instruct doctors not to start measures that promote dying or to remove measures that prolong dying.
- *Durable power of attorney for health care.* This gives the power to make health care decisions to another person. When a person cannot make health care decisions, the person with durable power of attorney can do so.
- *"Do Not Resuscitate" (DNR) order.* This means the person will not be resuscitated. The person is allowed to die with peace and dignity. The orders are written after consulting with the person and family.

- You may not agree with care and resuscitation decisions. However, you must follow the person's or family's wishes and the doctor's orders. These may be against your personal, religious, and cultural values. If so, discuss the matter with the nurse. An assignment change may be needed.

Signs of Death
- There are signs that death is near.
  - Movement, muscle tone, and sensation are lost.
  - Abdominal distention, fecal incontinence, nausea, and vomiting are common.
  - Body temperature rises. The person feels cool, looks pale, and perspires heavily.
  - The pulse is fast or slow, weak, and irregular. Blood pressure starts to fall.
  - Slow or rapid and shallow respirations are observed. Mucus collects in the airway. This causes the death rattle that is heard.
  - Pain decreases as the person loses consciousness. Some people are conscious until the moment of death.
- The signs of death include no pulse, no respirations, and no blood pressure. The pupils are dilated and fixed.

Care of the Body After Death
- Post-mortem care is done to maintain a good appearance of the body.
- Moving the body when giving post-mortem care can cause remaining air in the lungs, stomach, and intestines to be expelled. When air is expelled, sounds are produced.
- When giving post-mortem care, follow Standard Precautions and the Bloodborne Pathogen Standard.

CHAPTER 55 REVIEW QUESTIONS

Circle the BEST answer.

1. Which statement is *false?*
   a. Adults fear dying alone.
   b. Older persons usually have fewer fears about dying than younger adults.
   c. Adults often resent death.
   d. All adults welcome death.
2. Persons in the denial stage of dying
   a. Are angry
   b. Bargain with God
   c. Refuse to believe that they are dying
   d. Are calm and at peace
3. When caring for a person who is dying, you should do the following *except*
   a. Listen to the person
   b. Talk about your feelings about death
   c. Provide privacy during spiritual moments
   d. Use touch to show care and concern

4. When caring for a dying person, you provide all of the following *except*
   a. Eye care
   b. Oral hygiene
   c. Good skin care
   d. Physical exercise

5. When giving post-mortem care, you should wear gloves.
   a. True
   b. False

6. A document that states a person's wishes about health care when that person cannot make his or her own decisions is a
   a. Living will
   b. Advance directive
   c. Durable power of attorney for health care
   d. "Do Not Resuscitate" order

Answers to these questions are on p. 517.

Practice Examination 1

This test contains 75 questions. For each question, circle the BEST answer.

1. A nurse asks you to give a person his drug when he is done in the bathroom. Your response to the nurse is
   A. "I will give the drug for you."
   B. "I will ask the other nursing assistant to give the drug."
   C. "I am sorry but I cannot give that drug. I will let you know when he is out of the bathroom."
   D. "I refuse to give that drug."

2. An ethical person
   A. Does not judge others
   B. Avoids persons whose standards and values are different from his or hers
   C. Is prejudiced and biased
   D. Causes harm to another person

3. You smell alcohol on the breath of a co-worker. You
   A. Ignore the situation
   B. Tell the co-worker to get counseling
   C. Take a break and drink some alcohol too
   D. Tell the nurse at once

4. A person's call light goes unanswered. He gets out of bed and falls. His leg is broken. This is
   A. Neglect
   B. Emotional abuse
   C. Physical abuse
   D. Malpractice

5. Your mom asks you about a person on your unit. How should you respond?
   A. "She is walking better now that she is receiving physical therapy."
   B. "I'm sorry but I cannot talk about her. It is unprofessional and violates her privacy and confidentiality."
   C. "Don't tell anyone I told you but she is getting worse."
   D. "She has been very sad recently and needs visitors."

6. You are going off duty. The nursing assistant coming on duty is on the unit with you. A person puts her call light on. Your response is
   A. "I'm ready to go. I will let you answer that light."
   B. "I've been here all day so I am not answering that light."
   C. "No one helped me answer lights when I came on duty."
   D. "I will answer that light so you can get organized for the shift."

7. When recording in the medical record, you
   A. Write in pencil
   B. Spell words incorrectly
   C. Use only center-approved abbreviations
   D. Record what your co-worker did

8. You are answering the phone in the nurses' station. You
   A. Answer in a rushed manner
   B. Give a courteous greeting
   C. End the conversation and hang up without saying good-bye
   D. Give confidential information about a resident to the caller

9. A person who was admitted to the nursing center yesterday does not feel safe. You
   A. Are rude as you care for the person
   B. Ignore the person's requests for information
   C. Show the person around the nursing center
   D. Act rushed as you care for the person

10. A person is angry and is shouting at you. You should
    A. Yell back at the person
    B. Stay calm and professional
    C. Put the person in a room away from others
    D. Call the family

11. When speaking with another person, you
    A. Use medical terms that may not be familiar to the person
    B. Mumble your words as you talk
    C. Ask several questions at a time
    D. Speak clearly and distinctly

12. To use a transfer or gait belt safely, you should
    A. Ignore the manufacturer's instructions
    B. Leave the excess strap dangling
    C. Apply the belt over bare skin
    D. Apply the belt under the breasts

13. When you are listening to a person, you
    A. Look around the room
    B. Sit with your arms crossed
    C. Act rushed and not interested in what the person is saying
    D. Have good eye contact with the person

14. When caring for a person who is comatose, you
    A. Make jokes about how sick the person is
    B. Care for the person without talking to him or her
    C. Explain what you are doing to him or her
    D. Discuss your problems with the other nursing assistant in the room with you

15. You need to give care to a person when a visitor is present. You
    A. Politely ask the visitor to leave the room
    B. Do the care in the presence of the visitor
    C. Expose the person's body in front of the visitor
    D. Rudely tell the visitor where to wait while you care for the person

16. A person tells you he wants to talk with a minister. You
    A. Ignore the request
    B. Tell the nurse
    C. Ask what the person wants to discuss with the minister
    D. Tell the person there is no need to talk with a minister

17. When you care for a person who has a restraint, you
    A. Observe the person every 15 minutes
    B. Remove the restraint and re-position the person every 4 hours
    C. Apply the restraint tightly
    D. Apply the restraint incorrectly

18. As a person ages
    A. The skin becomes less dry
    B. Muscle strength increases
    C. Reflexes are faster
    D. Bladder muscles weaken
19. A person you are caring for touches your buttocks several times. You
    A. Tell the person you like being touched
    B. Ask the person not to touch you again
    C. Tell the person's daughter
    D. Tell the person's girlfriend
20. You are transporting a person in a wheelchair. You
    A. Pull the chair backward
    B. Let the person's feet touch the floor
    C. Push the chair forward
    D. Rest the footplates on the person's leg
21. You cannot read the person's name on the identification (ID) bracelet. You
    A. Tell the nurse so a new bracelet can be made
    B. Ignore the fact that you cannot read the name
    C. Ask another nursing assistant to identify the person
    D. Tell the family the person needs a new ID bracelet
22. The universal sign of choking is
    A. Holding your breath
    B. Clutching at the throat
    C. Waving your hands
    D. Coughing
23. A person is on a diabetic diet. You
    A. Serve the person's meals late
    B. Let the person eat whenever he or she is hungry
    C. Sometimes check the tray to see what was eaten
    D. Tell the nurse about changes in the person's eating habits
24. With mild airway obstruction
    A. The person is usually unconscious
    B. The person cannot speak
    C. Forceful coughing often does not remove the object
    D. Forceful coughing often can remove the object
25. To relieve severe airway obstruction in a conscious adult, you do
    A. Abdominal thrusts
    B. Back thrusts
    C. Chest compressions
    D. A finger sweep
26. Faulty electrical equipment
    A. Can be used in a nursing center
    B. Should be given to the nurse
    C. Should be taken home by you for repair
    D. Should be used only with alert persons
27. A warning label has been removed from a hazardous substance container. You
    A. May use the substance if you know what is in the container
    B. Leave the container where it is
    C. Take the container to the nurse and explain the problem
    D. Tell another nursing assistant about the missing label

28. A person's beliefs and values are different from your views. What should you do?
    A. Refuse to care for the person.
    B. Delegate care to another nursing assistant.
    C. Tell the nurse about your concerns.
    D. Tell the person how you feel.
29. You find a person smoking in the nursing center. You should
    A. Ignore the situation
    B. Tell the person to leave
    C. Tell another nursing assistant
    D. Ask the person to put out the cigarette and show him or her where smoking is permitted
30. During a fire, the first thing you do is
    A. Rescue persons in immediate danger
    B. Sound the nearest fire alarm
    C. Close doors and windows to confine the fire
    D. Extinguish the fire
31. A person with Alzheimer's disease has increased restlessness and confusion as daylight ends. You should
    A. Try to reason with the person
    B. Ask the person to tell you what is bothering him or her
    C. Provide a calm, quiet setting late in the day
    D. Complete the person's treatments and activities late in the day
32. To prevent suffocation, you should
    A. Make sure dentures fit loosely
    B. Cut food into large pieces
    C. Make sure the person can chew and swallow the food served
    D. Ignore loose teeth or dentures
33. When using a wheelchair, you should
    A. Lock both wheels before you transfer a person to and from the wheelchair
    B. Lock only 1 wheel before you transfer a person to and from the wheelchair
    C. Let the person's feet touch the floor when the chair is moving
    D. Let the person stand on the footplates
34. A person begins to fall while you are walking him or her. You should
    A. Try to prevent the fall
    B. Ease the person to the floor
    C. Let the person fall to avoid injury to yourself
    D. Tell the nurse at the end of the shift
35. A person has a restraint on. You know that
    A. Restraints are used for staff convenience
    B. Death from strangulation is a risk factor from using a restraint
    C. Restraints may be used to punish a person
    D. A written nurse's order is required for a restraint
36. Before feeding a person, you
    A. Tell the other nursing assistant
    B. Go to the restroom
    C. Wash your hands
    D. Tell the nurse

37. When wearing gloves, you remember to
    A. Wear them several times before discarding them
    B. Wear the same ones from room to room
    C. Wear gloves with a tear or puncture
    D. Change gloves when they become contaminated with urine
38. When washing your hands, you
    A. Use hot water
    B. Let your uniform touch the sink
    C. Keep your watch at your wrist
    D. Keep your hands and forearms lower than your elbows
39. You need to move a box from the floor to the counter in the utility room. You
    A. Bend from your waist to pick up the box
    B. Hold the box away from your body as you pick it up
    C. Bend your knees and squat to lift the box
    D. Stand with your feet close together as you pick up the box
40. The nurse asks you to place a person in Fowler's position. You
    A. Put the bed flat
    B. Raise the head of the bed between 45 and 60 degrees
    C. Raise the head of the bed between 80 and 90 degrees
    D. Raise the head of the bed 15 degrees
41. You accidentally scratch a person. This is
    A. Neglect
    B. Negligence
    C. Malpractice
    D. Physical abuse
42. You positioned a person in a chair. For good body alignment, you
    A. Have the person's back and buttocks against the back of the chair
    B. Leave the person's feet unsupported
    C. Have the backs of the person's knees touch the edge of the chair
    D. Have the person sit on the edge of the chair
43. You need to transfer a person with a weak left leg from the bed to the wheelchair. You
    A. Get the person out of bed on the left side
    B. Get the person out of bed on the right side
    C. Keep the person in bed
    D. Ask the person what side moves first
44. A person tries to scratch and kick you. You should
    A. Protect yourself from harm
    B. Argue with the person
    C. Become angry with the person
    D. Ignore the person
45. When moving a person up in bed
    A. Window coverings may be left open so people can look in
    B. Body parts may be exposed
    C. Ask the person to help
    D. Ask the person to lie still
46. For comfort, most older persons prefer
    A. Rooms that are cold
    B. Restrooms that smell of urine
    C. Loud talking and laughter at the nurses' station
    D. Lighting that meets their needs

47. Call lights are
    A. Placed on the person's strong side
    B. Answered when time permits
    C. Kept on the bedside table
    D. Kept on the person's weak side
48. A nurse asks you to inspect a person's closet. You
    A. Tell the nurse you cannot do this
    B. Inspect the closet when the person is in the dining room
    C. Ask the person if you can inspect his or her closet
    D. Tell the nurse to inspect the closet
49. When changing bed linens, you
    A. Hold the linens close to your uniform
    B. Shake the sheet when putting it on the bed
    C. Take only needed linens into the person's room
    D. Put used linens on the floor
50. To use a fire extinguisher, you
    A. Keep the safety pin in the extinguisher
    B. Direct the hose or nozzle at the top of the fire
    C. Squeeze the lever to start the stream
    D. Sweep the stream at the top of the fire
51. When doing mouth care for an unconscious person, you
    A. Do not need to wear gloves
    B. Give mouth care at least every 2 hours
    C. Place the person in a supine position
    D. Keep the mouth open with your fingers
52. A person is angry because he did not get to the activity room on time because a co-worker did not come to work. How should you respond to him?
    A. "It's not my fault. A co-worker called off today and we are short-staffed."
    B. "I'm sorry you were late for activities. I will try to plan better."
    C. "I am doing the best I can."
    D. "I'm just too busy."
53. You are asked to clean a person's dentures. You
    A. Use hot water
    B. Hold the dentures firmly and line the basin with a towel
    C. Wrap the dentures in tissues after cleaning
    D. Store the dentures in a denture cup with the person's room number on it
54. When bathing a person, you notice a rash that was not there before. You
    A. Do nothing
    B. Tell the person
    C. Tell the nurse and record it in the medical record
    D. Tell the person's daughter
55. When washing a person's eyes, you
    A. Use soap
    B. Clean the eye near you first
    C. Wipe from the inner to the outer aspect of the eye
    D. Wipe from the outer aspect to the inner aspect of the eye
56. When giving a back massage, you
    A. Use cold lotion
    B. Use light strokes
    C. Massage reddened bony areas
    D. Look for bruises and breaks in the skin

57. You need to give perineal care to a female. You
    A. Separate the labia and clean downward from front to back
    B. Separate the labia and clean upward from back to front
    C. Wear gloves only if there is drainage
    D. Only use water
58. When giving a person a tub bath or shower, you
    A. Do not give the person a call light
    B. Turn the hot water on first, then the cold water
    C. Stay within hearing distance if the person can be left alone
    D. Direct water toward the person while adjusting the water temperature
59. A person is on an anticoagulant. You
    A. Use a safety razor
    B. Use an electric razor
    C. Let him grow a beard
    D. Let him choose which type of razor to use
60. A person with a weak left arm wants to remove his or her sweater. You
    A. Let the person do it without any assistance
    B. Help the person remove the sweater from his or her right arm first
    C. Help the person remove the sweater from his or her left arm first
    D. Tell the person to keep the sweater on
61. When talking with a person, you should call the person
    A. "Honey"
    B. By his or her first name
    C. By his or her title—Mr. or Mrs. or Miss
    D. "Grandpa" or "Grandma"
62. A person has an indwelling catheter. You
    A. Let the person lie on the tubing
    B. Disconnect the catheter from the drainage tubing every 8 hours
    C. Secure the catheter to the lower leg
    D. Measure and record the amount of urine in the drainage bag
63. A person needs to eat a diet that contains carbohydrates. Carbohydrates
    A. Are needed for tissue repair and growth
    B. Provide energy and fiber for bowel elimination
    C. Add flavor to food and help the body use certain vitamins
    D. Are needed for nerve and muscle function
64. You are taking a rectal temperature with an electronic thermometer. You
    A. Insert the thermometer before lubricating it
    B. Leave the privacy curtain open
    C. Insert the thermometer 1 inch into the rectum
    D. Insert the thermometer ½ inch into the rectum
65. A person has a blood pressure (BP) of 86/58 mm Hg. You
    A. Report the BP to the nurse at once
    B. Record the BP but do not tell the nurse
    C. Ask the unit secretary to tell the nurse
    D. Retake the BP in 30 minutes before telling the nurse

66. On which person would you take an oral temperature?
    A. An unconscious person
    B. The person receiving oxygen
    C. The person who breathes through his or her mouth
    D. A conscious person
67. When caring for a person who is blind or visually impaired, you
    A. Offer the person your arm and have the person walk a half step behind you
    B. Do as much for the person as possible
    C. Shout at the person when talking with him or her
    D. Touch the person before indicating your presence
68. You are caring for a person with dementia. You
    A. Misplace the person's clothes
    B. Choose the activities the person attends
    C. Send personal items home
    D. Let the family make choices if the person cannot
69. When providing rehabilitation and restorative care for a person, you
    A. Can shout or scream at the person
    B. Can hit or strike the person
    C. Can call the person names
    D. Discuss your anger with the nurse
70. While bathing a person, you
    A. Keep doors and windows open
    B. Wash from the dirtiest areas to the cleanest areas
    C. Encourage the person to help as much as possible
    D. Rub the skin dry
71. When a person is dying
    A. Assume that the person can hear you
    B. Oral care is done every 5 hours
    C. Skin care is done weekly
    D. Re-position the person every 3 hours
72. A person is on intake and output. You
    A. Measure only liquids such as water and juice
    B. Measure ice cream and gelatin as part of intake
    C. Measure intravenous (IV) fluids
    D. Measure tube feedings
73. A person has been on bedrest. You need to have the person walk. What will you do first?
    A. Help the person move quickly.
    B. Have the person dangle before getting out of bed.
    C. Have the person sit in a chair.
    D. Walk with the person as soon as he or she gets out of bed.
74. Your ring accidentally causes a skin tear on an elderly person. You
    A. Tell yourself to be more careful the next time
    B. Tell the nurse at once
    C. Do nothing
    D. Hope no one finds out
75. To protect a person's privacy, you should
    A. Keep all information about the person confidential
    B. Discuss the person's treatment with another nursing assistant in the lunch room
    C. Open the person's mail
    D. Keep the privacy curtain open when providing care to the person

Practice Examination 2

This test contains 75 questions. For each question, circle the BEST answer.

1. You can refuse to do a delegated task when
   A. You are too busy
   B. You do not like the task
   C. The task is not in your job description
   D. It is the end of the shift
2. Mr. Smith does not want life-saving measures. You
   A. Explain to Mr. Smith why he should have life-saving measures
   B. Respect his decision
   C. Explain to Mr. Smith's family why life-saving measures are needed
   D. Tell your friend about Mr. Smith's decision
3. You are walking by a resident's room. You hear a nurse shouting at a person. This is
   A. Battery
   B. Malpractice
   C. Verbal abuse
   D. Neglect
4. When communicating with a foreign-speaking person, you
   A. Speak loudly or shout
   B. Use medical terms the person may not understand
   C. Use words the person seems to understand
   D. Speak quickly and mumble
5. To protect a person from getting burned, you
   A. Allow smoking in bed
   B. Turn hot water on first, then cold water
   C. Assist the person with drinking or eating hot food
   D. Let the person sleep with a heating pad
6. To prevent equipment accidents, you should
   A. Use 2-pronged plugs on all electrical devices
   B. Follow the manufacturer's instructions
   C. Wipe up spills when you have time
   D. Use unfamiliar equipment without training
7. To prevent a person from falling, you should
   A. Ignore call lights
   B. Use throw rugs on the floor
   C. Keep the bed in a high position
   D. Use grab bars in showers
8. You need to wash your hands
   A. Before you document a procedure
   B. After you remove gloves
   C. After you talk with a person
   D. After you talk with a co-worker
9. You need to move a person weighing 250 pounds in bed. You
   A. Do the procedure alone
   B. Keep the privacy curtain open
   C. Ask the person to lie still
   D. Ask for assistance from at least 2 other staff members
10. When transferring a person from a bed to a wheelchair, you never
    A. Ask a co-worker to help you
    B. Use a transfer or gait belt
    C. Have the person put his or her arms around your neck
    D. Lock the wheels on the wheelchair
11. When making a bed, you
    A. Keep the bed in the low position
    B. Wear gloves when removing linens
    C. Raise the head of the bed
    D. Raise the foot of the bed
12. To give perineal care to a male, you
    A. Use a circular motion and work toward the meatus
    B. Use a circular motion and start at the meatus and work outward
    C. Wear gloves only if there is drainage
    D. Use only water
13. A person with a weak left arm wants to put on his or her sweater. You
    A. Let the person do it without any assistance
    B. Help the person put the sweater on his or her right arm first
    C. Help the person put the sweater on his or her left arm first
    D. Tell the person to keep the sweater off
14. A person has an indwelling catheter. You
    A. Let the drainage bag touch the floor
    B. Keep the drainage bag higher than the bladder
    C. Hang the drainage bag on a bed rail
    D. Have the drainage bag hang from the bed frame or chair
15. A person needs to eat a diet that contains protein. Protein
    A. Is needed for tissue repair and growth
    B. Provides energy and fiber for bowel elimination
    C. Adds flavor to food and helps the body use certain vitamins
    D. Is needed for nerve and muscle function
16. Older persons
    A. Have an increased sense of thirst
    B. Need less water than younger persons
    C. May not feel thirsty
    D. Seldom need to have water offered to them
17. A person is NPO. You
    A. Post a sign in the bathroom
    B. Keep the water pitcher filled at the bedside
    C. Remove the water pitcher and glass from the room
    D. Provide oral hygiene every day
18. A person drank 3 oz of milk at lunch. He or she drank
    A. 30 mL
    B. 60 mL
    C. 90 mL
    D. 120 mL
19. When feeding a person, you
    A. Offer fluids at the end of the meal
    B. Use forks
    C. Do not talk to the person
    D. Allow time for chewing and swallowing
20. You need to do range of motion (ROM) to a person's right shoulder. You
    A. Force the joint beyond its present ROM
    B. Move the joint quickly
    C. Force the joint to the point of pain
    D. Support the part being exercised

21. A person has a weak left leg. The person should
    A. Hold the cane in his or her left hand
    B. Hold the cane in his or her right hand
    C. Hold the cane in either hand
    D. Use a walker
22. To promote comfort and relieve pain, you
    A. Keep wrinkles in the bed linens
    B. Position the person in good alignment
    C. Talk loudly to the person
    D. Use sudden and jarring movements of the bed or chair
23. A person is receiving oxygen through a nasal cannula. You
    A. Turn the oxygen higher when he or she is short of breath
    B. Fill the humidifier when it is not bubbling
    C. Check behind the ears and under the nose for signs of irritation
    D. Remove the cannula when the person goes to the dining room
24. You accidentally dropped a mercury glass thermometer and broke it. You
    A. Tell the nurse at once
    B. Put the mercury in your pocket
    C. Pick up the pieces of glass with your hands
    D. Touch the mercury
25. When taking a person's pulse, you
    A. Use the brachial pulse
    B. Take the pulse for 30 seconds if it is irregular
    C. Tell the nurse if the pulse is less than 60
    D. Use your thumb to take a pulse
26. You are counting respirations on a person. You
    A. Tell the person you are counting his or her respirations
    B. Count for 1 minute if an abnormal breathing pattern is noted
    C. Report a rate of 16 to the nurse at once
    D. Count for 30 seconds if an abnormal breathing pattern is noted
27. You are taking blood pressures on people assigned to you. An older person has a blood pressure (BP) of 158/96 mm Hg. You
    A. Report the BP to the nurse at once
    B. Finish taking all the blood pressures before telling the nurse
    C. Retake the BP in 30 minutes before telling the nurse
    D. Ask the unit secretary to tell the nurse about the BP
28. When would you take a rectal temperature?
    A. The person has diarrhea.
    B. The person is confused.
    C. The person is unconscious.
    D. The person is agitated.
29. A person has been admitted to the nursing center recently. You
    A. Look through his or her belongings
    B. Ignore his or her questions
    C. Speak in a gentle, calm voice
    D. Enter the person's room without knocking

30. When taking a person's height and weight, you
    A. Let the person wear shoes
    B. Have the person void before being weighed
    C. Weigh the person at different times of the day
    D. Balance the scale every 6 months
31. A person is bedfast. To prevent pressure ulcers, you
    A. Re-position the person at least every 3 hours
    B. Massage reddened areas
    C. Let heels and ankles touch the bed
    D. Keep the skin free of moisture from urine, stools, or perspiration
32. A person has a hearing problem. When talking with the person, you
    A. Keep the TV or radio on
    B. Shout
    C. Face the person
    D. Speak quickly
33. When caring for a person who is blind or visually impaired, you
    A. Place furniture and equipment where the person walks
    B. Keep the lights off
    C. Explain the location of food and beverages
    D. Re-arrange furniture and equipment
34. You are caring for a person with dementia. You
    A. Share information about the person's care
    B. Share information about the person's condition
    C. Protect confidential information
    D. Expose the person's body when you provide care
35. When caring for a confused person, you
    A. Call the person "Honey"
    B. Do not need to explain what you are doing
    C. Ask clear, simple questions
    D. Remove the calendar from the person's room
36. A person with Alzheimer's disease likes to wander. You
    A. Keep the person in his or her room
    B. Restrain the person
    C. Argue with the person who wants to leave
    D. Exercise the person as ordered
37. Restorative nursing programs
    A. Help maintain the lowest level of function
    B. Promote self-care measures
    C. Focus on the disability, not the person
    D. Help the person lose strength and independence
38. When caring for a person with a disability, you
    A. Focus on his or her limitations
    B. Expect progress in a rehabilitation program to be fast
    C. Remind the person of his or her progress in the rehabilitation program
    D. Deny the disability
39. After a person dies, you
    A. Can expose his or her body unnecessarily
    B. Can discuss the person's diagnosis with your family
    C. Can talk about the family's reactions to your friends
    D. Respect the person's right to privacy

40. You enter a person's room and find a fire in the wastebasket. Your first action is to
    A. Remove the person from the room
    B. Close the door
    C. Call for help
    D. Activate the fire alarm

41. You leave a person lying in urine and he or she develops a bedsore. This is
    A. Fraud
    B. Neglect
    C. Assault
    D. Battery

42. A nurse asks you to place a drug and a sterile dressing on a small foot wound. You
    A. Agree to do the task
    B. Ask another nursing assistant to do the task
    C. Politely tell the nurse you cannot do that task
    D. Report the nurse to the director of nursing

43. You observe a person's urine is foul-smelling and dark amber. Your first action is to
    A. Tell the other nursing assistant
    B. Tell the person
    C. Tell the nurse
    D. Record the observation

44. A daughter asks you for water for her mom. Your response is
    A. "I am not caring for your mom. I will get her nursing assistant for you."
    B. "I do not have time to do that."
    C. "That's not my job."
    D. "I will be happy to do that."

45. A person has a restraint on. You
    A. Observe the person for breathing and circulation complications every 30 minutes
    B. Know that unnecessary restraint is false imprisonment
    C. Use the most restrictive type of restraint
    D. Know that restraints decrease confusion and agitation

46. The nurse asks you to place a person in the supine position. You
    A. Elevate the head of the bed 45 degrees
    B. Elevate the foot of the bed 15 degrees
    C. Place the person on his or her back with the bed flat
    D. Place the person on his or her abdomen

47. The most important way to prevent or avoid spreading infection is to
    A. Wash hands
    B. Cover your nose when coughing
    C. Use disposable gloves
    D. Wear a mask

48. You are eating lunch and a nursing assistant begins to gossip about another person. You
    A. Join the conversation and talk about the person
    B. Remove yourself from the group
    C. Tell your roommate about the gossip you heard at lunch
    D. Tell another nursing assistant about the gossip you heard

49. When moving a person up in bed, you should
    A. Raise the head of the bed
    B. Ask the person to keep his or her legs straight
    C. Cause friction and shearing
    D. Ask a co-worker to help you

50. A person is on a sodium-controlled diet. This means
    A. Canned vegetables are omitted from his or her diet
    B. Salt may be added to food at the table
    C. Large amounts of salt are used in cooking
    D. Ham is eaten regularly

51. Elastic stockings
    A. Are applied after a person gets out of bed
    B. Should not have wrinkles or creases after being applied
    C. Come in 1 size only
    D. Are forced on the person

52. While walking, the person begins to fall. You
    A. Call for help
    B. Reach for a chair
    C. Ease the person to the floor
    D. Ask a visitor to help

53. Before bathing a person, you should
    A. Offer the bedpan or urinal
    B. Partially undress the person
    C. Raise the head of the bed
    D. Open the privacy curtain

54. When taking a rectal temperature with an electronic thermometer, you insert the thermometer
    A. ½ inch
    B. 1½ inches
    C. 2 inches
    D. 2½ inches

55. Touch
    A. Is a form of nonverbal communication
    B. Is a form of verbal communication
    C. Means the same thing to everyone
    D. Should be used for all persons

56. You may share information about a person's care and condition with
    A. The staff caring for the person
    B. The person's daughter
    C. Your family members
    D. The volunteer in the gift shop

57. A person tells you he or she has pain upon urination. You
    A. Tell the nurse
    B. Let the nurse document this information
    C. Ask the person to tell you if it happens again
    D. Tell the person's son

58. A person's culture and religion are different from yours. You
    A. Laugh about the person's customs
    B. Tell your family about the person's customs
    C. Ask the person to explain his or her beliefs and practices to you
    D. Tell the person his or her beliefs and customs are silly

59. You need to wear gloves when you
    A. Do range-of-motion exercises
    B. Feed a person
    C. Give perineal care
    D. Walk a person

60. An older person is normally alert. Today he or she is confused. What should you do?
    A. Ask the person why he or she is confused.
    B. Ignore the confusion.
    C. Check to see if the person is confused later in the day.
    D. Tell the nurse.
61. While walking with a person, he tells you he feels faint. What do you do first?
    A. Have the person sit down.
    B. Call for the nurse.
    C. Open the window.
    D. Ask the person to take a deep breath.
62. You are asked to encourage fluids for a person. You
    A. Increase the person's fluid intake
    B. Decrease the person's fluid intake
    C. Limit fluids to meal times
    D. Keep fluids where the person cannot reach them
63. Communication fails when you
    A. Use words the other person understands
    B. Talk too much
    C. Let others express their feelings and concerns
    D. Talk about a topic that is uncomfortable
64. During bathing, a person may
    A. Decide what products to use
    B. Be exposed in the shower room
    C. Have visitors present without his or her permission
    D. Have no personal choices
65. People in late adulthood need to
    A. Adjust to increased income
    B. Adjust to their health being better
    C. Develop new friends and relationships
    D. Adjust to increased strength
66. When measuring blood pressure, you should do the following except
    A. Apply the cuff to a bare upper arm
    B. Turn off the TV
    C. Locate the brachial artery
    D. Use the arm with an intravenous (IV) infusion
67. You find clean linens on the floor in a person's room. You
    A. Use the linens to make the bed
    B. Return the linens to the linen cart
    C. Put the linens in the laundry
    D. Tell the nurse

68. When doing mouth care on an unconscious person, you
    A. Use a large amount of fluid
    B. Position the person on his or her side
    C. Do the task without telling the person what you are doing
    D. Insert his or her dentures when done
69. When brushing or combing a person's hair, you
    A. Cut matted or tangled hair
    B. Encourage the person to do as much as possible
    C. Style the hair as you want
    D. Perform the task weekly
70. When providing nail and foot care, you
    A. Cut fingernails with scissors
    B. Trim toenails for a diabetic person
    C. Trim toenails for a person with poor circulation
    D. Check between the toes for cracks and sores
71. An indwelling catheter becomes disconnected from the drainage system. You
    A. Reconnect the tubing to the catheter quickly without gloves
    B. Tell the nurse at once
    C. Get a new drainage system
    D. Touch the ends of the catheter
72. Urinary drainage bags are
    A. Hung on the bed rail
    B. Emptied and measured at the end of each shift
    C. Kept on the floor
    D. Kept higher than the person's bladder
73. A person needs a condom catheter applied. You remember to
    A. Apply it to a penis that is red and irritated
    B. Use adhesive tape to secure the catheter
    C. Use elastic tape to secure the catheter
    D. Act in an unprofessional manner
74. For comfort during bowel elimination
    A. Have the person use the bedpan rather than the bathroom or commode if possible
    B. Permit visitors to stay
    C. Keep the door and privacy curtain open
    D. Leave the person alone if possible
75. You are transferring a person with a weak right side from the wheelchair to the bed. You
    A. Place the wheelchair on the left side of the bed
    B. Place the wheelchair on the right side of the bed
    C. Keep the person in the wheelchair
    D. Ask the person what side moves first

Skills Evaluation Review

Each state has its own policies and procedures for the skills test. The following information is an overview of what to expect.

- To pass the skills evaluation, you will need to perform 5 of all the skills available.
- To pass the skills evaluation, you must perform all 5 skills correctly.
- A nurse evaluates your performance of certain skills. Having someone watch as you work is not a new experience. Your instructor evaluated your performance during your training program. While you are working, your supervisor evaluates your skills.
- Mannequins and people are used as "patients" or "residents," depending on the skills you are performing. Speak to the person as you would a patient or resident.
- If you make a mistake, tell the evaluator what you did wrong. Then perform the skill correctly. Do not panic.
- Take whatever equipment you normally take to or use at work. Wear a watch with a second hand. You may need it to measure vital signs and check how much time you have left.

Before and During the Procedure

- Hand-washing is evaluated at the beginning of the skills test. You are expected to know when to wash your hands. Therefore you may not be told to do so. Follow the rules for hand hygiene during the test.
- Before entering a person's room, knock on the door. Greet the person by name and introduce yourself before beginning a procedure. Check the identification (ID) or the photo ID to make certain you are giving care to the right person.
- Explain what you are going to do before beginning the procedure and as needed throughout the procedure.
- Always follow the rules of medical asepsis. For example, remove gloves and dispose of them properly. Keep clean linens separated from used linens.
- Always protect the person's rights throughout the skills test.
- Communicate with the person as you give care. Focus on the person's needs and interests. Always treat the person with respect. Do not talk about yourself or your personal problems.
- Provide privacy. This involves pulling the privacy curtain around the bed, closing doors, and asking visitors to leave the room.
- Promote safety for the person. For example, lock the wheelchair when you transfer a person to and from it. Place the bed in the lowest horizontal position when the person must get out of bed or when you are done giving care.

- Make sure the call light is within the person's reach. Attaching it to the bed or bed rail does not mean the person can reach it.
- Use good body mechanics. Raise the bed and over-bed table to a good working height.
- Provide for comfort.
  - Make sure the person and linens are clean and dry. The person may have become incontinent during the procedure.
  - Change or straighten bed linens as needed.
  - Position the person for comfort and in good alignment.
  - Provide pillows as directed by the nurse and the care plan.
  - Raise the head of the bed as the person prefers and allowed by the nurse and the care plan.
  - Provide for warmth. The person may need an extra blanket, a lap blanket, a sweater, socks, and so on.
  - Adjust lighting to meet the person's needs.
  - Make sure eyeglasses, hearing aids, and other devices are in place as needed.
  - Ask the person if he or she is comfortable.
  - Ask the person if there is anything else you can do for him or her.
  - Make sure the person is covered for warmth and privacy.

Skills

Ask your instructor to tell you which of the following skills are tested in your state. Place a checkmark in the box in front of each tested skill so it will be easy for you to reference. The skills marked with an asterisk (*) are used with permission of National Council of State Boards of Nursing (NCSBN). These skills are offered as a study guide to you. The word "client" refers to the resident or person receiving care. You are responsible for following the most current standards, practices, and guidelines in your state.

The steps in boldface type are critical element steps. Critical element steps must be done correctly to pass the skill. If you miss a critical element step, you will not pass the skills evaluation. For example, you are to transfer a client from the bed to a wheelchair. You will fail if you do not lock the wheels on the wheelchair before transferring the person. An automatic failure is one that could potentially cause harm to a person. Your state may mark critical element steps in another way—underline or italics. If your state has one, review the candidate's handbook.

❏ *Hand Hygiene (Hand-Washing) (Chapter 16)

1. Addresses client by name and introduces self to client by name
2. Turns on water at sink
3. Wets hands and wrists thoroughly
4. Applies soap to hands
5. **Lathers all surfaces of wrists, hands, and fingers, producing friction for at least 20 (twenty) seconds keeping hands lower than the elbows and the fingertips down**
6. Cleans fingernails by rubbing fingertips against palms of the opposite hand
7. **Rinses all surfaces of wrists, hands, and fingers, keeping hands lower than the elbows and the fingertips down**
8. Uses clean, dry paper towel/towels to dry all surfaces of hands, wrists, and fingers then disposes of paper towel/towels into waste container
9. Uses clean, dry paper towel/towels to turn off faucet then disposes of paper towel/towels into waste container or uses knee/foot control to turn off faucet
10. Does not touch inside of sink at any time

❏ *Applies One Knee-High Elastic Stocking (Chapter 35)

1. Explains procedure, speaking clearly, slowly, and directly, maintaining face-to-face contact whenever possible
2. Privacy is provided with a curtain, screen, or door
3. Client is in supine position (lying down in bed) while stocking is applied
4. Turns stocking inside-out, at least to heel
5. Places foot of stocking over toes, foot, and heel
6. Pulls top of stocking over foot, heel, and leg
7. Moves foot and leg gently and naturally, avoiding force and over-extension of limb and joints
8. **Finishes procedure with no twists or wrinkles and heel of stocking (if present) is over heel and opening in toe area (if present) is either under or over toe area**
9. Signaling device is within reach and bed is in low position
10. After completing skill, washes hands

❏ *Assists to Ambulate Using a Transfer Belt (Chapter 19)

1. Explains procedure, speaking clearly, slowly, and directly, maintaining face-to-face contact whenever possible
2. **Before assisting to stand, client is wearing shoes**
3. Before assisting to stand, bed is at a safe level
4. Before assisting to stand, checks and/or locks bed wheels

5. **Before assisting to stand, client is assisted to sitting position with feet flat on the floor**
6. Before assisting to stand, applies transfer belt securely at the waist over clothing/gown
7. Before assisting to stand, provides instructions to enable client to assist in standing including prearranged signal to alert client to begin standing
8. Stands facing client positioning self to ensure safety of candidate and client during transfer. Counts to three (or says other prearranged signal) to alert client to begin standing
9. On signal, gradually assists client to stand by grasping transfer belt on both sides with an upward grasp (candidate's hands are in upward position), and maintaining stability of client's legs
10. Walks slightly behind and to one side of client for a distance of ten (10) feet, while holding onto the belt
11. After ambulation, assists client to bed and removes transfer belt
12. Signaling device is within reach and bed is in low position
13. After completing skill, washes hands

❏ *Assists With Use of Bedpan (Chapter 24)

1. Explains procedure speaking clearly, slowly, and directly, maintaining face-to-face contact whenever possible
2. Privacy is provided with a curtain, screen, or door
3. Before placing bedpan, lowers head of bed
4. Puts on clean gloves before handling bedpan
5. **Places bedpan correctly under client's buttocks**
6. Removes and disposes of gloves (without contaminating self) into waste container and washes hands
7. After positioning client on bedpan and removing gloves, raises head of bed
8. Toilet tissue is within reach
9. Hand wipe is within reach and client is instructed to clean hands with hand wipe when finished
10. Signaling device within reach and client is asked to signal when finished
11. Puts on clean gloves before removing bedpan
12. Head of bed is lowered before bedpan is removed
13. Avoids overexposure of client
14. Empties and rinses bedpan and pours rinse into toilet
15. After rinsing bedpan, places bedpan in designated dirty supply area
16. After placing bedpan in designated dirty supply area, removes and disposes of gloves (without contaminating self) into waste container and washes hands
17. Signaling device is within reach and bed is in low position

*Reproduced and used with permission from the *Nurse Assistant Candidate Handbook* from National Council of State Boards of Nursing (NCSBN), Chicago, Ill, © 2011.

❑ *Cleans Upper or Lower Denture
(Chapter 22)

1. Puts on clean gloves before handling dentures
2. Bottom of sink is lined and/or sink is partially filled with water before denture is held over sink
3. Rinses denture in moderate temperature running water before brushing them
4. Applies toothpaste to toothbrush
5. Brushes surfaces of denture
6. Rinses surfaces of denture under moderate temperature running water
7. Before placing denture into cup, rinses denture cup and lid
8. Places denture in denture cup with moderate temperature water solution and places lid on cup
9. Rinses toothbrush and places in designated toothbrush basin/container
10. Maintains clean technique with placement of toothbrush and denture
11. Sink liner is removed and disposed of appropriately and/or sink is drained
12. After rinsing equipment and disposing of sink liner, removes and disposes of gloves (without contaminating self) into waste container and washes hands

❑ *Counts and Records Radial Pulse
(Chapter 29)**

1. Explains procedure, speaking clearly, slowly, and directly, maintaining face-to-face contact whenever possible
2. Places fingertips on thumb side of client's wrist to locate radial pulse
3. Counts beats for one full minute
4. Signaling device is within reach
5. Before recording, washes hands
6. **After obtaining pulse by palpating in radial artery position, records pulse rate within plus or minus 4 beats of evaluator's reading**

❑ *Counts and Records Respirations
(Chapter 29)†

1. Explains procedure (for testing purposes), speaking clearly, slowly, and directly, maintaining face-to-face contact whenever possible
2. Counts respirations for one full minute
3. Signaling device is within reach
4. Washes hands
5. **Records respiration rate within plus or minus 2 breaths of evaluator's reading**

❑ *Dresses Client With Affected (Weak) Right
Arm (Chapter 23)

1. Explains procedure, speaking clearly, slowly, and directly, maintaining face-to-face contact whenever possible
2. Privacy is provided with a curtain, screen, or door
3. Asks which shirt he/she would like to wear and dresses him/her in shirt of choice
4. While avoiding overexposure of client, removes gown from the unaffected side first, then removes gown from the affected side and disposes of gown into soiled linen container
5. **Assists to put the right (affected/weak) arm through the right sleeve of the shirt before placing garment on left (unaffected) arm**
6. While putting on shirt, moves body gently and naturally, avoiding force and over-extension of limbs and joints
7. Finishes with clothing in place
8. Signaling device is within reach and bed is in low position
9. After completing skill, washes hands

❑ *Feeds Client Who Cannot Feed Self
(Chapter 27)

1. Explains procedure to client, speaking clearly, slowly, and directly, maintaining face-to-face contact whenever possible
2. Before feeding, candidate looks at name card on tray and asks client to state name
3. **Before feeding client, client is in an upright sitting position (75–90 degrees)**
4. Places tray where the food can be easily seen by client
5. Candidate cleans client's hands with hand wipe before beginning feeding
6. Candidate sits facing client during feeding
7. Tells client what foods are on tray and asks what client would like to eat first
8. Using spoon, offers client one bite of each type of food on tray, telling client the content of each spoonful
9. Offers beverage at least once during meal
10. Candidate asks client if they are ready for next bite of food or sip of beverage
11. At end of meal, candidate cleans client's mouth and hands with wipes
12. Removes food tray and places tray in designated dirty supply area
13. Signaling device is within client's reach
14. After completing skill, washes hands

*Reproduced and used with permission from the *Nurse Assistant Candidate Handbook* from National Council of State Boards of Nursing (NCSBN), Chicago, Ill, © 2011.
**Count for 1 full minute.
†Count for 1 full minute. For testing purposes you may explain to the client that you will be counting the respirations.

❏*Gives Modified Bed Bath (Face and One Arm, Hand, and Underarm) (Chapter 22)

1. Explains procedure, speaking clearly, slowly, and directly, maintaining face-to-face contact whenever possible
2. Privacy is provided with a curtain, screen, or door
3. Removes gown and places in soiled linen container while avoiding over exposure of the client
4. Before washing, checks water temperature for safety and comfort and asks client to verify comfort of water
5. Puts on clean gloves before washing client
6. **Beginning with eyes, washes eyes with wet washcloth (no soap), using a different area of the washcloth for each stroke, washing inner aspect to outer aspect, then proceeds to wash face**
7. Dries face with towel
8. Exposes one arm and places towel underneath arm
9. Applies soap to wet washcloth
10. Washes arm, hand, and underarm, keeping rest of body covered
11. Rinses and dries arm, hand, and underarm
12. Moves body gently and naturally, avoiding force and over-extension of limbs and joints
13. Puts clean gown on client
14. Empties, rinses, and dries basin
15. After rinsing and drying basin, places basin in designated dirty supply area
16. Disposes of linen into soiled linen container
17. Avoids contact between candidate clothing and used linens
18. After placing basin in designated dirty supply area, and disposing of used linen, removes and disposes of gloves (without contaminating self) into waste container and washes hands
19. Signaling device is within reach and bed is in low position

❏ Makes an Occupied Bed (Client Does Not Need Assistance to Turn) (Chapter 21)

1. Explains procedure, speaking clearly, slowly, and directly, maintaining face-to-face contact whenever possible
2. Privacy is provided with a curtain, screen, or door
3. Lowers head of bed before moving client
4. Client is covered while linens are changed
5. Loosens top linen from the end of the bed
6. Raises side rail on side to which client will move and client moves toward raised side rail
7. Loosens bottom used linen on working side and moves bottom used linen toward center of bed
8. Places and tucks in clean bottom linen or fitted bottom sheet on working side and tucks under client
9. Before going to other side, client moves back onto clean bottom linen
10. Raises side rail then goes to other side of bed
11. Removes used bottom linen

12. Pulls and tucks in clean bottom linen, finishing with bottom sheet free of wrinkles
13. Client is covered with clean top sheet and bath blanket/used top sheet has been removed
14. Changes pillowcase
15. Linen is centered and tucked at foot of bed
16. Avoids contact between candidate's clothing and used linens
17. Disposes of used linens into soiled linen container and avoids putting linens on floor
18. Signaling device is within reach and bed is in low position
19. Washes hands

❏*Measures and Records Blood Pressure (Chapter 29)

1. Explains procedure, speaking clearly, slowly, and directly, maintaining face-to-face contact whenever possible
2. Before using stethoscope, wipes bell/diaphragm and earpieces of stethoscope with alcohol
3. Client's arm is positioned with palm up and upper arm is exposed
4. Feels for brachial artery on inner aspect of arm, at bend of elbow
5. Places blood pressure cuff snugly on client's upper arm with sensor/arrow over brachial artery site
6. Earpieces of stethoscope are in ears and bell/diaphragm is over brachial artery site
7. Candidate inflates cuff between 160 mm Hg to 180 mm Hg. (If beat heard immediately upon cuff deflation, completely deflate cuff.) Re-inflate cuff to no more than 200 mm Hg.
8. Deflates cuff slowly and notes the **first sound** (systolic reading), and **last sound** (diastolic reading) (If rounding needed, measurements are rounded **UP** to the nearest 2 mm of mercury)
9. Removes cuff
10. Signaling device is within reach
11. Before recording, washes hands
12. **After obtaining reading using BP cuff and stethoscope, records both systolic and diastolic pressures each within plus or minus 8 mm Hg of evaluator's reading**

❏*Measures and Records Urinary Output (Chapter 27)

1. Puts on clean gloves before handling bedpan
2. Pours the contents of the bedpan into measuring container without spilling or splashing urine outside of container
3. Measures the amount of urine at eye level with container on flat surface
4. After measuring urine, empties contents of measuring container into toilet

*Reproduced and used with permission from the *Nurse Assistant Candidate Handbook* from National Council of State Boards of Nursing (NCSBN), Chicago, Ill, © 2011.

5. Rinses measuring container and pours rinse water into toilet
6. Rinses bedpan and pours rinse into toilet
7. After rinsing equipment, and before recording output, removes and disposes of gloves (without contaminating self) into waste container and washes hands
8. **Records contents of container within plus or minus 25 mL/cc of evaluator's reading**

❑ *Measures and Records Weight of Ambulatory Client (Chapter 32)*

1. Explains procedure, speaking clearly, slowly, and directly, maintaining face-to-face contact whenever possible
2. Client has shoes on before walking to scale
3. Before client steps on scale, candidate sets scale to zero
4. While client steps onto scale, candidate stands next to scale and assists client, if needed, onto center of the scale; then obtains client's weight
5. While client steps off scale, candidate stands next to scale and assists client, if needed, off scale before recording weight
6. Before recording, washes hands
7. **Records weight based on indicator on scale. Weight is within plus or minus 2 lbs of evaluator's reading (If weight recorded in kg, weight is within plus or minus 0.9 kg of evaluator's reading)**

❑ *Positions on Side (Chapter 18)*

1. Explains procedure, speaking clearly, slowly, and directly, maintaining face-to-face contact whenever possible
2. Privacy is provided with a curtain, screen, or door
3. Before turning, lowers head of bed
4. Raises side rail on side to which body will be turned
5. Slowly rolls onto side as one unit toward raised side rail
6. Places or adjusts pillow under head for support
7. Candidate positions client so that client is not lying on arm
8. Supports top arm with supportive device
9. Places supportive device behind client's back
10. Places supportive device between legs with top knee flexed; knee and ankle supported
11. Signaling device is within reach and bed is in low position
12. After completing skill, washes hands

❑ *Provides Catheter Care for Female (Chapter 25)*

1. Explains procedure, speaking clearly, slowly, and directly, maintaining face-to-face contact whenever possible

2. Privacy is provided with a curtain, screen, or door
3. Before washing checks water temperature for safety and comfort and asks client to verify comfort of water
4. Puts on clean gloves before washing
5. Places linen protector under perineal area before washing
6. Exposes area surrounding catheter while avoiding overexposure of client
7. Applies soap to wet washcloth
8. **While holding catheter at meatus without tugging, cleans at least four inches of catheter from meatus, moving in only one direction (i.e., away from meatus) using a clean area of the cloth for each stroke**
9. **While holding catheter at meatus without tugging, rinses at least four inches of catheter from meatus, moving only in one direction, away from meatus, using a clean area of the cloth for each stroke**
10. While holding catheter at meatus without tugging, dries at least four inches of catheter moving away from meatus
11. Empties, rinses, and dries basin
12. After rinsing and drying basin, places basin in designated dirty supply area
13. Disposes of used linen into soiled linen container and disposes of linen protector appropriately
14. Avoids contact between candidate clothing and used linen
15. After disposing of used linen and cleaning equipment, removes and disposes of gloves (without contaminating self) into waste container and washes hands
16. Signaling device is within reach and bed is in low position

❑ *Provides Fingernail Care on One Hand (Chapter 23)*

1. Explains procedure, speaking clearly, slowly, and directly, maintaining face-to-face contact whenever possible
2. Before immersing fingernails, checks water temperature for safety and comfort and asks client to verify comfort of water
3. Basin is in a comfortable position for client
4. Puts on clean gloves before cleaning fingernails
5. Fingernails are immersed in basin of water
6. Cleans under each fingernail with orangewood stick
7. Wipes orangewood stick on towel after each nail
8. Dries fingernail area
9. Candidate feels each nail and files as needed
10. Disposes of orangewood stick and emery board into waste container (for testing purposes)
11. Empties, rinses, and dries basin
12. After rinsing basin, places basin in designated used supply area
13. Disposes of used linens into used linens container

*Reproduced and used with permission from the *Nurse Assistant Candidate Handbook* from National Council of State Boards of Nursing (NCSBN), Chicago, Ill, © 2011.

14. After cleaning nails and equipment and disposing of used linens, removes and disposes of gloves (without contaminating self) into waste container and washes hands
15. Signaling device is within reach

❑*Provides Foot Care on One Foot (Chapter 23)

1. Explains procedure, speaking clearly, slowly, and directly, maintaining face-to-face contact whenever possible
2. Privacy is provided with a curtain, screen, or door
3. Before washing, checks water temperature for safety and comfort and asks client to verify comfort of water
4. Basin is in a comfortable position for client and on protective barrier
5. Puts on clean gloves before washing foot
6. Client's bare foot is placed into the water
7. Applies soap to wet washcloth
8. Lifts foot from water and washes foot (including between the toes)
9. Foot is rinsed (including between the toes)
10. Dries foot (including between the toes)
11. Applies lotion to top and bottom of foot, removing excess (if any) with a towel
12. Supports foot and ankle during procedure
13. Empties, rinses, and dries basin
14. After rinsing and drying basin, places basin in designated dirty supply area
15. Disposes of used linen into soiled linen container
16. After cleaning foot and equipment, and disposing of used linen, removes and disposes of gloves (without contaminating self) into waste container and washes hands
17. Signaling device is within reach

❑*Provides Mouth Care (Chapter 22)

1. Explains procedure, speaking clearly, slowly, and directly, maintaining face-to-face contact whenever possible
2. Privacy is provided with a curtain, screen, or door
3. Before providing mouth care, client is in upright sitting position (75–90 degrees)
4. Puts on clean gloves before cleaning mouth
5. Places clothing protector across chest before providing mouth care
6. Secures cup of water and moistens toothbrush
7. Before cleaning mouth applies toothpaste to moistened toothbrush
8. **Cleans mouth (including tongue and surfaces of teeth) using gentle motions**
9. Maintains clean technique with placement of toothbrush
10. Candidate holds emesis basin to chin while client rinses mouth

11. Candidate wipes mouth and removes clothing protector
12. After rinsing toothbrush, empty, rinse, and dry the basin and place used toothbrush in designated basin/container
13. Places basin and toothbrush in designated dirty supply area
14. Disposes of used linen into soiled linen container
15. After placing basin and toothbrush in designated dirty supply area, and disposing of used linen, removes and disposes of gloves (without contaminating self) into waste container and washes hands
16. Signaling device is within reach and bed is in low position

❑*Provides Perineal Care (Peri-Care) for Female (Chapter 22)

1. Explains procedure, speaking clearly, slowly, and directly, maintaining face-to-face contact whenever possible
2. Privacy is provided with a curtain, screen, or door
3. Before washing checks water temperature for safety and comfort and asks client to verify comfort of water
4. Puts on clean gloves before washing perineal area
5. Places pad/linen protector under perineal area before washing
6. Exposes perineal area while avoiding overexposure of client
7. Applies soap to wet washcloth
8. **Washes genital area, moving from front to back, while using a clean area of the washcloth for each stroke**
9. **Using clean washcloth, rinses soap from genital area, moving from front to back, while using a clean area of the washcloth for each stroke**
10. Dries genital area moving from front to back with towel
11. **After washing genital area, turns to side, then washes and rinses rectal area moving from front to back using a clean area of washcloth for each stroke. Dries with towel**
12. Repositions client
13. Empties, rinses, and dries basin
14. After rinsing and drying basin, places basin in designated dirty supply area
15. Disposes of used linen into soiled linen container and disposes of linen protector appropriately
16. Avoids contact between candidate clothing and used linen
17. After disposing of used linen, and placing used equipment in designated dirty supply area, removes and disposes of gloves (without contaminating self) into waste container and washes hands
18. Signaling device is within reach and bed is in low position

❏ *Transfers From Bed to Wheelchair Using Transfer Belt (Chapter 19)

1. Explains procedure, speaking clearly, slowly, and directly, maintaining face-to-face contact whenever possible
2. Privacy is provided with a curtain, screen, or door
3. Before assisting to stand, wheelchair is positioned along side of bed, at head of bed, facing the foot, or foot of bed facing head
4. Before assisting to stand, footrests are folded up or removed
5. Before assisting to stand, bed is at a safe level
6. **Before assisting to stand, locks wheels on wheelchair**
7. Before assisting to stand, checks and/or locks bed wheels
8. **Before assisting to stand, client is assisted to a sitting position with feet flat on the floor**
9. Before assisting to stand, client is wearing shoes
10. Before assisting to stand, applies transfer belt securely at the waist over clothing/gown
11. Before assisting to stand, provides instructions to enable client to assist in transfer including prearranged signal to alert when to begin standing
12. Stands facing client, positioning self to ensure safety of candidate and client during transfer. Counts to three (or says other prearranged signal) to alert client to begin standing
13. On signal, gradually assists client to stand by grasping transfer belt on both sides with an upward grasp (candidates hands are in upward position) and maintaining stability of client's legs
14. Assists client to turn to stand in front of wheelchair with back of client's legs against wheelchair
15. Lowers client into wheelchair
16. Positions client with hips touching back of wheelchair and transfer belt is removed
17. Positions feet on footrests
18. Signaling device is within reach
19. After completing skill, washes hands

❏ *Performs Modified Passive Range-of-Motion (PROM) for One Knee and One Ankle (Chapter 30)

1. Explains procedure, speaking clearly, slowly, and directly, maintaining face-to-face contact whenever possible
2. Privacy is provided with a curtain, screen, or door
3. Instructs client to inform candidate if pain is experienced during exercise
4. Supports leg at knee and ankle while performing range of motion for knee
5. Bends the knee then returns leg to client's normal position (extension/flexion) (AT LEAST 3 TIMES unless pain is verbalized)

6. Supports foot and ankle close to the bed while performing range of motion for ankle
7. Pushes/pulls foot toward head (dorsiflexion), and pushes/pulls foot down, toes point down (plantar flexion) (AT LEAST 3 TIMES unless pain is verbalized)
8. **While supporting the limb, moves joints gently, slowly, and smoothly through the range of motion, discontinuing exercise if client verbalizes pain**
9. Signaling device is within reach and bed is in low position
10. After completing skill, washes hands

❏ *Performs Modified Passive Range-of-Motion (PROM) for One Shoulder (Chapter 30)

1. Explains procedure, speaking clearly, slowly, and directly, maintaining face-to-face contact whenever possible
2. Privacy is provided with a curtain, screen, or door
3. Instructs client to inform candidate if pain is experienced during exercise
4. Supports client's upper and lower arm while performing range of motion for shoulder
5. **Raises client's straightened arm from side position upward toward head to ear level and returns arm down to side of body (flexion/extension) (AT LEAST 3 TIMES unless pain is verbalized). Supporting the limb, moves joint gently, slowly, and smoothly through the range of motion, discontinuing exercise if client verbalizes pain**
6. **Moves client's straightened arm away from the side of body to shoulder level and returns to side of body (abduction/adduction) (AT LEAST 3 TIMES unless pain is verbalized). Supporting the limb, moves joint gently, slowly, and smoothly through the range of motion, discontinuing exercise if client verbalizes pain**
7. Signaling device is within reach and bed is in low position
8. After completing skill, washes hands

❏ Performs Passive Range-of-Motion of Lower Extremity (Hip, Knee, Ankle) (Chapter 30)

1. Washes hands before contact with client
2. Identifies self to client by name and addresses client by name
3. Explains procedure to client, speaking clearly, slowly, and directly, maintaining face-to-face contact whenever possible
4. Provides for client's privacy during procedure with curtain, screen, or door
5. Positions client supine and in good body alignment
6. Supports client's leg by placing one hand under knee and other hand under heel
7. Moves entire leg away from body (performs AT LEAST 3 TIMES unless pain occurs)

*Reproduced and used with permission from the *Nurse Assistant Candidate Handbook* from National Council of State Boards of Nursing (NCSBN), Chicago, Ill, © 2011.

8. Moves entire leg toward body (performs AT LEAST 3 TIMES unless pain occurs)
9. Bends client's knee and hip toward client's trunk (performs AT LEAST 3 TIMES unless pain occurs)
10. Straightens knee and hip (performs AT LEAST 3 TIMES unless pain occurs)
11. Flexes and extends ankle through range-of-motion exercises (performs AT LEAST 3 TIMES unless pain occurs)
12. Rotates ankle through range-of-motion exercises (performs AT LEAST 3 TIMES unless pain occurs)
13. **While supporting limb, moves joints gently, slowly, and smoothly through range-of-motion to point of resistance, discontinuing exercise if pain occurs**
14. Provides for comfort
15. Before leaving client, places signaling device within client's reach
16. Washes hands

❏ *Performs Passive Range-of-Motion of Upper Extremity (Shoulder, Elbow, Wrist, Finger) (Chapter 30)*
1. Washes hands before contact with client
2. Identifies self to client by name and addresses client by name
3. Explains procedure to client, speaking clearly, slowly, and directly, maintaining face-to-face contact whenever possible
4. Provides for client's privacy during procedure with curtain, screen, or door
5. Supports client's extremity above and below joints while performing range-of-motion
6. Raises client's straightened arm toward ceiling and back toward head of bed and returns to flat position (flexion/extension) (performs AT LEAST 3 TIMES unless pain occurs)
7. Moves client's straightened arm away from client's side of body toward head of bed, and returns client's straightened arm to midline of client's body (abduction/adduction) (performs AT LEAST 3 TIMES unless pain occurs)
8. Moves client's shoulder through rotation range-of-motion exercises (performs AT LEAST 3 TIMES unless pain occurs)
9. Flexes and extends elbow through range-of-motion exercises (performs AT LEAST 3 TIMES unless pain occurs)
10. Provides range-of-motion exercises to wrist (performs AT LEAST 3 TIMES unless pain occurs)
11. Moves finger and thumb joints through range-of-motion exercises (performs AT LEAST 3 TIMES unless pain occurs)
12. **While supporting body part, moves joint gently, slowly, and smoothly through range-of-motion to point of resistance, discontinuing exercise if pain occurs**

13. Before leaving client, places signaling device within client's reach
14. Washes hands

❏ *Makes an Unoccupied (Closed) Bed (Chapter 21)*
1. Washes hands
2. Collects clean linens
3. Places clean linens on a clean surface
4. Raises the bed for good body mechanics
5. Puts on gloves
6. Removes linens without contaminating uniform. Rolls each piece away from self
7. Discards linens into laundry bag
8. Moves the mattress to the head of the bed
9. Applies mattress pad
10. Applies bottom sheet, keeping it smooth and free of wrinkles
11. Places the top sheet and bedspread on the bed, keeping them smooth and free of wrinkles
12. Tucks in top linens at the foot of the bed. Makes mitered corners
13. Applies clean pillowcase with zippers and/or tags to inside of pillowcase
14. Lowers the bed to its lowest position. Locks the bed wheels
15. Washes hands

❏ **Donning and Removing PPE (Gown and Gloves) (Chapter 16)*
1. Picks up gown and unfolds
2. Facing the back opening of gown, places arms through each sleeve
3. Fastens the neck opening
4. Secures gown at waist making sure that back of clothing is covered by gown (as much as possible)
5. Puts on gloves
6. Cuffs of gloves overlap cuffs of gown
7. **Before removing gown, with one gloved hand, grasps the other glove at the palm, removes glove**
8. **Slips fingers from ungloved hand underneath cuff of remaining glove at wrist, and removes glove turning it inside out as it is removed**
9. Disposes of gloves into designated waste container without contaminating self
10. After removing gloves, unfastens gown at neck and at waist
11. After removing gloves, removes gown without touching outside of gown
12. While removing gown, holds gown away from body, without touching the floor, turns gown inward and keeps it inside out
13. Disposes of gown in designated container without contaminating self
14. After completing skill, washes hands

*Reproduced and used with permission from the *Nurse Assistant Candidate Handbook* from National Council of State Boards of Nursing (NCSBN), Chicago, Ill, © 2011.

❑ *Performs Abdominal Thrusts (Chapter 13)*

1. Asks client if he or she is choking
2. Stands behind the client
3. Wraps arms around client's waist
4. Makes a fist with one hand
5. Places thumb side of fist against the client's abdomen
6. Positions fist in middle above navel and well below sternum (breastbone)
7. Grasps fist with other hand
8. Presses fist and other hand into client's abdomen with quick upward thrusts
9. Repeats thrusts until object is expelled or client becomes unresponsive

❑ *Ambulation With Cane or Walker (Chapter 30)*

1. Explains procedure to client, speaking clearly, slowly, and directly, maintaining face-to-face contact whenever possible
2. Locks bed wheels or wheelchair brakes
3. Assists client to a sitting position
4. **Before ambulating, puts on and properly fastens non-skid footwear**
5. Positions cane or walker correctly. Cane is on the client's strong side
6. Assists client to stand, using correct body mechanics
7. Stabilizes cane or walker and ensures that client stabilizes cane or walker
8. Stands behind and slightly to the side of client on the person's weak side
9. Ambulates client at least 10 steps
10. Assists client to pivot and sit, using correct body mechanics
11. Before leaving client, places signaling device within client's reach
12. Washes hands

❑ *Fluid Intake (Chapter 27)*

1. Observes dinner tray
2. Determines, in milliliters (mL), the amount of fluid consumed from each container
3. Determines total fluid consumed in mL
4. Records total fluid consumed on intake and output (I&O) sheet
5. Calculated total is within required range of evaluator's reading

❑ *Brushes or Combs Client's Hair (Chapter 23)*

1. Explains procedure to client, speaking clearly, slowly, and directly, maintaining face-to-face contact whenever possible
2. Collects brush or comb and bath towel
3. Places towel across client's back and shoulders or across the pillow
4. Asks client how he or she wants his or her hair styled
5. Combs/brushes hair gently and completely
6. Leaves hair neatly brushed, combed, and/or styled
7. Removes towel
8. Removes hair from comb or brush
9. Before leaving client, places signaling device within client's reach
10. Washes hands

❑ *Transfers a Client Using a Mechanical Lift (Chapter 19)*

1. Assembles required equipment; performs safety check of slings, straps, hooks, and chains
2. Checks client's weight to ensure it does not exceed the lift's capacity
3. Asks a co-worker to help
4. Explains procedure to client, speaking clearly, slowly, and directly, maintaining face-to-face contact whenever possible
5. Provides for privacy during procedure with curtain, screen, or door
6. Locks the bed wheels
7. Raises the bed for proper body mechanics
8. Lowers the head of the bed to a level appropriate for the client
9. Stands on one side of the bed; co-worker stands on the other side
10. Lowers the bed rails if up
11. Centers the sling under the client following the manufacturer's instructions
12. Ensures that the sling is smooth
13. Positions the client in semi-Fowler's position
14. Positions a chair to lower the client into it
15. Lowers the bed to its lowest position
16. Raises the lift to position it over the client
17. Positions the lift over the client
18. Attaches the sling to the sling hooks and checks fasteners for security
19. Crosses the client's arms over the chest
20. Raises the lift high enough until the client and sling are free of the bed
21. Instructs co-worker to support the client's legs as candidate moves the lift and the client away from the bed
22. Positions the lift so the client's back is toward the chair
23. Slowly lowers the client into the chair
24. Places client in comfortable position, in correct body alignment
25. Lowers the sling hooks and unhooks the sling
26. Removes the sling from under the client unless otherwise indicated. Moves lift away from client
27. Puts footwear on the client
28. Covers the client's lap and legs with a lap blanket
29. Positions the chair as the client prefers
30. Places signaling device within client's reach
31. Washes hands

❑ *Provides Mouth Care for an Unconscious Client (Chapter 22)*

1. Explains procedure to client, speaking clearly, slowly, and directly, maintaining face-to-face contact whenever possible
2. Provides for privacy during procedure with curtain, screen, or door
3. Washes hands
4. Positions client on side with head turned well to one side
5. Puts on gloves
6. Places the towel under the client's face
7. Places the kidney basin under the chin
8. Uses swabs or toothbrush and toothpaste or other cleaning solution
9. Cleans inside of mouth including the gums, tongue, and teeth
10. Cleans and dries face
11. Removes the towel and kidney basin
12. Applies lubricant to the lips
13. Positions client for comfort and safety
14. Removes and discards the gloves
15. Places signaling device within the client's reach
16. Washes hands

❑ *Provides Drinking Water (Chapter 27)*

1. Washes hands
2. Assembles equipment—ice, scoop, pitcher, cup, straw
3. Explains procedure to client, speaking clearly, slowly, and directly, maintaining face-to-face contact whenever possible
4. Uses the scoop to fill the pitcher with ice; does not let the scoop touch the rim or inside of the pitcher
5. Places scoop in appropriate receptacle after each use
6. Adds water to pitcher
7. Places the pitcher, disposable cup, and straw (if used) on the over-bed table, within the person's reach
8. Before leaving, places signaling device within client's reach
9. Washes hands

❑ *Provides Perineal Care for Uncircumcised Male (Chapter 22)*

1. Explains procedure to client, speaking clearly, slowly, and directly, maintaining face-to-face contact whenever possible
2. Provides for privacy during procedure with curtain, screen, or door
3. Washes hands
4. Fills basin with comfortably warm water
5. Puts on gloves
6. Elevates bed to working height
7. Places waterproof pad under buttocks
8. Gently grasps penis
9. Retracts the foreskin
10. Using a circular motion, cleans the tip by starting at the meatus of the urethra and working outward

11. Rinses the area with another washcloth
12. Returns the foreskin to its natural position
13. Cleans the shaft of the penis with firm, downward strokes and rinses the area
14. Cleans the scrotum
15. Pats dry the penis and the scrotum
16. Cleans the rectal area
17. Removes the waterproof pad
18. Lowers the bed
19. Removes and discards the gloves
20. Washes hands
21. Before leaving, places signaling device within client's reach

❑ *Empties and Records Content of Urinary Drainage Bag (Chapter 25)*

1. Explains procedure to client, speaking clearly, slowly, and directly, maintaining face-to-face contact whenever possible
2. Washes hands
3. Puts on gloves
4. Places a paper towel on the floor
5. Places the graduate on the paper towel
6. Places the graduate under the collection bag
7. Ensures that the bag is below the bladder and the drainage tube is not kinked
8. Opens the clamp on the drain
9. Lets all urine drain into the graduate—does not let the drain touch the graduate
10. Closes and positions the clamp
11. Measures urine
12. Removes and discards the paper towel
13. Empties the contents of the graduate into the toilet and flushes
14. Rinses the graduate
15. Returns the graduate to its proper place
16. Removes the gloves
17. Washes hands
18. Records the time and amount on the intake and output (I&O) record
19. Provides for client comfort
20. Places the signaling device within reach of client

❑ *Applies a Vest Restraint (Chapter 15)*

1. Obtains the correct type and size of restraint
2. Checks straps for tears or frays
3. Washes hands
4. Explains procedure to client, speaking clearly, slowly, and directly, maintaining face-to-face contact whenever possible
5. Provides for privacy during procedure with curtain, screen, or door
6. Makes sure the client is comfortable and in good alignment
7. Assists the person to a sitting position
8. Applies the restraint following the manufacturer's instructions—the "V" part of the vest crosses in front

9. Makes sure the vest is free of wrinkles in the front and back
10. Brings the straps through the slots
11. Makes sure the client is comfortable and in good alignment
12. Secures the straps to the chair or to the movable part of the bed frame
13. Uses a secure knot that can be released with one pull
14. Makes sure the vest is snug—slide an open hand between the restraint and the client
15. Places the signaling device within the client's reach
16. Washes hands

❏ *Performs a Back Rub (Massage) (Chapter 31)*

1. Washes hands
2. Explains procedure to client, speaking clearly, slowly, and directly, maintaining face-to-face contact whenever possible
3. Provides for privacy during procedure with curtain, screen, or door
4. Raises the bed for good body mechanics
5. Lowers the bed rail near the candidate, if up
6. Positions the person in the prone or side-lying position
7. Exposes the back, shoulders, upper arms, and buttocks
8. Warms the lotion
9. Rubs entire back in upward, outward motion for approximately 2 to 3 minutes; does not massage reddened bony areas
10. Straightens and secures clothing or sleepwear
11. Returns client to comfortable and safe position
12. Places the signaling device within reach
13. Lowers the bed to its lowest position
14. Washes hands

❏ *Positions a Foley Catheter (Chapter 25)*

1. Explains procedure to client, speaking clearly, slowly, and directly, maintaining face-to-face contact whenever possible
2. Washes hands
3. Puts on gloves
4. Secures catheter and drainage tubing according to facility procedure
5. Places tubing over leg
6. Positions drainage tubing so urine flows freely into drainage bag and has no kinks
7. Attaches bag to bed frame, below level of bladder
8. Washes hands

❏ *Applies a Cold Pack or Warm Compress (Chapter 38)*

1. Washes hands
2. Collects needed equipment

3. Explains procedure to client, speaking clearly, slowly, and directly, maintaining face-to-face contact whenever possible
4. Provides for privacy during procedure with curtain, screen, or door
5. Positions the client for the procedure
6. Covers cold pack or warm compress with towel or other protective cover
7. Properly places cold pack or warm compress on site
8. Checks the client for complications every 5 minutes
9. Checks the cold pack or warm compress every 5 minutes
10. Removes the application at the specified time—usually after 15 to 20 minutes
11. Provides for comfort
12. Places the signaling device within reach
13. Washes hands

❏ *Positions for an Enema (Chapter 26)*

1. Washes hands
2. Explains procedure to client, speaking clearly, slowly, and directly, maintaining face-to-face contact whenever possible
3. Provides for privacy
4. Positions the client in Sims' position or in a left side-lying position
5. Covers client appropriately
6. Provides for comfort
7. Places the signaling device within reach
8. Washes hands

❏ *Positions Client for Meals (Chapter 27)*

1. Washes hands
2. Explains procedure to client, speaking clearly, slowly, and directly, maintaining face-to-face contact whenever possible
3. If the person will eat in bed:
   a. Raises the head of the bed to a comfortable position—usually Fowler's or high-Fowler's position is preferred
   b. Removes items from the over-bed table and cleans the over-bed table
   c. Adjusts the over-bed table in front of the person
   d. Places the client in proper body alignment
4. If the person will sit in a chair:
   a. Positions the person in a chair or wheelchair
   b. Provides support for the client's feet
   c. Removes items from the over-bed table and cleans the table
   d. Adjusts the over-bed table in front of the person
   e. Places the client in proper body alignment
5. Places the signaling device within reach
6. Washes hands

Takes and Records Axillary Temperature, Pulse, and Respirations (Chapter 29)

1. Washes hands before contact with client
2. Identifies self to client by name and addresses client by name
3. Explains procedure to client, speaking clearly, slowly, and directly, maintaining face-to-face contact whenever possible
4. Provides for client's privacy during procedure with curtain, screen, or door
5. Turns on digital oral thermometer
6. Dries axilla and places thermometer in the center of the axilla
7. Holds thermometer in place for appropriate length of time
8. Removes and reads thermometer
9. Records temperature on pad of paper
10. **Recorded temperature is within required range**
11. Discards sheath from thermometer
12. Places fingertips on thumb side of client's wrist to locate radial pulse
13. Counts beats for 1 full minute
14. Records pulse rate on pad of paper
15. **Recorded pulse is within required range**
16. Counts respirations for 1 full minute
17. Records respirations on pad of paper
18. **Recorded respirations are within required range**
19. Before leaving client, places signaling device within client's reach
20. Washes hands

Transfers Client From Wheelchair to Bed (Chapter 19)

1. Washes hands before contact with client
2. Identifies self to client by name and addresses client by name
3. Explains procedure to client, speaking clearly, slowly, and directly, maintaining face-to-face contact whenever possible
4. Provides for client's privacy during procedure with curtain, screen, or door
5. Positions wheelchair close to bed with arm of wheelchair almost touching bed
6. Before transferring client, ensures client is wearing non-skid footwear
7. Before transferring client, folds up footplates
8. Before transferring client, places bed at safe and appropriate level for client
9. **Before transferring client, locks wheels on wheelchair and locks bed brakes**
10. a. *With transfer (gait) belt:* Stands in front of client, positioning self to ensure safety of candidate and client during transfer (for example, knees bent, feet apart, back straight), places belt around client's waist, and grasps belt. Tightens belt so that fingers of candidate's hand can be slipped between transfer/gait belt and client

b. *Without transfer belt:* Stands in front of client, positioning self to ensure safety of candidate and client during transfer (for example, knees bent, feet apart, back straight, arms around client's torso under arms)
11. Provides instructions to enable client to assist in transfer, including prearranged signal to alert client to begin standing
12. Braces client's lower extremities to prevent slipping
13. Counts to three (or says other prearranged signal) to alert client to begin transfer
14. On signal, gradually assists client to stand
15. Assists client to pivot and sit on bed in manner that ensures safety
16. Removes transfer belt, if used
17. Assists client to remove non-skid footwear
18. Assists client to move to center of bed
19. Provides for comfort and good body alignment
20. Before leaving client, places signaling device within client's reach
21. Washes hands

Applies an Incontinence Brief (Chapter 24)

1. Washes hands before contact with client
2. Identifies self to client by name and addresses client by name
3. Explains procedure to client, speaking clearly, slowly, and directly, maintaining face-to-face contact whenever possible
4. Starts with scale balanced at zero before weighing client
5. Chooses correct brief and size per facility instructions
6. Provides privacy for the resident
7. Elevates bed to comfortable working height
8. Puts on gloves
9. Places waterproof pad under client, asking client to raise buttocks or turning the client to the side
10. Loosens tabs on each side of the product
11. Turns the client away from you
12. Removes the product from front to back, rolling the product up and placing the product into trash bag
13. Opens the new brief, folding it in half, length-wise along the center, and inserts it between the client's legs from front to back; unfolds and spreads the back panel
14. Turns the client onto his or her back, with the product under buttocks with top of absorbent pad aligned just above the buttocks crease
15. Grasps and stretches the leg portion of front panel to extend elastic for groin placement
16. Rolls ruffles away from groin
17. Snuggly places bottom tabs angled toward abdomen on both sides
18. Places top tabs on each side angled toward bottom tabs
19. Removes gloves
20. Washes hands
21. Covers client appropriately and provides for comfort
22. Places signaling device within reach

After the Procedure

After you demonstrate a skill, complete a safety check of the room.

- The person is wearing eyeglasses, hearing aids, and other devices as needed.
- The call light is plugged in and within reach.
- Bed rails are up or down according to the care plan.
- The bed is in the lowest horizontal position.
- The bed position is locked if needed.
- Manual bed cranks are in the down position.
- Bed wheels are locked.
- Assistive devices are within reach. Walker, cane, and wheelchair are examples.
- The over-bed table, filled water pitcher and cup, tissues, phone, TV controls, and other needed items are within reach.

- Unneeded equipment is unplugged or turned off.
- Harmful substances are stored properly. Lotion, mouthwash, shampoo, after-shave, and other personal care products are examples.

After the Test

- Celebrate—you have completed the competency evaluation! The length of time for you to get your test results varies with each state. In the meantime, try to relax. Continue your daily routine and be the best nursing assistant you can be.

Answers to Review Questions in Textbook Chapters Review

Chapter 1
1. c
2. b
3. a

Chapter 2
1. d
2. b
3. a
4. b

Chapter 3
1. a
2. a
3. b
4. a

Chapter 4
1. b
2. b
3. b

Chapter 5
1. c
2. c
3. b
4. a
5. d
6. b
7. c
8. a

Chapter 6
1. c
2. c
3. a
4. d
5. d
6. b

Chapter 7
1. a
2. c
3. d

Chapter 8
1. d
2. a

Chapter 9
1. b
2. d
3. d
4. c
5. d
6. b
7. a
8. c
9. d
10. c
11. c
12. d
13. a
14. b

Chapter 11
1. a
2. b
3. b

Chapter 12
1. d
2. c
3. c
4. d
5. c
6. d

Chapter 13
1. b
2. d
3. a
4. d
5. c
6. c
7. b
8. b
9. c
10. b

Chapter 14
1. a
2. d
3. b
4. c
5. c
6. c

Chapter 15
1. a
2. b

3. a
4. a
5. b
6. b

Chapter 16
1. b
2. d
3. d
4. a
5. a
6. c

Chapter 17
1. c
2. b
3. c
4. d

Chapter 18
1. c
2. a
3. c

Chapter 19
1. b
2. a
3. d

Chapter 20
1. a
2. a
3. a
4. c
5. b
6. c
7. d

Chapter 21
1. b
2. a
3. a
4. d
5. c

Chapter 22
1. c
2. d

3. b
4. d
5. c
6. b
7. a
8. c
9. a
10. a

Chapter 23
1. a
2. b
3. a
4. a
5. b
6. a
7. a
8. a
9. b
10. b
11. d

Chapter 24
1. b
2. d
3. c
4. a
5. c

Chapter 25
1. b
2. b
3. d
4. c

Chapter 26
1. b
2. d
3. d
4. a

Chapter 27
1. d
2. a
3. b
4. a
5. d
6. d
7. a
8. c
9. c

Chapter 29
1. b
2. a
3. b
4. b

Chapter 30
1. c
2. a
3. b
4. a

Chapter 31
1. d
2. c
3. d
4. a
5. d

Chapter 32
1. b
2. d
3. d
4. a

Chapter 35
1. a
2. a

Chapter 36
1. d
2. c
3. d

Chapter 37
1. c
2. c
3. a
4. b

Chapter 38
1. d
2. c

Chapter 39
1. c
2. b
3. a
4. c
5. d

Chapter 41
1. a
2. a
3. d
4. a
5. b

Chapter 42
1. d
2. b
3. c
4. c

Chapter 43
1. b
2. c

3. a
4. b

Chapter 44
1. a
2. a
3. a
4. b
5. d

Chapter 45
1. d
2. c
3. a
4. c

Chapter 46
1. b
2. a
3. d

Chapter 47
1. c
2. a
3. b

Chapter 48
1. a
2. a
3. a
4. c

5. b
6. d

Chapter 49
1. c
2. d
3. a
4. d

Chapter 51
1. d
2. b

Chapter 54
1. c
2. a

3. c
4. b
5. b

Chapter 55
1. d
2. c
3. b
4. d
5. a
6. b

1. **C** You never give drugs. You may politely refuse to do a task that you have not been trained to do. However, you need to tell the nurse. Do not ignore a request to do something. Page 26, Chapter 3.

2. **A** An ethical person does not judge others or cause harm to another person. Ethical behavior involves not being prejudiced or biased. Ethical behavior also involves not avoiding persons whose standards and values are different from your own. Page 39, Chapter 5.

3. **D** An ethical person is knowledgeable of what is right conduct and wrong conduct. Health care workers do not drink alcohol before coming to work and do not drink alcohol while working. Page 39, Chapter 5.

4. **A** Neglect is failure to provide a person with the goods or services needed to avoid physical harm, mental anguish, or mental illness. Page 46, Chapter 5.

5. **B** The person's information is confidential. Information about the patient or resident is shared only among health team members involved in his or her care. Page 39, Chapter 5.

6. **D** End-of-shift is a time for good teamwork. Continue to do your job. Your attitude is important. Page 74, Chapter 7.

7. **C** Write in ink, spell words correctly, and use only center-approved abbreviations. Page 75, Chapter 7.

8. **B** Give a courteous greeting. End the conversation politely and say good-bye. Confidential information about a resident or employee is not given to any caller. Page 77, Chapter 7.

9. **C** Safety and security needs relate to feeling safe from harm, danger, and fear. Health care agencies are strange places with strange routines and equipment. People feel safer if they know what to expect. Be kind and understanding. Show the person the nursing center, listen to his or her concerns, and explain routines and procedures. Page 94, Chapter 9.

10. **B** When a person is angry or hostile, stay calm and professional. The person is usually not angry with you. He or she may be angry at another person or situation. Page 105, Chapter 9.

11. **D** Use words that are familiar to the person. Speak clearly, slowly, and distinctly. Also, ask 1 question at a time and wait for an answer. Page 98, Chapter 9.

12. **D** Follow the manufacturer's instructions. The excess strap should be tucked under the belt. The belt is applied over clothing and under the breasts. Pages 194–195, Chapter 14.

13. **D** Listening requires that you care and have interest in the other person. Have good eye contact with the person. Focus on what the person is saying. Page 100, Chapter 9.

14. **C** Assume that a comatose person hears and understands you. Talk to the person and tell him or her what you are going to do. Page 103, Chapter 9.

15. **A** Protect a person's right to privacy when giving care. Politely ask visitors to leave the room. Do not expose the person's body in front of them. Show visitors where to wait. Page 103, Chapter 9.

16. **B** If a person wants to talk with a minister or spiritual leader, tell the nurse. Many people gain comfort and strength from prayer and religious practices. Page 95, Chapter 9.

17. **A** Observe the person with a restraint at least every 15 minutes. Remove the restraint and re-position the person every 2 hours. Apply a restraint so it is snug and firm but not tight. You could be negligent if the restraint is not applied properly. Page 204, Chapter 15.

18. **D** The skin becomes more dry, muscle strength decreases, reflexes are slower, and bladder muscles weaken. Page 143, Chapter 12.

19. **B** Always act in a professional manner. Page 798, Chapter 51.

20. **C** Push the chair forward when transporting the person. Do not pull the chair backward unless going through a doorway. Page 284, Chapter 19.

21. **A** Tell the nurse at once. It is important to do the correct procedure on the right person. You have to be able to read the person's name on the ID bracelet or use the photo ID to identify the person. Page 157, Chapter 13.

22. **B** Clutching at the throat is the "universal sign of choking." Page 165, Chapter 13.

23. **D** When a person is on a diabetic diet, tell the nurse about changes in the person's eating habits. The person's meals and snacks need to be served on time. The person needs to eat at regular intervals to maintain a certain blood sugar. Always check the tray to see what was eaten. Page 453, Chapter 27.

24. **D** With mild airway obstruction, the person is conscious and can speak. Often forceful coughing can remove the object. Page 163, Chapter 13.

25. **A** Abdominal thrusts are used to relieve severe airway obstruction. Page 165, Chapter 13.

26. **B** Do not use faulty electrical equipment in nursing centers. Take the item to the nurse. Page 169, Chapter 13.

27. **C** If a warning label is removed or damaged, do not use the substance. Take the container to the nurse and explain the problem. Page 171, Chapter 13.

28. **C** An ethical person realizes that a person's values and standards may be different from his or hers. Page 39, Chapter 5.

29. **D** Remind a person not to smoke inside the center. Page 175, Chapter 13.

30. **A** During a fire, remember the word *RACE*. Page 175, Chapter 13.

31. **C** If a person with Alzheimer's disease has sundowning (increased restlessness and confusion as daylight ends), provide a calm, quiet setting late in the day. Do not try to reason with the person because he or she cannot understand what you are saying. Do not ask the person to tell you what is bothering him or her. Communication is impaired. Complete treatments and activities early in the day. Pages 778–779, Chapter 49.

32. **C** Make sure dentures fit properly. Cut food into small pieces and make sure the person can chew and swallow the food served. Report loose teeth or dentures to the nurse. Page 164, Chapter 13.

33. **A** Lock both wheels before you transfer a person to and from the wheelchair. The person's feet are on the footplates before moving the chair. Do not let the person stand on the footplates. Page 284, Chapter 19.

34. **B** Ease the person to the floor. Do not try to prevent the fall or yell at the person. The person should not get up before the nurse checks for injuries. Therefore the nurse needs to be told as soon as the fall occurs. Page 196, Chapter 14.

35. **B** Death from strangulation is the most serious risk factor from using a restraint. Restraints are not used for staff convenience or to punish a person. A written doctor's order is required before a restraint can be applied. Page 203, Chapter 15.

36. **C** Wash your hands before and after giving care to a person. Page 222, Chapter 16.

37. **D** Gloves need to be changed when they become contaminated with blood, body fluids, secretions, and excretions. Page 223, Chapter 16.

38. **D** When washing your hands, keep your hands and forearms lower than your elbows. Do not use hot water or let your uniform touch the sink. Push your watch up your arm so you can wash past your wrist. Page 223, Chapter 16.

39. **C** Bend your knees and squat to lift a heavy object. Hold items close to your body when lifting a heavy object. For a wider base of support and more balance, stand with your feet apart. Do not bend from your waist when lifting objects. Pages 250, 253, Chapter 17.

40. **B** The head of the bed is raised between 45 and 60 degrees for Fowler's position. Page 256, Chapter 17.

41. **B** Negligence—an unintentional wrong in which a person did not act in a reasonable and careful manner and causes harm to a person or the person's property. Page 41, Chapter 5.

42. **A** Have the person's back and buttocks against the back of the chair. Feet are flat on the floor or on the wheelchair footplates. The backs of the person's knees and calves are slightly away from the edge of the seat. Page 259, Chapter 17.

43. **B** Help the person out of bed on his or her strong side. In transferring, the strong side moves first. It pulls the weaker side along. Page 287, Chapter 19.

44. **A** When a person tries to bite, scratch, pinch, or kick you, you need to protect the person, others, and yourself from harm. Page 104, Chapter 9.

45. **B** Protect the person's right to privacy at all times. Screen the person properly and do not expose body parts. Page 263, Chapter 18.

46. **D** For comfort, adjust lighting to meet the person's changing needs. Nursing centers maintain a temperature range of 71°F to 81°F. Unpleasant odors may be offensive or embarrassing to people. Many older persons are sensitive to noise. Page 304, Chapter 20.

47. **A** Call lights are placed on the person's strong side and kept within the person's reach. Call lights are answered promptly. Page 313, Chapter 20.

48. **C** You must have the person's permission to open or search closets or drawers. Page 315, Chapter 20.

49. **C** When handling linens, do not take unneeded linens to a person's room. Once in the room, extra linens are considered contaminated. Because your uniform is considered dirty, always hold linens away from your body. To prevent the spread of microbes, never shake linens. Never put clean or used linens on the floor. Page 320, Chapter 21.

50. **C** To use a fire extinguisher, remember the word *PASS*. P—pull the safety pin, A—aim low, S—squeeze the lever, S—sweep back and forth. Page 176, Chapter 13.

51. **B** Mouth care is given at least every 2 hours for an unconscious person. To prevent aspiration, you position the person on 1 side with the head turned well to the side. Use a padded tongue blade to keep the person's mouth open. Wear gloves. Page 342, Chapter 22.

52. **B** A good attitude is needed at work. Be willing to help others. Be pleasant and respectful of others. Page 59, Chapter 6.

53. **B** During cleaning, firmly hold dentures over a basin of water lined with a towel. This prevents them from falling onto a hard surface and breaking. Clean and store dentures in cool water. Hot water causes dentures to lose their shape. To prevent losing dentures, label the denture cup with the person's name. Page 344, Chapter 22.

54. **C** Report and record the location and description of the rash. Page 348, Chapter 22.

55. **C** Gently wipe the eye from the inner aspect to the outer aspect of the eye. Clean the far eye first. Do not use soap. Page 350, Chapter 22.

56. **D** When giving a back massage, wear gloves if the person's skin has open areas. Warm the lotion before applying it to the person. Use firm strokes. Do not massage reddened bony areas. This can lead to more tissue damage. Page 537, Chapter 31.

57. **A** Separate the labia and clean downward from front to back. Wear gloves and use soap. Pages 360–361, Chapter 22.

58. **C** Stay within hearing distance if the person can be left alone. Place the call light within the person's reach. Cold water is turned on first, then hot water. Direct water away from the person while adjusting the water temperature. Page 354, Chapter 22.

59. **B** Electric razors are used when a person is on an anticoagulant. An anticoagulant prevents or slows down blood clotting. Bleeding occurs easily. A nick or cut from a safety razor can cause bleeding. Page 374, Chapter 23.

60. **B** Remove clothing from the strong or "good" (unaffected) side first. Page 379, Chapter 23.

61. **C** Address a person with dignity and respect. Call the person by his or her title—Mr. or Mrs. or Miss. Address a person by his or her first name, or another name, if the person asks you to do so. Page 93, Chapter 9.

62. **D** Measure and record the amount of urine in the drainage bag. The catheter is secured to the person's thigh or abdomen. Do not disconnect the catheter from the drainage tubing. Do not let the person lie on the tubing. Page 409, Chapter 25.

63. **B** Carbohydrates provide energy and fiber for bowel elimination. Page 447, Chapter 27.

64. **D** When taking a rectal temperature with an electronic thermometer, the thermometer is inserted ½ inch into the rectum. A glass thermometer is inserted 1 inch. Lubricate the bulb end of the thermometer for easy insertion and to prevent tissue damage. Provide for privacy. An electronic thermometer remains in place until the temperature registers on the display. Page 492, Chapter 29.

65. **A** Report any systolic pressure below 90 mm Hg and any diastolic pressure below 60 mm Hg at once. Record the BP. It is your responsibility to tell the nurse. Page 506, Chapter 29.

66. **D** Oral temperatures are not taken on unconscious persons, persons receiving oxygen, or persons who breathe through their mouth. Page 487, Chapter 29.

67. **A** To assist with walking, offer the person your arm and have the person walk a half step behind you. When caring for a person who is blind or visually impaired, let the person do as much for himself or herself as possible. Use a normal voice tone. Do not shout at the person. Identify yourself when you enter the room. Do not touch the person until you have indicated your presence. Pages 686–687, Chapter 42.

68. **D** The person with confusion and dementia has the right to personal choice. He or she also has the right to keep and use personal items. The family makes choices if the person cannot. Page 782, Chapter 49.

69. **D** Discuss your feelings with the nurse. No one can shout, scream, or hit the person. Nor can they call the person names. The person did not choose loss of function. Pages 671, 673, Chapter 41.

70. **C** Encourage the person to help as much as possible. Doors and windows are closed to reduce drafts. You wash from the cleanest areas to the dirtiest areas. Pat the skin dry to avoid irritating or breaking the skin. Page 347, Chapter 22.

71. **A** When a person is dying, always assume that the person can hear you. Re-position the person every 2 hours to promote comfort. Skin care, personal hygiene, back massages, oral hygiene, and good body alignment promote comfort. Pages 854–855, Chapter 55.

72. **B** Foods that melt at room temperature (ice cream, sherbet, custard, pudding, gelatin, and Popsicles) are measured and recorded as intake. The nurse measures and records IV fluids and tube feedings. Page 456, Chapter 22.

73. **B** After bedrest, activity increases slowly and in steps. First the person dangles. Sitting in a chair follows. Next the person walks in the room and then in the hallway. Page 276, Chapter 18.

74. **B** Tell the nurse at once if you find or cause a skin tear. Page 607, Chapter 36.

75. **A** Treat the resident with respect and ensure privacy. The resident has a right not to have his or her private affairs exposed or made public without giving consent. Only staff involved in the resident's care should see, handle, or examine his or her body. Page 15, Chapter 2.

1. **C** You may politely refuse to do a task that is not in your job description. Pages 35–36, Chapter 4.
2. **B** An ethical person realizes that a person's values and standards may be different from his or hers. You may not agree with advance directives or resuscitation decisions. However, you must respect the person's wishes. Page 39, Chapter 5, and Page 855, Chapter 55.
3. **C** Verbal abuse is using oral or written words or statements that speak badly of, sneer at, criticize, or condemn a person. Page 46, Chapter 5.
4. **C** Speak in a normal tone. Use words the person seems to understand and speak slowly and distinctly. Page 102, Chapter 9.
5. **C** Do not allow smoking in bed. Turn cold water on first, then hot water. Assist the person with drinking or eating hot food. Do not let the person sleep with a heating pad. Page 158, Chapter 13.
6. **B** Use 3-pronged plugs on all electrical devices and follow the manufacturer's instructions on equipment. Wipe up spills right away. Do not use unfamiliar equipment. Ask for training if you are unfamiliar with something. Page 169, Chapter 13.
7. **D** Answer call lights promptly. Throw rugs, scatter rugs, and area rugs are not used. The person's bed should be in the lowest horizontal position, except when giving care. Grab bars should be used when the person showers. Pages 188–189, Chapter 14.
8. **B** Decontaminate your hands after removing gloves. Page 223, Chapter 16.
9. **D** Sometimes multiple people or a mechanical lift is needed for moving and turning persons in bed. If the person weighs more than 200 pounds, at least 3 staff members help with the move. Page 265, Chapter 18.
10. **C** A person must not put his or her arms around your neck. He or she can pull you forward or cause you to lose your balance. Neck, back, and other injuries from falls are possible. Ask a co-worker to help you. Also, you should use a transfer or gait belt. Lock the wheels on the wheelchair. Page 287, Chapter 19.
11. **B** Wear gloves when removing linens. Linens may contain blood, body fluids, secretions, or excretions. Raise the bed for good body mechanics. The bed is flat when you place clean linens on it. Page 324, Chapter 21.
12. **B** Use a circular motion, start at the meatus, and work outward. Gloves are worn. Soap is used. Page 362, Chapter 22.
13. **C** Put clothing on the weak (affected) side first. Page 379, Chapter 23.
14. **D** The drainage bag hangs from the bed frame or chair. It must not touch the floor. The bag is always kept lower than the person's bladder. The drainage bag does not hang on the bed rail. Page 409, Chapter 25.
15. **A** Protein is needed for tissue repair and growth. Page 447, Chapter 27.
16. **C** Older persons may not feel thirsty (decreased sense of thirst). Offer water often. Page 456, Chapter 27.
17. **C** NPO means nothing by mouth. An NPO sign is posted above the bed. The water pitcher and glass are removed from the room. Oral hygiene is performed frequently. Page 456, Chapter 27.
18. **C** 1 oz equals 30 mL. 3 oz equals 90 mL. Page 456, Chapter 27.
19. **D** Allow time for chewing and swallowing. Fluids are offered during the meal. A teaspoon, rather than a fork, is used for feeding. Sit and talk with the person. Page 463, Chapter 27.
20. **D** Support the part being exercised. Do not force a joint beyond its present ROM. Move the joint slowly, smoothly, and gently. Do not force the joint to the point of pain. Page 517, Chapter 30.
21. **B** A cane is held on the strong side of the body. If the left leg is weak, the cane is held in the right hand. Pages 522–523, Chapter 30.
22. **B** Position the person in good alignment. Bed linens are kept tight and wrinkle-free. Talk softly and gently. Avoid sudden and jarring movements of the bed or chair. Page 536, Chapter 31.
23. **C** Check behind the ears and under the nose for signs of irritation. Never remove an oxygen device. Do not adjust the oxygen flow rate. Do not fill the humidifier. Page 656, Chapter 39.
24. **A** Tell the nurse at once. Mercury is a hazardous substance. Do not touch the mercury. Follow special procedures for handling hazardous materials. Page 491, Chapter 29.
25. **C** Record and report at once a pulse rate less than 60 or more than 100 beats per minute. The radial pulse is used for routine vital signs. If the pulse is irregular, count it for 1 minute. Do not use your thumb to take a pulse. Page 499, Chapter 29.
26. **B** Count the respirations for 1 minute if an abnormal breathing pattern is noted. People change their breathing patterns when they know respirations are being counted. Therefore the person should not know that you are counting respirations. The healthy adult has 12 to 20 respirations per minute. Page 505, Chapter 29.
27. **A** Report at once any systolic pressure above 120 mm Hg and any diastolic pressure above 80 mm Hg. Record the BP. It is your responsibility to tell the nurse. Page 506, Chapter 29.
28. **C** Rectal temperatures are not taken if a person has diarrhea, is confused, or is agitated. Page 488, Chapter 29.
29. **C** Residents must be cared for in a manner that promotes dignity and self-esteem. Use the right tone of voice. Respect private space and property. Listen to the person with interest. Knock on the door and wait to be asked in before entering. Page 17, Chapter 2.

30. **B** Have the person void before being weighed. A full bladder adds weight. No footwear is worn. Footwear adds to the weight and height measurements. Weigh the person at the same time of day, usually before breakfast. Balance the scale before weighing the person. Page 552, Chapter 32.

31. **D** Keep the skin free of moisture from urine, stools, or perspiration. Re-position the person at least every 2 hours. Do not massage reddened areas. Keep the heels and ankles off the bed. Page 627, Chapter 37.

32. **C** Face the person when speaking. Reduce or eliminate background noise. Speak in a normal voice tone. Speak clearly, distinctly, and slowly. Page 680, Chapter 42.

33. **C** Explain the location of food and beverages. Keep furniture and equipment out of areas where the person walks. Provide lighting as the person prefers. Do not re-arrange furniture and equipment. Pages 686–687, Chapter 42.

34. **C** The person with confusion and dementia has the right to privacy and confidentiality. Information about the person's care and condition is shared only with those involved in providing the care. Protect the person from exposure. Page 784, Chapter 49.

35. **C** Ask clear, simple questions. Explain what you are going to do and why. Call the person by name every time you are in contact with him or her. Keep calendars and clocks in the person's room. Page 770, Chapter 49.

36. **D** Exercise the person as ordered. Adequate exercise often reduces wandering. Do not keep the person in his or her room. Involve the person in activities. Do not restrain the person or argue with the person who wants to leave. Page 778, Chapter 49.

37. **B** Restorative nursing programs promote self-care measures. They help maintain the person's highest level of function. The programs focus on the whole person. The care helps the person regain health, strength, and independence. Page 667, Chapter 41.

38. **C** Remind the person of his or her progress in the rehabilitation program. Focus on the person's abilities and strengths. Progress may be slow. Do not deny the disability. Page 671, Chapter 41.

39. **D** Respect the person's right to privacy. Do not expose the person's body unnecessarily. Only those involved in the person's care need to know the person's diagnosis. The final moments of death are kept confidential. So are family reactions. Page 859, Chapter 55.

40. **A** Remember the word *RACE*. Your first action is to Rescue the person in immediate danger. Then sound the Alarm, Confine the fire, and Extinguish the fire. Page 175, Chapter 13.

41. **B** Failure to provide a person with the goods or services needed to avoid physical harm or mental anguish is neglect. Page 46, Chapter 5.

42. **C** You have not been trained to give drugs or to perform sterile procedures. Do not perform tasks that are not in your job description. Page 26, Chapter 3.

43. **C** Ask the nurse to observe urine that looks or smells abnormal. Then record your observation. Page 409, Chapter 25.

44. **D** A good attitude is needed at work. People rely on you to give good care. You are expected to be pleasant and respectful. Always be willing to help others. Page 59, Chapter 6.

45. **B** Unnecessary restraint is false imprisonment. Observe the person for complications every 15 minutes. The least restrictive type of restraint is ordered by the doctor. Restraints can increase confusion and agitation. Pages 204–205, Chapter 15.

46. **C** The supine position is the back-lying position. For good alignment, the bed is flat and the head and shoulders are supported on a pillow. Place arms and hands at the sides. Page 256, Chapter 17.

47. **A** Hand-washing is the most important way to prevent or avoid spreading infection. Page 222, Chapter 16.

48. **B** To gossip means to spread rumors or talk about the private matters of others. Gossiping is unprofessional and hurtful. If others are gossiping, you need to remove yourself from the group. Do not make or repeat any comment that can hurt another person. Pages 56, 59, Chapter 6.

49. **D** Ask a co-worker to help you. The head of the bed is lowered. The person flexes both knees. Friction and shearing cause skin tears and need to be prevented. Pages 267–269, Chapter 18.

50. **A** On a sodium-controlled diet, high-sodium foods such as ham and canned vegetables are omitted. Salt is not added to food at the table. The amount of salt used in cooking is limited. Pages 452–453, Chapter 27.

51. **B** Elastic stockings should not have wrinkles or creases after being applied. Wrinkles and creases can cause skin breakdown. Apply stockings before the person gets out of bed. Apply the correct size. Page 598, Chapter 35.

52. **C** When a person begins to fall, ease him or her to the floor. Also protect the person's head. Page 196, Chapter 14.

53. **A** Before bathing, allow the person to use the bathroom, bedpan, or urinal. Page 349, Chapter 22.

54. **A** Insert an electronic thermometer ½ inch into the rectum. Page 492, Chapter 29.

55. **A** Touch is a form of nonverbal communication. It conveys comfort and caring. Touch means different things to different people. Some people do not like to be touched. Page 99, Chapter 9.

56. **A** A person's information is confidential. The information is shared only among health team members involved in the person's care. Pages 59–60, Chapter 6.

57. **A** Report and record complaints of urgency, burning, dysuria, or other urinary problems. Page 400, Chapter 24.

58. **C** Respect a person's culture and religion. Learn about his or her beliefs and practices. This helps you understand the person and give better care. Page 94, Chapter 9.

59. **C** Wear gloves when giving perineal care. Gloves are needed whenever contact with blood, body fluids, secretions, excretions, mucous membranes, and non-intact skin is likely. Pages 229, 233, Chapter 16.

60. **D** Report any changes from normal or changes in the person's condition to the nurse at once. Then record your observation. Page 73, Chapter 7.

61. **A** If a person is standing, have him or her sit before fainting occurs. Page 843, Chapter 54.

62. **A** The person drinks an increased amount of fluid. Keep fluids within the person's reach. Offer fluids regularly. Page 456, Chapter 27.

63. **B** Communication fails when you talk too much and fail to listen. Page 103, Chapter 9.

64. **A** During bathing, a person has the right to privacy and the right to personal choice. Page 347, Chapter 22.

65. **C** People in late adulthood need to develop new friends and relationships. They need to adjust to retirement and reduced income, decreased strength, and loss of health. They need to cope with a partner's death and prepare for their own death. Page 137, Chapter 11.

66. **D** Blood pressure is not taken on an arm with an IV infusion. When taking a blood pressure, apply the cuff to the bare upper arm. Make sure the room is quiet. Talking, TV, radio, and sounds from the hallway can affect an accurate measurement. Place the diaphragm of the stethoscope over the brachial artery. Page 508, Chapter 29.

67. **C** Never put clean or used linens on the floor. The floor is dirty. You cannot use the linens. Page 323, Chapter 21.

68. **B** To prevent aspiration, position the unconscious person on 1 side when you do mouth care. Use a small amount of fluid to clean the mouth. Tell the person what you are doing. Dentures are not worn when the person is unconscious. Page 342, Chapter 22.

69. **B** Encourage people to do their own hair care. Do not cut matted or tangled hair. The person chooses his or her hairstyle. Brushing and combing are done with morning care and whenever needed. Page 369, Chapter 23.

70. **D** Check between the toes for cracks and sores. These areas are often overlooked. If left untreated, a serious infection could occur. Fingernails are cut with nail clippers, not scissors. You do not trim or cut toenails if a person has diabetes or has poor circulation. Page 377, Chapter 23.

71. **B** If an indwelling catheter becomes disconnected from the drainage system, you tell the nurse at once. Page 412, Chapter 25.

72. **B** Urinary drainage bags are emptied and the contents measured at the end of each shift. Drainage bags must not touch the floor. The bag is always kept lower than the person's bladder. Page 409, Chapter 25.

73. **C** Use elastic tape to secure a condom catheter. Elastic tape expands when the penis changes size and adhesive tape does not. Do not apply a condom catheter if the penis is red and irritated. Always act in a professional manner. Page 418, Chapter 25.

74. **D** For comfort during bowel elimination, leave the person alone if possible. Provide for privacy. Help the person to the toilet or commode if possible. Page 426, Chapter 26.

75. **A** Help the person from the wheelchair to the bed on his or her strong side. In transferring, the strong side moves first. It pulls the weaker side along. Page 287, Chapter 19.